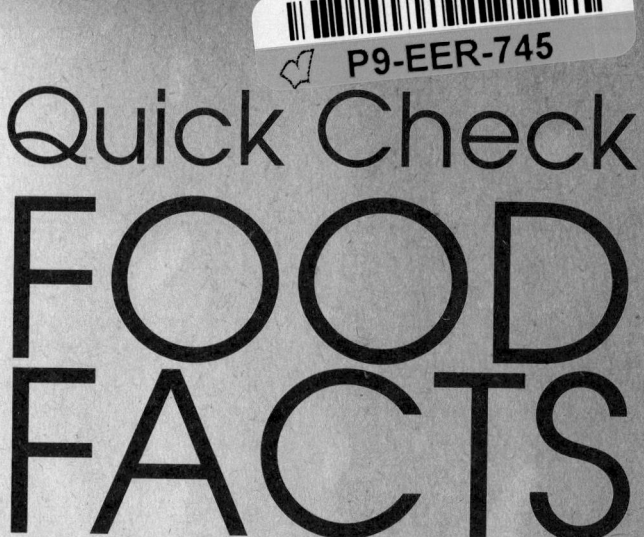

Quick Check
FOOD FACTS

Fourth Edition

Compiled by the Editorial Staff
of Barron's Educational Series, Inc.

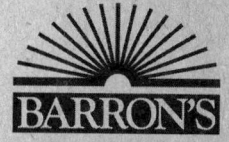

BARRON'S

Acknowledgment

The publisher gratefully acknowledges the participating national restaurant chains for allowing inclusion of nutritional data of selected menu items in this edition.

Nutritional data for Dunkin' Donuts® and Applebee's® current as of 2015.

McDonald's® trademarks and nutritional information used with permission from McDonald's Corporation.

Subway® trademarks and nutritional information used with permission from Subway.

Wendy's® nutrition information is based on standard product formulations. Variations may occur due to differences in suppliers, ingredient substitutions, recipe revisions, product assembly at the restaurant level, and/or season of the year. Nutrition calculations follow federal regulations regarding the rounding of nutritional data. This information is effective as of June 2011. For the most comprehensive and up-to-date information, or to calculate nutrition facts, visit **www.wendys.com**.

About the Author

Amy Shapiro, RD, CDN, CPT, is a registered dietitian and professional speaker promoting wellness in corporate, clinical, and private settings. With degrees in both Psychology and Nutrition, Amy's focus is on behavior modification and lifestyle management. Additionally, Amy is a personal trainer certified by the American Council on Exercise and a wellness coach. Utilizing years of experience educating and coaching clients and worksite wellness groups to achieve weight loss success, Amy published her first book *Lose It for the Last Time*.

© Copyright 2016, 2012, 2006, 1999 by Barron's Educational Series, Inc.

All rights reserved.
No part of this publication may be reproduced or distributed in any form or by any means without the written permission of the copyright owner.

All inquiries should be addressed to:
Barron's Educational Series, Inc.
250 Wireless Boulevard
Hauppauge, New York, 11788
www.barronseduc.com

ISBN: 978-1-4380-0692-5

Library of Congress Control Number: 2015941624

Printed in the United States of America

9 8 7 6 5 4 3 2 1

10%
POST-CONSUMER WASTE
Paper contains a minimum of 10% post-consumer waste (PCW). Paper used in this book was derived from certified, sustainable forestlands.

Contents

Preface

The information in this book (excluding the nutritional counts of selected menu items from national restaurant chains) is based on the USDA National Nutrient Database for Standard Reference, Release 23, published in computer-readable form by the U.S. Department of Agriculture. The original database is very large and unwieldy, and we have extracted just the most useful information for publication here.

For each food we list serving size, and then, per serving:

Total calories (kcal)   **Cholesterol** (milligrams)   **Sugar** (grams)
Total fat (grams)   **Carbohydrates** (grams)   **Protein** (grams)
Saturated fat (grams)   **Fiber** (grams)   **Sodium** (milligrams)

In a very few cases, numbers were missing from the USDA database. They are left blank here.

Introduction

Our food choices have a great impact on our health and well-being. Often our decisions about food are based on likes and dislikes, but also what is within our budget, convenient, or available. In fact, the availability of food in our environment, at home, at work, and on the street, means we have to make food decisions many times a day. And our food choices can also affect the people around us, including family, friends, and coworkers. We make decisions not only about what to eat, but how much to eat as well. This book is a guide to making healthy food decisions. Here are some tips to get started:

Healthy Eating Tips

1. Vary Food Choices

There are over 40 essential nutrients that you can only get from the foods you eat. Since each food contains only a few of these nutrients in limited amounts, you can see why eating a variety of foods is important. Not only do you need to eat foods from each of the food categories—grains, vegetables, fruits, dairy, proteins—but within each food category, you should eat a variety of foods. For instance, eating a rainbow of colors of fruits and vegetables will provide a variety of different nutrients—vitamins, minerals, and antioxidants.

2. Slash Sodium

The U.S. Dietary Guidelines for Americans and the American Heart Association recommend limiting sodium to less than 2,300 mg a day (the amount in 1 teaspoon of salt) for healthy adults and 1,500 mg per day for those who are salt sensitive—individuals who have high blood pressure, are 40 years of age or older, or who are African-Americans. More than two-thirds of the adult population falls into one or more of these categories. Most adults consume 3,400 mg of sodium each day, twice the amount suitable for at risk adults, the majority of which comes from processed foods and restaurant meals. Many snack foods, canned soups, canned vegetables, processed tomato products, and salad dressings are high in sodium. Check the nutrition facts on the label; 140 mg or less per serving is considered low sodium.

3. Choose Healthy Fats

Research has shown that it is the type of fat, not the amount, that has the biggest effect on your health. Fats are an important part of every diet because

- They deliver essential fatty acids that your body cannot manufacture
- They are a delivery system for the fat-soluble vitamins A, D, E, and K, meaning the body can't digest and make use of these vitamins without fat
- They contribute to our feeling of fullness, which helps with portion control and weight maintenance

However, fats are high in calories and should be enjoyed in moderation. Heart-healthy fats include monounsaturated (for example, olive oil) and polyunsaturated (for example, omega-3 fatty acids). Trans fats are unhealthy and should be avoided. Research is ongoing to determine the impact of saturated fats on heart health so for now it is recommended to consume them in moderation.

4. Practice Portion Control

Most people eat more than they need. And most people gain weight from eating and drinking more calories than the body is using for energy. Use the serving sizes recommended by the ChooseMyPlate program. You can also make use of the serving sizes listed in the Nutrition Facts Box on food labels. Keep in mind that serving sizes listed by manufacturers are not standard and may not be appropriate for adults consuming fewer than 2,000 calories per day or those on special diets. Other useful tools are measuring cups and spoons, food scales, and premeasured bowls and plates. Follow the guidelines from ChooseMyPlate to fill half your plate with fruits and vegetables, one quarter with grains, and the remaining quarter with lean protein. Use the suggested portion sizes given in this book to help you with portion control.

5. Go for Whole Grains

The U.S. Dietary Guidelines recommend that at least half of the grains you consume be whole grains, meaning minimally processed. All grains contain three components—the germ, endosperm, and bran. During processing, one or more of these components are lost. The bran is full of fiber, while the germ and endosperm contain valuable micronutrients (vitamins, minerals, and antioxidants). Eating more whole grains reduces risk of heart disease, diabetes, high blood pressure, and high cholesterol. Research has shown that eating 2½ servings of grains daily is enough to lower your chance of developing heart disease. Check the nutrition facts to see that the amount of fiber is at least 10% or more of total carbohydrates. A healthy carbohydrate alternative to processed grains are starchy vegetables. Potatoes, peas, corn, and winter squash are good sources of fiber as well. Eat the whole grain for the best nutrition.

6. Cut Added Sugar

Sugar occurs naturally in varying amounts in all carbohydrates including fruit, vegetables, dairy, and whole grains. These foods fuel the body and the sugar they contain does not cause unhealthy spikes in blood glucose (sugar) levels due to the presence of fiber and/or protein. Most sugars in the American diet are added to foods during processing and preparation and cause unhealthy blood glucose highs and lows. Natural and added sugars are not listed separately on food labels. The USDA recommends limiting added sugar to 10 teaspoons (40 grams) per day. The average person consumes 20 teaspoons of added sugar each day mostly from soda, sports drinks, sugar-sweetened fruit drinks, desserts, and candy. Added sugar is a major contributor to weight gain and obesity. Check the ingredients list for added sugars.

7. Bone Up on Calcium

Research suggests milk and milk products improve bone health (including teeth) especially in children and teens. By age 20, the body has built about 90% of the bone it will ever have. Calcium intake is very important to preserve that bone for a lifetime. Consumption of milk and milk products is also associated with reduced risk of heart disease, type 2 diabetes, and high blood pressure. Most people consume less than the recommended amounts and intake declines with age. Almost half of the milk products consumed in the U.S. come from cheese. Choosing low-fat dairy products provides the same amount of calcium, vitamin D, and potassium with fewer calories and less unhealthy fat than cheese.

8. Go Fish

Seafood contains a variety of nutrients, notably the omega-3 fatty acids, EPA, and DHA. The U.S. Dietary Guidelines recommend eating about 8–12 ounces per week. Eating seafood contributes to the prevention of heart disease. Studies have shown omega-3 fatty acids may lower triglycerides and LDL-cholesterol, reduce risk of inflammation, depression, arthritis, ADHD, and dementia. To reduce exposure to mercury in the fish supply, limit intake of white (albacore) tuna to 6 oz per week. Seafood varieties commonly consumed that are higher in EPA and DHA and lower in mercury include skip jack tuna, salmon, anchovies, herring, sardines, mussels, Pacific oysters, farm-raised trout, and Atlantic and Pacific mackerel. Federal agencies warn pregnant and nursing mothers as well as young children to avoid high-mercury fish including tuna, swordfish, tilefish, king mackerel, and shark. Other high-mercury fish includes seabass, halibut, and orange roughy.

9. Slow Down

Americans lead an ever increasing fast-paced lifestyle with more responsibilities and less free time, contributing to more eating on the run. Eating too fast (and with distractions) leads to eating larger portions than is appropriate and to digestive difficulties. Providing time for family meals is also important since it is an opportunity to eat more nutritious foods—time to enjoy the flavors and textures of the meal and model healthy eating behaviors to children. Fast eaters can slow down by putting the utensil down between bites, using a smaller fork, eating with the non-dominant hand, or keeping pace with the slowest eater at the table.

10. Create a Healthy Space

When and what we eat is often dictated by the foods in our environment. We are surrounded daily by opportunities to eat. Creating a healthy space at home and work helps reduce the likelihood of eating in the absence of hunger or reaching for an unhealthy food. Keep all snack foods off the counter or desk except for fruit. Break down large containers into servings before the foods are stored for portion control. Place vegetables, fruits, and yogurts at eye level in the fridge.

11. Use ChooseMyPlate

The U.S. Dietary Guidelines form the basis for the federal government's nutrition education program, ChooseMyPlate. This program uses a portioned plate logo to divide food choices into five food groups. This logo shows that half your plate should be fruits and vegetables, one quarter grain, and the last quarter protein with a glass of milk. The ChooseMyPlate program provides recommended food plans, food lists, serving sizes, health benefits, nutrients, and tips for making wise choices. Find ChooseMyPlate diet recommendations, serving sizes, and tips throughout this book.

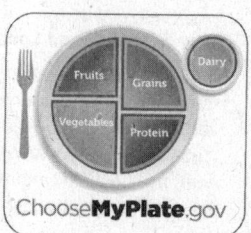

Healthy Shopping Tips

1. Shop with a List

Planning ahead is important for saving money and eating healthy. Plan meals for a week at a time and keep a running grocery list in a central location where family members can add items as they are needed. Organize your list in categories based on the way you travel through the supermarket.

2. Comparison Shop

Compare the prices of similar items. Most shelf tags have a total price and a price per unit that provides an easy way to compare apples to apples. Should you buy apples in a 3 lb bag for $4.99 or individual apples that are $0.99 each? Scan supermarket ads, circulars, and the Internet for specials and coupons. Use coupons only for foods that are on your list.

3. Start on the Perimeter

Most fresh foods are on the perimeter of the supermarket—fresh fruits and vegetables; meats, poultry, and fish; dairy products; and the bakery. This is where you can be assured of natural nutrients without many preservatives or artificial ingredients. Some fresh items are in the interior—grains, rice, flours, and nuts. Make the majority of your purchases from the perimeter before shopping the aisles.

4. Organic vs. Conventionally Grown

Organic agriculture produces food products using methods that preserve the environment while avoiding chemicals and additives such as pesticides, hormones, and antibiotics. Foods labeled organic are free of genetically modified ingredients (GMOs). The organic standards apply to both animals and crops and are defined by the USDA. While organically produced foods may not contain a higher nutrient content than their conventionally raised equivalents, some individuals prefer to buy organic to reduce the exposure to chemicals that may prove to be a health risk.

5. Buy Seasonal and Locally

Seasonal and locally grown products are usually cheaper and healthier. They maintain more nutrients because they have not traveled as far from picking to store. They are cheaper because there are more available. Stay attuned to the season so that you can purchase fruits and vegetables that are the most economical, the freshest, and the cheapest. When produce is not in season, buy canned or frozen without sauces and added salt.

6. Buy in Bulk

Buying foods in bulk can often save you money, but only if you can use the larger amount. Packaging costs money, so the less package the more you save. Check out the unit price to see how much you are saving buying the larger size. For instance, steel-cut oats in bulk (50 lb bag) are $1.02 a pound, while a 4 lb tin runs $2.75 a pound. Other items you can save on by buying in bulk are grains, lentils, dried beans, and rice. Be careful when purchasing more perishable items like fruit and dairy products. Always check the expiration and sell-by dates.

7. Read Nutrition Facts Labels and Ingredients Lists

The front of a package may make claims like "Healthy," "Natural," and "Contains" but the back or side of the package will give you the real scoop. Check out the Nutrition Facts Box that gives you the amount of individual nutrients. Compare these nutrients between products to see which is better. Read the ingredients list to check for partially hydrogenated fats, which mean "trans fats" and added sugars.

8. Avoiding Common Allergens

Approximately 4% of adults and children living in the U.S. have food allergies. The Food Allergen Labeling and Consumer Protection Act (FALCPA), which took effect January 2006 mandates that foods containing any of the eight major food allergens (milk, eggs, fish, crustacean shellfish, peanuts, tree nuts, wheat, and soy) be clearly stated on the label. More recently, the FDA issued a rule defining the term "gluten-free" to mean the food is inherently gluten-free or does not have an ingredient that is derived from a grain containing gluten or an ingredient that has been processed from a gluten containing grain in an amount greater than 20 parts per million (ppm) of gluten. This law affects an estimated 3 million Americans diagnosed with celiac disease as well as individuals who choose a gluten-free diet for other health reasons. Although clear labeling of allergens makes it easier to live with food allergies, you are advised to continue to thoroughly read ingredients to avoid an incident.

9. Understand Health and Nutrition Claims

You'll find a variety of health and nutrition claims on labels. These can be a help to those who need to find foods that are heart healthy or low in sodium, but be sure to check the Nutrition Facts numbers to make sure the food fits into your food plan.

10. Store Brands vs. National Brands

It used to be that store brands were cheaper and lower quality versions of national brands. Now store brands are quality lines of products that can save you money. Statistics say that store brands can save 30% over nationally branded products. In some supermarkets, store brands account for as much as 35% of total sales. Check out the store brands and compare them to their national counterparts.

What Does "Healthy" Mean?

Food labeling allows manufacturers to make a "healthy" claim on a food or beverage label if it meets specific nutrient criteria. The basic requirements are:

- Low in fat: 3 g or less or 30% or less fat calories
- Low in sodium: must be 140 mg or less with the exception of meal-type products (6 oz or more); the limit then is 360 mg for individual foods and 480 mg for meal-type foods
- 10% or more of at least one of the following:

  - Vitamin A
  - Vitamin C
  - Iron
  - Calcium
  - Protein
  - Fiber

How to Use This Book

This book can help you plan your menus and make a shopping list.

- Read the ChooseMyPlate recommendations for each food category for number of servings and serving sizes. The servings listed are appropriate for an adult consuming 2,000 calories per day. For a personalized foodplan based on your age, gender, weight, and activity level, go to *www.choosemyplate.gov*.
- Consider the number of people you are feeding when you create your shopping list. You will need to estimate those nutrient needs along with your own. Keep in mind it is important not to overfeed. Children's, as well as adult's, needs change with age and physical activity level. A moderately active adult female may need 2,000 calories but 1,800 calories or less if sedentary. A sedentary male may maintain his weight with 2,200 calories but, if very active, calories need to rise 2,400–3,000 a day. To calculate nutrition needs for each family member use *www.choosemyplate.gov*.
- Check the list of foods in each category provided in this book and choose a variety of items.
- Compare nutrients within categories for the best choices of nutrient dense foods such as protein, fiber, calcium, vitamins, and minerals. Nutrient dense foods supply more nutrients for the same amount of calories. Also check foods for unhealthy ingredients such as saturated fat, cholesterol, and sodium.
- Read the Shopping Tips and Shopping List Essentials for each category and include these suggestions into your meal planning and shopping list.
- Highlight the foods that are presently in your food plan and use a different color highlighter for the foods you want to try. Make a goal to try a new food each week. Remember that variety is important for healthy eating.
- Take this book to the supermarket for a quick check on the nutrients in foods that may not have nutrition facts—fruits, vegetables, bulk items, meat, poultry, and fish.

Using Nutrition Facts

1. Serving Size shows you how many servings are in the package, and how big the serving is. Keep in mind that a package of food often contains more than one serving!
2. Make sure you know how many servings are in the whole container and try to limit your intake to the suggested serving size.
3. Choose the food with the lower percent daily value of total fat. 20% DV or more of total fat is high. Limit intake of foods high in saturated fat.
4. Most trans fats are made from "hydrogenated" oils. Aim to keep your intake of trans fat as low as possible.
5. A balanced diet contains protein in the form of grains, lean meats, fish, legumes, and eggs.
6. Choose foods that have vitamins that make them higher in nutritional value.
7. The calories listed are for one serving of food.
8. This section tells you the percentage of a nutrient found in one serving of food, based on the established standard of 2,000 calories per day.
9. Foods that are high in fiber aid in digestion, can lower you cholesterol, and prevent against diseases such as diabetes. Whole grains, beans, fruits, and vegetables are good sources of fiber.

Nutrition Facts		
1. Serving Size 5 oz. (144g)		
2. Servings Per Container 4		
Amount Per Serving		
7. Calories 310 Calories from Fat 100		
		% Daily Value*
3. **Total Fat** 15g		21%
4. Saturated Fat 2.6g		17%
Trans Fat 1g		
Cholesterol 118mg		39%
Sodium 560mg		28%
Total Carbohydrate 12g		4%
9. Dietary Fiber 1g		4%
Sugars 1g		
5. **Protein** 24g		
6. Vitamin A 1% • Vitamin C 2%		
Calcium 2% • Iron 5%		

*Percent Daily Values are based on a 2,000 calorie diet. Your daily values may be higher or lower depending on your calorie needs:
Calories   2,000   2,500

ChooseMyPlate Key Messages

Small changes in your food habits result in improved nutrition. Use the Dietary Guidelines to choose steps that work for you and begin your journey to better health today.

To Balance Calories

- Enjoy your food, but eat less.
- Avoid oversized portions.

To Increase Healthy Food Choices

- Make half your plate fruits and vegetables.
- Switch to fat-free or low-fat (1%) milk.
- Make at least half your grains whole grains.

To Reduce Unhealthy Food Choices

- Compare sodium in foods like soup, bread, and frozen meals—and choose foods with lower numbers.
- Drink water instead of sugary drinks.
- Avoid foods with trans fats.

Go to *www.choosemyplate.gov* for a personalized food plan based on your age, gender, weight, and activity level. Find food lists and specific serving size photos.

Healthy Weight Chart

Male		Female	
Height	Ideal Weight	Height	Ideal Weight
4'6"	63–77 lbs.	4'6"	63–77 lbs.
4'7"	68–84 lbs.	4'7"	68–83 lbs.
4'8"	74–90 lbs.	4'8"	72–88 lbs.
4'9"	79–97 lbs.	4'9"	77–94 lbs.
4'10"	85–103 lbs.	4'10"	81–99 lbs.
4'11"	90–110 lbs.	4'11"	86–105 lbs.
5'0"	95–117 lbs.	5'0"	90–110 lbs.
5'1"	101-123 lbs.	5'1"	95–116 lbs.
5'2"	106–130 lbs.	5'2"	99–121 lbs.
5'3"	112–136 lbs.	5'3"	104–127 lbs.
5'4"	117–143 lbs.	5'4"	108–132 lbs.
5'5"	122–150 lbs.	5'5"	113–138 lbs.
5'6"	128–156 lbs.	5'6"	117–143 lbs.
5'7"	133–163 lbs.	5'7"	122–149 lbs.
5'8"	139–169 lbs.	5'8"	126–154 lbs.
5'9"	144–176 lbs.	5'9"	131–160 lbs.
5'10"	149–183 lbs.	5'10"	135–165 lbs.
5'11"	155–189 lbs.	5'11"	140-171 lbs.
6'0"	160–196 lbs.	6'0"	144–176 lbs.
6'1"	166–202 lbs.	6'1"	149–182 lbs.
6'2"	171–209 lbs.	6'2"	153–187 lbs.
6'3"	176–216 lbs.	6'3"	158–193 lbs.
6'4"	182–222 lbs.	6'4"	162–198 lbs.
6'5"	187–229 lbs.	6'5"	167–204 lbs.
6'6"	193–235 lbs.	6'6"	171–209 lbs.
6'7"	198–242 lbs.	6'7"	176–215 lbs.
6'8"	203–249 lbs.	6'8"	180–220 lbs.
6'9"	209–255 lbs.	6'9"	185–226 lbs.
6'10"	214–262 lbs.	6'10"	189–231 lbs.
6'11"	220–268 lbs.	6'11"	194–237 lbs.
7'0"	225–275 lbs.	7'0"	198–242 lbs.

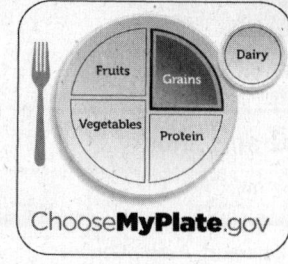

ChooseMyPlate.gov

Grains

Why Eat Grains?

Grains are important sources of many nutrients, including dietary fiber, several B vitamins (thiamin, riboflavin, niacin, and folate), and minerals (iron, magnesium, potassium, and selenium). Eating whole grains as part of a healthy diet may reduce the risk of heart disease and type 2 diabetes, and help with weight management. Additionally, consuming foods containing fiber, such as whole grains, may reduce constipation and diverticulitis. B vitamins play a role in metabolism, helping the body use energy from proteins, fats, and carbohydrates, and are essential for a healthy nervous system. Folate (folic acid), a B vitamin, is important before and during pregnancy because it helps prevent birth defects.

Daily Goal

6 one-ounce servings (1 ounce equivalents) for an adult on a 2,000-calorie diet
48 grams of whole grains
One-ounce equivalents:

1 slice bread	½ cup cooked rice or pasta
1 cup dry cereal	1 six-inch tortilla

Shopping Tips

- Make at least half your grains whole grains.
- Look for a whole grain as the first ingredient—whole wheat, brown rice, oatmeal, bulgur, or whole corn meal are examples of whole grains.
- Substitute whole wheat flour for up to half of regular flour in baking.
- Use barley and quinoa as alternatives to rice.

Shopping List Essentials

Whole wheat bread	Whole wheat flour	Whole grain cereal	Popcorn
Wild or Brown rice	Whole wheat pasta	Oatmeal	

Red Flags

"Wheat flour" or "corn starch" are not whole grains. If a product claims "whole grain" or sounds like it is made with whole grains, look for the amount of whole grains on the label or the Whole Grain Stamp found on many but not all whole grain foods.

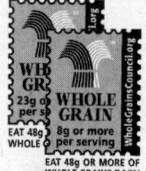

THE BASIC STAMP

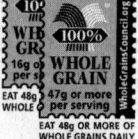

THE 100% STAMP

Preparation Pointer

When cooking grains such as barley, quinoa, brown and wild rice, replace water with low sodium, low fat vegetable or chicken broth for added flavor.

1

Food Serving size	Cal.	(g) Total Fat	(g) Sat. Fat	(mg) Chol.	(g) Carb.	(g) Fiber	(g) Sug.	(g) Prot.	(mg) Sod.
Grains, flour									
Acorn Flour, Full Fat 1 oz (28.35g)	140	8	1	0	15	0	0	2	0
Amaranth Grain, Cooked 1 cup (246g)	251	4	0	0	46	5.2	0	9	15
Arrowroot Flour 1 cup (128g)	457	0	0	0	113	4.4	0	0	3
Barley Flour or Meal 1 cup (148g)	511	2	0	0	110	14.9	1	16	6
Barley Malt Flour 1 cup (162g)	585	3	1	0	127	11.5	1	17	18
Barley, Hulled 1 cup (184g)	651	4	1	0	135	31.8	1	23	22
Barley, Pearled, Cooked 1 cup (157g)	193	1	0	0	44	6	0	4	5
Buckwheat 1 cup (170g)	583	6	1	0	122	17	0	23	2
Buckwheat Flour, Whole Groat 1 cup (120g)	402	4	1	0	85	12	3	15	13
Buckwheat Groats, Roasted, Cooked 1 cup (168g)	155	1	0	0	33	4.5	2	6	7
Buckwheat Groats, Roasted, Dry 1 cup (164g)	567	4	1	0	123	16.9	0	19	18
Bulgur, Cooked 1 tbsp (8.4g)	7	0	0	0	2	0.4	0	0	0
Bulgur, Dry 1 cup (140g)	479	2	0	0	106	25.6	1	17	24
Carob Flour 1 tbsp (6g)	13	0	0	0	5	2.4	3	0	2
Chickpea Flour (Besan) 1 cup (92g)	356	6	1	0	53	9.9	10	21	59
Corn Bran, Crude 1 cup (76g)	170	1	0	0	65	60	0	6	5
Corn Flour, Degermed, Unenriched, Yellow 1 cup (126g)	473	2	0	0	104	2.4	1	7	1

Food Serving size	Cal.	(g) Total Fat	(g) Sat. Fat	(mg) Chol.	(g) Carb.	(g) Fiber	(g) Sug.	(g) Prot.	(mg) Sod.
Corn Flour, Masa, Enriched, White									
1 cup (114g)	416	4	1	0	87	7.3	2	11	6
Corn Flour, Masa, Enriched, Yellow									
1 cup (114g)	416	4	1	0	87	7.3	0	11	6
Corn Flour, Masa, Unenriched, White									
1 cup (114g)	416	4	1	0	87	7.3	2	11	6
Corn Flour, Whole-grain, Blue (Harina de Maiz Morado)									
1 tbsp (6.9g)	25	0	0	0	5	0.6	0	1	0
Corn Flour, Whole-grain, White									
1 cup (117g)	422	5	1	0	90	8.5	1	8	6
Corn Flour, Whole-grain, Yellow									
1 cup (117g)	422	5	1	0	90	8.5	1	8	6
Cornmeal, Degermed, Enriched, White									
1 cup (157g)	581	3	0	0	125	6.1	3	11	11
Cornmeal, Degermed, Enriched, Yellow									
1 cup (157g)	581	3	0	0	125	6.1	3	11	11
Cornmeal, Degermed, Unenriched, White									
1 cup (157g)	581	3	0	0	125	6.1	3	11	11
Cornmeal, Degermed, Unenriched, Yellow									
1 cup (157g)	581	3	0	0	125	6.1	3	11	11
Cornmeal, Self-rising, Bolted, Plain, Enriched, White									
1 cup (122g)	407	4	1	0	86	8.2	0	10	1521
Cornmeal, Self-rising, Bolted, Plain, Enriched, Yellow									
1 cup (122g)	407	4	1	0	86	8.2	0	10	1521
Cornmeal, Self-rising, Bolted, with Wheat Flour, Enriched, White									
1 cup (170g)	592	5	1	0	125	10.7	0	14	2242
Cornmeal, Self-rising, Bolted, with Wheat Flour, Enriched, Yellow									
1 cup (170g)	592	5	1	0	125	10.7	0	14	2242
Cornmeal, Self-rising, Degermed, Enriched, White									
1 cup (138g)	490	2	0	0	103	9.8	0	12	1860
Cornmeal, Self-rising, Degermed, Enriched, Yellow									
1 cup (138g)	490	2	0	0	103	9.8	0	12	1860
Cornmeal, Whole-grain, White									
1 cup (122g)	442	4	1	0	94	8.9	1	10	43

Food Serving size	Cal.	(g) Total Fat	(g) Sat. Fat	(mg) Chol.	(g) Carb.	(g) Fiber	(g) Sug.	(g) Prot.	(mg) Sod.
Cornmeal, Whole-grain, Yellow 1 cup (122g)	442	4	1	0	94	8.9	1	10	43
Cottonseed Flour, Low Fat (Glandless) 1 oz (28.35g)	94	0	0	0	10	0	0	14	10
Cottonseed Flour, Part Defatted (Glandless) 1 tbsp (5g)	18	0	0	0	2	0.2	0	2	2
Cottonseed Kernels, Roasted (Glandless) 1 tbsp (10g)	51	4	1	0	2	0.6	0	3	3
Cottonseed Meal, Part Defatted (Glandless) 1 oz (28.35g)	104	1	0	0	11	0	0	14	10
Couscous, Cooked 1 cup, dry, yields (528g)	591	1	0	0	123	7.4	1	20	26
Couscous, Dry 1 cup (173g)	650	1	0	0	134	8.7	0	22	17
Hominy, Canned, White 1 cup (165g)	119	1	0	0	24	4.1	3	2	347
Hominy, Canned, Yellow 1 cup (160g)	115	1	0	0	23	4	0	2	336
Incaparina, Dry Mix (Corn & Soy Flours), Unprepared 1 cup (128g)	485	7	0	0	77	12.7	0	28	5
Leavening Agents, Baking Powder, Double-acting, Sodium Aluminum Sulfate .5 tsp (2.3g)	1	0	0	0	1	0	0	0	244
Leavening Agents, Baking Powder, Double-acting, Straight Phosphate .5 tsp (2.3g)	1	0	0	0	1	0	0	0	182
Leavening Agents, Baking Powder, Low Sodium .5 tsp (2.5g)	2	0	0	0	1	0.1	0	0	2
Leavening Agents, Baking Soda .5 tsp (2.3g)	0	0	0	0	0	0	0	0	629
Leavening Agents, Yeast, Baker's, Active Dry 1 tbsp (12g)	39	1	0	0	5	3.2	0	5	6
Millet Flour 1 cup (119g)	444	5	1	0	87	4.2	2	13	5
Miso 1 cup (275g)	547	17	3	0	73	14.9	17	32	10252

Food Serving size	Cal.	(g) Total Fat	(g) Sat. Fat	(mg) Chol.	(g) Carb.	(g) Fiber	(g) Sug.	(g) Prot.	(mg) Sod.
Oat Bran, Cooked 1 cup (219g)	88	2	0	0	25	5.7	0	7	2
Oats 1 cup (156g)	607	11	2	0	103	16.5	0	26	3
Pancakes Plain, Frozen, Ready-to-heat (Includes Buttermilk) 1 pancake (41g)	92	2	0	7	16	1	4	2	207
Pancakes, Blueberry, Prepared from Recipe 1 pancake (4″ dia) (38g)	84	3	1	21	11	0	0	2	157
Pancakes, Buttermilk, Prepared from Recipe 1 pancake (4″ dia) (38g)	86	4	1	22	11	0	0	3	198
Pancakes, Plain, Dry Mix, Complete (Includes Buttermilk) 1 cup, poured from box (130g)	489	6	1	27	93	3.5	0	13	1580
Pancakes, Plain, Dry Mix, Complete, Prepared 1 pancake (4″ dia) (38g)	74	1	0	5	14	0.5	0	2	239
Pancakes, Plain, Dry Mix, Incomplete (Includes Buttermilk) 1 cup, poured from box (112g)	398	2	0	0	82	6	2	11	1220
Pancakes, Plain, Dry Mix, Incomplete, Prepared 1 pancake (4″ dia) (38g)	83	3	1	27	11	0.7	0	3	192
Pancakes, Plain, Frozen, Ready-to-heat, Microwave (Including Buttermilk) 1 pancake (38g)	91	2	0	0	16	1	3	2	215
Pancakes, Plain, Prepared from Recipe 1 pancake (4″ dia) (38g)	86	4	1	22	11	0	0	2	167
Pancakes, Whole Wheat, Dry Mix, Incomplete, Prepared 1 pancake (4″ dia) (44g)	92	3	1	27	13	1.2	0	4	252
Rice Flour, Brown 1 cup (158g)	574	4	1	0	121	7.3	1	11	13
Rice Flour, White 1 cup (158g)	578	2	1	0	127	3.8	0	9	0
Rye 1 cup (169g)	571	3	0	0	128	25.5	2	17	3
Rye Flour, Dark 1 cup (128g)	416	3	0	0	88	30.5	3	20	3
Rye Flour, Light 1 cup (102g)	364	1	0	0	78	8.2	1	10	2

Food Serving size	Cal.	(g) Total Fat	(g) Sat. Fat	(mg) Chol.	(g) Carb.	(g) Fiber	(g) Sug.	(g) Prot.	(mg) Sod.
Rye Flour, Medium 1 cup (102g)	356	2	0	0	77	12	1	11	2
Semolina, Enriched 1 cup (167g)	601	2	0	0	122	6.5	0	21	2
Semolina, Unenriched 1 cup (167g)	601	2	0	0	122	6.5	0	21	2
Sesame Flour, High Fat 1 oz (28.35g)	149	11	1	0	8	0	0	9	12
Sesame Flour, Low Fat 1 oz (28.35g)	93	0	0	0	10	0	0	14	11
Sesame Flour, Part Defatted 1 oz (28.35g)	107	3	0	0	10	0	0	11	11
Sesame Meal, Part Defatted 1 oz (28.35g)	159	13	2	0	7	0	0	5	11
Sesame Sticks, Wheat-based, Salted 2 oz (57g)	308	21	4	0	27	1.6	0	6	848
Sesame Sticks, Wheat-based, Unsalted 2 oz (57g)	308	21	4	0	27	0	0	6	17
Sorghum 1 cup (192g)	651	6	1	0	143	12.1	0	22	12
Sorghum Flour 1 cup (121g)	437	4	1	0	94	8	2	10	5
Soy Flour, Defatted 1 tbsp (6.6g)	22	0	0	0	3	1.2	1	3	1
Soy Flour, Defatted, Crude Protein Basis (N x 6.25) 1 cup, stirred (100g)	372	9	1	0	31	16	15	50	9
Soy Flour, Full-fat, Roasted 1 cup, stirred (85g)	375	19	3	0	29	8.2	6	30	10
Soy Flour, Full-fat, Roasted, Crude Protein Basis (N x 6.25) 1 cup, stirred (85g)	373	19	3	0	26	0	0	32	10
Soy Flour, Low Fat 1 tbsp (5.5g)	21	0	0	0	2	0.9	1	3	0
Soy Flour, Low Fat, Crude Protein Basis (N x 6.25) 1 cup, stirred (88g)	325	6	1	0	30	9	17	45	16

Food Serving size	Cal.	(g) Total Fat	(g) Sat. Fat	(mg) Chol.	(g) Carb.	(g) Fiber	(g) Sug.	(g) Prot.	(mg) Sod.
Spelt, Cooked 1 cup (194g)	246	2	0	0	51	7.6	0	11	10
Spelt, Uncooked 1 cup (174g)	588	4	1	0	122	18.6	12	25	14
Teff, Cooked 1 cup (252g)	255	2	0	0	50	7.1	0	10	20
Teff, Uncooked 1 cup (193g)	708	5	1	0	141	15.4	4	26	23
Tortillas, Ready-to-bake or Fry, Flour 1 tortilla, medium (approx 6″ dia) (30g)	94	2	1	0	15	0.9	1	2	191
Tortillas, Ready-to-bake or Fry, Flour, Without Calcium 1 tortilla, medium (approx 6″ dia) (32g)	104	2	1	0	18	1.1	0	3	153
Triticale 1 cup (192g)	645	4	1	0	138	0	0	25	10
Triticale Flour, Whole Grain 1 cup (130g)	439	2	0	0	95	19	0	17	3
Wheat Bran, Crude 1 cup (58g)	125	2	0	0	37	24.8	0	9	1
Wheat Flour, Bread, Unenriched 1 cup, unsifted, dipped (137g)	495	2	0	0	99	3.3	0	16	3
Wheat Flour, White, All Purpose, Enriched, Bleached 1 cup (125g)	455	1	0	0	95	3.4	0	13	3
Wheat Flour, White, All Purpose, Enriched, Calcium-fortified 1 cup (125g)	455	1	0	0	95	3.4	0	13	3
Wheat Flour, White, All Purpose, Enriched, Unbleached 1 cup (125g)	455	1	0	0	95	3.4	0	13	3
Wheat Flour, White, All Purpose, Self-rising, Enriched 1 cup (125g)	443	1	0	0	93	3.4	0	12	1491
Wheat Flour, White, All Purpose, Unenriched 1 cup (125g)	455	1	0	0	95	3.4	0	13	3
Wheat Flour, White, Bread, Enriched 1 cup (137g)	495	2	0	0	99	3.3	0	16	3

Food Serving size	Cal.	(g) Total Fat	(g) Sat. Fat	(mg) Chol.	(g) Carb.	(g) Fiber	(g) Sug.	(g) Prot.	(mg) Sod.
Wheat Flour, White, Cake, Enriched 1 cup, unsifted, dipped (137g)	496	1	0	0	107	2.3	0	11	3
Wheat Flour, White, Tortilla, Mix, Enriched 1 cup (111g)	450	12	5	0	75	0	0	11	751
Wheat Flour, Whole Grain 1 cup (120g)	408	3	1	0	86	12.8	0	16	2
Wheat Germ, Crude 1 cup (115g)	414	11	2	0	60	15.2	0	27	14
Wheat, Durum 1 cup (192g)	651	5	1	0	137	0	0	26	4
Wheat, Hard Red Spring 1 cup (192g)	632	4	1	0	131	23.4	1	30	4
Wheat, Hard Red Winter 1 cup (192g)	628	3	1	0	137	23.4	1	24	4
Wheat, Hard White 1 cup (192g)	657	3	1	0	146	23.4	1	22	4
Wheat, Soft Red Winter 1 cup (168g)	556	3	0	0	125	21	1	17	3
Wheat, Soft White 1 cup (168g)	571	3	1	0	127	21.3	1	18	3
Wheat, Sprouted 1 cup (108g)	214	1	0	0	46	1.2	0	8	17
Whelk, Unspecified, Cooked, Moist Heat 3 oz (85g)	234	1	0	111	13	0	0	41	350
Whey, Acid, Dried 1 tbsp (2.9g)	10	0	0	0	2	0	2	0	28
Whey, Acid, Fluid 1 quart (984g)	236	1	1	10	50	0	50	7	472
Whey, Sweet, Dried 1 tbsp (7.5g)	26	0	0	0	6	0	6	1	81
Whey, Sweet, Fluid 1 quart (984g)	266	4	2	20	51	0	51	8	531
Yeast Extract Spread 1 tsp (6g)	9	0	0	0	1	0.2	0	2	216

Food Serving size	Cal.	(g) Total Fat	(g) Sat. Fat	(mg) Chol.	(g) Carb.	(g) Fiber	(g) Sug.	(g) Prot.	(mg) Sod.
Pastas and Pasta Products									
Campbell SpaghettiOs Plus Calcium 1 cup (1 serving) (252g)	169	1	0	5	35	3	90	6	600
Campbell SpaghettiOs with Sliced Franks 1 cup (1 serving) (252g)	219	6	2	20	32	4	56	9	600
Campbell SpaghettiOs, Mini Beef Ravioli in Meat Sauce 1 serving (259g)	256	5	2	10	43	4.9	89	11	1059
Campbell SpaghettiOs, Raviolios Beef Ravioli in Meat Sauce 1 cup (1 serving) (252g)	267	8	4	20	38	4	55	11	1091
Campbell SpaghettiOs, Spaghetti in Tomato and Cheese Sauce 1 cup (1 serving) (252g)	202	2	0	5	40	3	9	7	950
Campbell SpaghettiOs A to Z with Meatballs 1 cup (1 serving) (252g)	239	7	2	20	32	4	0	11	600
Campbell Supper Bakes Meal Kits, Herb Chicken with Rice .167 box (NLEA serving) (94g)	185	1	1	5	40	1	0	4	780
Campbell Supper Bakes Meal Kits, Savory Pork Chops with Herb Stuffing .167 box (85g)	154	1	1	5	31	2	29	5	784
Campbell's Red & White, Goldfish Pasta with Meatballs 1 serving, 1/2 cup (126g)	89	3	1	10	11	1	1	4	480
Kamut, Cooked 1 cup (172g)	251	2	0	0	52	6.7	0	11	10
Macaroni and Cheese, Canned Entrée 1 serving (244g)	200	6	2	15	28	1.2	12	8	737
Macaroni, Cooked, Enriched 1 cup, spiral shaped (134g)	212	1	0	0	41	2.4	1	8	1
Macaroni, Cooked, Unenriched 1 cup, elbow shaped (140g)	221	1	0	0	43	2.5	1	8	1
Macaroni, Dry, Enriched 1 cup, spiral shaped (84g)	312	1	0	0	63	2.7	2	11	5
Macaroni, Dry, Unenriched 2 oz (57g)	211	1	0	0	43	1.8	2	7	3
Macaroni, Protein-fortified, Cooked, Enriched (N x 5.70) 1 cup, small shells (115g)	189	0	0	0	36	0	0	9	6

Food Serving size	Cal.	(g) Total Fat	(g) Sat. Fat	(mg) Chol.	(g) Carb.	(g) Fiber	(g) Sug.	(g) Prot.	(mg) Sod.
Macaroni, Protein-fortified, Cooked, Enriched (N x 6.25)									
1 cup, small shells (115g)	189	0	0	0	36	1.7	0	10	6
Macaroni, Protein-fortified, Dry, Enriched (N x 5.70)									
2 oz (57g)	214	1	0	0	39	1.4	0	11	5
Macaroni, Protein-fortified, Dry, Enriched (N x 6.25)									
2 oz (57g)	213	1	0	0	37	1.4	0	12	5
Macaroni, Vegetable, Cooked, Enriched									
1 cup, spiral shaped (134g)	172	0	0	0	36	5.8	2	6	8
Macaroni, Vegetable, Dry, Enriched									
2 oz (57g)	209	1	0	0	43	2.5	0	7	25
Macaroni, Whole Wheat, Cooked									
1 cup, elbow shaped (140g)	174	1	0	0	37	3.9	1	7	4
Macaroni, Whole Wheat, Dry									
2 oz (57g)	198	1	0	0	43	4.7	0	8	5
Noodles, Chinese, Cellophane or Long Rice (Mung Beans), Dehydrated									
1 cup (140g)	491	0	0	0	121	0.7	0	0	14
Noodles, Chinese, Chow Mein									
1.5 oz (43g)	227	13	2	0	25	1.7	0	4	189
Noodles, Egg, Cooked, Enriched									
1 cup (160g)	221	3	1	46	40	1.9	1	7	8
Noodles, Egg, Cooked, Enriched, with Salt									
1 cup (160g)	221	3	1	46	40	1.9	1	7	264
Noodles, Egg, Cooked, Unenriched, with Salt									
1 cup (160g)	221	3	1	46	40	1.9	1	7	264
Noodles, Egg, Cooked, Unenriched, Without Salt									
1 cup (160g)	221	3	1	46	40	1.9	1	7	8
Noodles, Egg, Dry, Enriched									
2 oz (57g)	219	3	1	48	41	1.9	1	8	12
Noodles, Egg, Dry, Unenriched									
1 cup (38g)	146	2	0	32	27	1.3	1	5	8
Noodles, Egg, Spinach, Cooked, Enriched									
1 cup (160g)	211	3	1	53	39	3.7	1	8	19
Noodles, Egg, Spinach, Dry, Enriched									
2 oz (57g)	218	3	1	54	40	3.9	0	8	41

Food Serving size	Cal.	(g) Total Fat	(g) Sat. Fat	(mg) Chol.	(g) Carb.	(g) Fiber	(g) Sug.	(g) Prot.	(mg) Sod.
Noodles, Japanese, Soba, Cooked									
1 cup (114g)	113	0	0	0	24	0	0	6	68
Noodles, Japanese, Soba, Dry									
2 oz (57g)	192	0	0	0	43	0	0	8	451
Noodles, Japanese, Somen, Cooked									
1 cup (176g)	231	0	0	0	48	0	0	7	283
Noodles, Japanese, Somen, Dry									
2 oz (57g)	203	0	0	0	42	2.5	0	6	1049
Pasta with Meatballs in Tomato Sauce, Canned Entrée									
1 cup (255g)	273	13	5	23	28	6.9	6	11	742
Pasta with Sliced Franks in Tomato Sauce, Canned Entrée									
1 serving (1 cup) (252g)	227	6	2	23	32	4	10	11	600
Pasta with Tomato Sauce, No Meat, Canned									
1 serving, 1 cup (252g)	189	2	1	3	37	3.3	10	6	630
Pasta, Corn, Cooked									
1 cup (140g)	176	1	0	0	39	6.7	0	4	0
Pasta, Corn, Dry									
2 oz (57g)	203	1	0	0	45	6.3	0	4	2
Pasta, Fresh-refrigerated, Plain, as Purchased									
4.5 oz (128g)	369	3	0	93	70	0	0	14	33
Pasta, Fresh-refrigerated, Plain, Cooked									
2 oz (57g)	75	1	0	19	14	0	0	3	3
Pasta, Fresh-refrigerated, Spinach, as Purchased									
4.5 oz (128g)	370	3	1	93	71	0	0	14	35
Pasta, Fresh-refrigerated, Spinach, Cooked									
2 oz (57g)	74	1	0	19	14	0	0	3	3
Pasta, Homemade, Made with Egg, Cooked									
2 oz (57g)	74	1	0	23	13	0	0	3	47
Pasta, Homemade, Made Without Egg, Cooked									
2 oz (57g)	71	1	0	0	14	0	0	2	42
Spaghetti with Meat Sauce, Frozen Entrée									
1 oz (28.35g)	26	0	0	2	4	0.5	1	1	60
Spaghetti with Meatballs, Canned									
1 cup (255g)	273	13	5	23	28	0	8	11	1035

Food Serving size	Cal.	(g) Total Fat	(g) Sat. Fat	(mg) Chol.	(g) Carb.	(g) Fiber	(g) Sug.	(g) Prot.	(mg) Sod.
Spaghetti, Cooked, Enriched, with Salt 1 cup (140g)	220	1	0	0	43	2.5	1	8	183
Spaghetti, Cooked, Enriched, Without Salt 1 cup (140g)	221	1	0	0	43	2.5	1	8	1
Spaghetti, Cooked, Unenriched, with Salt 1 cup (140g)	220	1	0	0	43	2.5	1	8	183
Spaghetti, Cooked, Unenriched, Without Salt 1 cup (140g)	221	1	0	0	43	2.5	1	8	1
Spaghetti, Dry, Enriched 2 oz (57g)	211	1	0	0	43	1.8	2	7	3
Spaghetti, Dry, Unenriched 2 oz (57g)	211	1	0	0	43	1.8	2	7	3
Spaghetti, Protein-fortified, Cooked, Enriched (N x 5.70) 1 cup (140g)	230	0	0	0	44	2.4	0	11	7
Spaghetti, Protein-fortified, Cooked, Enriched (N x 6.25) 1 cup (140g)	230	0	0	0	43	2.8	0	12	7
Spaghetti, Protein-fortified, Dry, Enriched (N x 5.70) 2 oz (57g)	214	1	0	0	39	0	0	11	5
Spaghetti, Protein-fortified, Dry, Enriched (N x 6.25) 2 oz (57g)	213	1	0	0	37	1.4	0	12	5
Spaghetti, Spinach, Cooked 1 cup (140g)	182	1	0	0	37	0	0	6	20
Spaghetti, Spinach, Dry 2 oz (57g)	212	1	0	0	43	6	2	8	21
Spaghetti, Whole Wheat, Cooked 1 cup (140g)	174	1	0	0	37	6.3	1	7	4
Spaghetti, Whole Wheat, Dry 2 oz (57g)	198	1	0	0	43	0	0	8	5
Tortellini, Pasta with Cheese Filling, Fresh-refrigerated .75 cup (81g)	249	6	3	34	38	1.5	2	11	499
Vermicelli, Made from Soy 1 cup (140g)	463	0	0	0	115	5.5	0	0	6
Wonton Wrappers (Including Egg Roll Wrappers) 1 wrapper, egg roll (7" square) (32g)	93	0	0	3	19	0.6	0	3	183

Food Serving size	Cal.	(g) Total Fat	(g) Sat. Fat	(mg) Chol.	(g) Carb.	(g) Fiber	(g) Sug.	(g) Prot.	(mg) Sod.
Rice									
Rice Bowl with Chicken, Frozen Entrée, Prepared 1 bowl (340g)	428	5	1	54	76	2.4	80	19	1132
Rice Bran, Crude 1 cup (118g)	373	25	5	0	59	24.8	1	16	6
Rice Cake, Cracker (Including Hain Mini Rice Cakes) 1 cubic inch (4.2g)	16	0	0	0	3	0.2	0	0	3
Rice Cakes, Brown Rice, Buckwheat 2 cakes (18g)	68	1	0	0	14	0.7	0	2	21
Rice Cakes, Brown Rice, Buckwheat, Unsalted 2 cakes (18g)	68	1	0	0	14	0	0	2	1
Rice Cakes, Brown Rice, Multi-grain 2 cakes (18g)	70	1	0	0	14	0.5	0	2	45
Rice Cakes, Brown Rice, Multi-grain, Unsalted 2 cakes (18g)	70	1	0	0	14	0	0	2	1
Rice Cakes, Brown Rice, Plain 2 cakes (18g)	70	1	0	0	15	0.8	0	1	59
Rice Cakes, Brown Rice, Plain, Unsalted 2 cakes (18g)	70	1	0	0	15	0.8	0	1	5
Rice Cakes, Brown Rice, Rye 2 cakes (18g)	69	1	0	0	14	0.7	0	1	20
Rice Cakes, Brown Rice, Sesame Seed 2 cakes (18g)	71	1	0	0	15	1	0	1	41
Rice Cakes, Brown Rice, Sesame Seed, Unsalted 2 cakes (18g)	71	1	0	0	15	0	0	1	1
Rice Noodles, Cooked 1 cup (176g)	192	0	0	0	44	1.8	0	2	33
Rice Noodles, Dry 2 oz (57g)	207	0	0	0	47	0.9	0	2	104
Rice, Brown, Long-grain, Cooked 1 cup (195g)	216	2	0	0	45	3.5	1	5	10
Rice, Brown, Medium-grain, Cooked 1 cup (195g)	218	2	0	0	46	3.5	0	5	2
Rice, White, Glutinous, Cooked 1 cup (174g)	169	0	0	0	37	1.7	0	4	9

Food Serving size	Cal.	(g) Total Fat	(g) Sat. Fat	(mg) Chol.	(g) Carb.	(g) Fiber	(g) Sug.	(g) Prot.	(mg) Sod.
Rice, White, Long-grain, Parboiled, Enriched, Cooked 1 cup (158g)	194	1	0	0	41	1.4	0	5	3
Rice, White, Long-grain, Parboiled, Enriched, Dry 1 cup (185g)	692	2	1	0	150	3.3	1	14	4
Rice, White, Long-grain, Parboiled, Unenriched, Cooked 1 cup (158g)	194	1	0	0	41	1.4	0	5	3
Rice, White, Long-grain, Parboiled, Unenriched, Dry 1 cup (185g)	692	2	1	0	150	3.3	1	14	4
Rice, White, Long-grain, Precooked or Instant, Enriched, Dry 1 cup (95g)	361	1	0	0	78	1.8	0	7	10
Rice, White, Long-grain, Precooked or Instant, Enriched, Prepared 1 cup (165g)	193	1	0	0	41	1	0	4	7
Rice, White, Long-grain, Regular, Cooked 1 cup (158g)	205	0	0	0	45	0.6	0	4	2
Rice, White, Long-grain, Regular, Cooked, Enriched, with Salt 1 cup (158g)	205	0	0	0	45	0.6	0	4	604
Rice, White, Long-grain, Regular, Cooked, Unenriched, with Salt 1 cup (158g)	205	0	0	0	45	0.6	0	4	604
Rice, White, Long-grain, Regular, Cooked, Unenriched, Without Salt 1 cup (158g)	205	0	0	0	45	0.6	0	4	2
Rice, White, Medium-grain, Cooked 1 cup (186g)	242	0	0	0	53	0.6	0	4	0
Rice, White, Medium-grain, Cooked, Unenriched 1 cup (186g)	242	0	0	0	53	0	0	4	0
Rice, White, Short-grain, Cooked 1 cup (186g)	242	0	0	0	53	0	0	4	0
Rice, White, Short-grain, Cooked, Unenriched 1 cup (205g)	267	0	0	0	59	0	0	5	0
Rice, White, with Pasta, Cooked 1 cup (202g)	246	6	1	2	43	5.1	0	5	1147
Rice, White, with Pasta, Dry 1 cup (163g)	600	4	1	3	123	0	0	15	3042
Wild Rice, Cooked 1 cup (164g)	166	1	0	0	35	3	1	7	5

Food Serving size	Cal.	(g) Total Fat	(g) Sat. Fat	(mg) Chol.	(g) Carb.	(g) Fiber	(g) Sug.	(g) Prot.	(mg) Sod.
Cereals and Cereal Bars									
Amaranth Flakes 1 cup (38g)	134	3	1	0	27	3.6	5	6	13
Breakfast Bar, Corn Flake Crust with Fruit 1 oz (28.35g)	107	2	0	0	21	0.6	0	1	47
Cereal Ready-to-eat, Crispy Brown Rice 1 cup (32g)	124	1	0	0	28	2.3	0	2	4
Cereals Ready-to-eat, Familia 1 cup (122g)	473	8	1	0	90	10.4	0	12	61
Cereals Ready-to-eat, Frosted Oat Cereal, with Marshmallows .75 cup (30g)	116	1	0	0	25	1.3	0	2	150
Cereals Ready-to-eat, Marshmallow Alpha-Bits 1 cup (1 NLEA serving) (29g)	115	1	0	0	25	0.5	0	2	206
Cereals Ready-to-eat, Muesli, Dried Fruits and Nuts 1 cup (85g)	289	4	1	0	66	6.2	0	8	196
Cereals Ready-to-eat, Oat Bran Flakes, Health Valley 1 cup (47g)	166	1	0	0	37	6.1	0	5	17
Cereals Ready-to-eat, Post Banana Nut Crunch 1 cup (1 NLEA serving) (59g)	249	6	1	0	44	4	2	5	230
Cereals Ready-to-eat, Post Great Grains, Raisin, Date and Pecan .667 cup (1 NLEA serving) (54g)	204	5	1	0	40	4	0	4	160
Cereals Ready-to-eat, Post Honey Bunches of Oats, Honey Roasted .75 cup (1 NLEA serving) (30g)	118	1	0	0	25	1.4	2	2	150
Cereals Ready-to-eat, Post Honey Bunches of Oats, with Almonds .75 cup (1 NLEA serving) (31g)	126	3	0	0	24	1.4	0	2	136
Cereals Ready-to-eat, Weetabix, Whole Wheat Cereal 1 biscuit (18g)	67	1	0	0	14	2.1	0	2	70
Cereals Ready-to-eat, Wheat and Bran, Presweetened with Nuts and Fruits 1 cup (1 NLEA serving) (55g)	212	3	0	0	42	5.3	1	4	280
Cereals Ready-to-eat, Whole Wheat, Rolled Oats, Presweetened with Pecans .667 cup (1 NLEA serving) (53g)	216	6	1	0	38	3.7	0	5	214
Cereals, Corn Grits, White, Regular and Quick, Enriched, Cooked with Water, with Salt 1 tablespoon (16g)	11	0	0	0	2	0.1	0	0	36

Food Serving size	Cal.	(g) Total Fat	(g) Sat. Fat	(mg) Chol.	(g) Carb.	(g) Fiber	(g) Sug.	(g) Prot.	(mg) Sod.
Cereals, Corn Grits, White, Regular and Quick, Enriched, Cooked with Water, Without Salt 1 tbsp (16g)	11	0	0	0	2	0.1	0	0	0
Cereals, Corn Grits, White, Regular and Quick, Enriched, Dry 1 cup (156g)	577	3	1	0	123	7.2	1	12	2
Cereals, Corn Grits, White, Regular and Quick, Unenriched, Cooked with Water, with Salt 1 tablespoon (16g)	11	0	0	0	2	0.1	0	0	36
Cereals, Corn Grits, White, Regular and Quick, Unenriched, Cooked with Water, Without Salt .75 cup (182g)	107	0	0	0	23	0.5	0	3	4
Cereals, Corn Grits, White, Regular and Quick, Unenriched, Dry 1 tbsp (9.7g)	36	0	0	0	8	0.2	0	1	0
Cereals, Corn Grits, Yellow, Regular and Quick, Enriched, Cooked with Water, with Salt 1 cup (233g)	151	1	0	0	32	1.6	0	3	520
Cereals, Corn Grits, Yellow, Regular and Quick, Enriched, Cooked with Water, Without Salt 1 tbsp (16g)	151	1	0	0	32	1.6	0	3	5
Cereals, Corn Grits, Yellow, Regular and Quick, Enriched, Dry 1 cup (170g)	626	3	0	0	136	6.6	1	11	3
Cereals, Corn Grits, Yellow, Regular and Quick, Unenriched, Cooked with Water, with Salt .75 cup (182g)	151	1	0	0	32	1.6	0	3	520
Cereals, Corn Grits, Yellow, Regular and Quick, Unenriched, Cooked with Water, Without Salt .75 cup (182g)	107	0	0	0	23	0.5	0	3	4
Cereals, Corn Grits, Yellow, Regular and Quick, Unenriched, Dry 1 cup (156g)	579	2	0	0	124	2.5	1	14	2
Cereals, Cream of Rice, Cooked with Water, with Salt .75 cup (183g)	95	0	0	0	21	0.2	0	2	317
Cereals, Cream of Rice, Cooked with Water, Without Salt 1 tbsp (15g)	8	0	0	0	2	0	0	0	0
Cereals, Cream of Rice, Dry .25 cup (1 NLEA serving) (46g)	167	0	0	0	37	0.3	0	3	3

Food Serving size	Cal.	(g) Total Fat	(g) Sat. Fat	(mg) Chol.	(g) Carb.	(g) Fiber	(g) Sug.	(g) Prot.	(mg) Sod.
Cereals, Cream of Wheat, 1 Minute Cook Time, Dry									
1 tbsp (13.7g)	49	0	0	0	10	0.6	0	2	1
Cereals, Cream of Wheat, 1 Minute, Cooked with Water, Microwaved, Without Salt									
1 cup (237g)	130	1	0	0	25	3.6	7	5	9
Cereals, Cream of Wheat, 1 Minute, Cooked with Water, Stove-top, Without Salt									
1 cup (245g)	137	1	0	0	27	1	0	4	10
Cereals, Cream of Wheat, 2 1/2 Minutes, Cooked with Water, Microwaved									
1 cup (231g)	120	1	0	0	23	1.6	1	4	104
Cereals, Cream of Wheat, 2 1/2 Minutes, Cooked, Dry									
1 tbsp (13.8g)	49	0	0	0	10	0.6	0	2	45
Cereals, Cream of Wheat, 2 1/2 Minutes, Cooked, Stove-top, Without Salt									
1 cup (244g)	137	0	0	0	29	1.7	0	4	83
Cereals, Cream of Wheat, Instant, Dry									
1 cup (178g)	651	2	0	0	134	5.9	1	19	1016
Cereals, Cream of Wheat, Instant, Prepared with Water, with Salt (Wheat)									
.75 cup (181g)	112	0	0	0	24	1.1	0	3	273
Cereals, Cream of Wheat, Instant, Prepared with Water, Without Salt									
1 tbsp (15g)	9	0	0	0	2	0.1	0	0	15
Cereals, Cream of Wheat, Mix 'n Eat, Apple, Banana and Maple Flavors, Dry									
1 packet (35g)	131	0	0	0	29	0.9	0	2	238
Cereals, Cream of Wheat, Mix 'n Eat, Apple, Banana and Maple Flavors, Prepared									
1 packet, prepared (150g)	132	0	0	0	29	0.5	0	2	242
Cereals, Cream of Wheat, Mix 'n Eat, Plain, Dry									
1 packet (28g)	101	0	0	0	21	0.6	0	3	238
Cereals, Cream of Wheat, Mix 'n Eat, Plain, Prepared with Water									
1 packet, prepared (142g)	102	0	0	0	21	0.4	0	3	241
Cereals, Cream of Wheat, Regular (10 Minutes), Cooked with Water, with Salt									
1 cup (1 serving) (251g)	126	1	0	0	27	1.3	0	4	324
Cereals, Cream of Wheat, Regular (10 Minutes), Cooked with Water, Without Salt									
1 tbsp (16g)	8	0	0	0	2	0.1	0	0	1
Cereals, Cream of Wheat, Regular, 10 Minutes Cooking, Dry									
1 serving (3 tbsp) (33g)	122	0	0	0	25	1.3	0	3	2
Cereals, Farina, Enriched, Assorted Brands, Dry									
1 cup (176g)	634	2	0	0	129	7.4	1	20	218

Food Serving size	Cal.	(g) Total Fat	(g) Sat. Fat	(mg) Chol.	(g) Carb.	(g) Fiber	(g) Sug.	(g) Prot.	(mg) Sod.
Cereals, Farina, Enriched, Assorted Brands, Quick, Cooked with Water, Without Salt 1 tbsp (14.9g)	8	0	0	0	2	0.1	0	0	3
Cereals, Farina, Enriched, Cooked with Water, with Salt 1 cup (233g)	123	1	0	0	25	1.9	2	4	294
Cereals, Farina, Enriched, Cooked with Water, Without Salt 1 tbsp (15g)	8	0	0	0	2	0.1	0	0	3
Cereals, Farina, Unenriched, Dry 1 cup (176g)	649	1	0	0	137	3.3	0	19	5
Cereals, Kashi GoLean Hot Cereal, Hearty Honey and Cinnamon, Dry 1 packet (1 NLEA serving) (40g)	147	2	0	0	27	4.8	7	7	109
Cereals, Kashi, Heart to Heart, Instant Oatmeal, Apple Cinnamon, Dry 1 packet (1 NLEA serving) (43g)	152	2	0	0	32	5.4	11	5	89
Cereals, Kashi, Heart to Heart, Instant Oatmeal, Maple, Dry 1 packet (1 NLEA serving) (43g)	162	2	0	0	33	5	12	5	99
Cereals, Kashi, Kashi GoLean Hot Cereal, Truly Vanilla, Dry 1 packet (1 NLEA serving) (40g)	144	2	0	0	24	7.4	6	9	110
Cereals, Maltex, Cooked with Water, with Salt .75 cup (187g)	142	1	0	0	30	1.7	0	4	142
Cereals, Maltex, Cooked with Water, Without Salt 1 tbsp (16g)	12	0	0	0	3	0.1	0	0	1
Cereals, Maltex, Dry .25 cup (38g)	134	1	0	0	29	1.6	0	4	6
Cereals, Malt-O-Meal, Chocolate, Dry 1 tbsp (10.3g)	127	0	0	0	28	1	6	4	4
Cereals, Malt-O-Meal, Chocolate, Prepared with Water, Without Salt 1 serving (3 T dry cereal plus 1 cup water) (268g)	126	0	0	0	25	1.1	6	4	3
Cereals, Malt-O-Meal, Farina Hot Wheat Cereal, Dry 3 tbsp (35g)	127	0	0	0	26	1.4	0	5	4
Cereals, Malt-O-Meal, Original, Plain, Dry 1 tbsp (10.3g)	128	0	0	0	27	1	0	4	1
Cereals, Malt-O-Meal, Original, Plain, Prepared with Water, Without Salt 1 serving (3 T dry cereal plus 1 cup water) (268g)	129	0	0	0	25	1.1	0	4	0

Food Serving size	Cal.	(g) Total Fat	(g) Sat. Fat	(mg) Chol.	(g) Carb.	(g) Fiber	(g) Sug.	(g) Prot.	(mg) Sod.
Cereals, Maypo, Cooked with Water, with Salt .75 cup (180g)	128	2	0	0	24	3.6	11	4	194
Cereals, Maypo, Cooked with Water, Without Salt 1 tbsp (15g)	11	0	0	0	2	0.4	1	0	1
Cereals, Maypo, Dry 5 cup (47g)	181	2	0	0	34	5.1	16	6	9
Cereals, Oats, Instant, Fortified, Plain, Dry 1 packet (28g)	101	2	0	0	19	2.8	0	3	62
Cereals, Oats, Instant, Fortified, Plain, Prepared with Water 1 cup, dry, yields (501g)	341	7	1	0	58	8.5	2	12	245
Cereals, Oats, Instant, Fortified, with Cinnamon and Spice, Dry 1 packet (46g)	170	2	0	0	35	3	16	4	222
Cereals, Oats, Instant, Fortified, with Cinnamon and Spice, Prepared with Water 1 tbsp (15g)	16	0	0	0	3	0.3	1	0	20
Cereals, Oats, Instant, Fortified, with Raisins and Spice, Dry 1 packet (43g)	158	2	0	0	34	2.5	16	4	203
Cereals, Oats, Instant, Fortified, with Raisins and Spice, Prepared with Water 1 tbsp (15g)	13	0	0	0	3	0.2	1	0	17
Cereals, Oats, Regular and Quick and Instant, Not Fortified, Dry .333 cup (27g)	102	2	0	0	18	2.7	0	4	2
Cereals, Oats, Regular and Quick and Instant, Unenriched, Cooked with Water, with Salt 75 cup (175g)	124	3	1	0	21	3	0	4	124
Cereals, Oats, Regular and Quick and Instant, Unenriched, Cooked with Water, Without Salt 1 tbsp (14.6g)	10	0	0	0	2	0.2	0	0	1
Cereals, Quaker, Corn Grits, Instant, Butter Flavor, Dry 1 packet (28g)	103	2	1	0	21	1.3	0	2	335
Cereals, Quaker, Corn Grits, Instant, Cheddar Cheese Flavor, Dry 1 packet (28g)	102	2	0	1	20	1.2	1	3	460
Cereals, Quaker, Corn Grits, Instant, Cheddar Cheese Flavor, Prepared with Water 1 packet, prepared (142g)	102	2	0	0	20	1.1	1	2	508
Cereals, Quaker, Corn Grits, Instant, Country Bacon (Imitation Bacon Bits) Prepared with Water 1 packet, prepared (141g)	97	0	0	0	21	1.4	0	3	413

Food Serving size	Cal.	(g) Total Fat	(g) Sat. Fat	(mg) Chol.	(g) Carb.	(g) Fiber	(g) Sug.	(g) Prot.	(mg) Sod.
Cereals, Quaker, Corn Grits, Instant, Plain, Dry 1 tbsp (7g)	24	0	0	0	5	0.3	0	1	78
Cereals, Quaker, Corn Grits, Instant, Plain, Prepared Without Salt 1 cup (219g)	162	1	0	0	35	2.4	0	3	497
Cereals, Quaker, Corn Grits, Instant, with Imitation Bacon Bits, Dry 1 packet (28g)	98	0	0	0	22	1.5	0	3	341
Cereals, Quaker, Farina, Creamy Wheat, Enriched, Dry .25 cup (1 NLEA serving) (44g)	154	0	0	0	33	1.3	0	5	1
Cereals, Quaker, Hominy Grits, White, Quick, Dry .25 cup (37g)	129	0	0	0	29	1.8	0	3	0
Cereals, Quaker, Hominy Grits, White, Regular, Dry .25 cup (41g)	148	1	0	0	32	0.7	0	4	0
Cereals, Quaker, Hominy Grits, Yellow, Quick, Dry .25 cup (37g)	125	1	0	0	29	2.1	0	3	1
Cereals, Quaker, Instant Grits Product with American Cheese Flavor, Dry 1 packet (28g)	101	1	0	0	21	1.2	1	2	425
Cereals, Quaker, Instant Grits Product with Ham-n-Cheese 1 packet (28g)	99	1	0	0	20	1.2	1	3	540
Cereals, Quaker, Instant Grits Product with Imitation Bacon Bits and Cheddar Flavor, Dry 1 packet (28g)	102	1	0	0	20	1.3	1	3	436
Cereals, Quaker, Instant Grits, with Redeye Gravy and Imitation Ham Bits, Dry 1 packet (28g)	96	0	0	0	21	1.3	0	3	505
Cereals, Quaker, Instant Oat, Maple and Brown Sugar, Prepared with Boiling Water 1 packet, prepared (155g)	157	2	0	0	31	2.8	13	4	253
Cereals, Quaker, Instant Oatmeal Express Cinnamon Roll, Dry 1 cup (54g)	200	3	0	0	41	3.6	17	5	246
Cereals, Quaker, Instant Oatmeal Express, Baked Apple, Dry 1 cup (54g)	198	2	0	0	42	3.9	19	4	319
Cereals, Quaker, Instant Oatmeal, Apples and Cinnamon, Prepared with Boiling Water 1 packet, prepared (149g)	130	1	0	0	26	2.7	12	3	165
Cereals, Quaker, Instant Oatmeal, Apples and Cinnamon, Reduced Sugar 1 packet (35g)	111	2	0	0	22	3	6	3	166

Food Serving size	Cal.	(g) Total Fat	(g) Sat. Fat	(mg) Chol.	(g) Carb.	(g) Fiber	(g) Sug.	(g) Prot.	(mg) Sod.
Cereals, Quaker, Instant Oatmeal, Baked Apple, Prepared with Boiling Water									
1 packet, prepared (159g)	153	2	0	0	31	2.9	14	3	229
Cereals, Quaker, Instant Oatmeal, Banana Bread, Dry									
1 packet (41g)	151	2	0	0	31	2.7	12	4	287
Cereals, Quaker, Instant Oatmeal, Cinnamon Roll, Prepared with Boiling Water									
1 packet, prepared (173g)	209	3	0	0	41	3.6	17	5	249
Cereals, Quaker, Instant Oatmeal, Cinnamon Spice, Reduced Sugar									
1 packet (46g)	122	2	0	0	24	3	4	4	258
Cereals, Quaker, Instant Oatmeal, Cinnamon Spice, Prepared with Boiling Water									
1 tbsp (15g)	14	0	0	.0	3	0.3	1	0	17
Cereals, Quaker, Instant Oatmeal, Dinosaur Eggs with Dinosaur Bones, Brown Sugar Cinnamon, Dry									
1 packet (50g)	195	4	2	0	38	2.8	20	4	262
Cereals, Quaker, Instant Oatmeal, Dinosaur Eggs with Dinosaur Bones, Brown Sugar Cinnamon, Prepared with Boiling Water									
1 packet, prepared (167g)	199	4	2	0	38	2.8	19	4	261
Cereals, Quaker, Instant Oatmeal, Express Baked Apple, Prepared with Boiling Water									
1 packet, prepared (173g)	208	3	0	0	42	4	19	4	322
Cereals, Quaker, Instant Oatmeal, Express, Golden Brown Sugar, Dry									
1 cup (54g)	192	4	1	0	37	3.2	14	4	250
Cereals, Quaker, Instant Oatmeal, Express, Golden Brown Sugar, Prepared with Boiling Water									
1 packet, prepared (173g)	209	3	0	0	42	3.5	18	5	294
Cereals, Quaker, Instant Oatmeal, French Vanilla, Prepared with Boiling Water									
1 packet, prepared (162g)	165	2	0	0	33	2.9	13	4	249
Cereals, Quaker, Instant Oatmeal, Fruit and Cream, Prepared with Boiling Water									
1 packet, prepared (193g)	139	3	1	0	26	2.1	11	3	178
Cereals, Quaker, Instant Oatmeal, Fruit and Cream Variety, Reduced Sugar									
1 packet (35g)	124	2	1	0	24	2.7	6	3	184
Cereals, Quaker, Instant Oatmeal, Honey Nut, Prepared with Boiling Water									
1 packet, prepared (162g)	173	4	0	0	31	2.8	13	4	238
Cereals, Quaker, Instant Oatmeal, Low Sodium, Dry									
1 packet (28g)	102	2	0	0	19	2.7	0	4	78
Cereals, Quaker, Instant Oatmeal, Maple and Brown Sugar, Dry									
1 packet (43g)	158	2	0	0	33	3.1	13	4	217

Food Serving size	Cal.	(g) Total Fat	(g) Sat. Fat	(mg) Chol.	(g) Carb.	(g) Fiber	(g) Sug.	(g) Prot.	(mg) Sod.
Cereals, Quaker, Instant Oatmeal, Nutrition for Women, Apple Spice, Prepared with Boiling Water									
1 packet, prepared (166g)	178	2	0	0	35	3.2	16	5	319
Cereals, Quaker, Instant Oatmeal, Nutrition for Women, Brown Sugar, Prepared with Boiling Water									
1 packet, prepared (165g)	173	2	0	0	33	2.8	13	5	328
Cereals, Quaker, Instant Oatmeal, Raisin and Spice, Dry									
1 packet (43g)	155	2	0	0	33	2.5	15	4	189
Cereals, Quaker, Instant Oatmeal, Raisin and Spice, Prepared with Boiling Water									
1 packet, prepared (162g)	162	2	0	0	33	2.6	16	3	211
Cereals, Quaker, Instant Oatmeal, Raisins, Dates, and Walnuts, Dry									
1 packet (37g)	137	3	0	0	27	2.6	11	3	191
Cereals, Quaker, Instant Oatmeal, Treasure Hunt, Prepared with Boiling Water									
1 packet, prepared (166g)	179	2	1	0	36	2.7	17	4	257
Cereals, Quaker, Mother's Instant Oatmeal (Non-fortified), Dry									
.25 cup (1 NLEA serving) (40g)	144	3	1	0	26	3.8	1	5	1
Cereals, Quaker, Multigrain Oatmeal, Dry									
.5 cup (1 NLEA serving) (40g)	134	1	0	0	29	4.8	1	5	3
Cereals, Quaker, Oat Bran, Quaker/Mother's Oat Bran, Dry									
.5 cup (1 NLEA serving) (40g)	146	3	1	0	25	5.7	1	7	2
Cereals, Quaker, Quick Oats with iron, Dry									
.5 cup (40g)	148	3	0	0	27	3.8	1	5	.1
Cereals, Ralston, Cooked with Water, with Salt									
.75 cup (190g)	101	1	0	0	21	4.6	0	4	357
Cereals, Ralston, Cooked with Water, Without Salt									
1 tbsp (16g)	8	0	0	0	2	0.4	0	0	0
Cereals, Ralston, Dry									
.25 cup (30g)	102	1	0	0	22	4	0	4	3
Cereals, Ready-to-eat, Alpen									
1 cup (113g)	398	4	1	0	86	10.3	0	13	241
Cereals, Ready-to-eat, Apple Cinnamon Squares Mini-Wheats									
.75 cup (1 NLEA serving) (55g)	182	1	0	0	44	4.7	12	4	20
Cereals, Ready-to-eat, Bran Flakes, Single Brand									
.75 cup (1 NLEA serving) (30g)	96	1	0	0	24	5.3	6	3	220

Food Serving size	Cal.	(g) Total Fat	(g) Sat. Fat	(mg) Chol.	(g) Carb.	(g) Fiber	(g) Sug.	(g) Prot.	(mg) Sod.
Cereals, Ready-to-eat, Chocolate-flavored Frosted Puffed Corn									
1 cup (30g)	122	1	0	0	26	1.1	13	1	160
Cereals, Ready-to-eat, Corn Flakes									
1 oz (28.35g)	113	0	0	0	25	0.3	2	2	3
Cereals, Ready-to-eat, Cranberry Macadamia Nut Cereal									
1 cup (60g)	245	6	1	0	46	3.6	17	4	251
Cereals, Ready-to-eat, General Mills Cinnamon Chex									
.75 cup (1 NLEA serving) (30g)	121	2	0	0	25	0.7	8	1	184
Cereals, Ready-to-eat, General Mills Peanut Butter Toast Crunch									
.75 cup (30g)	130	4	1	0	23	1	13	2	135
Cereals, Ready-to-eat, General Mills, Apple Cinnamon Cheerios									
.75 cup (1 NLEA serving) (30g)	116	2	0	0	24	2	10	2	117
Cereals, Ready-to-eat, General Mills, Basic 4									
1 cup (1 NLEA serving) (55g)	197	2	1	0	44	3.7	12	4	285
Cereals, Ready-to-eat, General Mills, Berry Berry Kix									
.75 cup (1 NLEA serving) (26g)	124	1	0	0	28	1.9	7	2	171
Cereals, Ready-to-eat, General Mills, Berry Burst Cheerios, All Flavors									
.75 cup (1 NLEA serving) (27g)	99	1	0	0	22	2	8	3	173
Cereals, Ready-to-eat, General Mills, Boo Berry									
1 cup (1 NLEA serving) (33g)	127	1	0	0	28	1.4	9	2	151
Cereals, Ready-to-eat, General Mills, Cheerios									
1 cup (1 NLEA serving) (28g)	105	2	0	0	21	2.6	1	3	139
Cereals, Ready-to-eat, General Mills, Cheerios, Banana Nut									
.75 cup (1 NLEA serving) (28g)	105	1	0	0	24	1.7	9	2	149
Cereals, Ready-to-eat, General Mills, Cheerios, Chocolate									
.75 cup (1 NLEA serving) (27g)	103	1	0	0	23	1.7	9	2	150
Cereals, Ready-to-eat, General Mills, Cheerios, Yogurt Burst									
.75 cup (1 NLEA serving) (30g)	120	2	1	0	25	2	10	2	175
Cereals, Ready-to-eat, General Mills, Chocolate Chex									
.75 cup (1 NLEA serving) (32g)	132	3	1	0	26	0.6	8	2	205
Cereals, Ready-to-eat, General Mills, Chocolate Lucky Charms									
.75 cup (1 NLEA serving) (28g)	107	1	0	0	24	1.5	10	2	151
Cereals, Ready-to-eat, General Mills, Cinnamon Grahams									
.75 cup (30g)	113	1	0	0	26	1	11	2	237

Food Serving size	Cal.	(g) Total Fat	(g) Sat. Fat	(mg) Chol.	(g) Carb.	(g) Fiber	(g) Sug.	(g) Prot.	(mg) Sod.
Cereals, Ready-to-eat, General Mills, Cinnamon Toast Crunch									
.75 cup (1 NLEA serving) (31g)	127	3	0	0	24	2.1	9	2	177
Cereals, Ready-to-eat, General Mills, Cocoa Puffs, 25% Reduced Sugar									
.75 cup (1 NLEA serving) (27g)	92	1	0	0	20	1.4	6	1	125
Cereals, Ready-to-eat, General Mills, Cookie Crisp									
1 oz (28.35g)	99	1	0	0	22	1.3	9	1	119
Cereals, Ready-to-eat, General Mills, Corn Chex									
1 cup (1 NLEA serving) (31g)	115	1	0	0	26	1.7	3	2	236
Cereals, Ready-to-eat, General Mills, Count Chocula									
.75 cup (1 NLEA serving) (27g)	103	1	0	0	23	1.4	9	1	132
Cereals, Ready-to-eat, General Mills, Dora the Explorer									
.75 cup (1 NLEA serving) (27g)	99	2	0	0	22	2.8	6	2	152
Cereals, Ready-to-eat, General Mills, Fiber One									
.5 cup (1 NLEA serving) (30g)	60	1	0	0	25	14.2	0	2	106
Cereals, Ready-to-eat, General Mills, Fiber One, Caramel Delight									
1 cup (1 NLEA serving) (50g)	172	3	1	0	41	9.6	10	3	235
Cereals, Ready-to-eat, General Mills, Fiber One, Frosted Shredded Wheat									
1 cup (1 NLEA serving) (60g)	193	1	0	0	49	9	12	5	1
Cereals, Ready-to-eat, General Mills, Fiber One, Honey Clusters									
1 cup (1 NLEA serving) (52g)	168	1	0	0	44	10	9	4	220
Cereals, Ready-to-eat, General Mills, Fiber One, Raisin Bran Clusters									
1 cup (1 NLEA serving) (55g)	174	1	0	0	46	10	14	3	199
Cereals, Ready-to-eat, General Mills, Franken Berry									
1 cup (1 NLEA serving) (33g)	127	1	0	0	28	1.4	9	2	151
Cereals, Ready-to-eat, General Mills, French Toast Crunch									
.75 cup (1 NLEA serving) (31g)	136	3	0	0	24	1	11	2	223
Cereals, Ready-to-eat, General Mills, Frosted Cheerios									
.75 cup (1 NLEA serving) (28g)	106	1	0	0	23	1.8	9	2	171
Cereals, Ready-to-eat, General Mills, Frosted Chex									
.75 cup (1 NLEA serving) (30g)	110	1	0	0	27	0	10	1	180
Cereals, Ready-to-eat, General Mills, Fruity Cheerios									
.75 cup (1 NLEA serving) (27g)	103	1	0	0	23	1.6	9	2	135
Cereals, Ready-to-eat, General Mills, Golden Grahams									
.75 cup (1 NLEA serving) (30g)	116	1	0	0	26	1.7	11	2	239

Food Serving size	Cal.	(g) Total Fat	(g) Sat. Fat	(mg) Chol.	(g) Carb.	(g) Fiber	(g) Sug.	(g) Prot.	(mg) Sod.
Cereals, Ready-to-eat, General Mills, Harmony									
1.25 cup (55g)	201	1	0	0	43	2.2	13	6	355
Cereals, Ready-to-eat, General Mills, Honey Nut Cheerios									
.75 cup (1 NLEA serving) (28g)	105	1	0	0	22	2	9	2	158
Cereals, Ready-to-eat, General Mills, Honey Nut Chex									
.75 cup (1 NLEA serving) (32g)	120	1	0	0	28	1.2	9	2	192
Cereals, Ready-to-eat, General Mills, Honey Nut Clusters									
1 cup (1 NLEA serving) (57g)	213	1	0	0	49	3.6	14	4	294
Cereals, Ready-to-eat, General Mills, Kaboom									
1.25 cup (1 NLEA serving) (30g)	120	1	0	0	26	1	6	1	190
Cereals, Ready-to-eat, General Mills, Kix									
1 cup (24g)	107	1	0	0	25	2.6	3	2	179
Cereals, Ready-to-eat, General Mills, Lucky Charms									
1 cup (35g)	103	1	0	0	22	1.4	1	2	175
Cereals, Ready-to-eat, General Mills, Multi-Bran Chex									
.75 cup (1 NLEA serving) (47g)	154	1	0	0	40	5.7	10	3	265
Cereals, Ready-to-eat, General Mills, Multi-Grain Cheerios									
1 cup (1 NLEA serving) (29g)	107	1	0	0	24	2.5	6	2	116
Cereals, Ready-to-eat, General Mills, Nature Valley Low Fat Fruit Granola									
.667 cup (1 NLEA serving) (55g)	210	3	0	0	44	2.8	18	4	273
Cereals, Ready-to-eat, General Mills, Oatmeal Crisp with Almonds									
1 cup (1 NLEA serving) (60g)	234	4	1	0	47	4.9	14	6	127
Cereals, Ready-to-eat, General Mills, Oatmeal Crisp, Apple Cinnamon									
1 cup (1 NLEA serving) (55g)	210	2	1	0	46	4	19	4	270
Cereals, Ready-to-eat, General Mills, Oatmeal Crisp, Raisin									
1 cup (1 NLEA serving) (62g)	237	2	0	0	52	4.7	20	5	122
Cereals, Ready-to-eat, General Mills, Raisin Nut Bran									
.75 cup (1 NLEA serving) (49g)	180	3	0	0	40	4.9	14	3	223
Cereals, Ready-to-eat, General Mills, Reese's Puffs									
.75 cup (1 NLEA serving) (29g)	120	3	1	0	22	1.4	10	2	161
Cereals, Ready-to-eat, General Mills, Rice Chex									
1 cup (1 NLEA serving) (27g)	101	0	0	0	23	1.2	2	2	242
Cereals, Ready-to-eat, General Mills, Total Blueberry Pomegranate									
1 cup (1 NLEA serving) (49g)	173	2	0	0	38	3.9	11	5	96

Food Serving size	Cal.	(g) Total Fat	(g) Sat. Fat	(mg) Chol.	(g) Carb.	(g) Fiber	(g) Sug.	(g) Prot.	(mg) Sod.
Cereals, Ready-to-eat, General Mills, Total Corn Flakes 1.333 cup (1 NLEA serving) (30g)	112	0	0	0	26	0.8	3	2	209
Cereals, Ready-to-eat, General Mills, Total Cranberry Crunch 1.25 cup (1 NLEA serving) (58g)	194	1	0	0	46	4.2	16	4	194
Cereals, Ready-to-eat, General Mills, Total Raisin Bran 1 cup (1 NLEA serving) (53g)	165	1	0	0	41	4.8	17	3	180
Cereals, Ready-to-eat, General Mills, Trix 1 cup (1 NLEA serving) (32g)	123	1	0	0	27	1.4	10	2	178
Cereals, Ready-to-eat, General Mills, Trix, Reduced Sugar, Bowlpak 1 bowlpak (21g)	84	1	0	0	18	1	6	1	120
Cereals, Ready-to-eat, General Mills, Wheat Chex .75 cup (1 NLEA serving) (47g)	119	0	0	0	27	0.6	13	1	249
Cereals, Ready-to-eat, General Mills, Wheaties .75 cup (1 NLEA serving) (27g)	95	1	-0	0	22	2.7	4	2	198
Cereals, Ready-to-eat, General Mills, Wheaties FUEL .75 cup (1 NLEA serving) (55g)	206	3	0	0	46	5.3	14	3	152
Cereals, Ready-to-eat, General Mills, Wheaties Raisin Bran 1 cup (1 NLEA serving) (55g)	183	1	0	0	45	5	18	4	251
Cereals, Ready-to-eat, General Mills, Whole Grain Total .75 cup (1 NLEA serving) (30g)	96	1	0	0	22	2.7	5	3	141
Cereals, Ready-to-eat, Granola, Homemade 1 oz (28.35g)	139	7	1	0	15	2.6	6	4	7
Cereals, Ready-to-eat, Health Valley, Fiber 7 Flakes .75 cup (1 NLEA serving) (31g)	109	0	0	0	24	4.4	6	4	62
Cereals, Ready-to-eat, Just Right with Crunchy Nuggets 1 cup (1 NLEA serving) (55g)	204	1	0	0	46	2.8	12	4	338
Cereals, Ready-to-eat, Kashi, Cinna-Raisin Crunch 1 cup (50g)	165	1	0	0	41	7.6	13	4	104
Cereals, Ready-to-eat, Kashi 7 Whole Grain Flakes 1 cup (1 NLEA serving) (50g)	169	1	0	0	41	5.9	6	6	146
Cereals, Ready-to-eat, Kashi 7 Whole Grain Honey Puffs 1 cup (1 NLEA serving) (30g)	105	1	0	0	24	1.8	7	3	2
Cereals, Ready-to-eat, Kashi 7 Whole Grain Nuggets .5 cup (1 NLEA serving) (58g)	206	2	0	0	47	6.8	3	7	260

Food Serving size	Cal.	(g) Total Fat	(g) Sat. Fat	(mg) Chol.	(g) Carb.	(g) Fiber	(g) Sug.	(g) Prot.	(mg) Sod.
Cereals, Ready-to-eat, Kashi GoLean									
1 cup (1 NLEA serving) (52g)	162	1	0	0	35	10.5	9	13	92
Cereals, Ready-to-eat, Kashi GoLean Crunch!									
1 cup (1 NLEA serving) (53g)	195	3	0	0	38	7.7	13	9	99
Cereals, Ready-to-eat, Kashi GoLean Crunch!, Honey Almond Flax									
1 cup (1 NLEA serving) (53g)	201	5	1	0	35	8	12	9	142
Cereals, Ready-to-eat, Kashi Good Friends									
1 cup (1 NLEA serving) (53g)	158	2	0	0	42	11.5	10	5	108
Cereals, Ready-to-eat, Kashi Granola, Cocoa Beach Cereal									
.5 cup (1 NLEA serving) (55g)	226	9	2	0	34	7	11	6	138
Cereals, Ready-to-eat, Kashi Granola, Mountain Medley Cereal									
.5 cup (1 NLEA serving) (55g)	218	7	1	0	37	6.3	12	6	121
Cereals, Ready-to-eat, Kashi Granola, Orchard Spice Cereal									
.5 cup (1 NLEA serving) (55g)	222	7	1	0	37	6.3	11	6	132
Cereals, Ready-to-eat, Kashi Granola, Summer Berry Cereal									
.5 cup (1 NLEA serving) (55g)	215	6	1	0	37	6.8	9	7	132
Cereals, Ready-to-eat, Kashi Heart to Heart Warm Cinnamon									
.75 cup (1 NLEA serving) (33g)	120	2	0	0	26	4.4	5	4	83
Cereals, Ready-to-eat, Kashi Heart to Heart, Honey Toasted Oat									
.75 cup (1 NLEA serving) (33g)	120	2	0	0	26	4.5	5	4	88
Cereals, Ready-to-eat, Kashi Mighty Bites, Honey Crunch Cereal									
1 cup (1 NLEA serving) (33g)	116	1	0	0	23	3	6	6	159
Cereals, Ready-to-eat, Kashi Organic Promise Cinnamon Harvest									
1 cup (1 NLEA serving) (54g)	185	1	0	0	43	5.9	9	6	2
Cereals, Ready-to-eat, Kashi Organic Promise Island Vanilla Biscuit									
27 biscuits (1 NLEA serving) (55g)	193	1	0	0	44	5.9	9	6	7
Cereals, Ready-to-eat, Kashi Organic Promise Strawberry Fields									
1 cup (1 NLEA serving) (32g)	197	0	0	0	46	2.8	11	5	185
Cereals, Ready-to-eat, Kashi Heart to Heart Wild Blueberry									
1 cup (1 NLEA serving) (55g)	204	3	0	0	42	3.9	12	6	133
Cereals, Ready-to-eat, Kashi Kashi U									
1 cup (1 NLEA serving) (55g)	207	4	0	0	43	6.7	11	6	126
Cereals, Ready-to-eat, Kashi Organic Promise Autumn Wheat									
1 cup (1 NLEA serving) (54g)	191	1	0	0	45	6	7	5	0

Food Serving size	Cal.	(g) Total Fat	(g) Sat. Fat	(mg) Chol.	(g) Carb.	(g) Fiber	(g) Sug.	(g) Prot.	(mg) Sod.
Cereals, Ready-to-eat, Kellogg's Corn Flakes									
1 cup (1 NLEA serving) (28g)	100	0	0	0	24	0.9	3	2	204
Cereals, Ready-to-eat, Kellogg's Frosted Mini-Wheats, Original									
5 biscuits (1 NLEA serving) (51g)	175	1	0	0	42	5.1	11	5	5
Cereals, Ready-to-eat, Kellogg's Fruit Harvest Strawberry/Blueberry									
.75 cup (1 NLEA serving) (29g)	107	0	0	0	25	1.3	10	2	137
Cereals, Ready-to-eat, Kellogg's Honey Crunch Corn Flakes									
.75 cup (1 NLEA serving) (30g)	116	1	0	0	26	1	10	2	210
Cereals, Ready-to-eat, Kellogg's Mini-Wheats, Frosted Strawberry Delight									
24 biscuit (1 NLEA serving) (52g)	194	1	0	0	47	5.6	12	5	2
Cereals, Ready-to-eat, Kellogg's Special K, Low Carb Lifestyle Protein Plus									
.75 cup (1 NLEA serving) (29g)	101	3	1	0	14	4.9	2	10	110
Cereals, Ready-to-eat, Kellogg's Special K, Vanilla Almond									
.75 cup (1 NLEA serving) (30g)	113	1	0	0	25	2.8	9	2	171
Cereals, Ready-to-eat, Kellogg's, All-Bran Buds									
.333 cup (1 NLEA serving) (30g)	77	1	0	0	24	12.8	8	3	206
Cereals, Ready-to-eat, Kellogg's, All-Bran Strawberry Medley									
1 cup (1 NLEA serving) (55g)	175	2	0	0	44	9.9	10	6	231
Cereals, Ready-to-eat, Kellogg's, All-Bran with Extra Fiber									
.5 cup (1 NLEA serving) (26g)	50	1	0	0	20	13	0	3	124
Cereals, Ready-to-eat, Kellogg's, All-Bran Yogurt Bites									
1.25 cup (1 NLEA serving) (56g)	192	3	2	0	44	10.1	7	6	235
Cereals, Ready-to-eat, Kellogg's, All-Bran, Original									
.5 cup (1 NLEA serving) (31g)	81	2	0	0	23	9.1	5	4	80
Cereals, Ready-to-eat, Kellogg's, Apple Jacks									
1 cup (1 NLEA serving) (28g)	105	1	1	0	25	2.6	12	1	130
Cereals, Ready-to-eat, Kellogg's, Berry Rice Krispies									
1 cup (1 NLEA serving) (30g)	115	0	0	0	26	0.1	9	2	218
Cereals, Ready-to-eat, Kellogg's, Cinnabon Cereal									
1 cup (1 NLEA serving) (30g)	123	2	0	0	25	1.2	12	2	116
Cereals, Ready-to-eat, Kellogg's, Cinnamon Mini Swirlz									
1 cup (1 NLEA serving) (30g)	122	2	0	0	25	1	3	2	116

Food Serving size	Cal.	(g) Total Fat	(g) Sat. Fat	(mg) Chol.	(g) Carb.	(g) Fiber	(g) Sug.	(g) Prot.	(mg) Sod.
Cereals, Ready-to-eat, Kellogg's, Cocoa Krispies									
.75 cup (1 NLEA serving) (31g)	121	1	1	0	27	0.4	12	1	131
Cereals, Ready-to-eat, Kellogg's, Complete Oat Bran Flakes									
.75 cup (1 NLEA serving) (30g)	105	1	0	0	23	3.9	6	3	210
Cereals, Ready-to-eat, Kellogg's, Complete Wheat Flakes									
.75 cup (1 NLEA serving) (29g)	95	1	0	0	24	5	5	3	208
Cereals, Ready-to-eat, Kellogg's, Corn Pops									
1 cup (1 NLEA serving) (32g)	116	0	0	0	27	2.5	9	1	107
Cereals, Ready-to-eat, Kellogg's, Cracklin' Oat Bran									
.75 cup (1 NLEA serving) (49g)	194	7	3	0	34	6.2	14	5	137
Cereals, Ready-to-eat, Kellogg's, Crispix									
1 cup (laboratory weight) (30g)	107	0	0	0	25	0.8	3	2	177
Cereals, Ready-to-eat, Kellogg's, Eggo Crunch Cereal, Maple Flavor									
1 cup (1 NLEA serving) (31g)	117	1	0	0	26	1.8	12	2	146
Cereals, Ready-to-eat, Kellogg's, Froot Loops									
1 cup (1 NLEA serving) (29g)	109	1	1	0	26	2.7	12	2	136
Cereals, Ready-to-eat, Kellogg's, Frosted Flakes									
1 cup (42g)	155	1	0	0	37	0.9	15	2	197
Cereals, Ready-to-eat, Kellogg's, Frosted Mini-Wheats, Bite-size									
24 biscuits (1 NLEA serving) (59g)	189	1	0	0	45	5.8	11	5	1
Cereals, Ready-to-eat, Kellogg's, Frosted Mini-Wheats, Bite-size Strawberry									
24 biscuits (1 NLEA serving) (52g)	180	1	0	0	43	5	12	4	0
Cereals, Ready-to-eat, Kellogg's, Frosted Mini-Wheats, Maple and Brown Sugar, Bite-size									
24 biscuits (1 NLEA serving) (52g)	193	1	0	0	47	5.7	12	5	3
Cereals, Ready-to-eat, Kellogg's, Frosted Rice Krispies									
.75 cup (1 NLEA serving) (30g)	115	0	0	0	27	0.2	12	1	111
Cereals, Ready-to-eat, Kellogg's, Honey Smacks									
.75 cup (1 NLEA serving) (27g)	103	1	0	0	24	1.4	15	2	38
Cereals, Ready-to-eat, Kellogg's, Just Right Fruit and Nut									
.75 cup (1 NLEA serving) (53g)	194	2	0	0	43	2.8	13	4	243
Cereals, Ready-to-eat, Kellogg's, Low Fat Granola with Raisins									
.667 cup (1 NLEA serving) (60g)	229	3	1	0	48	4.4	17	5	149

Food Serving size	Cal.	(g) Total Fat	(g) Sat. Fat	(mg) Chol.	(g) Carb.	(g) Fiber	(g) Sug.	(g) Prot.	(mg) Sod.
Cereals, Ready-to-eat, Kellogg's, Low Fat Granola Without Raisins									
.5 cup (1 NLEA serving) (49g)	191	3	1	0	40	3.4	14	4	126
Cereals, Ready-to-eat, Kellogg's, Marshmallow Froot Loops									
1 cup (1 NLEA serving) (30g)	109	1	0	0	26	2.1	14	1	114
Cereals, Ready-to-eat, Kellogg's, Mueslix									
.667 cup (1 NLEA serving) (55g)	195	3	0	0	41	4.6	14	5	139
Cereals, Ready-to-eat, Kellogg's, Product 19									
1 cup (1 NLEA serving) (30g)	112	0	0	0	25	0.8	4	3	218
Cereals, Ready-to-eat, Kellogg's, Puffed Wheat									
.75 cup (1 NLEA serving) (9g)	29	0	0	0	7	1.4	0	1	0
Cereals, Ready-to-eat, Kellogg's, Raisin Bran									
1 cup (1 NLEA serving) (59g)	191	1	0	0	47	8.1	19	4	225
Cereals, Ready-to-eat, Kellogg's, Raisin Bran Crunch									
1 cup (1 NLEA serving) (53g)	188	1	0	0	45	4.2	19	3	200
Cereals, Ready-to-eat, Kellogg's, Reduced Sugar Froot Loops									
1.25 cup (1 NLEA serving) (32g)	126	1	0	0	27	3.3	10	2	179
Cereals, Ready-to-eat, Kellogg's, Reduced Sugar Frosted Flakes Cereal									
1 cup (1 NLEA serving) (31g)	107	0	0	0	26	3	7	2	158
Cereals, Ready-to-eat, Kellogg's, Rice Krispies									
1 cup (29g)	110	1	0	0	25	0.1	3	2	153
Cereals, Ready-to-eat, Kellogg's, Rice Krispies Treats Cereal									
.75 cup (1 NLEA serving) (30g)	119	1	0	0	26	0.1	9	1	170
Cereals, Ready-to-eat, Kellogg's, Shredded Wheat Miniatures									
30 biscuits (1 NLEA serving) (30g)	102	1	0	0	24	3.9	1	3	0
Cereals, Ready-to-eat, Kellogg's, Smart Start Antioxidants Cereal									
1 cup (1 NLEA serving) (50g)	186	1	0	0	44	2.9	14	4	213
Cereals, Ready-to-eat, Kellogg's, Smart Start Strong Heart, Original									
1.25 cup (1 NLEA serving) (60g)	220	2	0	0	47	5.3	17	6	140
Cereals, Ready-to-eat, Kellogg's, Smart Start, Maple Brown Sugar									
1.25 cup (I NLEA serving) (60g)	220	2	0	0	47	5.1	17	6	138

Food Serving size	Cal.	(g) Total Fat	(g) Sat. Fat	(mg) Chol.	(g) Carb.	(g) Fiber	(g) Sug.	(g) Prot.	(mg) Sod.
Cereals, Ready-to-eat, Kellogg's, Smorz									
1 cup (1 NLEA serving) (30g)	122	2	1	0	25	0.8	13	1	138
Cereals, Ready-to-eat, Kellogg's, Special K									
1 cup (1 NLEA serving) (31g)	117	1	0	0	23	0.3	4	6	220
Cereals, Ready-to-eat, Kellogg's, Special K, Low Fat Granola									
.75 cup (1 NLEA serving) (52g)	195	3	1	0	39	5.9	9	7	114
Cereals, Ready-to-eat, Kellogg's, Special K, Red Berries									
1 cup (1 NLEA serving) (31g)	111	0	0	0	27	2.6	9	2	190
Cereals, Ready-to-eat, Kellogg's, Special K, Blueberry									
.75 cup (1 NLEA serving) (30g)	109	0	0	0	26	2.6	8	2	144
Cereals, Ready-to-eat, Kellogg's, Special K, Chocolatey Delight									
.75 cup (1 NLEA serving) (31g)	118	2	2	0	25	3.3	9	2	180
Cereals, Ready-to-eat, Kellogg's, Special K, Cinnamon Pecan									
.75 cup (1 NLEA serving) (30g)	113	2	0	0	24	3.1	7	2	195
Cereals, Ready-to-eat, Kellogg's, Special K, Fruit and Yogurt									
.75 cup (1 NLEA serving) (32g)	117	1	0	0	27	2.6	10	2	145
Cereals, Ready-to-eat, Malt-O-Meal, Apple Zings									
1 cup (33g)	130	1	0	0	28	0.7	16	2	144
Cereals, Ready-to-eat, Malt-O-Meal, Berry Colossal Crunch									
.75 cup (1 NLEA serving) (30g)	122	1	0	0	26	0.5	13	1	210
Cereals, Ready-to-eat, Malt-O-Meal, Blueberry Muffin Tops Cereal									
.75 cup (30g)	133	3	0	0	24	1.4	11	1	139
Cereals, Ready-to-eat, Malt-O-Meal, Cinnamon Toasters									
.75 cup (30g)	129	3	0	0	24	1.4	10	2	138
Cereals, Ready-to-eat, Malt-O-Meal, Cocoa Dyno-Bites									
.75 cup (29g)	117	1	1	0	26	0.3	13	1	150
Cereals, Ready-to-eat, Malt-O-Meal, Coco-Roos									
.75 cup (1 NLEA serving) (30g)	119	1	1	0	26	0.9	15	1	110
Cereals, Ready-to-eat, Malt-O-Meal, Colossal Crunch									
.75 cup (30g)	113	1	0	0	24	0.7	13	1	179
Cereals, Ready-to-eat, Malt-O-Meal, Corn Bursts									
1 cup (31g)	119	0	0	0	27	0.6	13	1	249
Cereals, Ready-to-eat, Malt-O-Meal, Crispy Rice									
1 cup (1 NLEA serving) (33g)	126	0	0	0	29	0.3	3	2	300

Food Serving size	Cal.	(g) Total Fat	(g) Sat. Fat	(mg) Chol.	(g) Carb.	(g) Fiber	(g) Sug.	(g) Prot.	(mg) Sod.
Cereals, Ready-to-eat, Malt-O-Meal, Frosted Flakes									
1 cup (40g)	120	0	0	0	28	0.7	12	1	140
Cereals, Ready-to-eat, Malt-O-Meal, Frosted Mini Spooners									
1 cup (55g)	213	1	0	0	46	5.8	10	5	10
Cereals, Ready-to-eat, Malt-O-Meal, Fruity Dyno-Bites									
.75 cup (27g)	109	1	0	0	24	0.3	12	1	170
Cereals, Ready-to-eat, Malt-O-Meal, Golden Puffs									
1 cup (37g)	147	0	0	0	33	1	19	2	89
Cereals, Ready-to-eat, Malt-O-Meal, Honey Buzzers									
1.333 cup (29g)	115	1	0	0	25	0.8	11	2	220
Cereals, Ready-to-eat, Malt-O-Meal, Honey Graham Squares									
.75 cup (1 NLEA serving) (30g)	119	3	0	0	22	1.3	10	1	251
Cereals, Ready-to-eat, Malt-O-Meal, Honey Nut Toasty O's Cereal									
1 cup (30g)	117	1	0	0	25	1.7	12	3	251
Cereals, Ready-to-eat, Malt-O-Meal, Maple & Brown Sugar Hot Wheat Cereal, Dry									
.25 cup (45g)	166	0	0	0	36	0.8	13	4	2
Cereals, Ready-to-eat, Malt-O-Meal, Marshmallows Mateys									
1 cup (30g)	118	1	0	0	25	1.4	13	2	200
Cereals, Ready-to-eat, Malt-O-Meal, Puffed Rice Cereal									
1 cup (15g)	60	0	0	0	14	0.2	0	1	1
Cereals, Ready-to-eat, Malt-O-Meal, Puffed Wheat Cereal									
1 cup (15g)	59	0	0	0	12	1.1	0	2	2
Cereals, Ready-to-eat, Malt-O-Meal, Raisin Bran Cereal									
1 cup (59g)	189	1	0	0	46	8.1	19	5	340
Cereals, Ready-to-eat, Malt-O-Meal, Toasty O's									
1 cup (1 NLEA serving) (30g)	121	2	0	0	22	3.2	1	4	269
Cereals, Ready-to-eat, Malt-O-Meal, Tootie Fruities									
1 cup (1 NLEA serving) (32g)	128	1	0	0	28	0.8	15	2	148
Cereals, Ready-to-eat, Nature's Path, Optimum									
1 cup (55g)	190	3	0	0	40	10	16	8	230
Cereals, Ready-to-eat, Nature's Path, Optimum Slim									
1 cup (55g)	180	3	0	0	38	11	10	9	290
Cereals, Ready-to-eat, Oat, Corn & Wheat Squares, Presweetened, Maple Flavor									
1 cup (1 NLEA serving) (30g)	129	3	0	0	24	0.5	11	2	130

Food Serving size	Cal.	(g) Total Fat	(g) Sat. Fat	(mg) Chol.	(g) Carb.	(g) Fiber	(g) Sug.	(g) Prot.	(mg) Sod.
Cereals, Ready-to-eat, Post, Blueberry Morning 1.25 cup (1 NLEA serving) (55g)									
	211	2	0	0	44	2.1	11	4	260
Cereals, Ready-to-eat, Post Raisin Bran Cereal 1 cup (1 NLEA serving) (59g)	187	1	0	0	45	7.1	17	6	250
Cereals, Ready-to-eat, Post Selects Cranberry Almond Crunch .75 cup (1 NLEA serving) (51g)	197	3	0	0	40	3.1	13	4	115
Cereals, Ready-to-eat, Post Shredded Wheat n' Bran, Spoon-size 1.25 cup (1 NLEA serving) (59g)									
	197	1	0	0	47	7.9	9	7	3
Cereals, Ready-to-eat, Post Toasties Corn Flakes 1 box, single serving (.75 oz) (21g)	76	0	0	0	18	0.9	1	1	150
Cereals, Ready-to-eat, Post, 100% Bran Cereal .333 cup (1 NLEA serving) (29g)	83	1	0	0	23	8.3	7	4	121
Cereals, Ready-to-eat, Post, Alpha-Bits .67 cup (1 serving for children under 4 years)									
	78	1	0	0	16	1.4	4	2	118
Cereals, Ready-to-eat, Post, Cocoa Pebbles .75 cup (1 NLEA serving) (30g)	115	1	1	0	25	0.5	10	1	172
Cereals, Ready-to-eat, Post, Fruity Pebbles .75 cup (1 NLEA serving) (30g)	109	1	1	0	23	0.2	9	1	144
Cereals, Ready-to-eat, Post, Golden Crisp .75 cup (1 NLEA serving) (27g)	103	0	0	0	24	1.4	14	1	26
Cereals, Ready-to-eat, Post, Grape-Nuts Cereal 1 cup (115g)	212	1	0	0	47	7	5	6	275
Cereals, Ready-to-eat, Post, Grape-Nuts Flakes .75 cup (1 NLEA serving) (29g)	109	1	0	0	24	3	4	3	136
Cereals, Ready-to-eat, Post, Great Grains Crunchy Pecan Cereal .667 cup (1 NLEA serving) (53g)									
	216	6	1	0	38	3.7	8	5	214
Cereals, Ready-to-eat, Post, Honey Nut Shredded Wheat 1 cup (1 NLEA serving) (52g)	220	2	0	0	49	6.3	12	5	60
Cereals, Ready-to-eat, Post, Honeycomb Cereal 1.5 cup (1 NLEA serving) (32g)	127	1	0	0	28	1	10	2	132
Cereals, Ready-to-eat, Post, Oreo O's Cereal .75 cup (27g)	112	2	0	0	22	1.5	13	1	128

Food Serving size	Cal.	(g) Total Fat	(g) Sat. Fat	(mg) Chol.	(g) Carb.	(g) Fiber	(g) Sug.	(g) Prot.	(mg) Sod.
Cereals, Ready-to-eat, Post, Shredded Wheat, Bite-size									
1 cup (1 NLEA serving) (52g)	183	1	0	0	44	5	12	4	10
Cereals, Ready-to-eat, Post, Shredded Wheat, Original Big Biscuit									
1 serving (46g)	155	1	0	0	36	5.5	0	5	3
Cereals, Ready-to-eat, Post, Shredded Wheat, Spoon-size									
1 box, single serving (.875 oz) (25g)	183	1	0	0	44	5	12	4	10
Cereals, Ready-to-eat, Puffed Kashi									
1 cup (1 NLEA serving) (19g)	64	0	0	0	15	1.5	1	2	2
Cereals, Ready-to-eat, Quaker, Apple Zaps									
.75 cup (1 NLEA serving) (30g)	118	1	0	0	27	0.7	14	1	135
Cereals, Ready-to-eat, Quaker, Cocoa Blasts									
1 cup (1 NLEA serving) (33g)	130	1	0	0	29	0.8	16	1	135
Cereals, Ready-to-eat, Quaker, Fruitangy Oh!s									
1 cup (1 NLEA serving) (31g)	122	1	0	0	27	0.8	13	2	152
Cereals, Ready-to-eat, Quaker, Cinnamon Life									
.75 cup (1 NLEA serving) (32g)	120	1	0	0	25	2	8	3	148
Cereals, Ready-to-eat, Quaker, 100% Natural Cereal with Oats, Honey and Raisins									
.5 cup (1 NLEA serving) (51g)	213	3	1	1	44	5.3	14	5	129
Cereals, Ready-to-eat, Quaker, 100% Natural Granola Oats and Honey									
.5 cup (1 NLEA serving) (48g)	202	6	1	1	35	4.9	10	5	24
Cereals, Ready-to-eat, Quaker, Cap'n Crunch									
.75 cup (1 NLEA serving) (27g)	107	1	1	0	23	0.7	12	1	204
Cereals, Ready-to-eat, Quaker, Cap'n Crunch with Crunchberries									
.75 cup (1 NLEA serving) (26g)	103	1	1	0	22	0.7	11	1	189
Cereals, Ready-to-eat, Quaker, Cap'n Crunch's Peanut Butter Crunch									
.75 cup (1 NLEA serving) (27g)	113	2	1	0	21	0.7	9	2	200
Cereals, Ready-to-eat, Quaker, Cinnamon Oatmeal Squares									
1 cup (1 NLEA serving) (60g)	227	3	0	0	48	4.9	13	6	263
Cereals, Ready-to-eat, Quaker, Honey Graham Life Cereal									
.75 cup (1 NLEA serving) (32g)	119	1	0	0	25	2	7	3	156
Cereals, Ready-to-eat, Quaker, Honey Graham Oh!s									
.75 cup (1 NLEA serving) (27g)	111	2	2	0	23	0.6	12	1	183
Cereals, Ready-to-eat, Quaker, King Vitaman									
1.5 cup (1 NLEA serving) (31g)	118	1	0	0	26	1.1	6	2	256

Food Serving size	Cal.	(g) Total Fat	(g) Sat. Fat	(mg) Chol.	(g) Carb.	(g) Fiber	(g) Sug.	(g) Prot.	(mg) Sod.
Cereals, Ready-to-eat, Quaker, Kretschmer Honey Crunch Wheat Germ 1.667 tbsp (1 NLEA serving) (14g)									
	52	1	0	0	8	1.4	3	4	2
Cereals, Ready-to-eat, Quaker, Kretschmer Toasted Wheat Bran .25 cup (1 NLEA serving) (16g)	32	1	0	0	10	6.6	0	3	1
Cereals, Ready-to-eat, Quaker, Kretschmer Wheat Germ, Regular 1.67 tablespoon (14g)	51	1	0	0	7	1.7	0	4	1
Cereals, Ready-to-eat, Quaker, Low Fat 100% Natural Granola with Raisins .67 cup (1 NLEA serving) (55g)	215	3	1	0	45	3.1	18	4	139
Cereals, Ready-to-eat, Quaker, Marshmallow Safari .75 cup (1 NLEA serving) (30g)	119	2	0	0	25	1.3	14	2	192
Cereals, Ready-to-eat, Quaker, Mother's Cinnamon Oat Crunch 1 cup (1 NLEA serving) (60g)	229	3	0	0	48	4.9	15	6	165
Cereals, Ready-to-eat, Quaker, Mother's Cocoa Bumpers 1 cup (1 NLEA serving) (33g)	126	1	0	0	30	0.9	14	1	149
Cereals, Ready-to-eat, Quaker, Mother's Toasted Oat Bran Cereal, Brown Sugar .75 cup (1 NLEA serving) (32g)	119	2	0	0	24	2.8	5	4	209
Cereals, Ready-to-eat, Quaker, Oat Bran Cereal 1.25 cup (57g)	212	3	1	0	43	5.6	9	7	207
Cereals, Ready-to-eat, Quaker, Oatmeal Cereal, Brown Sugar Bliss 1 cup (49g)	188	3	1	0	39	3.6	0	4	249
Cereals, Ready-to-eat, Quaker, Oatmeal Squares 1 cup (1 NLEA serving) (56g)	212	3	0	0	44	4.6	9	6	194
Cereals, Ready-to-eat, Quaker, Puffed Rice 1 cup (1 NLEA serving) (14g)	54	0	0	0	12	0.2	0	1	1
Cereals, Ready-to-eat, Quaker, Puffed Wheat 1.25 cup (1 NLEA serving) (15g)	55	0	0	0	11	1.4	0	2	1
Cereals, Ready-to-eat, Quaker, Quaker Crunchy Bran .75 cup (1 NLEA serving) (27g)	89	1	1	0	23	4.1	6	2	205
Cereals, Ready-to-eat, Quaker, Quaker Oat Life, Plain .75 cup (1 NLEA serving) (32g)	79	1	0	0	16	1.4	4	2	105
Cereals, Ready-to-eat, Quaker, Sun Country Granola with Almonds .5 cup (1 NLEA serving) (57g)	266	10	1	0	38	3	12	7	19
Cereals, Ready-to-eat, Quaker, Sweet Crunch/Quisp 1 cup (1 NLEA serving) (27g)	110	2	1	0	23	0.6	12	1	200

Food Serving size	Cal.	(g) Total Fat	(g) Sat. Fat	(mg) Chol.	(g) Carb.	(g) Fiber	(g) Sug.	(g) Prot.	(mg) Sod.
Cereals, Ready-to-eat, Quaker, Sweet Puffs									
1 cup (34g)	133	1	0	0	30	1.2	16	2	80
Cereals, Ready-to-eat, Quaker, Toasted Oatmeal Cereal									
1 cup (1 NLEA serving) (49g)	188	2	1	0	39	2.7	12	5	274
Cereals, Ready-to-eat, Quaker, Toasted Oatmeal Cereal, Honey Nut									
1 cup (1 NLEA serving) (49g)	188	2	1	0	40	2.7	12	4	228
Cereals, Ready-to-eat, Ralston Corn Biscuits									
1 cup (31g)	110	0	0	0	26	0.8	3	2	230
Cereals, Ready-to-eat, Ralston Corn Flakes									
1 cup (31g)	100	0	0	0	25	0.8	2	2	160
Cereals, Ready-to-eat, Ralston Crispy Hexagons									
1 cup (28g)	110	0	0	0	25	0.4	4	2	150
Cereals, Ready-to-eat, Ralston Crispy Rice									
1 cup (28g)	110	0	0	0	24	0.2	3	2	153
Cereals, Ready-to-eat, Ralston Tasteeos									
1 cup (28g)	100	2	0	0	21	3	1	3	160
Cereals, Ready-to-eat, Ralston, Enriched Bran Flakes									
1 cup (42g)	130	1	0	0	34	7.1	7	4	246
Cereals, Ready-to-eat, Rice, Puffed, Fortified									
.5 oz (14.2g)	57	0	0	0	13	0.2	0	1	0
Cereals, Ready-to-eat, Rolled Oats, Whole Wheat, Rice, Maple flavor, with Pecans									
1 serving (1 NLEA serving) (52g)	219	5	2	0	40	3.1	13	4	145
Cereals, Ready-to-eat, Uncle Sam Cereal									
1 cup (1 serving) (55g)	190	6	1	0	36	11.2	1	9	113
Cereals, Ready-to-eat, USDA Commodity Corn and Rice (Includes All Brands)									
1 serving (NLEA serving = 1 cup) (29g)	110	0	0	0	25	0.4	3	2	231
Cereals, Ready-to-eat, Waffelos									
1 oz (28.35g)	115	1	0	0	24	0	0	2	118
Cereals, Ready-to-eat, Wheat and Malt Barley Flakes									
1 box, single serving (.75 oz) (21g)	77	1	0	0	17	1.8	4	2	101
Cereals, Ready-to-eat, Wheat Germ, Toasted, Plain									
1 cup (113g)	432	12	2	0	56	17.1	9	33	5

Food Serving size	Cal.	(g) Total Fat	(g) Sat. Fat	(mg) Chol.	(g) Carb.	(g) Fiber	(g) Sug.	(g) Prot.	(mg) Sod.
Cereals, Ready-to-eat, Wheat, Puffed, Fortified									
.5 oz (14.2g)	52	0	0	0	11	0.6	0	2	1
Cereals, Ready-to-eat, Wheat, Shredded, Plain, Sugar and Salt-free									
1 serving (46g)	155	1	0	0	36	5.5	0	5	3
Cereals, Roman Meal with Oats, Cooked with Water, with Salt									
.75 cup (180g)	128	1	0	0	26	6.1	0	5	405
Cereals, Roman Meal with Oats, Cooked with Water, Without Salt									
.75 cup (180g)	128	1	0	0	26	5.2	0	5	7
Cereals, Roman Meal, Plain, Cooked with Water, with Salt									
.75 cup (181g)	110	1	0	0	25	6.2	0	5	148
Cereals, Roman Meal, Plain, Cooked with Water, Without Salt									
.75 cup (181g)	110	1	0	0	25	6.2	0	5	2
Cereals, Roman Meal, Plain, Dry									
1 tbsp (5.8g)	19	0	0	0	4	1	0	1	0
Cereals, Wafer Straws, Kellogg's, Apple Jacks Cereal Straws									
3 straws (1 NLEA serving) (31g)	136	4	2	3	24	0	12	2	16
Cereals, Wafer Straws, Kellogg's, Cocoa Krispies Cereal Straws									
3 straws (1 NLEA serving) (31g)	136	4	2	0	24	0.5	12	2	16
Cereals, Wafer Straws, Kellogg's, Froot Loops Cereal Straws									
3 straws (1 NLEA serving) (31g)	136	4	2	5	24	1	12	2	15
Cereals, Wheatena, Cooked with Water									
.75 cup (182g)	102	1	0	0	21	4.9	0	4	4
Cereals, Wheatena, Cooked with Water, with Salt									
.75 cup (182g)	107	1	0	0	21	3.6	0	4	433
Cereals, Wheatena, Dry									
1 cup (141g)	503	4	1	0	107	18	2	18	18
Cereals, Whole Wheat Hot Natural Cereal, Cooked with Water, with Salt									
.75 cup (182g)	113	1	0	0	25	2.9	0	4	424
Cereals, Whole Wheat Hot Natural Cereal, Cooked with Water, Without Salt									
.75 cup (182g)	113	1	0	0	25	2.9	0	4	0
Cereals, Whole Wheat Hot Natural Cereal, Dry									
.333 cup (31g)	106	1	0	0	23	2.9	0	3	1
Crisped Rice Bar, Chocolate Chip									
1 bar (1 oz) (28g)	113	4	1	0	20	0.6	0	1	78

Food Serving size	Cal.	(g) Total Fat	(g) Sat. Fat	(mg) Chol.	(g) Carb.	(g) Fiber	(g) Sug.	(g) Prot.	(mg) Sod.
Granola Bars, Hard, Almond 1 bar (24g)	119	6	3	0	15	1.2	0	2	61
Granola Bars, Hard, Chocolate Chip 1 bar (24g)	105	4	3	0	17	1.1	0	2	83
Granola Bars, Hard, Peanut 1 oz (28.35g)	136	6	1	0	18	1.2	10	3	79
Granola Bars, Hard, Peanut Butter 1 bar (24g)	116	6	1	0	15	0.7	0	2	68
Granola Bars, Hard, Plain 1 bar (1 oz) (28g)	132	6	1	0	18	1.5	0	3	82
Granola Bars, Oats, Fruits and Nuts 1 oz (28.35g)	113	2	0	0	22	1.5	12	2	71
Granola Bars, Soft, Coated, Milk Chocolate Coating, Chocolate Chip 1 bar (1 oz) (28g)	130	7	4	1	18	1	0	2	56
Granola Bars, Soft, Coated, Milk Chocolate Coating, Peanut Butter 1 bar (37g)	188	12	6	4	20	1	0	4	71
Granola Bars, Soft, Milk Chocolate Coated, Peanut Butter 1 oz (28.35g)	152	9	5	3	15	1.1	0	3	55
Granola Bars, Soft, Uncoated, Chocolate Chip 1 bar (1 oz) (28g)	117	5	2	0	20	1.1	8	2	50
Granola Bars, Soft, Uncoated, Chocolate Chip, Graham and Marshmallow 1 bar (1 oz) (28g)	120	4	3	0	20	1.1	0	2	88
Granola Bars, Soft, Uncoated, Nut and Raisin 1 bar (1 oz) (28g)	127	6	3	0	18	1.6	0	2	71
Granola Bars, Soft, Uncoated, Peanut Butter 1 bar (1 oz) (28g)	119	4	1	0	18	1.2	0	3	115
Granola Bars, Soft, Uncoated, Peanut Butter and Chocolate Chip 1 bar (1 oz) (28g)	121	6	2	0	17	1.2	0	3	92
Granola Bars, Soft, Uncoated, Plain 1 bar (1 oz) (28g)	124	5	2	0	19	1.3	0	2	78
Granola Bars, Soft, Uncoated, Raisin 1 bar (1 oz) (28g)	125	5	3	0	19	1.2	0	2	79
Granola Bars, with Coconut, Chocolate Coated 1 oz (28.35g)	151	9	6	0	16	1.8	0	1	43

Food Serving size	Cal.	(g) Total Fat	(g) Sat. Fat	(mg) Chol.	(g) Carb.	(g) Fiber	(g) Sug.	(g) Prot.	(mg) Sod.
Kashi, GoLean Crisp, Toasted Berry Crumble									
.75 cup (1 NLEA serving) (51g)	188	4	1	0	35	7.6	11	9	124
Rice and Wheat Cereal Bar									
1 bar (22g)	90	2	0	0	16	0.4	7	2	110
Snacks, Granola Bars, Fruit-filled, Nonfat									
1 oz (28.35g)	97	0	0	0	22	2.1	16	2	5
Snacks, Granola Bars, Soft Almond, Confectioners Coating									
1 bar (35g)	159	7	2	1	21	1.5	0	3	170
Snacks, Granola Bites, Mixed Flavors									
1 package (20g)	90	4	2	0	13	1.1	0	1	7
Snacks, Kellogg, Kellogg's Rice Krispies Treats Square									
1 bar (37g)	153	3	1	0	30	0.2	0	1	130
Snacks, Kellogg's Low Fat Granola Bar, Crunchy Almond/Brown Sugar									
1 bar (37g)	144	3	0	0	29	2.3	0	3	108
Snacks, Rice Cakes, Brown Rice, Corn									
2 cakes (18g)	69	1	0	0	15	0.5	0	2	30

Breads

Food Serving size	Cal.	(g) Total Fat	(g) Sat. Fat	(mg) Chol.	(g) Carb.	(g) Fiber	(g) Sug.	(g) Prot.	(mg) Sod.
Bread, Banana, Prepared from Recipe, Made with Margarine									
1 individual, loaf (include Keebler Elfin Loaves) (57g)									
	186	6	1	25	31	0.6	0	2	172
Bread, Boston Brown, Canned									
1 slice (45g)	88	1	0	0	19	2.1	1	2	284
Bread, Cornbread, Dry Mix, Enriched (Including Corn Muffin Mix)									
1 package (8.5 oz) (241g)	1007	29	7	5	167	15.7	49	17	1969
Bread, Cornbread, Dry Mix, Prepared									
1 piece (60g)	188	6	2	37	29	1.4	0	4	467
Bread, Cornbread, Dry Mix, Unenriched (Including Corn Muffin Mix)									
1 package (8.5 oz) (241g)	1007	29	7	5	167	15.7	0	17	2678
Bread, Cornbread, Prepared from Recipe, Made with Low Fat (2%) Milk									
1 piece (65g)	173	5	1	26	28	0	0	4	428
Bread, Cracked Wheat									
1 cubic inch (3.2g)	8	0	0	0	2	0.2	0	0	17
Bread, Egg									
1 slice (5″ x 3″ x 1/2″) (40g)	113	2	1	20	19	0.9	1	4	165

Food Serving size	Cal.	(g) Total Fat	(g) Sat. Fat	(mg) Chol.	(g) Carb.	(g) Fiber	(g) Sug.	(g) Prot.	(mg) Sod.
Bread, Egg, Toasted 1 slice (5″ x 3″ x 1/2″) (37g)	117	2	1	21	19	0.9	1	4	200
Bread, French or Vienna (Includes Sourdough) 1 slice, small (2″ x 2-1/2″ x 1-3/4″) (32g)	92	1	0	0	18	0.8	1	4	164
Bread, French or Vienna, Toasted (Includes Sourdough) 1 slice, small (29g)	93	1	0	0	18	0.9	1	4	209
Bread, Irish Soda, Prepared from Recipe 1 oz (28.35g)	82	1	0	5	16	0.7	0	2	113
Bread, Italian 1 slice, large (4-1/2″ x 3-1/4″ x 3/4″) (30g)	81	1	0	0	15	0.8	0	3	175
Bread, Multi-grain (Includes Whole Grain) 1 slice, regular (26g)	69	1	0	0	11	1.9	2	3	109
Bread, Multi-grain, Toasted (Includes Whole Grain) 1 slice, regular (24g)	69	1	0	0	11	1.9	2	3	110
Bread, Oat Bran 1 slice (30g)	71	1	0	0	12	1.4	2	3	122
Bread, Oat Bran, Toasted 1 slice (27g)	70	1	0	0	12	1.3	2	3	121
Bread, Oatmeal 1 slice (27g)	73	1	0	0	13	1.1	2	2	127
Bread, Oatmeal, Toasted 1 slice (25g)	73	1	0	0	13	1.1	2	2	163
Bread, Pan Dulce, Sweet Yeast Bread 1 slice (average weight of 1 slice) (63g)	231	7	1	0	36	1.4	8	6	144
Bread, Pita, White, Enriched 1 pita, small (4″ dia) (28g)	77	0	0	0	16	0.6	0	3	150
Bread, Pita, White, Unenriched 1 pita, large (6-1/2″ dia) (60g)	165	1	0	0	33	1.3	0	5	322
Bread, Pita, Whole Wheat 1 pita, small (4″ dia) (28g)	74	1	0	0	15	2.1	0	3	149
Bread, Pound Cake Type, Pan de Torta Salvadoran 1 cake, square (622g)	2426	109	19	0	319	10.6	113	44	2426

Food Serving size	Cal.	(g) Total Fat	(g) Sat. Fat	(mg) Chol.	(g) Carb.	(g) Fiber	(g) Sug.	(g) Prot.	(mg) Sod.
Bread, Protein (Including Gluten)									
1 slice (19g)	47	0.	0	0	8	0.6	0	2	91
Bread, Protein, Toasted (Including Gluten)									
1 slice (17g)	46	0	0	0	8	0.6	0	2	102
Bread, Pumpernickel									
1 slice, regular (26g)	65	1	0	0	12	1.7	0	2	174
Bread, Pumpernickel, Toasted									
1 slice (5″ x 4″ x 3/8″) (29g)	80	1	0	0	15	2.1	0	3	214
Bread, Raisin, Enriched									
1 slice, large (32g)	88	1	0	0	17	1.4	2	3	100
Bread, Raisin, Toasted, Enriched									
1 slice, large (29g)	86	1	0	0	17	1.4	2	2	123
Bread, Raisin, Unenriched									
1 slice, large (32g)	88	1	0	0	17	1.4	0	3	125
Bread, Reduced-calorie, Oat Bran									
1 slice (23g)	46	1	0	0	9	2.8	1	2	132
Bread, Reduced-calorie, Oat Bran, Toasted									
1 slice (19g)	45	1	0	0	9	2.7	1	2	79
Bread, Reduced-calorie, Oatmeal									
1 slice (23g)	48	1	0	0	10	0	0	2	89
Bread, Reduced-calorie, Rye									
1 slice (23g)	47	1	0	0	9	2.8	1	2	118
Bread, Reduced-calorie, Wheat									
1 slice (23g)	46	1	0	0	10	2.8	1	2	118
Bread, Reduced-calorie, White									
1 slice (23g)	48	1	0	0	10	2.2	1	2	104
Bread, Rice Bran									
1 slice (27g)	66	1	0	0	12	1.3	1	2	82
Bread, Rice Bran, Toasted									
1 slice (25g)	66	1	0	0	12	1.3	1	2	120
Bread, Rye									
1 slice, regular (32g)	83	1	0	0	15	1.9	1	3	211
Bread, Rye, Toasted									
1 slice, large (29g)	82	1	0	0	15	1.9	1	3	210

Food Serving size	Cal.	(g) Total Fat	(g) Sat. Fat	(mg) Chol.	(g) Carb.	(g) Fiber	(g) Sug.	(g) Prot.	(mg) Sod.
Bread, Salvadoran Sweet Cheese (Quesadilla Salvadorena) 1 cake, square (average weight of whole item) (399g)									
	1492	68	18	235	191	2.8	99	28	2035
Bread, Wheat 1 slice (25g)	67	1	0	0	12	0.9	1	3	130
Bread, Wheat Bran 1 slice (36g)	89	1	0	0	17	1.4	3	3	175
Bread, Wheat Germ 1 slice (28g)	73	1	0	0	14	0.6	1	3	155
Bread, Wheat Germ, Toasted 1 slice (25g)	73	1	0	0	14	0.6	1	3	155
Bread, Wheat, Toasted 1 slice (24g)	75	1	0	0	13	1.1	2	3	147
Bread, White, Commercially Prepared (Including Soft Bread Crumbs) 1 cup, crumbs (45g)	120	1	0	0	23	1.1	2	3	230
Bread, White, Commercially Prepared, Low Sodium, No Salt 1 cup, crumbs (45g)	120	2	0	0	22	1	2	4	12
Bread, White, Commercially Prepared, Toasted 1 cup, crumbs (45g)	132	2	0	0	24	1.1	2	4	266
Bread, White, Commercially Prepared, Toasted, Low Sodium, No Salt 1 slice (23g)	67	1	0	0	13	0	0	2	7
Bread, White, Prepared from Recipe, Made with Low Fat (2%) Milk 1 slice (42g)	120	2	0	1	21	0.8	0	3	151
Bread, White, Prepared from Recipe, Made with Nonfat Dry Milk 1 slice (44g)	121	1	0	0	24	0.9	0	3	148
Bread, Whole Wheat, Commercially Prepared 1 slice (28g)	69	1	0	0	12	1.9	2	4	132
Bread, Whole Wheat, Commercially Prepared, Toasted 1 slice (25g)	77	1	0	0	13	2.3	1	4	146
Bread, Whole Wheat, Prepared from Recipe 1 slice, regular (4" x 5" x 3/4") (46g)									
	128	2	0	0	24	2.8	2	4	159
Bread, Whole Wheat, Prepared from Recipe, Toasted 1 slice (42g)	128	2	0	0	24	2.8	2	4	160

Food Serving size	Cal.	(g) Total Fat	(g) Sat. Fat	(mg) Chol.	(g) Carb.	(g) Fiber	(g) Sug.	(g) Prot.	(mg) Sod.
George Weston Bakeries, Thomas' English Muffins									
1 serving (57g)	132	1	0	0	26	0	0	5	197
Rolls, Dinner, Egg									
1 roll (2-1/2" dia) (35g)	107	2	1	18	18	1.3	2	3	161
Rolls, Dinner, Oat Bran									
1 roll (33g)	78	2	0	0	13	1.4	2	3	136
Rolls, Dinner, Plain, Commercially Prepared (Including Brown-n-Serve)									
1 each (pan, dinner, or small roll) (2" square, 2" high) (25g)									
	78	2	0	1	13	0.5	1	3	134
Rolls, Dinner, Plain, Prepared from Recipe, Made with Low Fat (2%) Milk									
1 large, roll or bun (3-1/2" dia) (43g)									
	136	3	1	15	23	0.8	0	4	178
Rolls, Dinner, Rye									
1 medium (36g)	103	1	0	0	19	1.8	0	4	234
Rolls, Dinner, Wheat									
1 roll (1 oz) (28g)	76	2	0	0	13	1.1	0	2	136
Rolls, Dinner, Whole Wheat									
1 roll (hamburger, frankfurter roll) (43g)									
	114	2	0	0	22	3.2	4	4	172
Rolls, French									
1 roll (38g)	105	2	0	0	19	1.2	0	3	193
Rolls, Hamburger or Hot Dog, Mixed-grain									
1 roll (43g)	113	3	1	0	19	1.6	3	4	197
Rolls, Hamburger or Hot Dog, Plain									
1 roll (43g)	120	2	0	0	21	0.9	3	4	206
Rolls, Hamburger or Hot Dog, Reduced-calorie									
1 roll (43g)	84	1	0	0	18	2.7	2	4	190
Rolls, Hard (Including Kaiser)									
1 roll (3-1/2" dia) (57g)	167	2	0	0	30	1.3	1	6	310
Rolls, Pumpernickel									
1 roll (pan, dinner, or small roll) (2" square, 2" high) (28g)									
	78	1	0	0	15	1.5	0	3	198
Shortening Bread, Soybean (Hydrogenated) and Cottonseed									
1 cup (205g)	1812	205	45	0	0	0	0	0	0

Food Serving size	Cal.	(g) Total Fat	(g) Sat. Fat	(mg) Chol.	(g) Carb.	(g) Fiber	(g) Sug.	(g) Prot.	(mg) Sod.
Baked Products									
Archway Home Style Cookies, Apple Filled Oatmeal									
1 serving (25g)	98	3	1	2	17	0.4	8	1	83
Archway Home Style Cookies, Apricot Filled									
1 serving (25g)	100	3	1	2	16	0.6	8	1	80
Archway Home Style Cookies, Cherry Filled									
1 serving (25g)	101	4	1	5	16	0.5	8	1	87
Archway Home Style Cookies, Chocolate Chip Drop									
1 serving (25g)	102	4	1	3	16	0.4	7	1	98
Archway Home Style Cookies, Chocolate Chip Ice Box									
1 serving (24g)	119	6	2	3	16	0.5	8	1	65
Archway Home Style Cookies, Coconut Macaroon									
1 serving (22g)	101	5	4	0	13	1.1	10	1	44
Archway Home Style Cookies, Cookies Jar Hermits									
1 serving (25g)	98	2	1	3	18	0.5	9	1	164
Archway Home Style Cookies, Dark Molasses									
1 serving (28g)	114	4	1	0	19	0.3	10	1	155
Archway Home Style Cookies, Date Filled Oatmeal									
1 serving (25g)	100	3	1	2	17	0.5	9	1	83
Archway Home Style Cookies, Dutch Cocoa									
1 serving (24g)	103	4	1	2	17	0.6	8	1	92
Archway Home Style Cookies, Fat-free Devil's Food Cookie									
1 serving (20g)	68	0	0	0	16	0.6	8	1	79
Archway Home Style Cookies, Fat-free Oatmeal Raisin									
1 serving (31g)	108	0	0	14	25	0.7	15	1	179
Archway Home Style Cookies, Frosty Lemon									
1 serving (26g)	112	4	2	0	17	0.2	9	1	117
Archway Home Style Cookies, Fruit & Honey Bar									
1 serving (26g)	106	3	1	4	18	0.5	10	1	107
Archway Home Style Cookies, Gourmet Apple 'n Raisin									
1 serving (26g)	113	4	1	2	17	0.7	9	1	137
Archway Home Style Cookies, Gourmet Oatmeal Pecan									
1 serving (28g)	132	6	2	2	17	0.9	8	2	97
Archway Home Style Cookies, Gourmet Rocky Road									
1 serving (28g)	129	6	1	3	18	0.7	10	1	79

Food Serving size	Cal.	(g) Total Fat	(g) Sat. Fat	(mg) Chol.	(g) Carb.	(g) Fiber	(g) Sug.	(g) Prot.	(mg) Sod.
Archway Home Style Cookies, Gourmet Ruth's Golden Oatmeal									
1 serving (28g)	121	5	1	2	18	0.8	9	2	109
Archway Home Style Cookies, Iced Molasses									
1 serving (28g)	118	4	1	3	19	0.3	11	1	169
Archway Home Style Cookies, Iced Oatmeal									
1 serving (28g)	122	5	1	2	19	0.6	10	1	106
Archway Home Style Cookies, Molasses									
1 serving (26g)	105	3	1	7	18	0.3	9	1	150
Archway Home Style Cookies, Oatmeal									
1 serving (25g)	105	4	1	3	17	0.7	9	1	99
Archway Home Style Cookies, Oatmeal Raisin									
1 serving (26g)	106	3	1	2	18	0.7	10	1	88
Archway Home Style Cookies, Old Fashioned Molasses									
1 serving (26g)	106	3	1	7	18	0.3	9	1	146
Archway Home Style Cookies, Old Fashioned Windmill Cookies									
1 serving (20g)	94	4	1	0	14	0.4	7	1	94
Archway Home Style Cookies, Peanut Butter									
1 serving (21g)	101	5	1	8	12	0.6	7	2	85
Archway Home Style Cookies, Pecan Ice Box									
1 serving (24g)	120	6	1	7	15	0.3	7	1	76
Archway Home Style Cookies, Raspberry Filled									
1 serving (25g)	100	3	1	2	16	0.6	8	1	84
Archway Home Style Cookies, Reduced-fat Ginger Snaps									
1 serving (32g)	136	4	1	0	24	0.4	12	1	130
Archway Home Style Cookies, Ruth's Oatmeal									
1 serving (26g)	111	4	1	4	17	0.7	9	2	114
Archway Home Style Cookies, Strawberry Filled									
1 serving (25g)	100	3	1	2	16	0.6	8	1	94
Archway Home Style Cookies, Sugar									
1 serving (24g)	99	3	1	4	17	0.4	0	1	154
Archway Home Style Cookies, Sugar Free Chocolate Chip									
1 serving (24g)	117	5	2	0	16	0.3	0	1	64
Archway Home Style Cookies, Sugar Free Oatmeal									
1 serving (24g)	106	5	1	0	16	0.5	0	1	74

Food Serving size	Cal.	(g) Total Fat	(g) Sat. Fat	(mg) Chol.	(g) Carb.	(g) Fiber	(g) Sug.	(g) Prot.	(mg) Sod.
Archway Home Style Cookies, Sugar Free Rocky Road 1 serving (24g)	112	5	1	0	15	0.7	0	1	68
Artificial Blueberry Muffin, Mix, Dry 1 muffin (31g)	126	3	1	0	24	0	0	1	236
Bagel, Plain, Toasted, Enriched with Calcium Propionate (Includes Onion, Poppy, Sesame) 1 small bagel (3″ dia) (69g)	177	1	0	0	35	1.5	3	7	357
Bagels, Cinnamon-raisin 1 small bagel (3″ dia) (69g)	188	1	0	0	38	1.6	4	7	299
Bagels, Cinnamon-raisin, Toasted 1 small bagel (3-1/2″ to 4″dia) (65g)	191	1	0	0	39	1.6	4	7	225
Bagels, Egg 1 mini bagel (2-1/2″ dia) (26g)	72	1	0	6	14	0.6	0	3	131
Bagels, Oat Bran 1 small bagel (3″ dia) (69g)	176	1	0	0	37	2.5	1	7	407
Bagels, Plain, Enriched, Without Calcium Propionate (Including Onion, Poppy, Sesame) 1 mini bagel (2-1/2″ dia) (26g)	72	0	0	0	14	0.6	0	3	139
Bagels, Plain, Toasted, Enriched with Calcium Propionate (Includes Onion, Poppy, Sesame) 1 small bagel (3″ dia) (65g)	187	1	0	0	37	1.7	4	7	312
Bagels, Plain, Unenriched, with Calcium Propionate (Including Onion, Poppy, Sesame) 1 mini bagel (2-1/2″ dia) (26g)	72	0	0	0	14	0.6	0	3	139
Bagels, Plain, Unenriched, Without Calcium Propionate (Including Onion, Poppy, Sesame) 1 mini bagel (2-1/2″ dia) (26g)	72	0	0	0	14	0.6	0	3	139
Baking Chocolate, Mars Snackfood US, M&M's Milk Chocolate Mini Baking Bits 1 serving, 0.5 oz, about 1 tbsp (14g)	70	3	2	2	10	0.4	9	1	10
Baking Chocolate, Mars Snackfood US, M&M's Semisweet Chocolate Mini Baking Bits 1 package (net weight, 12 oz) (340g)	1758	89	53	10	224	22.8	180	15	7
Baking Chocolate, Mexican, Squares 1 tablet (20g)	85	3	2	0	15	0.8	14	1	1

Food Serving size	Cal.	(g) Total Fat	(g) Sat. Fat	(mg) Chol.	(g) Carb.	(g) Fiber	(g) Sug.	(g) Prot.	(mg) Sod.
Baking Chocolate, Unsweetened, Liquid 1 oz (28.35g)	134	14	7	0	10	5.1	0	3	3
Baking Chocolate, Unsweetened, Squares 1 cup, grated (132g)	661	69	43	0	39	21.9	1	17	32
Biscuit, Plain or Buttermilk, Refrigerated Dough, Higher Fat 1 biscuit (43g)	138	6	2	0	19	0.3	3	3	430
Biscuits, Mixed Grain, Refrigerated Dough 1 biscuit (2-1/2" dia) (44g)	116	2	1	0	21	0	0	3	295
Biscuits, Plain or Buttermilk, Commercially Baked 1 large (77g)	281	13	2	1	37	1	3	5	607
Biscuits, Plain or Buttermilk, Dry Mix 1 cup, poured from box (128g)	548	20	5	3	81	2.7	15	10	1295
Biscuits, Plain or Buttermilk, Dry Mix, Prepared 1 oz (28.35g)	95	3	1	1	14	0.5	0	2	271
Biscuits, Plain or Buttermilk, Prepared from Recipe 1 biscuit (4" dia) (101g)	357	16	4	3	45	1.5	2	7	586
Biscuits, Plain or Buttermilk, Refrigerated Dough, Higher Fat, Baked 1 biscuit (2-1/2" dia) (27g)	95	4	1	0	13	0.2	2	2	292
Biscuits, Plain or Buttermilk, Refrigerated Dough, Lower Fat 1 biscuit (2" dia) (23g)	59	1	0	0	11	0.4	2	2	227
Biscuits, Plain or Buttermilk, Refrigerated Dough, Lower Fat, Baked 1 biscuit (2-1/4" dia) (21g)	63	1	0	0	12	0.4	2	2	305
Bread Sticks, Plain 1 stick, small (approx 4-1/4" long) (5g)	21	0	0	0	3	0.2	0	1	33
Bread Stuffing, Bread, Dry Mix 1 package (6 oz) (170g)	656	6	1	2	130	5.4	14	19	2389
Bread Stuffing, Bread, Dry Mix, Prepared .5 cup (100g)	177	9	2	0	22	2.9	2	3	524
Bread Stuffing, Cornbread, Dry Mix 1 package (6 oz) (170g)	661	7	2	0	130	24.3	8	17	2181
Bread Stuffing, Cornbread, Dry Mix, Prepared .5 cup (100g)	179	9	2	0	22	2.9	4	3	455
Cake, Angel Food, Commercially Prepared 1 cake (9" dia x 4") (340g)	877	3	0	0	197	5.1	0	20	2547

Food Serving size	Cal.	(g) Total Fat	(g) Sat. Fat	(mg) Chol.	(g) Carb.	(g) Fiber	(g) Sug.	(g) Prot.	(mg) Sod.
Cake, Angel Food, Dry Mix 1 package (14.5 oz) (411g)	1533	2	0	0	350	1.2	182	37	2006
Cake, Angel Food, Dry Mix, Prepared 1 tube, cake (10" dia, 4-3/8" high) (596g)	1532	2	0	0	350	1.2	182	36	3046
Cake, Boston Cream Pie, Commercially Prepared 1 piece (1/6 of pie) (92g)	232	8	2	34	39	1.3	33	2	234
Cake, Carrot, Dry Mix, Pudding Type 1 package (18 oz) (510g)	2117	50	8	0	404	0	0	26	2892
Cake, Cherry Fudge with Chocolate Frosting 1 piece (1/8 cake) (71g)	187	9	4	30	27	0.9	23	2	185
Cake, Chocolate, Commercially Prepared with Chocolate Frosting 1 piece (1/8 of 18 oz cake) (64g)	235	10	3	27	35	1.8	0	3	214
Cake, Chocolate, Dry Mix, Pudding Type 1 package (18.25 oz) (517g)	2047	48	10	0	407	18.1	238	24	4617
Cake, Chocolate, Dry Mix, Regular 1 package (18.50 oz) (524g)	2243	82	17	0	383	12.6	201	31	4323
Cake, Chocolate, Prepared from Recipe Without Frosting 1 piece (1/12 of 9" dia) (95g)	352	14	5	55	51	1.5	0	5	299
Cake, Fruit Cake, Commercially Prepared 1 piece (43g)	139	4	0	2	26	1.6	13	1	138
Cake, German Chocolate, Dry Mix, Pudding Type 1 package (18.25 oz) (517g)	2073	49	17	0	414	18.1	256	21	4203
Cake, Gingerbread, Dry Mix 1 package (14.5 oz) (411g)	1796	57	14	0	307	7	192	18	2700
Cake, Gingerbread, Prepared from Recipe 1 piece (1/9 of 8" square) (74g)	263	12	3	24	36	0	0	3	242
Cake, Marble, Dry Mix, Pudding Type 1 package (18.25 oz) (517g)	2151	60	13	0	410	15	298	18	3392
Cake, Pineapple Upside-down, Prepared from Recipe 1 piece (1/9 of 8" square) (115g)	367	14	3	25	58	0.9	0	4	367
Cake, Pound, Bimbo Bakeries USA, Panque Casero, Home Baked Style 1 loaf (311g)	1300	67	0	0	152	3.1	89	21	1110

Food Serving size	Cal.	(g) Total Fat	(g) Sat. Fat	(mg) Chol.	(g) Carb.	(g) Fiber	(g) Sug.	(g) Prot.	(mg) Sod.
Cake, Pound, Commercially Prepared, Butter									
1 piece (1/12 of 12 oz cake) (28g)	109	6	3	62	14	0.1	0	2	111
Cake, Pound, Commercially Prepared, Fat Free									
1 cake (340g)	962	4	1	0	207	3.7	117	18	1159
Cake, Pound, Commercially Prepared, Other than All Butter, Enriched									
1 piece (1/12 of 12 oz cake) (28g)	109	5	1	16	15	0.3	0	1	112
Cake, Pound, Commercially Prepared, Other than All Butter, Unenriched									
1 piece (1/12 of 12 oz cake) (28g)	109	5	1	16	15	0.3	0	1	112
Cake, Shortcake, Biscuit-type, Prepared from Recipe									
1 oz (28.35g)	98	4	1	1	14	0	0	2	143
Cake, Snack Cakes, Crème-filled, Chocolate with Frosting									
1 cupcake (50g)	200	8	2	0	30	1.6	19	2	166
Cake, Snack Cakes, Crème-filled, Sponge									
1 cake (42g)	157	5	2	17	27	0.4	16	1	215
Cake, Snack Cakes, Cupcakes, Chocolate with Frosting, Low Fat									
1 cupcake (43g)	131	2	0	0	29	1.8	0	2	178
Cake, Sponge, Commercially Prepared									
1 piece (1/12 of 16 oz cake) (38g)	110	1	0	39	23	0.2	14	2	54
Cake, Sponge, Prepared from Recipe									
1 piece (1/12 of 10 inch cake) (63g)	187	3	1	107	36	0	0	5	144
Cake, White, Dry Mix, Pudding Type, Enriched									
1 package (18.50 oz) (524g)	2217	50	12	0	424	3.7	256	20	3485
Cake, White, Dry Mix, Pudding Type, Unenriched									
1 package (18.50 oz) (524g)	2217	50	12	0	424	3.7	0	20	3485
Cake, White, Dry Mix, Regular									
1 package (18.50 oz) (524g)	2232	57	9	0	409	4.7	286	24	3479
Cake, White, Dry Mix, Special Dietary (Including Lemon-flavored)									
1 package (8 oz) (227g)	901	19	3	0	181	0	0	7	590
Cake, White, Prepared from Recipe with Coconut Frosting									
1 piece (1/12 of 9″ dia) (112g)	399	12	4	1	71	1.1	64	5	318
Cake, White, Prepared from Recipe, Without Frosting									
1 piece (1/12 of 9″ dia) (74g)	264	9	2	1	42	0.6	26	4	242

Food Serving size	Cal.	(g) Total Fat	(g) Sat. Fat	(mg) Chol.	(g) Carb.	(g) Fiber	(g) Sug.	(g) Prot.	(mg) Sod.
Cake, Yellow, Commercially Prepared, with Chocolate Frosting									
1 piece (1/8 of 18 oz cake) (64g)	243	11	3	35	35	1.2	0	2	216
Cake, Yellow, Commercially Prepared, with Vanilla Frosting									
1 piece (1/8 of 18 oz cake) (64g)	239	9	2	35	38	0.2	0	2	220
Cake, Yellow, Dry Mix, Light									
1 package (18.50 oz) (524g)	2117	29	7	0	441	6.8	0	25	3165
Cake, Yellow, Dry Mix, Pudding Type									
1 package (18.50 oz) (524g)	2217	51	13	0	419	3.7	232	21	3600
Cake, Yellow, Dry Mix, Regular, Enriched									
1 package (18.50 oz) (524g)	2264	61	9	10	409	5.8	227	23	3443
Cake, Yellow, Dry Mix, Regular, Unenriched									
1 package (18.50 oz) (524g)	2264	61	9	10	409	5.8	0	23	3443
Cake, Yellow, Prepared from Recipe, Without Frosting									
1 piece (1/12 of 8" dia) (68g)	245	10	3	37	36	0.5	0	4	233
Cheesecake, Commercially Prepared									
1 piece (1/6 of 17 oz cake) (80g)	257	18	8	44	20	0.3	17	4	166
Cheesecake, Prepared from Mix, No-bake-type									
1 piece (1/12 of 9" dia) (99g)	271	13	7	29	35	1.9	0	5	376
Coffee Cake, Cheese									
1 piece (1/6 of 16 oz cake) (76g)	258	12	4	65	34	0.8	0	5	258
Coffee Cake, Cinnamon with Crumb Topping, Commercially Prepared, Enriched									
1 individual, cake (57g)	238	13	3	18	27	1.1	0	4	200
Coffee Cake, Cinnamon with Crumb Topping, Commercially Prepared, Unenriched									
1 individual, cake (57g)	238	13	3	18	27	1.1	0	4	200
Coffee Cake, Cinnamon with Crumb Topping, Dry Mix									
1 package (10.5 oz) (298g)	1299	36	9	0	232	5.4	127	14	1776
Coffee Cake, Cinnamon with Crumb Topping, Dry Mix, Prepared									
1 piece (1/8 of 8" x 5-3/4" cake) (56g)	178	5	1	27	30	0.7	17	3	236
Coffee Cake, Crème-filled, with Chocolate Frosting									
1 piece (1/6 of 19 oz cake) (90g)	298	10	3	62	48	1.8	0	5	291

Food Serving size	Cal.	(g) Total Fat	(g) Sat. Fat	(mg) Chol.	(g) Carb.	(g) Fiber	(g) Sug.	(g) Prot.	(mg) Sod.
Coffee Cake, Fruit 1 piece (1/8 cake) (50g)	156	5	1	4	26	1.3	0	3	193
Cookies, Animal Crackers (Including Arrowroot, Tea Biscuits) 1 Arrowroot biscuit (include Arrowroot cookie) (4.9g)	22	1	0	0	4	0.1	1	0	24
Cookies, Brownies, Commercially Prepared 1 square, large (2-3/4" sq x 7/8") (56g)	227	9	2	10	36	1.2	21	3	144
Cookies, Brownies, Dry Mix, Regular 1 package (21.5 oz) (610g)	2647	91	15	0	467	0	0	24	1848
Cookies, Brownies, Dry Mix, Special Dietary 1 package (8.5 oz) (241g)	1027	30	5	0	194	10.1	0	7	200
Cookies, Brownies, Dry Mix, Special Dietary, Prepared 1 brownie (2" square) (22g)	84	2	1	0	16	0.8	0	1	21
Cookies, Brownies, Prepared from Recipe 1 brownie (2" square) (24g)	112	7	2	18	12	0	0	1	82
Cookies, Butter, Commercially Prepared, Enriched 1 cookie (5g)	23	1	1	6	3	0	1	0	12
Cookies, Butter, Commercially Prepared, Unenriched 1 cookie (5g)	23	1	1	6	3	0	0	0	18
Cookies, Chocolate Chip, Commercially Prepared, Regular, Higher Fat, Enriched 1 cookie, bite size (2.2g)	10	1	0	0	1	0.1	1	0	8
Cookies, Chocolate Chip, Commercially Prepared, Regular, Higher Fat, Unenriched 1 cookie, medium (2-1/4" dia) (10g)	48	2	1	0	7	0.3	0	1	32
Cookies, Chocolate Chip, Commercially Prepared, Regular, Lower Fat 1 cookie (10g)	45	2	0	0	7	0.4	0	1	38
Cookies, Chocolate Chip, Commercially Prepared, Soft-type 1 cookie (average weight of 1 cookie) (12.2g)	55	3	1	0	8	0.3	5	1	33
Cookies, Chocolate Chip, Commercially Prepared, Special Dietary 1 cookie, medium (1-5/8" dia) (7g)	32	1	0	0	5	0.1	3	0	1
Cookies, Chocolate Chip, Dry Mix 1 package (17.5 oz) (496g)	2465	125	41	0	328	0	0	23	1438

Food Serving size	Cal.	(g) Total Fat	(g) Sat. Fat	(mg) Chol.	(g) Carb.	(g) Fiber	(g) Sug.	(g) Prot.	(mg) Sod.
Cookies, Chocolate Chip, Prepared from Recipe, Made with Butter 1 cookie, medium (2-1/4″ dia) (16g)	78	5	2	11	9	0	0	1	55
Cookies, Chocolate Chip, Prepared from Recipe, Made with Margarine 1 bar (2″ square) (32g)	156	9	3	10	19	0.9	0	2	116
Cookies, Chocolate Chip, Refrigerated Dough 1 portion, dough spoon from roll (29g)	128	6	2	7	18	0.4	0	1	61
Cookies, Chocolate Chip, Refrigerated Dough, Baked 1 cookie, medium (2-1/4″ dia) (12g)	59	3	1	3	8	0.2	0	1	28
Cookies, Chocolate Sandwich, with Crème Filling, Regular 3 cookies (1 NLEA serving) (34g)	159	7	2	0	24	1	14	2	171
Cookies, Chocolate Sandwich, with Crème Filling, Regular, Chocolate-coated 1 cookie (17g)	82	4	1	0	11	0.9	11	1	55
Cookies, Chocolate Sandwich, with Crème filling, Special Dietary 1 cookie (10g)	46	2	0	0	7	0.4	2	0	24
Cookies, Chocolate Sandwich, with Extra Crème Filling 1 cookie (13g)	65	3	1	0	9	0.4	6	1	46
Cookies, Chocolate Wafers 1 cup, crumbs (112g)	485	16	5	2	81	3.8	33	7	773
Cookies, Coconut Macaroons, Prepared from Recipe 1 cookie, medium (2″ dia) (24g)	97	3	3	0	17	0.4	17	1	59
Cookies, Fig Bars 1 Figaroo (2 square halves) (43g)	150	3	0	0	30	2	20	2	151
Cookies, Fortune 1 cookie (8g)	30	0	0	0	7	0.1	4	0	22
Cookies, Fudge, Cake-type (Including Trolley Cakes) 1 cookie (21g)	73	1	0	0	16	0.6	0	1	40
Cookies, Ginger Snaps 1 cookie (7g)	29	1	0	0	5	0.2	1	0	39
Cookies, Graham Crackers, Chocolate-coated 1 cracker (2-1/2″ square) (14g)	68	3	2	0	9	0.4	6	1	36

Food Serving size	Cal.	(g) Total Fat	(g) Sat. Fat	(mg) Chol.	(g) Carb.	(g) Fiber	(g) Sug.	(g) Prot.	(mg) Sod.
Cookies, Graham Crackers, Plain or Honey (Including Cinnamon)									
1 cup, crushed (84g)	355	8	1	0	65	2.4	26	6	401
Cookies, Ladyfingers, with Lemon Juice and Rind									
1 anisette sponge (4″ x 1-1/8″ x 7/8″) (13g)	47	1	0	29	8	0.1	3	1	19
Cookies, Ladyfingers, Without Lemon Juice and Rind									
1 anisette sponge (4″ x 1-1/8″ x 7/8″) (13g)	47	1	0	29	8	0.1	0	1	19
Cookies, Marshmallow, Chocolate-coated (Including Marshmallow Pies)									
1 fudge marshmallow (28g)	118	5	1	0	19	0.6	13	1	47
Cookies, Molasses									
1 large (3-1/2″ to 4″ dia) (include Archway brand) (32g)	138	4	1	0	24	0.3	6	2	147
Cookies, Oatmeal, Commercially Prepared, Fat Free									
1 oz (28.35g)	92	0	0	0	22	2.1	12	2	62
Cookies, Oatmeal, Commercially Prepared, Regular									
1 cookie, big (3-1/2″ - 4″ dia) (include Archway brand, Grandma brand) (25g)	113	5	1	0	17	0.7	6	2	96
Cookies, Oatmeal, Commercially Prepared, Soft-type									
1 cookie (15g)	61	2	1	1	10	0.4	0	1	52
Cookies, Oatmeal, Commercially Prepared, Special Dietary									
1 cookie, medium (1-5/8″ dia) (7g)	31	1	0	0	5	0.2	2	0	1
Cookies, Oatmeal, Dry Mix									
1 package (17.5 oz) (496g)	2292	95	24	0	334	0	0	32	2346
Cookies, Oatmeal, Prepared from Recipe, with Raisins									
1 cookie (2-5/8″ dia) (15g)	65	2	0	5	10	0	0	1	81
Cookies, Oatmeal, Prepared from Recipe, Without Raisins									
1 cookie (2-5/8″ dia) (15g)	67	3	1	5	10	0	0	1	90
Cookies, Oatmeal, Refrigerated Dough									
1 portion, dough for 1 cookie (16g)	68	3	1	4	9	0.4	0	1	47
Cookies, Oatmeal, Refrigerated Dough, Baked									
1 cookie (12g)	57	3	1	3	8	0.3	0	1	39
Cookies, Peanut Butter Sandwich, Regular									
1 cookie (14g)	67	3	1	0	9	0.3	5	1	52

Food Serving size	Cal.	(g) Total Fat	(g) Sat. Fat	(mg) Chol.	(g) Carb.	(g) Fiber	(g) Sug.	(g) Prot.	(mg) Sod.
Cookies, Peanut Butter Sandwich, Special Dietary 1 cookie (10g)	54	3	0	0	5	0	0	1	41
Cookies, Peanut Butter, Commercially Prepared, Regular 1 cookie (15g)	72	4	1	0	9	0.3	5	1	62
Cookies, Peanut Butter, Commercially Prepared, Soft-type 1 cookie (15g)	69	4	1	0	9	0.3	0	1	50
Cookies, Peanut Butter, Prepared from Recipe 1 cookie (3″ dia) (20g)	95	5	1	6	12	0	0	2	104
Cookies, Peanut Butter, Refrigerated Dough 1 portion, dough for 1 cookie (16g)	73	4	1	4	8	0.2	0	1	64
Cookies, Peanut Butter, Refrigerated Dough, Baked 1 cookie (12g)	60	3	1	4	7	0.1	0	1	52
Cookies, Raisin, Soft-type 1 cookie (15g)	60	2	1	0	10	0.2	7	1	51
Cookies, Shortbread, Commercially Prepared, Pecan 1 cookie (2″ dia) (14g)	76	5	1	5	8	0.3	0	1	39
Cookies, Shortbread, Commercially Prepared, Plain 1 cookie (1-5/8″ square) (8g)	40	2	0	2	5	0.1	1	0	36
Cookies, Sugar Wafers with Crème Filling, Regular 1 cookie (10.1g)	51	2	1	0	7	0.2	4	0	10
Cookies, Sugar Wafers with Crème Filling, Special Dietary 1 wafer (4g)	20	1	0	0	3	0	0	0	0
Cookies, Sugar, Commercially Prepared, Regular (Including Vanilla) 1 cookie (15g)	72	3	1	8	10	0.1	6	1	54
Cookies, Sugar, Commercially Prepared, Special Dietary 1 cookie, medium (1-5/8″ dia) (7g)	30	1	0	0	5	0.1	2	0	0
Cookies, Sugar, Prepared from Recipe, Made with Margarine 1 cookie (3″ dia) (14g)	66	3	1	4	8	0.2	3	1	69
Cookies, Sugar, Refrigerated Dough 1 cookie, dough for 1 rolled cookie (17g)	74	4	1	5	10	0.1	4	1	72
Cookies, Sugar, Refrigerated Dough, Baked 1 cookie, 1 rolled cookie dough (15g)	73	3	1	5	10	0.1	4	1	70

Food Serving size	Cal.	(g) Total Fat	(g) Sat. Fat	(mg) Chol.	(g) Carb.	(g) Fiber	(g) Sug.	(g) Prot.	(mg) Sod.
Cookies, Vanilla Sandwich with Crème Filling									
1 cookie, oval (3-1/8" x 1-1/4" x 3/8") (15g)	72	3	0	0	11	0.2	6	1	52
Cookies, Vanilla Wafers, Higher Fat									
1 wafer (6g)	28	1	0	0	4	0.1	0	0	18
Cookies, Vanilla Wafers, Lower Fat									
1 cup, crumbs (80g)	353	12	3	41	59	1.5	30	4	310
Corn Cakes									
2 cakes (18g)	70	0	0	0	15	0.3	4	1	88
Corn Cakes, Very Low Sodium									
2 cakes (18g)	70	0	0	0	15	0	0	1	5
Corn-based, Extruded, Cones, Plain									
1 oz (28.35g)	145	8	6	0	18	0.3	0	2	290
Cornstarch									
1 cup (128g)	488	0	0	0	117	1.2	0	0	12
Cracker Meal									
1 cup (115g)	440	2	0	0	93	3	0	11	18
Crackers, Cheese, Low Sodium									
1 cup, Cheez-its (62g)	312	16	6	8	36	1.5	0	6	284
Crackers, Cheese, Regular									
1 cup, bite size (62g)	312	16	6	8	36	1.5	0	6	617
Crackers, Cheese, Sandwich-type with Cheese Filling									
1 sandwich (6.5g)	32	2	0	0	4	0.1	1	1	57
Crackers, Cheese, Sandwich-type, with Peanut Butter Filling									
1 cup, crushed (83g)	412	21	4	0	47	2.8	6	10	758
Crackers, Cream, Gamesa Sabrosas									
1 cracker (3.1g)	15	1	0	0	2	0.1	0	0	36
Crackers, Cream, La Moderna Rikis Cream Crackers									
1 cracker (3.1g)	13	1	0	0	2	0.1	0	0	23
Crackers, Crispbread, Rye									
1 cup, crushed (55g)	201	1	0	0	45	9.1	1	4	249
Crackers, Matzo, Egg									
1 matzo (28g)	109	1	0	23	22	0.8	0	3	6
Crackers, Matzo, Egg and Onion									
1 matzo (28g)	109	1	0	13	22	1.4	0	3	80

Food Serving size	Cal.	Total Fat (g)	Sat. Fat (g)	Chol. (mg)	Carb. (g)	Fiber (g)	Sug. (g)	Prot. (g)	Sod. (mg)
Crackers, Matzo, Plain 1 matzo (28g)	111	0	0	0	23	0.8	0	3	0
Crackers, Matzo, Whole Wheat 1 matzo (28g)	98	0	0	0	22	3.3	0	4	1
Crackers, Melba Toast, Plain 1 cup, pieces (30g)	117	1	0	0	23	1.9	0	4	179
Crackers, Melba Toast, Plain, Without Salt 1 cup, crushed (70g)	273	2	0	0	54	4.4	0	8	13
Crackers, Melba Toast, Rye (Including Pumpernickel) 1 toast (5g)	19	0	0	0	4	0.4	0	1	45
Crackers, Melba Toast, Wheat 1 toast (5g)	19	0	0	0	4	0.4	0	1	42
Crackers, Milk 1 cracker (11g)	50	2	0	1	8	0.2	2	1	65
Crackers, Rusk Toast 1 rusk (10g)	41	1	0	8	7	0	0	1	25
Crackers, Rye, Sandwich-type, with Cheese Filling 1 cracker, sandwich (7g)	34	2	0	1	4	0.3	0	1	73
Crackers, Rye, Wafers, Plain 1 cup, crushed (61g)	204	1	0	0	49	14	1	6	340
Crackers, Rye, Wafers, Seasoned 1 cracker, triple (22g)	84	2	0	0	16	4.6	0	2	195
Crackers, Saltines (Including Oyster, Soda, Soup) 1 cup, crushed (70g)	295	6	1	0	52	2	2	7	781
Crackers, Saltines, Fat Free, Low-sodium 6 saltines (30g)	118	0	0	0	25	0.8	0	3	215
Crackers, Saltines, Low Salt (Including Oyster, Soda, Soup) 1 cup, oyster crackers (45g)	189	4	1	0	33	1.3	1	4	89
Crackers, Saltines, Unsalted Tops (Including Oyster, Soda, Soup) 1 cracker (3g)	13	0	0	0	2	0.1	0	0	23
Crackers, Snack, Goya Crackers 1 cracker (12.7g)	55	2	1	0	8	0.5	0	2	84
Crackers, Standard Snack-type, Regular 1 cracker, round (3.2g)	16	1	0	0	2	0.1	0	0	28

Food Serving size	Cal.	(g) Total Fat	(g) Sat. Fat	(mg) Chol.	(g) Carb.	(g) Fiber	(g) Sug.	(g) Prot.	(mg) Sod.
Crackers, Standard Snack-type, Regular, Low Salt									
1 cup, bite size (62g)	311	16	2	0	38	1	1	5	134
Crackers, Standard Snack-type, Sandwich, with Cheese Filling									
1 cracker, sandwich (7g)	33	1	0	0	4	0.1	0	1	62
Crackers, Standard Snack-type, Sandwich, with Peanut Butter Filling									
1 cracker, sandwich (7g)	35	2	0	0	4	0.2	1	1	63
Crackers, Wheat, Low Salt									
1 cup, crushed (83g)	393	17	4	0	54	3.7	11	7	158
Crackers, Wheat, Reduced Fat									
1 cracker (1.8g)	8	0	0	0	1	0.1	0	0	16
Crackers, Wheat, Regular									
1 cracker, thin square (2g)	9	0	0	0	1	0.1	0	0	18
Crackers, Wheat, Sandwich, with Cheese Filling									
1 cracker, sandwich (7g)	35	2	0	0	4	0.2	0	1	64
Crackers, Wheat, Sandwich, with Peanut Butter Filling									
1 cracker, sandwich (7g)	35	2	0	0	4	0.3	0	1	56
Crackers, Whole Wheat									
6 crackers, Triscuits, regular size (28g)	120	4	1	0	19	2.9	0	3	197
Crackers, Whole Wheat, Low Salt									
1 cup, crushed (94g)	416	16	3	0	64	9.9	0	8	175
Crackers, Whole Wheat, Reduced Fat									
1 cracker (4.2g)	17	0	0	0	3	0.5	0	0	31
Cream Puffs, Prepared from Recipe, Shell (Including Éclair)									
1 eclair (5″ x 2″ x 1-3/4″) (48g)	174	12	3	94	11	0.4	0	4	267
Cream Puffs, Prepared from Recipe, Shell, with Custard Filling									
1 cream puff (130g)	335	20	5	174	30	0.5	12	9	443
Croissants, Apple									
1 croissant, medium (57g)	145	5	3	18	21	1.4	0	4	156
Croissants, Butter									
1 croissant, mini (28g)	114	6	3	19	13	0.7	3	2	97
Croissants, Cheese									
1 croissant, small (42g)	174	9	4	24	20	1.1	5	4	152

Food Serving size	Cal.	(g) Total Fat	(g) Sat. Fat	(mg) Chol.	(g) Carb.	(g) Fiber	(g) Sug.	(g) Prot.	(mg) Sod.
Croutons, Plain 1 cup (30g)	122	2	0	0	22	1.5	0	4	209
Croutons, Seasoned 1 cup (40g)	186	7	2	3	25	2	2	4	436
Danish Pastry, Cheese 1 pastry (71g)	266	16	5	16	26	0.7	5	6	229
Danish Pastry, Cinnamon, Enriched 1 large (approx 7″ dia) (142g)	572	32	8	30	63	1.8	28	10	527
Danish Pastry, Cinnamon, Unenriched 1 large (approx 7″ dia) (142g)	572	32	8	30	63	1.7	0	10	527
Danish Pastry, Fruit, Enriched 1 large (approx 7″ dia) (142g)	527	26	7	162	68	2.7	39	8	503
Danish Pastry, Fruit, Unenriched (Including Apple, Cinnamon, Raisin, Strawberry) 1 container (3 oz) (142g)	527	26	4	57	68	2.7	0	8	503
Danish Pastry, Lemon, Unenriched 1 pastry (71g)	263	13	2	28	34	1.3	0	4	251
Danish Pastry, Nut (Including Almond, Raisin Nut, Cinnamon Nut) 1 pastry (4-1/4″ dia) (65g)	280	16	4	30	30	1.3	17	5	194
Danish Pastry, Raspberry, Unenriched 1 pastry (4-1/4″ dia) (71g)	263	13	2	28	34	1.3	0	4	251
Desserts, Apple Crisp, Prepared from Recipe 1 recipe, yields (844g)	1359	29	6	0	260	11.8	166	15	2962
Desserts, Egg Custard, Baked, Prepared from Recipe 1 recipe, yields (563g)	586	26	12	473	62	0	62	28	343
Doughnuts, Cake-type, Chocolate, Sugared, or Glazed 1 doughnut (3-3/4″ dia) (60g)	250	12	3	34	34	1.3	19	3	238
Doughnuts, Cake-type, Plain (Includes Unsugared, Old-fashioned) 1 doughnut, stick (52g)	217	12	4	5	24	0.8	8	3	290
Doughnuts, Cake-type, Plain, Chocolate-coated, or Frosted 1 donettes (2″ dia) (18g)	81	5	2	3	9	0.3	5	1	59
Doughnuts, Cake-type, Plain, Sugared, or Glazed 1 doughnut, medium (approx 3″ dia) (45g)	192	10	3	14	23	0.7	0	2	181
Doughnuts, Cake-type, Wheat, Sugared, or Glazed 1 doughnut (2″ dia) (28g)	101	5	1	6	12	0.6	6	2	120

Food Serving size	Cal.	(g) Total Fat	(g) Sat. Fat	(mg) Chol.	(g) Carb.	(g) Fiber	(g) Sug.	(g) Prot.	(mg) Sod.
Doughnuts, French Crullers, Glazed									
1 cruller (3″ dia) (41g)	169	8	2	5	24	0.5	14	1	141
Doughnuts, Yeast-leavened, Glazed, Enriched (Including Honey Buns)									
1 doughnut, hole (13g)	52	2	1	4	7	0.3	3	1	41
Doughnuts, Yeast-leavened, Glazed, Unenriched (Including Honey Buns)									
1 doughnut, medium (3-1/4″ dia) (60g)	242	14	3	4	27	0.7	0	4	205
Doughnuts, Yeast-leavened, with Crème Filling									
1 doughnut, oval (3-1/2″ x 2-1/2″) (85g)	307	21	5	20	26	0.7	12	5	263
Doughnuts, Yeast-leavened, with Jelly Filling									
1 doughnut, oval (3-1/2″ x 2-1/2″) (85g)	289	16	4	22	33	0.8	18	5	204
Eclairs, Custard-filled, with Chocolate Glaze, Prepared from Recipe									
1 cream puff (3-1/2″ x 2″) (112g)	293	18	5	142	27	0.7	7	7	377
English Muffin, Plain, Enriched, with Calcium Propionate (Including Sourdough)									
1 muffin (57g)	129	1	0	0	25	2	2	5	206
English Muffin, Plain, Toasted, Enriched, with Calcium Propionate (including Sourdough)									
1 muffin (52g)	140	1	0	0	27	1.5	2	5	248
English Muffins, Mixed-grain (Including Granola)									
1 muffin (66g)	155	1	0	0	31	1.8	1	6	220
English Muffins, Mixed-grain, Toasted (Including Granola)									
1 muffin (61g)	156	1	0	0	31	1.8	1	6	276
English Muffins, Plain, Enriched, Without Calcium Propionate (Including Sourdough)									
1 muffin (57g)	134	1	0	0	26	1.5	0	4	264
English Muffins, Plain, Unenriched, with Calcium Propionate (Including Sourdough)									
1 muffin (57g)	134	1	0	0	26	1.5	0	4	264
English Muffins, Plain, Unenriched, Without Calcium Propionate (Including Sourdough)									
1 muffin (57g)	134	1	0	0	26	1.5	0	4	264
English Muffins, Raisin-cinnamon (Includes Apple-cinnamon)									
1 muffin (57g)	137	1	0	0	27	1.5	8	5	158

Food Serving size	Cal.	(g) Total Fat	(g) Sat. Fat	(mg) Chol.	(g) Carb.	(g) Fiber	(g) Sug.	(g) Prot.	(mg) Sod.
English Muffins, Raisin-cinnamon, Toasted (Including Apple-cinnamon)									
1 muffin (52g)	144	1	0	0	29	1.6	7	5	192
English Muffins, Wheat									
1 muffin (57g)	127	1	0	0	26	2.6	1	5	218
English Muffins, Wheat, Toasted									
1 muffin (52g)	126	1	0	0	25	2.6	1	5	216
English Muffins, Whole Wheat									
1 muffin (66g)	134	1	0	0	27	4.4	5	6	240
English Muffins, Whole Wheat, Toasted									
1 muffin (61g)	135	1	0	0	27	4.5	5	6	422
French Toast, Prepared from Recipe, Made with Low Fat (2%) Milk									
1 slice (65g)	149	7	2	75	16	0	0	5	311
General Mills, Betty Crocker Supermoist Yellow Cake Mix, Dry									
1 serving (43g)	178	3	1	0	35	0	19	2	289
Hush Puppies, Prepared from Recipe									
1 cup (152g)	512	21	3	68	70	4.3	3	12	1015
Interstate Brands Corp., Wonder Hamburger Rolls									
1 serving (43g)	117	2	0	0	22	1.1	5	3	210
Keebler, Keebler Chocolate Graham Selects									
1 serving (31g)	144	5	1	0	22	0	8	2	111
Keebler, Keebler Golden Vanilla Wafers, Artificially Flavored									
1 serving (31g)	147	6	1	0	22	0	8	2	120
Keikitos (Muffins), Latino Bakery Item									
1 piece (42g)	196	11	0	0	22	0.5	11	3	216
Kellogg's Eggo Low Fat Nutri-Grain Waffles									
1 serving (70g)	142	2	0	0	28	2.6	4	4	391
Kellogg's Low Fat Pop Tarts, Frosted Brown Sugar Cinnamon									
1 pastry (50g)	188	3	1	0	39	0.6	18	2	210
Kellogg's Low Fat Pop Tarts, Frosted Chocolate Fudge									
1 pastry (52g)	190	3	1	0	40	0.6	19	3	249
Kellogg's Low Fat Pop Tarts, Frosted Strawberry									
1 pastry (52g)	191	3	1	0	40	0.6	21	2	201
Kellogg's Low Fat Pop Tarts, Strawberry									
1 pastry (52g)	192	3	1	0	40	0.6	19	2	182

Food Serving size	Cal.	(g) Total Fat	(g) Sat. Fat	(mg) Chol.	(g) Carb.	(g) Fiber	(g) Sug.	(g) Prot.	(mg) Sod.
Kellogg's Nutri-Grain Cereal Bars, Mixed Berry									
1 bar (NLEA serving) (116g)	429	9	2	0	84	2.2	39	5	329
Kellogg's Pop-Tarts Pastry Swirls, Apple Cinnamon Danish									
1 pastry (62g)	256	11	3	0	37	0.9	11	3	190
Kellogg's Pop-Tarts Pastry Swirls, Cheese Danish									
1 pastry (62g)	252	11	3	1	37	0.3	12	3	180
Kellogg's Pop-Tarts Pastry Swirls, Strawberry Danish									
1 pastry (62g)	254	11	3	0	37	1.1	16	3	170
Kraft Foods, Shake 'N' Bake Original Recipe, Coating for Pork, Dry									
1 serving (28g)	106	1	0	0	22	0	0	2	611
Krusteaz Almond Poppyseed Muffin Mix, Artificially Flavored, Dry									
1 serving (40g)	167	4	1	0	30	0.7	16	2	236
Leavening Agents, Cream of Tartar									
.5 tsp (1.5g)	4	0	0	0	1	0	0	0	1
Leavening Agents, Yeast, Baker's, Compressed									
1 cake (0.6 oz) (17g)	18	0	0	0	3	1.4	0	1	5
Martha White Foods, Martha White's Buttermilk Biscuit Mix, Dry									
1 serving (41g)	159	5	2	1	24	0.6	2	3	531
Martha White Foods, Martha White's Chewy Fudge Brownie Mix									
1 serving (28g)	114	2	0	0	23	0.8	15	1	128
Millet, Cooked									
1 cup (174g)	207	2	0	0	41	2.3	0	6	3
Millet, Puffed									
1 cup (21g)	74	1	0	0	17	0.6	0	3	1
Mission Foods, Mission Flour Tortillas, Soft Taco, 8 Inch									
1 serving (51g)	146	3	0	0	25	0	0	4	458
Muffins, Blueberry, Commercially Prepared (Includes Mini-muffins)									
1 mini (1-1/4″ dia) (17g)	67	3	1	7	8	0.3	5	1	59
Muffins, Blueberry, Commercially Prepared, Low Fat									
1 oz (28.35g)	72	1	0	8	14	1.2	8	1	117
Muffins, Blueberry, Dry Mix									
1 package, mix + drained berries (356g)									
	1303	36	9	0	225	0	0	17	1951
Muffins, Blueberry, Prepared from Recipe, Made with Low Fat (2%) Milk									
1 muffin (57g)	162	6	1	21	23	0	0	4	251

Food Serving size	Cal.	(g) Total Fat	(g) Sat. Fat	(mg) Chol.	(g) Carb.	(g) Fiber	(g) Sug.	(g) Prot.	(mg) Sod.
Muffins, Blueberry, Toaster-type 1 muffin, toaster (33g)	103	3	0	2	18	0.6	2	2	82
Muffins, Blueberry, Toaster-type, Toasted 1 muffin, toaster (31g)	103	3	0	2	18	0.6	4	2	158
Muffins, Corn, Commercially Prepared 1 mini (17g)	52	1	0	4	9	0.6	1	1	109
Muffins, Corn, Dry Mix, Prepared 1 oz (28.35g)	91	3	1	18	14	0.7	0	2	225
Muffins, Corn, Prepared from Recipe, Made with Low Fat (2%) Milk 1 muffin (2-3/4" dia x 2") (57g)	180	7	1	24	25	0	0	4	333
Muffins, Corn, Toaster-type 1 muffin, toaster (33g)	114	4	1	4	19	0.5	0	2	142
Muffins, Oat Bran 1 mini (17g)	46	1	0	0	8	0.8	1	1	67
Muffins, Plain, Prepared from Recipe, Made with Low Fat (2%) Milk 1 muffin (57g)	169	6	1	22	24	1.5	0	4	266
Muffins, Wheat Bran, Dry Mix 1 package (7 oz) (198g)	784	24	6	0	145	0	0	14	1386
Muffins, Wheat Bran, Toaster-type with Raisins, Toasted 1 muffin, toaster (34g)	106	3	1	3	19	2.8	8	2	179
Muffins, Wheat Bran, Toaster-type, with Raisins 1 muffin, toaster (36g)	106	3	0	6	19	2.8	5	2	178
Nabisco Graham Crackers 1 serving (28g)	119	3	0	0	21	1	6	2	185
Nabisco Oreo Crunchies, Cookie Crumb Topping 1 serving (11g)	52	2	0	0	8	0.4	4	1	58
Nabisco Ritz Crackers 5 crackers (1 NLEA serving) (16g)	79	4	1	0	10	0.4	1	1	141
Nabisco Snackwell's Fat-free Devil's Food Cookie Cakes 1 serving (16g)	49	0	0	0	12	0.3	7	1	28
Noodles, Flat, Crunchy, Chinese Restaurant 1 cup (45g)	234	14	2	0	23	0.9	0	5	170

Food Serving size	Cal.	(g) Total Fat	(g) Sat. Fat	(mg) Chol.	(g) Carb.	(g) Fiber	(g) Sug.	(g) Prot.	(mg) Sod.
Pan Dulce, La Ricura, Salpora De Arroz, Cookie-like									
1 piece (1 serving) (42g)	187	7	0	0	28	0.5	9	4	187
Pastry, Pastelitos De Guava (Guava Pastries)									
1 piece (86g)	326	16	5	9	41	1.9	15	5	199
Phyllo Dough									
1 sheet, dough (19g)	57	1	0	0	10	0.4	0	1	92
Pie Crust, Cookie-type, Chocolate, Ready Crust									
1 crust (182g)	881	41	9	0	117	4.9	48	11	915
Pie Crust, Cookie-type, Graham Cracker, Ready Crust									
1 oz (28.35g)	142	7	1	0	18	0.5	5	1	94
Pie Crust, Cookie-type, Prepared from Recipe, Chocolate Wafer, Chilled									
1 piece (1/8 of 9″ crust) (28g)	142	9	2	0	15	0.4	6	1	188
Pie Crust, Cookie-type, Prepared from Recipe, Graham Cracker, Baked									
1 tart shell (22g)	109	5	1	0	14	0.3	8	1	126
Pie Crust, Cookie-type, Prepared from Recipe, Graham Cracker, Chilled									
1 piece (1/8 of 9″ crust) (30g)	145	7	2	0	19	0.5	11	1	168
Pie Crust, Cookie-type, Prepared from Recipe, Vanilla Wafer, Chilled									
1 crust, single 9″ (176g)	935	64	13	69	88	0.2	13	7	906
Pie Crust, Deep Dish, Frozen, Baked, Made with Enriched Flour									
1 pie crust (average weight) (202g)	1052	64	18	0	106	4.6	0	12	794
Pie Crust, Deep Dish, Frozen, Unbaked, Made with Enriched Flour									
1 pie crust (average weight) (225g)	1053	65	18	0	105	3.2	0	12	794
Pie Crust, Refrigerated, Regular, Baked									
1 pie crust (198g)	1002	57	22	0	116	2.8	0	7	935
Pie Crust, Standard-type, Dry Mix, Prepared, Baked									
1 piece (1/8 of 9″ crust) (20g)	100	6	2	0	10	0.4	0	1	146
Pie Crust, Standard-type, Frozen, Ready-to-bake, Enriched, Baked									
1 pie crust (average weight of 1 baked crust) (154g)	782	44	14	0	87	5.1	7	10	719
Pie Crust, Standard-type, Frozen, Ready-to-bake, Unenriched									
1 piece (1/8 of 9″ crust) (16g)	73	5	1	0	7	0.1	0	1	92
Pie Crust, Standard-type, Prepared from Recipe, Baked									
1 piece (1/8 of 9″ crust) (23g)	121	8	2	0	11	0.4	0	1	125

Food Serving size	Cal.	(g) Total Fat	(g) Sat. Fat	(mg) Chol.	(g) Carb.	(g) Fiber	(g) Sug.	(g) Prot.	(mg) Sod.
Pie Crust, Standard-type, Prepared from Recipe, Unbaked									
1 piece (1/8 of 9″ crust) (24g)	113	7	2	0	10	0.8	0	1	116
Pie, Apple, Commercially Prepared, Enriched Flour									
1 piece (1/8 of 9″ dia) (125g)	296	14	5	0	43	2	20	2	251
Pie, Apple, Commercially Prepared, Unenriched Flour									
1 piece (1/8 of 9″ dia) (125g)	296	14	5	0	43	2	0	2	333
Pie, Apple, Prepared from Recipe									
1 piece (1/8 of 9″ dia) (155g)	411	19	5	0	58	0	0	4	327
Pie, Banana Cream, Prepared from Mix, No-bake-type									
1 piece (1/8 of 9″ dia) (92g)	231	12	6	27	29	0.6	0	3	267
Pie, Banana Cream, Prepared from Recipe									
1 pie (9″ dia) (1186g)	3190	161	45	605	390	8.3	143	52	2846
Pie, Blueberry, Commercially Prepared									
1 piece (1/8 of 9″ dia) (125g)	290	13	2	0	44	1.3	12	2	274
Pie, Blueberry, Prepared from Recipe									
1 piece (1/8 of 9″ dia) (147g)	360	17	4	0	49	0	0	4	272
Pie, Cherry, Commercially Prepared									
1 piece (1/8 of 9″ dia) (125g)	325	14	3	0	50	1	18	3	308
Pie, Cherry, Prepared from Recipe									
1 piece (1/8 of 9″ dia) (180g)	486	22	5	0	69	0	0	5	344
Pie, Chocolate Creme, Commercially Prepared									
1 oz (28.35g)	100	6	4	3	11	0.2	8	1	75
Pie, Chocolate Mousse, Prepared from Mix, No-bake-type									
1 piece (1/8 of 9″ dia) (95g)	247	15	8	33	28	0	0	3	437
Pie, Coconut Crème, Commercially Prepared									
1 piece (1/6 of 7″ pie) (64g)	191	11	4	0	24	0.8	12	1	131
Pie, Coconut Creme, Prepared from Mix, No-bake-type									
1 piece (1/8 of 9″ dia) (94g)	259	17	8	22	27	0.5	0	3	309
Pie, Coconut Custard, Commercially Prepared									
1 piece (1/6 of 8″ pie) (104g)	270	14	6	36	31	1.9	0	6	348
Pie, Crust, Refrigerated, Regular, Unbaked									
1 pie crust (average weight) (229g)	1019	58	22	0	117	4.1	0	7	937
Pie, Dutch Apple, Commercially Prepared									
1 slice (137g)	397	16	3	0	61	2.2	30	3	274

Food Serving size	Cal.	(g) Total Fat	(g) Sat. Fat	(mg) Chol.	(g) Carb.	(g) Fiber	(g) Sug.	(g) Prot.	(mg) Sod.
Pie, Egg Custard, Commercially Prepared									
1 piece (1/6 of 8″ pie) (105g)	221	12	2	35	22	1.7	12	6	158
Pie, Fried Pies, Cherry									
1 pie (5″ x 3-3/4″) (128g)	404	21	3	0	55	3.3	0	4	479
Pie, Fried Pies, Fruit									
1 pie (5″ x 3-3/4″) (128g)	404	21	3	0	55	3.3	27	4	479
Pie, Fried Pies, Lemon									
1 pie (5″ x 3-3/4″) (128g)	404	21	3	0	55	3.3	0	4	479
Pie, Lemon Meringue, Commercially Prepared									
1 piece (1/6 of 8″ pie) (113g)	303	10	2	51	53	1.4	27	2	194
Pie, Lemon Meringue, Prepared from Recipe									
1 piece (1/8 of 9″ dia) (127g)	362	16	4	67	50	0	0	5	307
Pie, Mince, Prepared from Recipe									
1 piece (1/8 of 9″ dia) (165g)	477	18	4	0	79	4.3	47	4	419
Pie, Peach									
1 piece (1/6 of 8″ pie) (117g)	261	12	2	0	38	0.9	7	2	227
Pie, Pecan, Commercially Prepared									
1 slice (133g)	541	22	4	56	79	2.8	33	6	210
Pie, Pecan, Prepared from Recipe									
1 piece (1/8 of 9″ dia) (122g)	503	27	5	106	64	0	0	6	320
Pie, Pumpkin, Commercially Prepared									
1 slice (133g)	323	13	3	35	46	2.4	25	5	450
Pie, Pumpkin, Prepared from Recipe									
1 piece (1/8 of 9″ dia) (155g)	316	14	5	65	41	0	0	7	349
Pie, Vanilla Cream, Prepared from Recipe									
1 piece (1/8 of 9″ dia) (126g)	350	18	5	78	41	0.8	16	6	328
Pillsbury Golden Layer Buttermilk Biscuits, Artificially Flavored, Refrigerated Dough									
1 serving (34g)	104	5	1	0	14	0.4	2	2	360
Pillsbury Grands, Buttermilk Biscuits, Refrigerated Dough									
1 serving (61g)	193	8	3	0	25	0.7	4	4	631
Pillsbury, Buttermilk Biscuits, Artificially Flavored, Refrigerated Dough									
1 serving (64g)	150	2	0	0	29	1	4	4	570
Pillsbury, Chocolate Chip Cookies, Refrigerated Dough									
1 serving (28g)	135	7	2	5	17	0.6	10	1	85

Food Serving size	Cal.	(g) Total Fat	(g) Sat. Fat	(mg) Chol.	(g) Carb.	(g) Fiber	(g) Sug.	(g) Prot.	(mg) Sod.
Pillsbury, Cinnamon Rolls, with Icing, Refrigerated Dough									
1 serving (44g)	145	5	1	0	23	0.5	10	2	340
Pillsbury, Crusty French Loaf, Refrigerated Dough									
1 serving (62g)	149	2	1	0	29	1.1	2	5	358
Pillsbury, Traditional Fudge Brownie Mix, Dry									
1 serving (30g)	132	4	1	0	23	0	15	1	88
Puff Pastry, Frozen, Ready-to-bake, Baked									
1 sheet (245g)	1367	94	13	0	112	3.7	2	18	620
Lard									
1 cup (205g)	1849	205	80	195	0	0	0	0	0
Shortening Cake Mix, Soybean (Hydrogenated) and Cottonseed (Hydrogenated)									
1 cup (205g)	1812	205	56	0	0	0	0	0	0
Shortening Confectionery, Coconut (Hydrogenated) and/or Palm Kernel (Hydrogenated)									
1 cup (205g)	1812	205	187	0	0	0	0	0	0
Shortening Frying (Heavy Duty) Beef Tallow and Cottonseed									
1 cup (205g)	1845	205	92	205	0	0	0	0	0
Shortening Frying (Heavy Duty),.Palm (Hydrogenated)									
1 cup (205g)	1812	205	97	0	0	0	0	0	0
Shortening Frying Heavy Duty, Soybean Hydrogenated, Linoleic (Less than 1%)									
1 cup (205g)	1812	205	43	0	0	0	0	0	0
Shortening Household Soybean (Hydrogenated) and Palm									
1 cup (205g)	1812	205	62	0	0	0	0	0	0
Shortening Industrial, Lard and Vegetable Oil									
1 cup (205g)	1845	205	83	115	0	0	0	0	0
Shortening Industrial, Soy (Part Hydrogenated), for baking and confections									
1 cup (205g)	1812	205	39	0	0	0	0	0	.0
Shortening Industrial, Soybean (Hydrogenated) and Corn for frying									
1 cup (205g)	1812	205	36	0	0	0	0	0	0
Shortening, Confectionery, Fractionated Palm									
1 cup (218g)	1927	218	143	0	0	0	0	0	0
Shortening, Household, Lard and Vegetable Oil									
1 cup (205g)	1845	205	83	115	0	0	0	0	0
Shortening, Household, Partially Hydrogenated Soybean and Cottonseed									
1 cup (205g)	1812	205	51	0	0	0	0	0	0

Food Serving size	Cal.	(g) Total Fat	(g) Sat. Fat	(mg) Chol.	(g) Carb.	(g) Fiber	(g) Sug.	(g) Prot.	(mg) Sod.
Shortening, Special Purpose for Baking, Soybean (Hydrogenated) Palm and Cottonseed									
1 cup (205g)	1812	205	59	0	0	0	0	0	0
Shortening, Special Purpose for Cakes and Frostings, Soybean (Hydrogenated)									
1 cup (205g)	1812	205	41	0	0	0	0	0	0
Shortening, Vegetable, Household									
1 cup (205g)	1812	205	51	0	0	0	0	0	8
Strudel, Apple									
1 piece (71g)	195	8	1	4	29	1.6	18	2	111
Sweet Rolls, Cheese									
1 roll (66g)	238	12	4	50	29	0.8	0	5	236
Sweet Rolls, Cinnamon, Commercially Prepared with Raisins									
1 large (83g)	309	14	3	55	42	2	26	5	252
Sweet Rolls, Cinnamon, Refrigerated Dough with Frosting									
1 roll (30g)	100	4	1	0	15	0	0	2	230
Sweet Rolls, Cinnamon, Refrigerated Dough with Frosting, Baked									
1 roll (30g)	109	4	1	0	17	0	0	2	250
Taco Shells, Baked									
1 large (6-1/2″ dia) (21g)	98	4	1	0	13	1	0	1	82
Taco Shells, Baked, Without Salt									
1 medium (approx 5″ dia) (13g)	61	3	0	0	8	1	0	1	2
Toaster Pastries, Brown Sugar Cinnamon									
1 toaster pastry (50g)	206	7	2	0	34	0.5	0	3	212
Toaster Pastries, Fruit									
1 toaster pastry (54g)	211	6	1	0	37	0.6	15	3	180
Toaster Pastries, Fruit, Frosted									
1 oz (28.35g)	111	3	1	0	20	0.2	10	1	88
Toaster Pastries, Fruit, Toasted (Apple, Blueberry, Cherry, Strawberry)									
1 pastry (51g)	209	6	1	0	37	0.5	15	2	181
Toaster Pastries, Kellogg's Pop Tarts, Apple Cinnamon									
1 pastry (52g)	205	5	1	0	37	0.6	18	2	174
Toaster Pastries, Kellogg's Pop Tarts, Blueberry									
1 pastry (52g)	212	7	1	0	36	0.6	16	2	182
Toaster Pastries, Kellogg's Pop Tarts, Brown Sugar Cinnamon									
1 pastry (50g)	219	9	1	0	32	0.8	13	3	190

Food Serving size	Cal.	(g) Total Fat	(g) Sat. Fat	(mg) Chol.	(g) Carb.	(g) Fiber	(g) Sug.	(g) Prot.	(mg) Sod.
Toaster Pastries, Kellogg's Pop Tarts, Cherry									
1 pastry (52g)	204	5	1	0	37	0.6	16	2	220
Toaster Pastries, Kellogg's Pop Tarts, Frosted Blueberry									
1 pastry (52g)	203	5	1	0	37	0.6	16	2	166
Toaster Pastries, Kellogg's Pop Tarts, Frosted Brown Sugar Cinnamon									
1 pastry (50g)	211	7	1	0	34	0.7	15	3	175
Toaster Pastries, Kellogg's Pop Tarts, Frosted Cherry									
1 pastry (52g)	204	5	1	0	37	0.5	19	2	166
Toaster Pastries, Kellogg's Pop Tarts, Frosted Chocolate Fudge									
1 pastry (52g)	201	5	1	0	37	0.6	20	3	229
Toaster Pastries, Kellogg's Pop Tarts, Frosted Chocolate Vanilla Cream									
1 pastry (52g)	203	5	1	0	37	0.5	19	3	229
Toaster Pastries, Kellogg's Pop Tarts, Frosted Grape									
1 pastry (52g)	203	5	1	0	38	0.5	18	2	173
Toaster Pastries, Kellogg's Pop Tarts, Frosted Raspberry									
1 pastry (52g)	205	6	1	0	37	0.5	18	2	166
Toaster Pastries, Kellogg's Pop Tarts, Frosted Strawberry									
1 pastry (52g)	203	5	1	0	38	0.5	20	2	169
Toaster Pastries, Kellogg's Pop Tarts, Frosted Wild Berry									
1 pastry (54g)	210	5	1	0	39	0.5	21	2	168
Toaster Pastries, Kellogg's Pop Tarts, S'mores									
1 pastry (52g)	204	5	1	0	36	0.7	19	3	213
Toaster Pastries, Kellogg's Pop Tarts, Strawberry									
1 pastry (52g)	205	5	2	0	37	0.6	17	2	185

Vegetables

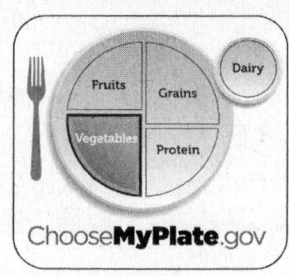

ChooseMyPlate.gov

Why Eat Vegetables?

Eating a diet rich in vegetables and fruits as part of an overall healthy diet may reduce the risk of heart disease, including heart attack, stroke, and type 2 diabetes. Most vegetables are naturally low in fat and calories, and none have cholesterol, although added sauces or seasonings may add fat, calories, or cholesterol. Vegetables are important sources of many nutrients, including potassium, dietary fiber, folate (folic acid), vitamin A, and vitamin C. Diets rich in potassium may help to maintain healthy blood pressure. Vitamin A keeps eyes and skin healthy and helps to protect against infections. Vitamin C helps heal cuts and wounds, keeps teeth and gums healthy, and aids in iron absorption. Vegetables fall into two categories; starchy and non-starchy. Starchy vegetables include white potatoes, sweet potatoes, yams, beets, parsnip, winter squash, peas, and beans. Starchy vegetables are nutritious and healthy when portion controlled. Non-starchy vegetables are high in nutrients (vitamins, minerals, and antioxidants) including fiber and low in carbohydrates and calories when compared to starchy vegetables. So, for the same calories you can eat much larger quantities of non-starchy vegetables. A list of common non-starchy vegetables include broccoli, spinach, cauliflower, cabbage, brussels sprouts, asparagus, eggplant, cucumber, leafy greens, mushrooms, snow peas, sugar snap peas, peppers, zucchini, onions, and herbs. Aim for 3–5 servings of non-starchy vegetables each day. Use starchy vegetables in place of highly processed carbohydrate food choices.

Daily Goal

2½ cups or more (cup equivalents) for an adult on a 2,000-calorie diet
One-cup equivalents:

1 cup cooked vegetable	1 three-inch tomato
2 cups raw vegetables	1 cup cooked dry peas or beans
2 medium carrots	1 cup starchy vegetable

Shopping Tips

- Choose vegetables rich in color—red, orange, or dark green.
- Buy fresh vegetables in season.
- Purchase locally grown vegetables when possible.
- Stock up on frozen or salt-free canned vegetables for fast preparation.
- Remember that over a quarter of your plate should be vegetables.

Shopping List Essentials

Tomatoes	Broccoli	Leafy Greens (Spinach,	Squash
Peppers	Cauliflower	Kale, Collard Greens)	Mushrooms
Carrots	Green beans	Sweet potatoes/yams	

Red Flags

Canned vegetables that are not salt-free can be high in sodium. Canned vegetables including canned beans should be rinsed before using. Frozen vegetables may have more intact nutrients than canned because they have been minimally processed. But be wary of frozen vegetables that contain sauces. Sauces add calories, fat, and salt; therefore, choose those without sauces and seasonings.

Preparation Pointer

Boost the nutrients and the flavor of fresh or frozen non-starchy vegetables. After steaming in the microwave or on the stove top, add fresh lemon juice to broccoli, spinach, or asparagus. Also add flavor to non-starchy vegetables with garlic, onion, or shallots, and fresh or dried herbs like thyme, parsley, oregano, and basil.

Food Serving size	Cal.	(g) Total Fat	(g) Sat. Fat	(mg) Chol.	(g) Carb.	(g) Fiber	(g) Sug.	(g) Prot.	(mg) Sod.
Vegetables									
Artichokes (Globe or French), Cooked, Boiled, Drained, with Salt									
.5 cup, hearts (84g)	45	0	0	0	10	7.2	1	2	50
Artichokes (Globe or French), Cooked, Boiled, Drained, Without Salt									
.5 cup, hearts (84g)	45	0	0	0	10	7.2	1	2	50
Artichokes (Globe or French), Frozen, Cooked, Boiled, Drained, with Salt									
1 package (9 oz) yields (240g)	108	1	0	0	22	11	2	7	694
Artichokes (Globe or French), Frozen, Cooked, Boiled, Drained, Without Salt									
1 package (9 oz) yields (240g)	108	1	0	0	22	11	2	7	127
Artichokes (Globe or French), Frozen, Unprepared									
1 package (9 oz) (255g)	97	1	0	0	20	9.9	0	7	120
Asparagus, Canned, Drained, Solids									
1 spear (about 5″ long) (18g)	3	0	0	0	0	0.3	0	0	52
Asparagus, Canned, No Salt, Solids and Liquids									
1 can (300 x 407) (411g)	62	1	0	0	10	4.1	4	7	107
Asparagus, Canned, Regular Package, Solids and Liquids									
1 can (300 x 407) (411g)	62	1	0	0	10	4.1	0	7	1167
Asparagus, Cooked, Boiled, Drained									
4 spears (1/2″ base) (60g)	13	0	0	0	2	1.2	1	1	8
Asparagus, Cooked, Boiled, Drained, with Salt									
4 spears (1/2″ base) (60g)	13	0	0	0	2	1.2	1	1	144
Asparagus, Frozen, Cooked, Boiled, Drained, with Salt									
1 package (10 oz) yields (293g)	53	1	0	0	6	4.7	1	9	703
Asparagus, Frozen, Cooked, Boiled, Drained, Without Salt									
1 package (10 oz) yields (293g)	53	1	0	0	6	4.7	1	9	9
Asparagus, Frozen, Unprepared									
1 package (10 oz) (284g)	68	1	0	0	12	5.4	0	9	23
Basil, Fresh									
2 tbsp, chopped (5.3g)	1	0	0	0	0	0.1	0	0	0
Broccoli, Cooked, Boiled, Drained, with Salt									
1 stalk, medium (7-1/2″ - 8″ long) (180g)	63	1	0	0	13	5.9	3	4	472
Broccoli, Cooked, Boiled, Drained, Without Salt									
1 stalk, medium (7-1/2″ - 8″ long) (180g)	63	1	0	0	13	5.9	3	4	74

Food Serving size	Cal.	(g) Total Fat	(g) Sat. Fat	(mg) Chol.	(g) Carb.	(g) Fiber	(g) Sug.	(g) Prot.	(mg) Sod.
Broccoli, Flower Clusters, Raw 1 floweret (11g)	3	0	0	0	1	0	0	0	3
Ginger Root, Raw .25 cup, slices (1″ dia) (24g)	19	0	0	0	4	0.5	0	0	3
Lemon Grass (Citronella), Raw 1 tbsp (4.8g)	5	0	0	0	1	0	0	0	0
Lentils, Mature Seeds, Cooked, Boiled, Without Salt 1 tbsp (12.3g)	14	0	0	0	2	1	0	1	0
Lentils, Pink, Raw 1 cup (192g)	662	4	1	0	114	20.7	0	48	13
Lettuce, Butterhead (Including Boston and Bibb Types), Raw 1 head (5″ dia) (163g)	21	0	0	0	4	1.8	2	2	8
Lettuce, Cos and Romaine, Raw 1 leaf, inner (6g)	1	0	0	0	0	0.1	0	0	0
Lettuce, Green Leaf, Raw 1 head (360g)	54	1	0	0	10	4.7	3	5	101
Lettuce, Red Leaf, Raw 1 leaf, inner (2.6g)	0	0	0	0	0	0	0	0	1
Lima Beans, Immature Seeds, Cooked, Boiled, Drained, with Salt 1 cup (170g)	209	1	0	0	40	9	3	12	430
Lima Beans, Immature Seeds, Frozen, Baby, Cooked, Boiled, Drained, with Salt 1 package (10 oz) yields (311g)	327	1	0	0	60	18.7	4	21	824
Lima Beans, Immature Seeds, Frozen, Fordhook, Cooked, Boiled, Drained, with Salt 1 package (10 oz) yields (311g)	320	1	0	0	60	18	4	19	899
Lima Beans, Large, Mature Seeds, Canned 1 cup (241g)	190	0	0	0	36	11.6	0	12	810
Lima Beans, Large, Mature Seeds, Cooked, Boiled, with Salt 1 cup (188g)	216	1	0	0	39	13.2	5	15	447
Lima Beans, Large, Mature Seeds, Cooked, Boiled, Without Salt 1 tbsp (11.7g)	13	0	0	0	2	0.8	0	1	0
Lima Beans, Thin Seeded (Baby), Mature Seeds, Cooked, Boiled, with Salt 1 cup (182g)	229	1	0	0	42	14	0	15	435

Food Serving size	Cal.	(g) Total Fat	(g) Sat. Fat	(mg) Chol.	(g) Carb.	(g) Fiber	(g) Sug.	(g) Prot.	(mg) Sod.
Lima Beans, Thin Seeded (Baby), Mature Seeds, Cooked, Boiled, Without Salt									
1 cup (182g)	229	1	0	0	42	14	0	15	5
Lotus Root, Cooked, Boiled, Drained, with Salt									
10 slices (2-1/2″ dia) (89g)	59	0	0	0	14	2.8	0	1	250
Lotus Root, Cooked, Boiled, Drained, Without Salt									
10 slices (2-1/2″ dia) (89g)	59	0	0	0	14	2.8	0	1	40
Malabar Spinach, Cooked									
1 bunch (17g)	4	0	0	0	0	0.4	0	1	9
Mountain Yam, Hawaii, Cooked, Steamed, with Salt									
1 cup, cubes (145g)	119	0	0	0	29	0	0	3	360
Mountain Yam, Hawaii, Cooked, Steamed, Without Salt									
1 cup, cubes (145g)	119	0	0	0	29	0	0	3	17
Mountain Yam, Hawaii, Raw									
1 yam (420g)	281	0	0	0	69	0	0	6	55
Mushrooms, Brown, Italian or Crimini, Raw									
1 cup, sliced (72g)	16	0	0	0	3	0.4	1	2	4
Mushrooms, Canned, Drained, Solid									
1 can (132g)	33	0	0	0	7	3.2	3	2	561
Mushrooms, Chanterelle, Raw									
1 piece (5.4g)	2	0	0	0	0	0.2	0	0	0
Mushrooms, Enoki, Raw									
1 medium (3g)	1	0	0	0	0	0.1	0	0	0
Mushrooms, Morel, Raw									
1 piece (12.9g)	4	0	0	0	1	0.4	0	0	3
Mushrooms, Oyster, Raw									
1 small (15g)	5	0	0	0	1	0.3	0	0	3
Mushrooms, Portobello, Exposed to Ultra-violet Light, Grilled									
1 cup, sliced (121g)	35	1	0	0	5	2.7	3	4	13
Mushrooms, Portobello, Exposed to Ultra-violet Light, Raw									
1 piece, whole (84g)	18	0	0	0	3	1.1	2	2	8
Mushrooms, Portobello, Grilled									
1 cup, sliced (121g)	35	1	0	0	5	2.7	3	4	13
Mushrooms, Portobello, Raw									
1 piece, whole (84g)	18	0	0	0	3	1.1	2	2	8

Food Serving size	Cal.	(g) Total Fat	(g) Sat. Fat	(mg) Chol.	(g) Carb.	(g) Fiber	(g) Sug.	(g) Prot.	(mg) Sod.
Mushrooms, Shiitake, Cooked, with Salt 4 mushrooms (72g)	40	0	0	0	10	1.5	3	1	173
Mushrooms, Shiitake, Cooked, Without Salt 4 mushrooms (72g)	40	0	0	0	10	1.5	3	1	3
Mushrooms, Shiitake, Dried 4 mushrooms (15g)	44	0	0	0	11	1.7	0	1	2
Mushrooms, Shiitake, Stir-fried 1 cup, sliced (97g)	38	0	0	0	7	3.5	0	3	5
Mushrooms, Straw, Canned, Drained, Solid 1 piece (5.5g)	2	0	0	0	0	0.1	0	0	21
Mushrooms, White, Cooked, Boiled, Drained, with Salt 1 tbsp (9.8g)	3	0	0	0	1	0.2	0	0	23
Mushrooms, White, Cooked, Boiled, Drained, Without Salt 1 tbsp (9.8g)	3	0	0	0	1	0.2	0	0	0
Mushrooms, White, Stir-fried 1 cup, sliced (108g)	28	0	0	0	4	1.9	0	4	13
Mussel, Blue, Cooked, Moist Heat 3 oz (85g)	146	4	1	48	6	0	0	20	314
Mustard Greens, Cooked, Boiled, Drained, with Salt 1 cup, chopped (140g)	21	0	0	0	3	2.8	0	3	353
Mustard Greens, Cooked, Boiled, Drained, Without Salt 1 cup, chopped (140g)	36	1	0	0	6	2.8	2	4	13
New Zealand Spinach, Cooked, Boiled, Drained, with Salt 1 cup, chopped (180g)	22	0	0	0	4	0	0	2	617
New Zealand Spinach, Cooked, Boiled, Drained, Without Salt 1 cup, chopped (180g)	22	0	0	0	4	0	0	2	193
Okra, Cooked, Boiled, Drained, with Salt 8 pods (3″ long) (85g)	19	0	0	0	4	2.1	2	2	205
Okra, Cooked, Boiled, Drained, Without Salt 8 pods (3″ long) (85g)	19	0	0	0	4	2.1	2	2	5
Okra, Frozen, Cooked, Boiled, Drained, with Salt .5 cup, slices (92g)	31	0	0	0	6	1.9	3	1	220
Okra, Frozen, Cooked, Boiled, Drained, Without Salt 1 package (10 oz) yields (255g)	74	1	0	0	16	5.4	7	4	8

Food Serving size	Cal.	(g) Total Fat	(g) Sat. Fat	(mg) Chól.	(g) Carb.	(g) Fiber	(g) Sug.	(g) Prot.	(mg) Sod.
Okra, Frozen, Unprepared 1 package (10 oz) (284g)	85	1	0	0	19	6.2	8	5	9
Onions, Raw 1 cup, sliced (115g)	46	0	0	0	11	2	5	1	5
Onions, Spring or Scallions (Including Tops and Bulb), Raw 1 tbsp, chopped (6g)	2	0	0	0	0	0.2	0	0	1
Onions, Sweet, Raw 1 onion (331g)	106	0	0	0	25	3	17	3	26
Onions, Young Green, Tops Only 1 stalk (12g)	3	0	0	0	1	0.2	1	0	2
Parsley, Raw 1 tbsp (3.8g)	1	0	0	0	0	0.1	0	0	2
Parsnips, Cooked, Boiled, Drained, with Salt 1 parsnip (9″ long) (160g)	114	0	0	0	27	6.4	8	2	394
Parsnips, Cooked, Boiled, Drained, Without Salt 1 parsnip (9″ long) (160g)	114	0	0	0	27	5.8	8	2	16
Peas and Carrots, Frozen, Cooked, Boiled, Drained, without Salt .5 cup (80g)	38	0	0	0	8	2.5	3	2	54
Peas, Edible-podded, Frozen, Unprepared 1 package (10 oz) (284g)	119	1	0	0	20	8.8	0	8	11
Peas, Edible-podded, Raw 1 cup, whole (63g)	26	0	0	0	5	1.6	3	2	3
Peas, Green, Frozen, Unprepared 1 package (284g)	219	1	0	0	39	12.8	14	15	307
Peas, Mature Seeds, Sprouted, Raw 1 cup (120g)	149	1	0	0	33	0	0	11	24
Peppers, Jalapeno, Raw 1 pepper (14g)	4	0	0	0	1	0.4	1	0	0
Peppers, Sweet, Green, Raw 1 cup, sliced (92g)	18	0	0	0	4	1.6	2	1	3
Peppers, Sweet, Yellow, Raw 10 strips (52g)	14	0	0	0	3	0.5	0	1	1
Poi 1 cup (240g)	269	0	0	0	65	1	1	1	29

Food Serving size	Cal.	(g) Total Fat	(g) Sat. Fat	(mg) Chol.	(g) Carb.	(g) Fiber	(g) Sug.	(g) Prot.	(mg) Sod.
Pumpkin, Raw 1 cup (1″ cubes) (116g)	30	0	0	0	8	0.6	2	1	1
Purslane, Cooked, Boiled, Drained, Without Salt 1 squash (431g)	78	1	0	0	15	0	0	6	190
Purslane, Raw 1 plant (3g)	0	0	0	0	0	0	0	0	1
Quinoa, Cooked 1 cup (185g)	222	4	0	0	39	5.2	0	8	13
Quinoa, Uncooked 1 cup (170g)	626	10	1	0	109	11.9	0	24	9
Radicchio, Raw 1 leaf (8g)	2	0	0	0	0	0.1	0	0	2
Radishes, Hawaiian Style, Pickled 1 cup (150g)	42	0	0	0	8	3.3	0	2	1184
Radishes, Oriental, Cooked, Boiled, Drained, with Salt 1 cup, slices (147g)	25	0	0	0	5	2.4	3	1	366
Radishes, Oriental, Cooked, Boiled, Drained, Without Salt 1 cup, sliced (147g)	25	0	0	0	5	2.4	3	1	19
Radishes, Oriental, Dried 1 cup (116g)	314	1	0	0	74	0	0	9	322
Refried Beans, Canned, Fat Free 1 can (445g)	352	2	0	0	60	20.9	3	24	1949
Refried Beans, Canned, Traditional Style 1 can (443g)	403	5	2	0	68	22.6	2	24	1989
Refried Beans, Canned, Vegetarian 1 can (444g)	369	4	1	0	60	20.9	3	23	1909
Rhubarb, Frozen, Cooked, with Sugar 1 cup (240g)	278	0	0	0	75	4.8	69	1	2
Rhubarb, Frozen, Uncooked 1 cup, diced (137g)	29	0	0	0	7	2.5	2	1	3
Rhubarb, Raw 1 stalk (51g)	11	0	0	0	2	0.9	1	0	2
Roughy, Orange, Cooked, Dry Heat 3 oz (85g)	89	1	0	68	0	0	0	19	59

Food Serving size	Cal.	(g) Total Fat	(g) Sat. Fat	(mg) Chol.	(g) Carb.	(g) Fiber	(g) Sug.	(g) Prot.	(mg) Sod.
Rutabagas, Cooked, Boiled, Drained, Without Salt									
1 cup, mashed (240g)	72	0	0	0	16	4.3	9	2	12
Salsify (Vegetable Oyster), Raw									
1 cup, slices (133g)	109	0	0	0	25	4.4	0	4	27
Salsify, Cooked, Boiled, Drained, with Salt									
1 cup, slices (135g)	92	0	0	0	21	4.2	4	4	340
Salsify, Cooked, Boiled, Drained, Without Salt									
1 cup, sliced (135g)	92	0	0	0	21	4.2	4	4	22
Shallots, Freeze-dried									
.25 cup (3.6g)	13	0	0	0	3	0	0	0	2
Spinach, Canned, No Salt, Solids and Liquids									
1 cup (234g)	44	1	0	0	7	5.1	0	5	176
Spinach, Canned, Regular Pack, Drained, Solid									
1 cup (214g)	49	1	0	0	7	5.1	1	6	689
Spinach, Canned, Regular Pack, Solids and Liquids									
1 cup (234g)	44	1	0	0	7	3.7	0	5	746
Spinach, Cooked, Boiled, Drained, with Salt									
1 cup (180g)	41	0	0	0	7	4.3	1	5	551
Spinach, Cooked, Boiled, Drained, Without Salt									
1 cup (180g)	41	0	0	0	7	4.3	1	5	126
Spinach, Frozen, Chopped or Leaf, Cooked, Boiled, Drained, with Salt									
.5 cup (95g)	32	1	0	0	5	3.5	0	4	306
Spinach, Frozen, Chopped or Leaf, Cooked, Boiled, Drained, Without Salt									
.5 cup (95g)	32	1	0	0	5	3.5	0	4	92
Spinach, Frozen, Chopped or Leaf, Unprepared									
1 package (10 oz) (284g)	82	2	0	0	12	8.2	2	10	210
Succotash (Corn and Limas), Canned, with Cream Style Corn									
1 cup (266g)	205	1	0	0	47	8	0	7	652
Succotash (Corn and Limas), Canned, with Whole Kernel Corn, Solids and Liquids									
1 cup (255g)	161	1	0	0	36	6.6	0	7	564
Succotash (Corn and Limas), Cooked, Boiled, Drained, with Salt									
1 cup (192g)	213	2	0	0	47	0	0	10	486
Succotash (Corn and Limas), Cooked, Boiled, Drained, Without Salt									
1 cup (192g)	221	2	0	0	47	8.6	0	10	33

Food Serving size	Cal.	(g) Total Fat	(g) Sat. Fat	(mg) Chol.	(g) Carb.	(g) Fiber	(g) Sug.	(g) Prot.	(mg) Sod.
Succotash (Corn and Limas), Frozen, Cooked, Boiled, Drained, with Salt									
1 cup (170g)	158	2	0	0	34	7	4	7	478
Succotash (Corn and Limas), Frozen, Cooked, Boiled, Drained, Without Salt									
1 cup (170g)	158	2	0	0	34	7	4	7	77
Succotash (Corn and Limas), Frozen, Unprepared									
1 package (10 oz) (284g)	264	3	0	0	57	11.4	0	12	128
Tapioca, Pearl, Dry									
1 cup (152g)	544	0	0	0	135	1.4	5	0	2
Taro Leaves, Cooked, Steamed, Without Salt									
1 cup (145g)	35	1	0	0	6	2.9	0	4	3
Taro Shoots, Cooked, Without Salt									
1 cup, slices (140g)	20	0	0	0	4	0	0	1	3
Taro, Cooked, with Salt									
1 cup, slices (132g)	187	0	0	0	46	6.7	1	1	331
Taro, Cooked, Without Salt									
1 cup, sliced (132g)	187	0	0	0	46	6.7	1	1	20
Taro, Leaves, Cooked, Steamed, with Salt									
1 cup (145g)	35	1	0	0	6	2.9	0	4	345
Taro, Shoots, Cooked, with Salt									
1 cup, slices (140g)	20	0	0	0	4	0	0	1	333
Taro, Tahitian, Cooked, with Salt									
1 cup, slices (137g)	60	1	0	0	9	0	0	6	397
Taro, Tahitian, Cooked, Without Salt									
1 cup, slices (137g)	60	1	0	0	9	0	0	6	74
Taro, Tahitian, Raw									
1 cup, slices (125g)	55	1	0	0	9	0	0	3	63
Tomatoes, Green, Raw									
1 large (182g)	42	0	0	0	9	2	7	2	24
Tomatoes, Red, Ripe, Cooked									
2 medium (246g)	44	0	0	0	10	1.7	6	2	27
Tomatoes, Red, Ripe, Cooked, Stewed									
1 recipe, yields (604g)	477	16	3	0	79	10.3	0	12	2748
Tomatoes, Red, Ripe, Cooked, with Salt									
.5 cup (120g)	22	0	0	0	5	0.8	3	1	296

Food Serving size	Cal.	(g) Total Fat	(g) Sat. Fat	(mg) Chol.	(g) Carb.	(g) Fiber	(g) Sug.	(g) Prot.	(mg) Sod.
Tomatoes, Red, Ripe, Raw, Year Round Average									
1 cup, chopped or sliced (180g)	32	0	0	0	7	2.2	5	2	9
Tomatoes, Sun-dried									
1 piece (2g)	5	0	0	0	1	0.2	1	0	42
Tomatoes, Sun-dried, Packed in Oil, Drained									
1 piece (3g)	6	0	0	0	1	0.2	0	0	8
Turnip Greens and Turnips, Frozen, Cooked, Boiled, Drained, with Salt									
.5 cup (86g)	29	0	0	0	4	2.7	1	3	219
Turnip Greens and Turnips, Frozen, Cooked, Boiled, Drained, Without Salt									
1 cup (163g)	57	1	0	0	8	5.1	2	5	31
Turnip Greens and Turnips, Frozen, Unprepared									
1 package (3 lb) (1361g)	286	3	0	0	46	32.7	0	33	245
Turnip Greens, Canned, No Salt									
1 cup (144g)	27	0	0	0	4	1.9	1	2	42
Turnip Greens, Canned, Solids and Liquids									
1 can, 15 oz (303 x 406) (425g)	60	1	0	0	10	7.2	0	6	1177
Turnip Greens, Cooked, Boiled, Drained, with Salt									
1 cup, chopped (144g)	29	0	0	0	6	5	1	2	382
Turnip Greens, Cooked, Boiled, Drained, Without Salt									
1 cup, chopped (144g)	29	0	0	0	6	5	1	2	42
Turnip Greens, Frozen, Cooked, Boiled, Drained, with Salt									
.5 cup (82g)	24	0	0	0	4	2.8	1	3	206
Turnip Greens, Frozen, Cooked, Boiled, Drained, Without Salt									
1 package (10 oz) yields (220g)	64	1	0	0	11	7.5	2	7	33
Turnip Greens, Frozen, Unprepared									
1 package (10 oz) (284g)	62	1	0	0	10	7.1	0	7	34
Turnips, Cooked, Boiled, Drained, with Salt									
1 cup, mashed (230g)	51	0	0	0	12	4.6	7	2	658
Turnips, Cooked, Boiled, Drained, Without Salt									
1 cup, mashed (230g)	51	0	0	0	12	4.6	7	2	37
Turnips, Frozen, Cooked, Boiled, Drained, without Salt									
1 cup (156g)	36	0	0	0	7	3.1	4	2	56
Turnips, Frozen, Unprepared									
1 package, mashed (10oz) (284g)	45	0	0	0	8	5.1	0	3	71

Food Serving size	Cal.	(g) Total Fat	(g) Sat. Fat	(mg) Chol.	(g) Carb.	(g) Fiber	(g) Sug.	(g) Prot.	(mg) Sod.
Water Chestnuts, Chinese (Matai), Raw									
4 water chestnuts (36g)	35	0	0	0	9	1.1	2	1	5
Water Chestnuts, Chinese, Canned, Solids and Liquids									
4 water chestnuts (28g)	14	0	0	0	3	0.7	1	0	2
Waxgourd (Chinese Preserving Melon), Cooked, Boiled, Drained, with Salt									
1 cup, cubes (175g)	19	0	0	0	4	1.8	2	1	600
Waxgourd (Chinese Preserving Melon), Cooked, Boiled, Drained, Without Salt									
1 cup, cubes (175g)	25	0	0	0	5	1.8	2	1	187
Waxgourd (Chinese Preserving Melon), Raw									
1 waxgourd (5700g)	741	11	1	0	171	165.3	0	23	6327
Yam, Cooked, Boiled, Drained, or Baked, Without Salt									
.5 cup, cubes (68g)	79	0	0	0	19	2.7	0	1	5
Yam, Cooked, Boiled, Drained, or Baked, with Salt									
.5 cup, cubes (68g)	78	0	0	0	18	2.7	0	1	166
Yardlong Bean, Cooked, Boiled, Drained, with Salt									
1 pod (14g)	7	0	0	0	1	0	0	0	34
Yardlong Bean, Cooked, Boiled, Drained, Without Salt									
1 pod (14g)	7	0	0	0	1	0	0	0	1
Yardlong Beans, Mature Seeds, Cooked, Boiled, with Salt									
1 cup (171g)	202	1	0	0	36	6.5	0	14	412
Yardlong Beans, Mature Seeds, Cooked, Boiled, Without Salt									
1 cup (171g)	202	1	0	0	36	6.5	0	14	9

Potatoes

Food Serving size	Cal.	Total Fat	Sat. Fat	Chol.	Carb.	Fiber	Sug.	Prot.	Sod.
Potato, Baked, Flesh and Skin, Without Salt									
1 potato, medium (173g)	161	0	0	0	37	3.8	2	4	17
Potato, Flesh and Skin, Raw									
1 potato, medium (2-1/4" to 3-1/4" dia) (213g)	164	0	0	0	37	4.7	2	4	13
Potatoes, Baked, Flesh, Without Salt									
1 potato (2-1/3" x 4-3/4") (156g)	145	0	0	0	34	2.3	3	3	8
Potatoes, Baked, Skin, with Salt									
1 skin (58g)	115	0	0	0	27	4.6	1	2	149

Food Serving size	Cal.	(g) Total Fat	(g) Sat. Fat	(mg) Chol.	(g) Carb.	(g) Fiber	(g) Sug.	(g) Prot.	(mg) Sod.
Potatoes, Baked, Skin, Without Salt									
1 skin (58g)	115	0	0	0	27	4.6	1	2	12
Potatoes, Boiled, Cooked in Skin, Flesh, with Salt									
1 potato (2-1/2″ dia, sphere) (136g)	118	0	0	0	27	2.7	1	3	326
Potatoes, Boiled, Cooked in Skin, Flesh, Without Salt									
1 potato (2-1/2″ dia, sphere) (136g)	118	0	0	0	27	2.4	1	3	5
Potatoes, Boiled, Cooked in Skin, with Salt									
1 skin (34g)	27	0	0	0	6	1.1	0	1	85
Potatoes, Boiled, Cooked in Skin, Without Salt									
1 skin (34g)	27	0	0	0	6	1.1	0	1	5
Potatoes, Boiled, Cooked Without Skin, Flesh, with Salt									
1 medium (2-1/4″ to 2-1/4″ dia.) (167g)	144	0	0	0	33	3.3	1	3	402
Potatoes, Boiled, Cooked Without Skin, Flesh, Without Salt									
1 medium (2-1/4″ to 3-1/4″ dia.) (167g)	144	0	0	0	33	3	1	3	8
Potatoes, Canned, Drained Solid									
1 potato (35g)	21	0	0	0	5	0.8	0	0	77
Potatoes, Canned, Drained Solid, No Salt									
1 cup (180g)	112	0	0	0	24	4.3	0	3	9
Potatoes, Canned, Solids and Liquids									
1 can (303 x 406) (454g)	200	0	0	0	45	6.4	0	5	985
Potatoes, Red, Flesh and Skin, Baked									
1 potato, medium (2-1/4″ to 3-1/4″ dia.) (173g)	154	0	0	0	34	3.1	2	4	21
Potatoes, Red, Flesh and Skin, Raw									
1 potato, medium (2-1/4″ to 3-1/4″ dia) (213g)	149	0	0	0	34	3.6	3	4	38
Potatoes, Russet, Flesh and Skin, Baked									
1 potato, medium (2-1/4″ to 3-1/4″ dia.) (173g)	168	0	0	0	37	4	2	5	24
Potatoes, Russet, Flesh and Skin, Raw									
1 potato, medium (2-1/4″ to 3-1/4″ dia) (213g)	168	0	0	0	38	2.8	1	5	11

Food Serving size	Cal.	(g) Total Fat	(g) Sat. Fat	(mg) Chol.	(g) Carb.	(g) Fiber	(g) Sug.	(g) Prot.	(mg) Sod.
Potatoes, White, Flesh and Skin, Baked 1 potato, medium (2-1/4″ to 3-1/4″ dia) (138g)	130	0	0	0	29	2.9	2	3	10
Potatoes, White, Flesh and Skin, Raw 1 potato, medium (2-1/4″ to 3-1/4″ dia) (213g)	147	0	0	0	33	5.1	2	4	34
Side Dishes, Potato Salad .333 cup (95g)	108	6	1	57	13	0	0	1	312
Sweet Potato Leaves, Cooked, Steamed, with Salt 1 cup (64g)	22	0	0	0	5	1.2	3	1	159
Sweet Potato Leaves, Cooked, Steamed, Without Salt 1 cup (64g)	22	0	0	0	5	1.2	3	1	8
Sweet Potato, Canned, Mashed 1 can (404 x 307) (496g)	501	1	0	0	115	8.4	27	10	372
Sweet Potato, Canned, Syrup packed, Drained, Solids 1 cup (196g)	212	1	0	0	50	5.9	11	3	76
Sweet Potato, Canned, Syrup Packed, Solids and Liquids 1 can (404 x 307) (638g)	568	1	0	0	134	16	98	6	281
Sweet Potato, Canned, Vacuum Pack 1 cup, pieces (200g)	182	0	0	0	42	3.6	10	3	106
Sweet Potato, Cooked, Baked in Skin, with Salt .5 cup, mashed (100g)	92	0	0	0	21	3.3	11	2	246
Sweet Potato, Cooked, Baked in Skin, Without Salt 1 large (180g)	162	0	0	0	37	5.9	12	4	65
Sweet Potato, Cooked, Boiled, Without Skin 1 medium (151g)	115	0	0	0	27	3.8	9	2	41
Sweet Potato, Cooked, Boiled, Without Skin, with Salt 1 medium (151g)	115	0	0	0	27	3.8	9	2	397
Sweet Potato, Cooked, Candied, Home-prepared 1 piece (2-1/2″ x 2″ dia) (105g)	151	3	1	8	29	2.5	0	1	74
Sweet Potato, Frozen, Cooked, Baked, with Salt 1 cup, cubes (176g)	176	0	0	0	41	3.2	0	3	429
Sweet Potato, Frozen, Cooked, Baked, Without Salt 1 cup, cubes (176g)	176	0	0	0	41	3.2	16	3	14

Food Serving size	Cal.	(g) Total Fat	(g) Sat. Fat	(mg) Chol.	(g) Carb.	(g) Fiber	(g) Sug.	(g) Prot.	(mg) Sod.
Sweet Potato, Frozen, Unprepared									
1 cup, cubes (176g)	169	0	0	0	39	3	0	3	11
Sweet Potato, Raw, Unprepared									
1 sweet potato, 5″ long (130g)	112	0	0	0	26	3.9	5	2	72

Vegetable Products

Food Serving size	Cal.	(g) Total Fat	(g) Sat. Fat	(mg) Chol.	(g) Carb.	(g) Fiber	(g) Sug.	(g) Prot.	(mg) Sod.
Alfalfa Seeds, Sprouted, Raw									
1 tbsp (3g)	1	0	0	0	0	0.1	0	0	0
Baked Beans, Canned, No Salt									
1 cup (253g)	266	1	0	0	52	13.9	0	12	3
Bamboo Shoots, Canned, Drained, Solids									
1 can (303 x 406) (262g)	50	1	0	0	8	3.7	5	5	18
Bamboo Shoots, Cooked, Boiled, Drained, with Salt									
1 shoot (144g)	16	0	0	0	2	1.4	0	2	346
Bamboo Shoots, Cooked, Boiled, Drained, Without Salt									
1 shoot (144g)	17	0	0	0	3	1.4	0	2	6
Beans, Adzuki, Mature Seeds, Canned, Sweetened									
1 cup (296g)	702	0	0	0	163	0	0	11	645
Beans, Adzuki, Mature Seeds, Cooked, Boiled, with Salt									
1 cup (230g)	294	0	0	0	57	16.8	0	17	561
Beans, Adzuki, Mature Seeds, Cooked, Boiled, Without Salt									
1 cup (230g)	294	0	0	0	57	16.8	0	17	18
Beans, Adzuki, Mature Seeds, Raw									
1 cup (197g)	648	1	0	0	124	25	0	39	10
Beans, Adzuki, Yokan, Mature Seeds									
1 slice (14g)	36	0	0	0	9	0	0	0	12
Beans, Baked, Canned, Plain or Vegetarian									
1 cup (254g)	239	1	0	0	54	10.4	20	12	871
Beans, Baked, Canned, with Beef									
1 cup (266g)	322	9	4	59	45	0	0	17	1264
Beans, Baked, Canned, with Franks									
1 cup (259g)	368	17	6	16	40	17.9	17	17	1114
Beans, Baked, Canned, with Pork									
1 cup (253g)	268	4	2	18	51	13.9	0	13	1047

Food Serving size	Cal.	(g) Total Fat	(g) Sat. Fat	(mg) Chol.	(g) Carb.	(g) Fiber	(g) Sug.	(g) Prot.	(mg) Sod.
Beans, Baked, Canned, with Pork and Sweet Sauce									
1 cup (253g)	283	4	1	18	53	10.6	22	13	845
Beans, Baked, Canned, with Pork and Tomato Sauce									
1 cup (246g)	231	2	1	17	46	9.8	14	13	1075
Beans, Baked, Home Prepared									
1 cup (253g)	392	13	5	13	55	13.9	0	14	1068
Beans, Black, Mature Seeds, Cooked, Boiled, with Salt									
1 cup (172g)	227	1	0	0	41	15	0	15	408
Beans, Black, Mature Seeds, Cooked, Boiled, Without Salt									
1 cup (172g)	227	1	0	0	41	15	0	15	2
Beans, Black, Turtle Soup, Mature Seeds, Canned									
1 cup (240g)	218	1	0	0	40	16.6	0	14	922
Beans, Black, Turtle Soup, Mature Seeds, Cooked, Boiled, with Salt									
1 cup (185g)	241	1	0	0	45	9.8	1	15	442
Beans, Black, Turtle Soup, Mature Seeds, Cooked, Boiled, Without Salt									
1 cup (185g)	241	1	0	0	45	9.8	1	15	6
Beans, Chili, Barbecue, Ranch Style, Cooked									
1 cup (253g)	245	3	0	0	43	10.6	0	13	1834
Beans, Cranberry (Roman), Mature Seeds, Canned									
1 cup (260g)	216	1	0	0	39	16.4	0	14	863
Beans, Cranberry (Roman), Mature Seeds, Cooked, Boiled, with Salt									
1 cup (177g)	241	1	0	0	43	17.7	0	17	419
Beans, Cranberry (Roman), Mature Seeds, Cooked, Boiled, Without Salt									
1 cup (177g)	241	1	0	0	43	17.7	0	17	2
Beans, Cranberry (Roman), Mature Seeds, Raw									
1 cup (195g)	653	2	1	0	117	48.2	0	45	12
Beans, French, Mature Seeds, Cooked, Boiled, with Salt									
1 cup (177g)	228	1	0	0	43	16.6	0	12	428
Beans, French, Mature Seeds, Cooked, Boiled, Without Salt									
1 cup (177g)	228	1	0	0	43	16.6	0	12	11
Beans, Great Northern, Mature Seeds, Canned									
1 cup (262g)	299	1	0	0	55	12.8	0	19	10
Beans, Great Northern, Mature Seeds, Cooked, Boiled, with Salt									
1 cup (177g)	209	1	0	0	37	12.4	0	15	421

Food Serving size	Cal.	(g) Total Fat	(g) Sat. Fat	(mg) Chol.	(g) Carb.	(g) Fiber	(g) Sug.	(g) Prot.	(mg) Sod.
Beans, Great Northern, Mature Seeds, Cooked, Boiled, Without Salt									
1 cup (177g)	209	1	0	0	37	12.4	0	15	4
Beans, Kidney, All Types, Mature Seeds, Canned									
1 cup (256g)	215	2	0	0	37	13.6	5	13	758
Beans, Kidney, All Types, Mature Seeds, Cooked, Boiled, with Salt									
1 cup (177g)	225	1	0	0	40	11.3	1	15	421
Beans, Kidney, All Types, Mature Seeds, Cooked, Boiled, Without Salt									
1 tbsp (11g)	14	0	0	0	3	0.7	0	1	0
Beans, Kidney, California Red, Mature Seeds, Cooked, Boiled, with Salt									
1 cup (177g)	219	0	0	0	40	16.5	0	16	425
Beans, Kidney, California Red, Mature Seeds, Cooked, Boiled, Without Salt									
1 cup (177g)	219	0	0	0	40	16.5	0	16	7
Beans, Kidney, Red, Mature Seeds, Canned									
1 tbsp (16g)	13	0	0	0	2	0.9	0	1	41
Beans, Kidney, Red, Mature Seeds, Cooked, Boiled, with Salt									
1 cup (177g)	225	1	0	0	40	13.1	1	15	421
Beans, Kidney, Red, Mature Seeds, Cooked, Boiled, Without Salt									
1 tbsp (11g)	14	0	0	0	3	0.8	0	1	0
Beans, Kidney, Royal Red, Mature Seeds, Cooked, Boiled with Salt									
1 cup (177g)	218	0	0	0	39	16.5	0	17	427
Beans, Kidney, Royal Red, Mature Seeds, Cooked, Boiled, Without Salt									
1 cup (177g)	218	0	0	0	39	16.5	0	17	9
Beans, Lima, Immature Seeds, Canned, Regular Packed, Solids and Liquids									
1 can (303 x 406) (454g)	322	1	0	0	61	16.3	0	18	1144
Beans, Lima, Immature Seeds, Cooked, Boiled, Drained, Without Salt									
1 cup (170g)	209	1	0	0	40	9	3	12	29
Beans, Lima, Immature Seeds, Fozen, Fordhook, Cooked, Boiled, Drained, Without Salt									
1 package (10 oz) yields (311g)	320	1	0	0	60	18	4	19	215
Beans, Lima, Immature Seeds, Frozen, Baby, Cooked, Boiled, Drained, Without Salt									
1 package (10 oz) yields (311g)	327	1	0	0	60	18.7	4	21	90
Beans, Lima, Immature Seeds, Frozen, Baby, Unprepared									
1 package (10 oz) (284g)	375	1	0	0	71	17	0	22	148

Food Serving size	Cal.	(g) Total Fat	(g) Sat. Fat	(mg) Chol.	(g) Carb.	(g) Fiber	(g) Sug.	(g) Prot.	(mg) Sod.
Beans, Lima, Immature Seeds, Frozen, Fordhook, Unprepared									
1 package (10 oz) (284g)	301	1	0	0	56	15.6	4	18	165
Beans, Liquid from Stewed Kidney Beans									
1 cup (240g)	113	8	3	10	7	0.2	0	4	5
Beans, Navy, Mature Seeds, Canned									
1 cup (262g)	296	1	0	0	54	13.4	1	20	1174
Beans, Navy, Mature Seeds, Cooked, Boiled, with Salt									
1 cup (182g)	255	1	0	0	47	19.1	1	15	431
Beans, Navy, Mature Seeds, Cooked, Boiled, Without Salt									
1 cup (182g)	255	1	0	0	47	19.1	1	15	0
Beans, Pink, Mature Seeds, Cooked, Boiled, with Salt									
1 cup (169g)	252	1	0	0	47	9	1	15	402
Beans, Pink, Mature Seeds, Cooked, Boiled, Without Salt									
1 cup (169g)	252	1	0	0	47	9	1	15	3
Beans, Pinto, Immature Seeds, Frozen, Cooked, Boiled, Drained, with Salt									
.333 package (10 oz) yields (94g)	152	0	0	0	29	8.1	0	9	300
Beans, Pinto, Immature Seeds, Frozen, Cooked, Boiled, Drained, Without Salt									
1 package (10 oz) yields (284g)	460	1	0	0	88	24.4	0	26	236
Beans, Pinto, Immature Seeds, Frozen, Unprepared									
1 package (10 oz) (284g)	483	1	0	0	92	16.2	0	28	261
Beans, Pinto, Mature Seeds, Canned									
1 cup (240g)	206	2	0	0	37	11	1	12	706
Beans, Pinto, Mature Seeds, Cooked, Boiled, with Salt									
1 cup (171g)	245	1	0	0	45	15.4	1	15	407
Beans, Pinto, Mature Seeds, Cooked, Boiled, Without Salt									
1 tbsp (10.6g)	15	0	0	0	3	1	0	1	0
Beans, Shellie, Canned, Solids and Liquids									
1 cup (245g)	74	0	0	0	15	8.3	2	4	818
Beans, Small White, Mature Seeds, Cooked, Boiled, with Salt									
1 cup (179g)	254	1	0	0	46	18.6	0	16	426
Beans, Small White, Mature Seeds, Cooked, Boiled, Without Salt									
1 cup (179g)	254	1	0	0	46	18.6	0	16	4

Food Serving size	Cal.	(g) Total Fat	(g) Sat. Fat	(mg) Chol.	(g) Carb.	(g) Fiber	(g) Sug.	(g) Prot.	(mg) Sod.
Beans, Snap, Canned, All Styles, Seasoned, Solids and Liquids									
1 can (303 x 406) (439g)	70	1	0	0	15	6.6	0	4	1637
Beans, Snap, Green Variety, Canned, Regular Packed, Solids and Liquids									
1 can, total can contents (423g)	63	1	0	0	14	6.3	5	3	812
Beans, Snap, Green, Canned, No Salt, Drained, Solid									
10 beans (62g)	14	0	0	0	3	1.2	0	1	143
Beans, Snap, Green, Canned, No Salt, Solids and Liquids									
1 can (303 x 406) (439g)	66	0	0	0	15	6.6	0	4	61
Beans, Snap, Green, Canned, Regular Packed, Drained, Solids									
10 beans (62g)	14	0	0	0	3	1.4	0	1	162
Beans, Snap, Green, Cooked, Boiled, Drained, with Salt									
1 cup (125g)	44	0	0	0	10	4	2	2	299
Beans, Snap, Green, Cooked, Boiled, Drained, Without Salt									
1 cup (125g)	44	0	0	0	10	4	2	2	1
Beans, Snap, Green, Frozen, All Styles, Microwaved									
1 cup (111g)	44	0	0	0	8	3.8	3	2	3
Beans, Snap, Green, Frozen, All Styles, Unprepared									
1 package (10 oz) (284g)	111	1	0	0	21	7.4	6	5	9
Beans, Snap, Green, Frozen, Cooked, Boiled, Drained, with Salt									
1 cup (135g)	35	0	0	0	8	4.1	2	2	331
Beans, Snap, Green, Frozen, Cooked, Boiled, Drained, Without Salt									
1 cup (135g)	38	0	0	0	9	4.1	2	2	1
Beans, Snap, Green, Microwaved									
1 cup, 1/2″ pieces (116g)	45	1	0	0	7	3.9	4	3	3
Beans, Snap, Yellow, Canned, No Salt, Drained, Solids									
10 beans (62g)	12	0	0	0	3	0.8	1	1	1
Beans, Snap, Yellow, Canned, No Salt, Solids and Liquids									
1 can (303 x 406) (439g)	66	0	0	0	15	6.6	0	4	61
Beans, Snap, Yellow, Canned, Regular Pack, Drained, Solids									
10 beans (62g)	12	0	0	0	3	0.8	1	1	156
Beans, Snap, Yellow, Canned, Regular Pack, Solids and Liquids									
1 can (303 x 406) (439g)	66	0	0	0	15	6.6	0	4	1137
Beans, Snap, Yellow, Cooked, Boiled, Drained, with Salt									
1 cup (125g)	44	0	0	0	10	4.1	2	2	299

Food Serving size	Cal.	(g) Total Fat	(g) Sat. Fat	(mg) Chol.	(g) Carb.	(g) Fiber	(g) Sug.	(g) Prot.	(mg) Sod.
Beans, Snap, Yellow, Cooked, Boiled, Drained, Without Salt									
1 cup (125g)	44	0	0	0	10	4.1	2	2	4
Beans, Snap, Yellow, Frozen, All Styles, Unprepared									
1 package (10 oz) (284g)	94	1	0	0	22	8	0	5	9
Beans, Snap, Yellow, Frozen, Cooked, Boiled, Drained, with Salt									
1 cup (135g)	35	0	0	0	8	4.1	2	2	331
Beans, Snap, Yellow, Frozen, Cooked, Boiled, Drained, Without Salt									
1 cup (135g)	38	0	0	0	9	4.1	2	2	12
Beans, White, Mature Seeds, Canned									
1 cup (262g)	299	1	0	0	56	12.6	1	19	13
Beans, White, Mature Seeds, Cooked, Boiled, with Salt									
1 cup (179g)	249	1	0	0	45	11.3	1	17	433
Beans, White, Mature Seeds, Cooked, Boiled, Without Salt									
1 tbsp (11.2g)	16	0	0	0	3	0.7	0	1	1
Beans, Yellow, Mature Seeds, Cooked, Boiled, with Salt									
1 cup (177g)	255	2	0	0	45	18.4	0	16	427
Beans, Yellow, Mature Seeds, Cooked, Boiled, Without Salt									
1 cup (177g)	255	2	0	0	45	18.4	0	16	9
Edamame, Frozen, Unprepared									
1 package (432g)	475	20	0	0	37	20.7	11	44	26
Beef Broth and Tomato Juice, Canned									
1 can (5.5 oz) (168g)	62	0	0	0	14	0.2	0	1	220
Beet Greens, Cooked, Boiled, Drained, with Salt									
1 cup (1″ pieces) (144g)	39	0	0	0	8	4.2	1	4	687
Beets Greens, Cooked, Boiled, Drained, Without Salt									
.5 cup (1″ pieces) (72g)	19	0	0	0	4	2.1	0	2	174
Beets, Canned, Drained, Solids									
1 cup, shredded (195g)	60	0	0	0	14	3.5	11	2	378
Beets, Canned, No Salt, Solids and Liquids									
1 cup (246g)	69	0	0	0	16	3	13	2	52
Beets, Canned, Regular Package, Solids and Liquids									
1 cup (246g)	74	0	0	0	18	3	16	2	352
Beets, Cooked, Boiled, Drained									
2 beets (2″ dia. sphere) (100g)	44	0	0	0	10	2	8	2	77

Food Serving size	Cal.	(g) Total Fat	(g) Sat. Fat	(mg) Chol.	(g) Carb.	(g) Fiber	(g) Sug.	(g) Prot.	(mg) Sod.
Beets, Cooked, Boiled, Drained, with Salt									
2 beets (2″ dia, sphere) (100g)	44	0	0	0	10	2	8	2	285
Beets, Harvard, Canned, Solids and Liquids									
1 cup, slices (246g)	180	0	0	0	45	6.2	0	2	399
Beets, Pickled, Canned, Solids and Liquids									
1 cup, slices (227g)	148	0	0	0	37	5.9	31	2	599
Broccoli, Chinese, Cooked									
1 cup (88g)	19	1	0	0	3	2.2	1	1	6
Broccoli, Frozen, Chopped, Cooked, Boiled, Drained, with Salt									
1 cup (184g)	52	0	0	0	10	5.5	3	6	478
Broccoli, Frozen, Chopped, Cooked, Boiled, Drained, Without Salt									
1 cup (184g)	52	0	0	0	10	5.5	3	6	20
Broccoli, Frozen, Chopped, Unprepared									
1 package (10 oz) (284g)	74	1	0	0	14	8.5	4	8	68
Broccoli, Frozen, Spears, Cooked, Boiled, Drained, with Salt									
.5 cup (92g)	26	0	0	0	5	2.8	1	3	239
Broccoli, Frozen, Spears, Cooked, Boiled, Drained, Without Salt									
.5 cup (92g)	26	0	0	0	5	2.8	1	3	22
Broccoli, Frozen, Spears, Unprepared									
1 package (2 lb) (907g)	263	3	0	0	49	27.2	13	28	154
Broccoli, Raab, Cooked									
1 NLEA serving (85g)	28	0	0	0	3	2.4	1	3	48
Broccoli, Raab, Raw									
1 stalk (19g)	4	0	0	0	1	0.5	0	1	6
Broccoli, Raw									
1 bunch (608g)	207	2	0	0	40	15.8	10	17	201
Brussels Sprouts, Cooked, Boiled, Drained, with Salt									
.5 cup (78g)	28	0	0	0	6	2	1	2	200
Brussels Sprouts, Cooked, Boiled, Drained, Without Salt									
.5 cup (78g)	28	0	0	0	6	2	1	2	16
Brussels Sprouts, Frozen, Cooked, Boiled, Drained, with Salt									
1 cup (155g)	65	1	0	0	13	6.4	3	6	401
Brussels Sprouts, Frozen, Cooked, Boiled, Drained, Without Salt									
1 cup (155g)	65	1	0	0	13	6.4	3	6	23

Food Serving size	Cal.	(g) Total Fat	(g) Sat. Fat	(mg) Chol.	(g) Carb.	(g) Fiber	(g) Sug.	(g) Prot.	(mg) Sod.
Brussels Sprouts, Frozen, Unprepared									
1 package (10 oz) (284g)	116	1	0	0	22	10.8	0	11	28
Cabbage, Chinese (Pak-choi), Cooked, Boiled, Drained, with Salt									
1 cup, shredded (170g)	20	0	0	0	3	1.7	1	3	459
Cabbage, Chinese (Pak-choi), Cooked, Boiled, Drained, Without Salt									
1 cup, shredded (170g)	20	0	0	0	3	1.7	1	3	58
Cabbage, Chinese (Pak-choi), Raw									
1 head (840g)	109	2	0	0	18	8.4	10	13	546
Cabbage, Chinese (Pe-tsai), Cooked, Boiled, Drained, with Salt									
1 leaf (14g)	2	0	0	0	0	0.2	0	0	34
Cabbage, Chinese (Pe-tsai), Cooked, Boiled, Drained, Without Salt									
1 leaf (14g)	2	0	0	0	0	0.2	0	0	1
Cabbage, Chinese (Pe-tsai), Raw									
1 cup, shredded (76g)	12	0	0	0	2	0.9	1	1	7
Cabbage, Common (Danish, Domestic and Pointed Types), Stored, Raw									
1 head (908g)	218	2	0	0	49	20.9	0	11	163
Cabbage, Common, Cooked, Boiled, Drained, with Salt									
1 head (1262g)	290	1	0	0	70	24	35	16	3218
Cabbage, Common, Freshly Harvest, Raw									
1 head (908g)	218	2	0	0	49	20.9	0	11	163
Cabbage, Cooked, Boiled, Drained, Without Salt									
1 head (1262g)	290	1	0	0	70	24	35	16	101
Cabbage, Japanese Style, Fresh, Pickled									
1 cup (150g)	45	0	0	0	9	4.7	1	2	416
Cabbage, Mustard, Salted									
1 cup (128g)	36	0	0	0	7	4	27	1	918
Cabbage, Napa, Cooked									
1 cup (109g)	13	0	0	0	2	0	0	1	12
Cabbage, Red, Cooked, Boiled, Drained, with Salt									
.5 cup, shredded (75g)	22	0	0	0	5	2	2	1	183
Cabbage, Red, Cooked, Boiled, Drained, Without Salt									
.5 cup, shredded (75g)	22	0	0	0	5	2	2	1	21
Cabbage, Savoy, Cooked, Boiled, Drained, with Salt									
1 cup, shredded (145g)	35	0	0	0	8	4.1	0	3	377

Food Serving size	Cal.	(g) Total Fat	(g) Sat. Fat	(mg) Chol.	(g) Carb.	(g) Fiber	(g) Sug.	(g) Prot.	(mg) Sod.
Cabbage, Savoy, Cooked, Boiled, Drained, Without Salt									
1 cup, shredded (145g)	35	0	0	0	8	4.1	0	3	35
Campbell's V8 100% Vegetable Juice									
1 serving (243g)	51	0	0	0	10	1.9	0	2	420
Carrot Juice, Canned									
1 fl oz (29.5g)	12	0	0	0	3	0.2	1	0	9
Carrot, Dehydrated									
1 cup (74g)	252	1	0	0	59	17.5	29	6	204
Carrots, Canned, No Salt, Drained Solid									
1 cup, sliced (146g)	37	0	0	0	8	2.2	4	1	61
Carrots, Canned, No Salt, Solids and Liquids									
1 can (303 x 406) (454g)	104	1	0	0	24	8.2	11	3	154
Carrots, Canned, Regular Packed, Drained Solids									
1 cup, mashed (228g)	57	0	0	0	13	3.4	6	1	552
Carrots, Canned, Regular Packed, Solids and Liquids									
1 can (303 x 406) (454g)	104	1	0	0	24	8.2	11	3	1090
Carrots, Cooked, Boiled, Drained, with Salt									
.5 cup, slices (78g)	27	0	0	0	6	2.3	3	1	236
Carrots, Cooked, Boiled, Drained, Without Salt									
.5 cup, slices (78g)	27	0	0	0	6	2.3	3	1	45
Carrots, Frozen, Cooked, Boiled, Drained, with Salt									
1 cup, slices (146g)	54	1	0	0	11	4.8	6	1	431
Carrots, Frozen, Cooked, Boiled, Drained, Without Salt									
1 cup, sliced (146g)	54	1	0	0	11	4.8	6	1	86
Carrots, Frozen, Unprepared									
1 package, (10 oz) (284g)	102	1	0	0	22	9.4	14	2	193
Cauliflower, Cooked, Boiled, Drained, with Salt									
3 flowerets (54g)	12	0	0	0	2	1.2	1	1	131
Cauliflower, Cooked, Boiled, Drained, Without Salt									
3 flowerets (54g)	12	0	0	0	2	1.2	1	1	8
Cauliflower, Frozen, Cooked, Boiled, Drained, with Salt									
1 cup (1" pieces) (180g)	31	0	0	0	6	4.9	1	3	457
Cauliflower, Frozen, Cooked, Boiled, Drained, Without Salt									
1 cup (1" pieces) (180g)	34	0	0	0	7	4.9	2	3	32

Food Serving size	Cal.	(g) Total Fat	(g) Sat. Fat	(mg) Chol.	(g) Carb.	(g) Fiber	(g) Sug.	(g) Prot.	(mg) Sod.
Cauliflower, Frozen, Unprepared 1 package (10 oz) (284g)	68	1	0	0	13	6.5	6	6	68
Cauliflower, Green, Cooked, No Salt Added .2 head (90g)	29	0	0	0	6	3	0	3	21
Cauliflower, Green, Cooked, with Salt .5 cup (1″ pieces) (62g)	20	0	0	0	4	2	0	2	161
Cauliflower, Green, Raw 1 floweret (25g)	8	0	0	0	2	0.8	1	1	6
Celery, Cooked, Boiled, Drained, with Salt 2 stalks (75g)	14	0	0	0	3	1.2	2	1	245
Celery, Cooked, Boiled, Drained, Without Salt 2 stalks (75g)	14	0	0	0	3	1.2	2	1	68
Chard, Swiss, Cooked, Boiled, Drained, with Salt 1 cup, chopped (175g)	35	0	0	0	7	3.7	2	3	726
Chard, Swiss, Cooked, Boiled, Drained, Without Salt 1 cup, chopped (175g)	35	0	0	0	7	3.7	2	3	313
Chives, Freeze-dried .25 cup (0.8g)	2	0	0	0	1	0.2	0	0	1
Cole Slaw, Home Prepared .5 cup (60g)	47	2	0	5	7	0.9	0	1	14
Collards, Cooked, Boiled, Drained, with Salt 1 cup, chopped (190g)	49	1	0	0	9	5.3	1	4	479
Collards, Frozen, Chopped, Cooked, Boiled, Drained, with Salt 1 cup, chopped (170g)	61	1	0	0	12	4.8	1	5	486
Collards, Frozen, Chopped, Unprepared 1 package (10 oz) (284g)	94	1	0	0	18	10.2	0	8	136
Coriander Leaf, Dried 1 tsp (0.6g)	2	0	0	0	0	0.1	0	0	1
Coriander Seed 1 tsp (1.8g)	5	0	0	0	1	0.8	0	0	1
Corn, Sweet, White 1 ear, medium (6-3/4″ to 7-1/2″ long) (90g)	77	1	0	0	17	2.4	3	3	14
Corn, Sweet, White, Canned, Cream Style, No Salt 1 can (303 x 406) (482g)	347	2	0	0	87	5.8	11	8	14

Food Serving size	Cal.	(g) Total Fat	(g) Sat. Fat	(mg) Chol.	(g) Carb.	(g) Fiber	(g) Sug.	(g) Prot.	(mg) Sod.
Corn, Sweet, White, Canned, Cream Style, Regular Pack									
1 can (303 x 406) (482g)	347	2	0	0	87	5.8	11	8	1374
Corn, Sweet, White, Canned, Vacuum Pack, No Salt									
1 can (303 x 406) (340g)	269	2	0	0	66	6.8	0	8	10
Corn, Sweet, White, Canned, Vacuum Pack, Regular Pack									
1 can (303 x 406) (340g)	269	2	0	0	66	6.8	0	8	925
Corn, Sweet, White, Canned, Whole Kernel, Drained, Solids									
1 can (303 x 406) (298g)	241	3	0	0	55	6	7	8	963
Corn, Sweet, White, Canned, Whole Kernel, No Salt, Solids and Liquids									
1 can (303 x 406) (482g)	308	2	0	0	74	3.4	0	9	58
Corn, Sweet, White, Canned, Whole Kernel, Regular Pack, Solids and Liquids									
1 can (303 x 406) (482g)	308	2	0	0	74	8.2	0	9	1027
Corn, Sweet, White, Cooked, Boiled, Drained, with Salt									
1 ear, medium (6-3/4" to 7-1/2" long) (103g)	100	1	0	0	22	2.8	8	3	261
Corn, Sweet, White, Cooked, Boiled, Drained, Without Salt									
1 ear, medium (6-3/4" to 7-1/2" long) (103g)	100	1	0	0	22	2.8	8	3	3
Corn, Sweet, White, Frozen, Kernels Cut Off Cob, Boiled, Drained, with Salt									
1 package (10 oz) yields (284g)	227	1	0	0	56	6.8	9	8	696
Corn, Sweet, White, Frozen, Kernels Cut Off Cob, Boiled, Drained, Without Salt									
1 package (10 oz) yields (284g)	227	1	0	0	56	6.8	9	8	14
Corn, Sweet, White, Frozen, Kernels Cut Off Cob, Unprepared									
1 package (10 oz) (284g)	250	2	0	0	59	6.8	0	9	9
Corn, Sweet, White, Frozen, Kernels On Cob, Cooked, Boiled, Drained, with Salt									
1 ear, yields (63g)	59	0	0	0	14	1.8	0	2	151
Corn, Sweet, White, Frozen, Kernels On Cob, Cooked, Boiled, Drained, Without Salt									
1 ear, yields (63g)	59	0	0	0	14	1.3	0	2	3
Corn, Sweet, White, Frozen, Kernels On Cob, Unprepared									
1 ear, yields (125g)	123	1	0	0	29	3.5	0	4	6
Corn, Sweet, Yellow, Canned, Brine, Regular Packed, Solids and Liquids									
1 can (303 x 406) (482g)	308	2	0	0	74	8.2	14	9	1027
Corn, Sweet, Yellow, Canned, Cream Style, No Salt									
1 can (303 x 406) (482g)	347	2	0	0	87	5.8	16	8	14

Food Serving size	Cal.	(g) Total Fat	(g) Sat. Fat	(mg) Chol.	(g) Carb.	(g) Fiber	(g) Sug.	(g) Prot.	(mg) Sod.
Corn, Sweet, Yellow, Canned, Cream Style, Regular Packed 1 can (303 x 406) (482g)	347	2	0	0	87	5.8	16	8	1374
Corn, Sweet, Yellow, Canned, No Salt, Solids and Liquids 1 can (303 x 406) (482g)	308	2	0	0	74	8.2	14	9	58
Corn, Sweet, Yellow, Canned, Vacuum Packed, No Salt 1 can (303 x 406) (340g)	269	2	0	0	66	6.8	12	8	10
Corn, Sweet, Yellow, Canned, Vacuum Packed, Regular Packed 1 can, 15 oz (303 x 406) (425g)	336	2	0	0	83	8.5	15	10	1156
Corn, Sweet, Yellow, Canned, Whole Kernel, Drained Solid 1 can (12 oz) yields (211g)	171	2	0	0	40	4	6	6	629
Corn, Sweet, Yellow, Cooked, Boiled, Drained, with Salt 1 ear, medium (6-3/4″ to 7-1/2″ long) (103g)	99	2	0	0	22	2.5	5	4	261
Corn, Sweet, Yellow, Cooked, Boiled, Drained, Without Salt 1 ear, medium (6-3/4″ to 7-1/2″ long) (103g)	9	2	0	0	22	2.5	5	4	1
Corn, Sweet, Yellow, Frozen, Kernels Cut Off Cob, Boiled, Drained, Without Salt 1 package (10 oz) yields (284g)	230	2	0	0	55	6.8	9	7	3
Corn, Sweet, Yellow, Frozen, Kernels Cut Off Cob, Unprepared 1 package (284g)	250	2	0	0	59	6	7	9	9
Corn, Sweet, Yellow, Frozen, Kernels On Cob, Cooked, Boiled, Drained, with Salt 1 ear, yields (63g)	59	0	0	0	14	1.8	2	2	151
Corn, Sweet, Yellow, Frozen, Kernels On Cob, Cooked, Boiled, Drained, Without Salt 1 ear, yields (63g)	59	0	0	0	14	1.8	2	2	3
Corn, Sweet, Yellow, Frozen, Kernels On Cob, Unprepared 1 ear, yields (125g)	123	1	0	0	29	3.5	5	4	6
Corn, Sweet, Yellow, Frozen, Kernels, Cut Off Cob, Boiled, Drained, with Salt 1 package (10 oz) yields (284g)	224	2	0	0	53	6.8	9	7	696
Corn, White 1 cup (166g)	606	8	1	0	123	0	0	16	58
Corn, with Red and Green Peppers, Canned, Solids and Liquids 1 cup (227g)	170	1	0	0	41	0	0	5	788
Corn, Yellow 1 cup (166g)	606	8	1	0	123	12.1	1	16	58

Food Serving size	Cal.	(g) Total Fat	(g) Sat. Fat	(mg) Chol.	(g) Carb.	(g) Fiber	(g) Sug.	(g) Prot.	(mg) Sod.
Corn, Yellow, Whole Kernel, Frozen, Microwaved									
1 cup (141g)	185	2	0	0	36	3.7	5	5	6
Cress, Garden, Cooked, Boiled, Drained, with Salt									
1 cup (135g)	31	1	0	0	5	0.9	4	3	329
Cress, Garden, Cooked, Boiled, Drained, Without Salt									
.5 cup (68g)	16	0	0	0	3	0.5	2	1	5
Dandelion Greens, Cooked, Boiled, Drained, with Salt									
1 cup, chopped (105g)	35	1	0	0	7	3	2	2	294
Dandelion, Greens, Cooked, Boiled, Drained, Without Salt									
1 cup, chopped (105g)	35	1	0	0	7	3	1	2	46
Dill Weed, Dried									
1 tsp (1g)	3	0	0	0	1	0.1	0	0	2
Dill Weed, Fresh									
5 sprigs (1g)	0	0	0	0	0	0	0	0	1
Eggplant, Cooked, Boiled, Drained, with Salt									
1 cup (1″ cubes) (99g)	33	0	0	0	8	2.5	3	1	237
Eggplant, Cooked, Boiled, Drained, Without Salt									
1 cup (1″ cubes) (99g)	35	0	0	0	9	2.5	3	1	1
Eggplant, Pickled									
1 cup (136g)	67	1	0	0	13	3.4	0	1	2277
Falafel, Home Prepared									
1 patty (approx 2-1/4″ dia) (17g)	57	3	0	0	5	0	0	2	50
Gardenburger, Black Bean Chipotle Burger									
1 patty (71g)	95	3	0	0	16	4.5	1	5	387
Gardenburger, Breaded Chik 'N Veggie Patties									
1 patty (71g)	155	9	1	0	13	3.6	1	9	493
Gardenburger, California Burger									
1 patty (71g)	102	4	0	0	15	2.6	1	4	400
Gardenburger, Flame Grilled Burger									
1 patty (71g)	87	3	0	0	6	5.1	0	12	501
Gardenburger, Garden Vegan									
1 patty (71g)	75	1	0	0	12	4.3	0	9	273
Gardenburger, Gourmet Baja Steak									
1 steak (156g)	192	6	2	6	36	9.7	3	7	688

Food Serving size	Cal.	(g) Total Fat	(g) Sat. Fat	(mg) Chol.	(g) Carb.	(g) Fiber	(g) Sug.	(g) Prot.	(mg) Sod.
Gardenburger, Gourmet Fire Dragon Steak									
1 steak (156g)	158	8	2	0	28	11.9	7	5	566
Gardenburger, Gourmet Hula Steak									
1 steak (156g)	253	8	6	0	48	10.8	12	6	602
Gardenburger, Gourmet Tuscany Steak									
1 steak (156g)	215	8	4	17	36	12.9	4	12	747
Gardenburger, Herb Crusted Cutlet									
1 patty (71g)	142	7	1	0	13	3.2	1	9	413
Gardenburger, Homestyle Classic Veggie Burger									
1 patty (71g)	121	6	0	0	8	4.5	0	12	493
Gardenburger, Malibu Burger, Made with Organic Whole Grains, Corn, and Carrots									
1 patty (91g)	171	8	1	0	21	4.6	2	5	611
Gardenburger, Original									
1 patty (71g)	103	3	1	9	18	4.6	1	5	401
Gardenburger, Savory Portobello Veggie Burger									
1 patty (71g)	99	3	1	3	17	5	1	4	493
Gardenburger, Sun-dried Tomato Basil Burger									
1 patty (71g)	97	3	1	3	17	3.7	2	4	275
Gardenburger, Veggie Medley Burger									
1 patty (71g)	96	3	0	0	17	5.2	1	3	376
Gourd, Dishcloth (Towelgourd), Cooked, Boiled, Drained, Without Salt									
.5 cup (1″ slices) (89g)	48	0	0	0	12	2.6	5	1	229
Gourd, Dishcloth (Towelgourd), Raw									
1 gourd (178g)	36	0	0	0	8	2	4	2	5
Gourd, White-flowered (Calabash), Raw									
1 gourd (771g)	108	0	0	0	26	3.9	0	5	15
Grape Leaves, Canned									
1 leaf (4g)	3	0	0	0	0	0	0	0	114
Green Giant, Harvest Burger, Original Flavor, All Vegetable Protein Patty, Frozen									
1 patty (90g)	138	4	1	0	7	5.7	5	18	411
Hearts of Palm, Canned									
1 piece (33g)	9	0	0	0	2	0.8	0	1	141
Horseradish, Prepared									
1 tbsp (15g)	7	0	0	0	2	0.5	1	0	63

Food Serving size	Cal.	(g) Total Fat	(g) Sat. Fat	(mg) Chol.	(g) Carb.	(g) Fiber	(g) Sug.	(g) Prot.	(mg) Sod.
Horseradish, Tree Leafy Tips, Cooked, Boiled, Drained, Without Salt									
1 cup, chopped (42g)	25	0	0	0	5	0.8	0	2	4
Horseradish, Tree Leafy Tips, Raw									
1 cup, chopped (21g)	13	0	0	0	2	0.4	0	2	2
Horseradish, Tree, Leafy Tips, Cooked, Boiled, Drained, with Salt									
1 cup, chopped (42g)	25	0	0	0	5	0.8	0	2	103
Horseradish, Tree, Pods, Cooked, Boiled, Drained, with Salt									
1 cup, slices (118g)	42	0	0	0	10	5	0	2	329
Horseradish, Tree, Pods, Cooked, Boiled, Drained, Without Salt									
1 cup, slices (118g)	42	0	0	0	10	5	0	2	51
Horseradish, Tree, Pods, Raw									
1 pod (15-1/3″ long) (11g)	4	0	0	0	1	0.4	0	0	5
Jerusalem Artichokes, Raw									
1 cup, slices (150g)	110	0	0	0	26	2.4	14	3	6
Kale, Cooked, Boiled, Drained, with salt									
1 cup, chopped (130g)	36	1	0	0	7	2.6	2	2	337
Kale, Cooked, Boiled, Drained, Without Salt									
1 cup, chopped (130g)	36	1	0	0	7	2.6	2	2	30
Kale, Frozen, Cooked, Boiled, Drained, with Salt									
1 cup, chopped (130g)	39	1	0	0	7	2.6	2	4	326
Kale, Frozen, Cooked, Boiled, Drained, Without Salt									
.5 cup, chopped or diced (65g)	20	0	0	0	3	1.3	1	2	10
Kale, Frozen, Unprepared									
1 package, (10 oz) (284g)	80	1	0	0	14	5.7	0	8	43
Kale, Scotch, Cooked, Boiled, Drained, with Salt									
1 cup, chopped (130g)	36	1	0	0	7	0	0	2	365
Kale, Scotch, Cooked, Boiled, Drained, Without Salt									
1 cup, chopped (130g)	36	1	0	0	7	1.6	0	2	59
Kohlrabi, Raw									
1 slice (16g)	4	0	0	0	1	0.6	0	0	3
Leeks (Bulb and Lower Leaf Portion), Cooked, Boiled, Drained, with Salt									
.25 cup, chopped (26g)	8	0	0	0	2	0.3	1	0	64
Leeks (Bulb and Lower Leaf Portion), Cooked, Boiled, Drained, Without Salt									
.25 cup, chopped or diced (26g)	8	0	0	0	2	0.3	1	0	3

Food Serving size	Cal.	(g) Total Fat	(g) Sat. Fat	(mg) Chol.	(g) Carb.	(g) Fiber	(g) Sug.	(g) Prot.	(mg) Sod.
Leeks (Bulb and Lower Leaf Portion), Freeze-dried									
.25 cup (0.8g)	3	0	0	0	1	0.1	0	0	0
Leeks (Bulb and Lower Leaf Portion), Raw									
1 leek (89g)	54	0	0	0	13	1.6	3	1	18
Lentils, Mature Seeds, Cooked, Boiled, with Salt									
1 cup (198g)	226	1	0	0	39	15.6	4	18	471
Lima Beans, Immature Seeds, Canned, No Salt, Solids and Liquids									
1 can (303 x 406) (454g)	322	1	0	0	61	16.3	4	18	18
Mixed Vegetable and Fruit Juice Drink, with Added Nutrition									
8 fl oz (247g)	72	0	0	0	18	0	5	0	52
Mustard Greens, Frozen, Cooked, Boiled, Drained, with Salt									
1 package (10 oz) yields (212g)	40	1	0	0	7	5.9	1	5	553
Mustard Greens, Frozen, Cooked, Boiled, Drained, Without Salt									
1 package (10 oz) yields (212g)	40	1	0	0	7	5.9	1	5	53
Mustard Greens, Frozen, Unprepared									
1 package (10 oz) (284g)	57	1	0	0	10	9.4	0	7	82
Mustard Spinach (Tendergreen), Cooked, Boiled, Drained, with Salt									
1 cup, chopped (180g)	29	0	0	0	5	3.6	0	3	450
Mustard Spinach (Tendergreen), Cooked, Boiled, Drained, Without Salt									
1 cup, chopped (180g)	29	0	0	0	5	3.6	0	3	25
Onion Rings, Breaded, Partially Fried, Frozen, Prepared, Heated in Oven									
10 rings, large (3-4" dia) (71g)	196	10	2	0	24	1.6	4	3	263
Onions, Canned, Solids and Liquids									
.5 cup, chopped or diced (112g)	21	0	0	0	5	1.3	2	1	416
Onions, Cooked, Boiled, Drained, with Salt									
1 tbsp, chopped (15g)	6	0	0	0	1	0.2	1	0	36
Onions, Cooked, Boiled, Drained, Without Salt									
1 tbsp, chopped (15g)	7	0	0	0	2	0.2	1	0	0
Onions, Dehydrated Flakes									
.25 cup (14g)	49	0	0	0	12	1.3	5	1	3
Onions, Frozen, Chopped, Cooked, Boiled, Drained, with Salt									
.5 cup, chopped or diced (105g)	27	0	0	0	6	1.8	3	1	260
Onions, Frozen, Chopped, Cooked, Boiled, Drained, Without Salt									
.5 cup, chopped or diced (105g)	29	0	0	0	7	1.9	3	1	13

Food Serving size	Cal.	(g) Total Fat	(g) Sat. Fat	(mg) Chol.	(g) Carb.	(g) Fiber	(g) Sug.	(g) Prot.	(mg) Sod.
Onions, Frozen, Chopped, Unprepared									
1 package (10 oz) (284g)	82	0	0	0	19	5.1	0	2	34
Onions, Frozen, Whole, Cooked, Boiled, Drained, with Salt									
1 cup (210g)	55	0	0	0	13	2.9	6	1	512
Onions, Frozen, Whole, Cooked, Boiled, Drained, Without Salt									
1 cup (210g)	59	0	0	0	14	2.9	6	1	17
Onions, Frozen, Whole, Unprepared									
1 package (10 oz) (284g)	99	0	0	0	24	4.8	11	3	28
Onions, Yellow, Sauteed									
1 cup, chopped (87g)	115	9	1	0	7	1.5	0	1	10
Parsley, Freeze-dried									
.25 cup (1.4g)	4	0	0	0	1	0.5	0	0	5
Peas and Carrots, Canned, No Salt, Solids and Liquids									
1 cup (255g)	97	1	0	0	22	8.4	7	6	10
Peas and Carrots, Canned, Regular Package, Solids and Liquids									
1 cup (255g)	97	1	0	0	22	5.1	0	6	663
Peas and Carrots, Frozen, Cooked, Boiled, Drained, with Salt									
.5 cup (80g)	38	0	0	0	8	2.5	3	2	243
Peas and Carrots, Frozen, Cooked, Boiled, Drained, Without Salt									
.5 cup (80g)	38	0	0	0	8	2.5	3	2	54
Peas and Carrots, Frozen, Unprepared									
1 package (10 oz) (284g)	151	1	0	0	32	9.7	0	10	224
Peas and Onions, Canned, Solids and Liquids									
1 cup (120g)	61	0	0	0	10	2.8	0	4	530
Peas and Onions, Frozen, Cooked, Boiled, Drained, Without Salt									
1 cup (180g)	81	0	0	0	16	4	7	5	67
Peas and Onions, Frozen, Unprepared									
1 package (10 oz) (284g)	199	1	0	0	38	9.9	0	11	173
Peas, Edible-podded, Boiled, Drained, Without Salt									
1 cup (160g)	67	0	0	0	11	4.5	6	5	6
Peas, Edible-podded, Cooked, Boiled, Drained, with Salt									
1 cup (160g)	64	0	0	0	10	4.5	6	5	384
Peas, Edible-podded, Frozen, Cooked, Boiled, Drained, with Salt									
1 package (10 oz) yields (253g)	64	0	0	0	10	4.5	6	5	384

Food Serving size	Cal.	(g) Total Fat	(g) Sat. Fat	(mg) Chol.	(g) Carb.	(g) Fiber	(g) Sug.	(g) Prot.	(mg) Sod.
Peas, Edible-podded, Frozen, Cooked, Boiled, Drained, Without Salt									
1 package (10 oz) yields (253g)	132	1	0	0	23	7.8	12	9	13
Peas, Edible-podded, Frozen, Unprepared									
1 package (10 oz) (284g)	119	1	0	0	20	8.8	0	8	11
Peas, Green (Includes Baby and Lesuer Types), Canned, Drained Solids, Unprepared									
1 can (303 x 406) (313g)	216	2	0	0	36	15.3	9	14	911
Peas, Green, Canned, No Salt, Drained Solids									
1 can (303 x 406) (313g)	216	1	0	0	39	12.8	13	14	6
Peas, Green, Canned, No Salt, Solids and Liquids									
1 can (303 x 406) (482g)	255	1	0	0	47	15.9	15	15	43
Peas, Green, Canned, Regular Package, Solids and Liquids									
1 can (303 x 406) (482g)	255	1	0	0	47	15.9	15	15	1205
Peas, Green, Canned, Seasoned, Solids and Liquids									
.5 cup (114g)	57	0	0	0	11	2.3	0	4	290
Peas, Green, Cooked, Boiled, Drained, with Salt									
1 cup (160g)	134	0	0	0	25	8.8	9	9	382
Peas, Green, Cooked, Boiled, Drained, Without Salt									
1 cup (160g)	134	0	0	0	25	8.8	9	9	5
Peas, Green, Frozen, Cooked, Boiled, Drained, with Salt									
1 package (10 oz) yields (253g)	197	1	0	0	36	13.9	12	13	817
Peas, Green, Frozen, Cooked, Boiled, Drained, Without Salt									
1 package (10 oz) yields (253g)	197	1	0	0	36	13.9	12	13	182
Peas, Split, Mature Seeds, Cooked, Boiled, with Salt									
1 cup (196g)	227	1	0	0	40	16.3	6	16	466
Peas, Split, Mature Seeds, Cooked, Boiled, Without Salt									
1 tbsp (12.2g)	14	0	0	0	3	1	0	1	0
Peppers, Chili, Ground, Canned									
1 cup (139g)	29	0	0	0	6	2.4	0	1	552
Peppers, Hot Chili, Green, Canned, Pods, Excluding Seeds, Solids and Liquids									
.5 cup, chopped or diced (68g)	14	0	0	0	3	0.9	2	1	798
Peppers, Hot Chili, Green, Raw									
.5 cup, chopped or diced (75g)	30	0	0	0	7	1.1	4	2	5

Food Serving size	Cal.	(g) Total Fat	(g) Sat. Fat	(mg) Chol.	(g) Carb.	(g) Fiber	(g) Sug.	(g) Prot.	(mg) Sod.
Peppers, Hot Chili, Red, Canned, Excluding Seeds, Solids and Liquids									
.5 cup, chopped or diced (68g)	14	0	0	0	3	0.9	2	1	798
Peppers, Hot Chili, Sun-dried									
1 pepper (0.5g)	2	0	0	0	0	0.1	0	0	0
Peppers, Jalapeno, Canned, Solids and Liquids									
1 cup, sliced (104g)	28	1	0	0	5	2.7	2	1	1738
Peppers, Pasilla, Dried									
1 pepper (7g)	24	1	0	0	4	1.9	0	1	6
Peppers, Sweet, Green, Canned, Solids and Liquids									
1 cup, halves (140g)	25	0	0	0	5	1.7	0	1	1917
Peppers, Sweet, Green, Cooked, Boiled, Drained, with Salt									
1 pepper (73g)	19	0	0	0	4	0.9	2	1	174
Peppers, Sweet, Green, Cooked, Boiled, Drained, Without Salt									
1 tbsp, chopped (11.6g)	3	0	0	0	1	0.1	0	0	0
Peppers, Sweet, Green, Freeze-dried									
.25 cup (1.6g)	5	0	0	0	1	0.3	1	0	3
Peppers, Sweet, Green, Frozen, Chopped, Cooked, Boiled, Drained, with Salt									
1 tbsp, chopped (11.6g)	2	0	0	0	0	0	0	0	28
Peppers, Sweet, Green, Frozen, Chopped, Unprepared									
1 package (10 oz) (284g)	57	1	0	0	13	4.5	0	3	14
Peppers, Sweet, Red, Canned, Solids and Liquids									
.5 cup, halves (70g)	13	0	0	0	3	0.8	0	1	958
Peppers, Sweet, Red, Cooked, Boiled, Drained, with Salt									
1 pepper (73g)	19	0	0	0	4	0.9	3	1	174
Peppers, Sweet, Red, Cooked, Boiled, Drained, Without Salt									
1 tbsp (11.6g)	3	0	0	0	1	0.1	1	0	0
Peppers, Sweet, Red, Freeze-dried									
.25 cup (1.6g)	5	0	0	0	1	0.3	1	0	3
Peppers, Sweet, Red, Frozen, Chopped, Cooked, Boiled, Drained, with Salt									
1 tbsp, chopped (11.6g)	2	0	0	0	0	0	0	0	28
Peppers, Sweet, Red, Frozen, Chopped, Cooked, Boiled, Drained, Without Salt									
1 tbsp, chopped (11.6g)	2	0	0	0	0	0	0	0	0
Peppers, Sweet, Red, Frozen, Chopped, Unprepared									
1 package (10 oz) (28g)	6	0	0	0	1	0.4	1	0	1

Food Serving size	Cal.	(g) Total Fat	(g) Sat. Fat	(mg) Chol.	(g) Carb.	(g) Fiber	(g) Sug.	(g) Prot.	(mg) Sod.
Pickle Relish, Hamburger .5 cup (122g)	157	1	0	0	42	3.9	0	1	1337
Pickle Relish, Hot Dog .5 cup (122g)	111	1	0	0	28	1.8	0	2	1331
Pickle Relish, Sweet 1 tbsp (15g)	20	0	0	0	5	0.2	4	0	122
Pickles, Chowchow, with Cauliflower Onion Mustard, Sweet 1 cup (245g)	296	2	0	0	65	3.7	59	4	1291
Pickles, Cucumber, Dill or Kosher Dill 1 slice (7g)	1	0	0	0	0.1	0	0	0	57
Pickles, Cucumber, Dill, Low Sodium 1 slice (6g)	1	0	0	0	0	0.1	0	0	1
Pickles, Cucumber, Sour 1 large (4″ long) (135g)	15	0	0	0	3	1.6	1	0	1631
Pickles, Cucumber, Sour, Low Sodium 1 cup (about 23 slices) (155g)	17	0	0	0	4	1.9	2	1	28
Pickles, Cucumber, Sweet (Includes Bread and Butter Pickles) 1 cup (153g)	139	1	0	0	32	1.5	28	1	699
Pickles, Cucumber, Sweet, Low Sodium (Includes Bread and Butter Pickles) 1 cup, sliced (170g)	207	0	0	0	57	1.9	45	1	31
Pimiento, Canned 1 cup (192g)	44	1	0	0	10	3.6	5	2	27
Potato Flour 1 cup (160g)	571	1	0	0	133	9.4	6	11	88
Potato Pancakes 1 medium, 3-1/4 in. x 3-5/8 in., 5/8 in. thick. (37g)	99	5	1	35	10	1.2	1	2	283
Potato Puffs, Frozen, Oven-heated 10 Crispy Crowns (60g)	115	5	1	0	16	1.2	0	1	278
Potato Puffs, Frozen, Unprepared 10 pieces (91g)	168	8	1	0	23	2.1	0	2	389
Potato Salad, Home-prepared 1 cup (250g)	358	21	4	170	28	3.3	0	7	1323
Potato Soup, Instant, Dry, Mix 1 serving, 1/3 cup (39g)	134	1	0	5	30	3	4	4	936

Food Serving size	Cal.	(g) Total Fat	(g) Sat. Fat	(mg) Chol.	(g) Carb.	(g) Fiber	(g) Sug.	(g) Prot.	(mg) Sod.
Potato Sticks .5 cup (18g)	94	6	2	0	10	0.6	0	1	45
Potatoes, au Gratin, Dry Mix, Prepared with Water, Whole Milk, and Butter 1 package, yield, 5.5 oz (822g)	764	34	21	123	106	7.4	0	19	3609
Potatoes, au Gratin, Dry Mix, Unprepared .167 package (5.5 oz) (26g)	82	1	1	0	19	1.1	0	2	545
Potatoes, au Gratin, Home-prepared from Recipe Using Butter 1 cup (245g)	323	19	12	56	28	4.4	0	12	1061
Potatoes, au Gratin, Home-prepared from Recipe Using Margarine 1 cup (245g)	323	19	9	37	28	4.4	0	12	1061
Potatoes, Baked, Flesh and Skin, with Salt 1 potato, medium (2-1/4" to 3-1/4" dia) (173g)	161	0	0	0	37	3.8	2	4	17
Potatoes, Baked, Flesh, with Salt 1 potato (2-1/3" x 4-3/4") (156g)	145	0	0	0	34	2.3	3	3	376
Potatoes, French Fries, All Types, Salt Added in Process, Frozen, Oven-heated 1 package (9 oz), yields (198g)	325	10	2	0	55	5.5	1	5	768
Potatoes, French Fries, All Types, Salt Added in Process, Frozen, Unprepared 1 package (9 oz) (255g)	375	12	3	0	63	4.8	1	6	847
Potatoes, French Fries, All Types, Salt Not Added in Processing, Frozen 1 package (9 oz) (255g)	383	12	2	0	63	4.8	1	6	59
Potatoes, French Fries, All Types, Salt Not Added in Processing, Frozen, Oven-heated 10 strips (74g)	127	4	1	0	21	1.9	0	2	24
Potatoes, French Fries, Crinkle/Regular Cut, Salt Added in Process, Frozen 10 strips (82g)	143	4	1	0	25	2.2	0	2	294
Potatoes, French Fries, Crinkle/Regular Cut, Salt Added in Process, Frozen, Oven-heated 10 strips (69g)	115	4	1	0	19	1.6	0	2	270
Potatoes, French Fries, Shoestring, Salt Added in Process, Frozen 10 strips (30g)	50	2	0	0	8	0.7	0	1	97
Potatoes, French Fries, Shoestring, Salt Added in Process, Frozen, Oven-heated 10 strips (21g)	42	1	0	0	7	0.6	0	1	84
Potatoes, French Fries, Steak Fries, Salt Added in Process, Frozen 10 strips (153g)	203	5	1	0	36	2.9	0	3	485

Food Serving size	Cal.	(g) Total Fat	(g) Sat. Fat	(mg) Chol.	(g) Carb.	(g) Fiber	(g) Sug.	(g) Prot.	(mg) Sod.
Potatoes, French Fries, Steak Fries, Salt Added in Process, Frozen, Oven-heated 10 strips (133g)	202	5	1	0	36	3.5	0	3	496
Potatoes, Frozen, French Fries, Partially Fried, Cottage-cut, Prepared, Heated in Oven, with Salt 1 package (9 oz) yields (198g)	432	16	8	0	67	6.3	0	7	556
Potatoes, Frozen, French Fries, Partially Fried, Cottage-cut, Prepared, Heated in Oven, Without Salt 1 package (9 oz) yields (198g)	432	16	8	0	67	6.3	0	7	89
Potatoes, Frozen, French Fries, Partially Fried, Cottage-cut, Unprepared 1 package (9 oz) (255g)	390	15	7	0	61	7.7	0	6	82
Potatoes, Frozen, French Fries, Partially Fried, Extruded, Prepared, Heated in Oven, Without Salt 1 package (9 oz) yields (198g)	659	37	12	0	79	6.3	0	7	1214
Potatoes, Frozen, French Fries, Partially Fried, Extruded, Unprepared 1 package (9 oz) (255g)	663	38	12	0	77	11.5	0	7	1250
Potatoes, Frozen, Whole, Unprepared 1 cup (182g)	142	0	0	0	32	2.2	1	4	46
Potatoes, Hash Brown, Frozen, Plain, Prepared .5 cup (78g)	170	9	4	0	22	1.6	1	2	27
Potatoes, Hash Brown, Frozen, Plain, Unprepared 1 package (12 oz) (340g)	279	2	1	0	60	4.8	0	7	75
Potatoes, Hash Brown, Frozen, with Butter Sauce, Unprepared 1 package (6 oz) (170g)	230	11	4	0	31	4.9	0	3	131
Potatoes, Hash Brown, Home-prepared 1 cup (156g)	413	20	3	0	55	5	2	5	534
Potatoes, Mashed, Dehydrated, Flakes Without Milk, Dry Form 1 cup (60g)	212	0	0	0	49	4	2	5	62
Potatoes, Mashed, Dehydrated, Granules with Milk, Dry Form 1 cup (200g)	714	2	1	4	155	13.2	7	22	164
Potatoes, Mashed, Dehydrated, Granules Without Milk, Dry Form 1 cup (200g)	744	1	0	0	171	14.2	7	16	134
Potatoes, Mashed, Dehydrated, Prepared from Flakes Without Milk, Whole Milk and Butter 1 cup (210g)	204	11	7	29	23	1.7	3	4	344

Food Serving size	Cal.	(g) Total Fat	(g) Sat. Fat	(mg) Chol.	(g) Carb.	(g) Fiber	(g) Sug.	(g) Prot.	(mg) Sod.
Potatoes, Mashed, Dehydrated, Prepared from Granules with Milk, Water and Margarine Added									
1 cup (210g)	244	10	2	4	34	2.7	4	4	361
Potatoes, Mashed, Dehydrated, Prepared from Granules Without Milk, Whole Milk and Butter									
1 cup (210g)	227	10	6	29	30	4.6	0	4	540
Potatoes, Mashed, Home-prepared, Whole Milk and Butter Added									
1 cup (210g)	237	9	5	23	35	3.2	3	4	666
Potatoes, Mashed, Home-prepared, Whole Milk and Margarine Added									
1 cup (210g)	233	9	2	2	36	3.2	3	4	699
Potatoes, Mashed, Home-prepared, Whole Milk Added									
1 cup (210g)	174	1	1	4	37	3.2	3	4	634
Potatoes, Mashed, Prepared from Flakes, Without Milk, Whole Milk and Margarine									
1 cup (210g)	237	12	3	8	32	4.8	0	4	697
Potatoes, Mashed, Prepared from Granules, Without Milk, Whole Milk and Margarine									
1 cup (210g)	227	10	3	6	30	4.6	0	4	552
Potatoes, Microwaved, Cooked in Skin, Flesh and Skin, Without Salt									
1 potato (2-3/4″ dia by 4-3/4″ long) (202g)	212	0	0	0	49	4.6	0	5	16
Potatoes, Microwaved, Cooked in Skin, Flesh, with Salt									
1 potato (2-1/3″ x 4-3/4″) (156g)	156	0	0	0	36	2.5	0	3	379
Potatoes, Microwaved, Cooked in Skin, Flesh, Without Salt									
1 potato (2-1/3″ x 4-3/4″) (156g)	156	0	0	0	36	2.5	0	3	11
Potatoes, Microwaved, Cooked in Skin, Without Salt									
1 skin (58g)	77	0	0	0	17	3.2	0	3	9
Potatoes, Microwaved, Cooked, in Skin, Flesh and Skin, with Salt									
1 potato (2-1/3″ x 4-3/4″) (202g)	212	0	0	0	49	4.6	0	5	493
Potatoes, Microwaved, Cooked, in Skin, with Salt									
1 skin (58g)	77	0	0	0	17	3.2	0	3	146
Potatoes, Scalloped, Dry Mix, Prepared with Water, Whole Milk, and Butter									
.167 package (5.5 oz) yields (137g)	127	6	4	15	17	1.5	0	3	467

Food Serving size	Cal.	(g) Total Fat	(g) Sat. Fat	(mg) Chol.	(g) Carb.	(g) Fiber	(g) Sug.	(g) Prot.	(mg) Sod.
Potatoes, Scalloped, Dry Mix, Unprepared									
.167 package (5.5 oz) (26g)	93	1	0	1	19	2.2	0	2	410
Potatoes, Scalloped, Home-prepared with Butter									
1 cup (245g)	216	9	6	29	26	4.7	0	7	821
Potatoes, Scalloped, Home-prepared with Margarine									
1 cup (245g)	216	9	3	15	26	4.7	0	7	821
Pumpkin and Squash Seed Kernels, Dried									
1 oz (28.35g)	158	14	2	0	3	1.7	0	9	2
Pumpkin and Squash Seed Kernels, Roasted, with Salt									
1 oz (28.35g)	163	14	2	0	4	1.8	0	8	73
Pumpkin and Squash Seed Kernels, Roasted, Without Salt									
1 oz (28.35g)	163	14	2	0	4	1.8	0	8	5
Pumpkin and Squash Seeds, Whole, Roasted, with Salt									
1 oz (85 seeds) (28.35g)	126	5	1	0	15	5.2	0	5	720
Pumpkin and Squash Seeds, Whole, Roasted, Without Salt									
1 oz (85 seeds) (28.35g)	126	5	1	0	15	5.2	0	5	5
Pumpkin Flowers, Cooked, Boiled, Drained, Without Salt									
1 cup (134g)	20	0	0	0	4	1.2	3	1	8
Pumpkin Leaves, Cooked, Boiled, Drained, with Salt									
1 cup (71g)	15	0	0	0	2	1.9	0	2	173
Pumpkin Leaves, Cooked, Boiled, Drained, Without Salt									
1 cup (71g)	15	0	0	0	2	1.9	0	2	6
Pumpkin Pie Mix, Canned									
1 cup (270g)	281	0	0	0	71	22.4	0	3	562
Pumpkin, Canned, with Salt									
1 cup (245g)	83	1	0	0	20	7.1	8	3	590
Pumpkin, Canned, Without salt									
1 cup (245g)	83	1	0	0	20	7.1	8	3	12
Pumpkin, Cooked, Boiled, Drained, with Salt									
1 cup, mashed (245g)	44	0	0	0	11	2.7	5	2	581
Pumpkin, Cooked, Boiled, Drained, Without Salt									
1 cup, mashed (245g)	49	0	0	0	12	2.7	2	2	2
Pumpkin, Flowers, Cooked, Boiled, Drained, with Salt									
1 cup (134g)	20	0	0	0	4	1.2	3	1	324

Food Serving size	Cal.	(g) Total Fat	(g) Sat. Fat	(mg) Chol.	(g) Carb.	(g) Fiber	(g) Sug.	(g) Prot.	(mg) Sod.
Sauerkraut, Canned, Low Sodium									
1 cup (142g)	31	0	0	0	6	3.6	1	1	437
Sauerkraut, Canned, Solids and Liquids									
1 cup, undrained (236g)	45	0	0	0	10	6.8	4	2	1560
Spinach Souffle									
1 recipe, yields (813g)	1398	105	50	959	48	5.7	15	64	4602
Tomatoes, Red, Ripe, Canned, Packed in Tomato Juice									
1 tbsp (15g)	3	0	0	0	1	0.2	0	0	21
Tomatoes, Red, Ripe, Canned, Packed in Tomato Juice, No Salt Added									
1 tbsp (15g)	3	0	0	0	1	0.2	0	0	2
Tomatoes, Red, Ripe, Canned, Stewed									
1 cup (255g)	66	0	0	0	16	2.6	9	2	564
Tomatoes, Red, Ripe, Canned, with Green Chilies									
1 cup (241g)	36	0	0	0	9	0	0	2	966
Turnips, Frozen, Cooked, Boiled, Drained, Without Salt									
1 cup (156g)	36	0	0	0	7	3.1	4	2	56
Vegetable Juice Cocktail, Canned									
6 fl oz (182g)	35	0	0	0	8	1.5	6	1	360
Vegetable Oil Spread, Unspecified Oils, Approximately 37% Fat, with Salt, with Added Vitamin D									
1 cup (232g)	47	5	1	0	0	0	0	0	82
Vegetable Oil, Palm Kernel									
1 cup (218g)	1879	218	178	0	0	0	0	0	0
Vegetable Oil-butter Spread, Reduced Calorie									
1 cup (207g)	963	110	37	112	0	0	0	0	1203
Vegetables, Mixed (Corn, Lima Beans, Peas, Green Beans, Carrots) Canned, No Salt									
1 cup (182g)	67	0	0	0	13	5.6	1	3	47
Vegetables, Mixed, Canned, Drained, Solids									
1 cup (163g)	80	0	0	0	15	4.9	4	4	349
Vegetables, Mixed, Canned, Solids and Liquids									
1 cup (245g)	88	1	0	0	17	9.3	0	3	549
Vegetables, Mixed, Frozen, Cooked, Boiled, Drained, with Salt									
.5 cup (91g)	55	0	0	0	12	4	3	3	247

Food Serving size	Cal.	(g) Total Fat	(g) Sat. Fat	(mg) Chol.	(g) Carb.	(g) Fiber	(g) Sug.	(g) Prot.	(mg) Sod.
Vegetables, Mixed, Frozen, Cooked, Boiled, Drained, Without Salt									
1 package (10 oz) yields (275g)	179	0	0	0	36	12.1	9	8	96
Vegetables, Mixed, Frozen, Unprepared									
1 package (10 oz) (284g)	204	1	0	0	38	11.4	0	9	133
Vegetarian Fillets									
1 fillet (85g)	247	15	2	0	8	5.2	0	20	417
Vegetarian Meatloaf or Patties									
1 slice (56g)	110	5	1	0	4	2.6	0	12	308
Vegetarian Stew									
1 cup (247g)	304	7	1	0	17	2.7	35	42	988
Veggie Burgers or Soy Burgers, Unprepared									
1 pattie (70g)	124	4	1	4	10	3.4	1	11	398
Worthington Vegetable Scallops, Canned, Unprepared									
.5 cup (85g)	93	1	0	0	4	2.9	0	17	391
Worthington Veja-links, Canned, Unprepared									
1 link (31g)	48	3	0	1	1	1	0	5	164

Spices/Seasonings

Food Serving size	Cal.	Total Fat	Sat. Fat	Chol.	Carb.	Fiber	Sug.	Prot.	Sod.
Allspice, Ground									
1 tbsp (6g)	16	1	0	0	4	1.3	0	0	5
Anise Seed									
1 tbsp, whole (6.7g)	23	1	0	0	3	1	0	1	1
Bread Crumbs, Dry, Grated, Plain									
1 cup (108g)	427	6	1	0	78	4.9	7	14	791
Bread Crumbs, Dry, Grated, Seasoned									
1 cup (120g)	460	7	2	1	82	5.9	7	17	2111
Caraway Seed									
1 tbsp (6.7g)	22	1	0	0	3	2.5	0	1	1
Capers, Canned									
1 tbsp, drained (8.6g)	2	0	0	0	0	0.3	0	0	188
Celery Seed									
1 tbsp (6.5g)	25	2	0	0	3	0.8	0	1	10
Chervil, Dried									
1 tbsp (1.9g)	5	0	0	0	1	0.2	0	0	2

Food Serving size	Cal.	(g) Total Fat	(g) Sat. Fat	(mg) Chol.	(g) Carb.	(g) Fiber	(g) Sug.	(g) Prot.	(mg) Sod.
Chili Powder 1 tbsp (8g)	23	1	0	0	4	2.8	1	1	229
Cinnamon, Ground 1 tbsp (7.9g)	20	0	0	0	6	4.2	0	0	1
Coriander Leaf, Dried 1 tbsp (1.8g)	5	0	0	0	1	0.2	0	0	4
Coriander Seed 1 tbsp (5g)	15	1	0	0	3	2.1	0	1	2
Cumin Seed 1 tbsp, whole (6g)	23	1	0	0	3	0.6	0	1	10
Curry Powder 1 tbsp (6.3g)	20	1	0	0	4	3.4	0	1	3
Cloves, Ground 1 tbsp (6.5g)	18	1	0	0	4	2.2	0	0	18
Dill Seed 1 tbsp (6.6g)	20	1	0	0	4	1.4	0	1	1
Dill Weed, Dried 1 tbsp (3.1g)	8	0	0	0	2	0.4	0	1	6
Dill Weed, Fresh 1 cup, sprigs (8.9g)	4	0	0	0	1	0.2	0	0	5
Fennel Seed 1 tbsp, whole (5.8g)	20	1	0	0	3	2.3	0	1	5
Fenugreek Seed 1 tbsp (11.1g)	36	1	0	0	6	2.7	0	3	7
Garlic Powder 1 tbsp (9.7g)	32	0	0	0	7	0.9	0	2	6
George Weston Bakeries, Brownberry Sage and Onion Stuffing Mix, Dry 1 serving (67g)	261	3	1	0	49	3.6	0	9	1126
Ginger, Ground 1 tbsp (5.2g)	17	0	0	0	4	0.7	0	0	1
Mace, Ground 1 tbsp (5.3g)	25	2	1	0	3	1.1	0	0	4
Marjoram, Dried 1 tbsp (1.7g)	5	0	0	0	1	0.7	0	0	1

Food Serving size	Cal.	(g) Total Fat	(g) Sat. Fat	(mg) Chol.	(g) Carb.	(g) Fiber	(g) Sug.	(g) Prot.	(mg) Sod.
Mustard, Prepared, Yellow 1 cup (249g)	149	8	1	0	15	10	2	9	2749
Nutmeg, Ground 1 tbsp (7g)	37	3	2	0	3	1.5	0	0	1
Onion Powder 1 tbsp (6.9g)	24	0	0	0	5	1	0	1	5
Paprika 1 tbsp (6.8g)	19	1	0	0	4	2.4	1	1	5
Parsley, Dried 1 tbsp (1.6g)	5	0	0	0	1	0.4	0	0	7
Pepper, Ancho, Dried 1 pepper (17g)	48	1	0	0	9	3.7	0	2	7
Pepper, Black 1 tbsp, ground (6.9g)	17	0	0	0	4	1.7	0	1	1
Pepper, Red or Cayenne 1 tbsp (5.3g)	17	1	0	0	3	1.4	1	1	2
Pepper, Serrano, Raw 1 pepper (6.1g)	2	0	0	0	0	0.2	0	0	1
Pepper, White 1 tbsp, ground (7.1g)	21	0	0	0	5	1.9	0	1	0
Peppermint, Fresh 2 tbsp (3.2g)	2	0	0	0	0	0.3	0	0	1
Poppy Seed 1 tbsp (8.8g)	46	4	0	0	2	1.7	0	2	2
Poultry Seasoning 1 tbsp (5.6g)	19	1	0	0	4	0.8	0	0	3
Pumpkin Pie Spice 1 tsp (1.7g)	6	0	0	0	1	0.3	0	0	1
Rosemary, Dried 1 tbsp (3.3g)	11	1	0	0	2	1.4	0	0	2
Rosemary, Fresh 1 tbsp (1.7g)	2	0	0	0	0	0.2	0	0	0
Saffron 1 tbsp (2.1g)	7	0	0	0	1	0.1	0	0	3

Food Serving size	Cal.	(g) Total Fat	(g) Sat. Fat	(mg) Chol.	(g) Carb.	(g) Fiber	(g) Sug.	(g) Prot.	(mg) Sod.
Sage, Ground 1 tbsp (2g)	6	0	0	0	1	0.8	0	0	0
Salt, Table 1 tbsp (18g)	0	0	0	0	0	0	0	0	6976
Savory, Ground 1 tbsp (4.4g)	12	0	0	0	3	2	0	0	1
Spearmint, Dried 1 tbsp (1.6g)	5	0	0	0	1	0.5	0	0	6
Spearmint, Fresh 2 tbsp (11.4g)	5	0	0	0	1	0.8	0	0	3
Spices, Basil, Dried 1 tbsp, leaves (2.1g)	5	0	0	0	1	0.8	0	0	2
Spices, Bay Leaf 1 tsp, crumbled (1.8g)	6	0	0	0	1	0.5	0	0	0
Spices, Cardamom 1 tsp, ground (5.8g)	18	0	0	0	4	1.6	0	1	1
Spices, Mustard Seed, Ground 1 tbsp (6.3g)	32	2	0	0	2	0.8	0	2	1
Spices, Oregano, Dried 1 tsp, ground (1.8g)	5	0	0	0	1	0.8	0	0	0
Spices, Tarragon, Dried 1 tbsp, leaves (1.8g)	5	0	0	0	1	0.1	0	0	1
Spices, Thyme, Dried 1 tbsp, leaves (2.7g)	7	0	0	0	2	1	0	0	1
Thyme, Fresh .5 tsp (0.4g)	0	0	0	0	0	0.1	0	0	0
Turmeric, Ground 1 tbsp (9.4g)	29	0	0	0	6	2.1	0	1	3

Fruits

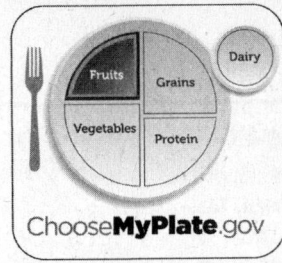

Choose**MyPlate**.gov

Why Eat Fruits?

Fruits provide nutrients vital for health and maintenance of your body. Most fruits are naturally low in fat, sodium, and calories. None have cholesterol. Fruits are sources of many essential nutrients that are under-consumed including potassium, dietary fiber, vitamin C, and folate (folic acid). Diets rich in potassium may help to maintain healthy blood pressure. Dietary fiber from fruits, as part of an overall healthy diet, helps reduce blood cholesterol levels and may lower risk of heart disease. Vitamin C is important for growth and repair of all body tissues, helps heal cuts and wounds, and keeps teeth and gums healthy. Fruits are also rich in antioxidants, substances that prevent or repair damage done to the body by oxidation. Although fruit contains the sugar fructose, fructose from whole fruit shows minimal changes in blood sugar and may in fact have a protective effect on the development of type 2 diabetes.

Daily Goal

Two cups for an adult on a 2,000-calorie diet
One-cup equivalents:

1 two-and-a-half-inch whole fruit	8 oz fruit juice (100%)
1 cup chopped or sliced fruit	32 seedless grapes
½ cup dried fruit	8 large strawberries

Shopping Tips

- Eat a variety of fruits.
- Choose fresh in season.
- Buy locally grown fruits when available.
- Buy fruits that are frozen and canned in water or 100% juice.
- Refrigerate or freeze cut-up fruit to store for later use.

Shopping List Essentials

Apples	Melon	Grapefruits	Plums
Bananas	Grapes	Prunes	Raisins
Berries	Oranges	Cherries	

Red Flags

Fruit juice concentrates calories and sugar and eliminates fiber. Eat the whole fruit for all the nutrients. Make sure that fruit drinks are 100% fruit and not sugar water with a little fruit juice. When purchasing frozen or canned fruit, be aware of extra sugar and calories in added sauces.

Preparation Pointer

Fruits make great snacks because they require very little preparation and most are portable for grab and go convenience. Some fruit can be washed and cut ahead of time like melons, others like berries will spoil faster and need to be prepped before eating. If you are looking to get more fruit into your diet, consider adding cut berries, grapes, or dried cranberries to your salad. Try pairing pork with apples, peaches, and apricots, chicken with citrus fruits, pears, peaches, prunes, or raisins.

Food Serving size	Cal.	(g) Total Fat	(g) Sat. Fat	(mg) Chol.	(g) Carb.	(g) Fiber	(g) Sug.	(g) Prot.	(mg) Sod.
Fruits									
Acerolas, (West Indian Cherry), Raw 1 fruit, without refuse (4.8g)	2	0	0	0	0	0.1	0	0	0
Apples, Canned, Sweetened, Sliced, Drained, Heated 1 cup, slices (204g)	137	1	0	0	34	4.1	30	0	6
Apples, Canned, Sweetened, Sliced, Drained, Unheated 1 cup, slices (204g)	137	1	0	0	34	3.5	31	0	6
Apples, Dehydrated (Low-moisture), Sulfured, Stewed 1 cup (193g)	143	0	0	0	38	5	0	1	50
Apples, Dehydrated (Low-moisture), Sulfured, Uncooked 1 cup (60g)	208	0	0	0	56	7.4	49	1	74
Apples, Dried, Sulfured, Stewed, with Sugar 1 cup (280g)	232	0	0	0	58	5.3	0	1	53
Apples, Dried, Sulfured, Stewed, Without Sugar 1 cup (255g)	145	0	0	0	39	5.1	34	1	51
Apples, Dried, Sulfured, Uncooked 1 ring (6.4g)	16	0	0	0	4	0.6	4	0	6
Apples, Frozen, Unsweetened, Heated 1 cup, slices (206g)	97	1	0	0	25	2.7	0	1	6
Apples, Frozen, Unsweetened, Unheated 1 cup, slices (173g)	83	1	0	0	21	2.2	17	0	5
Apples, Raw, Fuji, with Skin 1 large (236g)	149	0	0	0	36	5	28	0	2
Apples, Raw, Gala, with Skin 1 large (200g)	114	0	0	0	27	4.6	21	1	2
Apples, Raw, Golden Delicious, with Skin 1 large (215g)	123	0	0	0	29	5.2	22	1	4
Apples, Raw, Granny Smith, with Skin 1 large (206g)	119	0	0	0	28	5.8	20	1	2
Apples, Raw, Red Delicious, with Skin 1 large (260g)	153	1	0	0	37	6	27	1	3
Apples, Raw, with Skin 1 cup, slices (109g)	57	0	0	0	15	2.6	11	0	1

Food Serving size	Cal.	(g) Total Fat	(g) Sat. Fat	(mg) Chol.	(g) Carb.	(g) Fiber	(g) Sug.	(g) Prot.	(mg) Sod.
Apples, Raw, Without Skin									
1 large (3-1/4″ dia) (216g)	104	0	0	0	28	2.8	22	1	0
Apples, Raw, Without Skin, Cooked, Boiled									
1 cup, slices (171g)	91	1	0	0	23	4.1	19	0	2
Apples, Raw, Without Skin, Cooked, Microwave									
1 cup, slices (170g)	95	1	0	0	24	4.8	20	0	2
Applesauce, Canned, Sweetened, with Salt									
1 cup (255g)	194	0	0	0	51	3.1	0	0	71
Applesauce, Canned, Sweetened, Without Salt (Includes USDA Commodity)									
1 cup (246g)	167	0	0	0	43	3	36	0	5
Applesauce, Canned, Unsweetened, with Vitamin C									
1 cup (244g)	102	0	0	0	27	2.7	23	0	5
Applesauce, Canned, Unsweetened, Without Added Vitamin C (Includes USDA Commodity)									
1 cup (244g)	102	0	0	0	27	2.7	23	0	5
Apricot Nectar, Canned, Without Vitamin C									
1 fl oz (31.4g)	18	0	0	0	5	0.2	4	0	1
Apricots, Canned, Extra Heavy Syrup Packed, Without Skin, Solids and Liquids									
1 cup, whole, without pits (246g)	236	0	0	0	61	3.9	0	1	32
Apricots, Canned, Extra Light Syrup Packed, with Skin, Solids and Liquids									
1 cup, halves (247g)	121	0	0	0	31	4	0	1	5
Apricots, Canned, Heavy Syrup Packed, with Skin, Solids and Liquids									
1 cup, whole (240g)	199	0	0	0	52	3.8	48	1	10
Apricots, Canned, Heavy Syrup Packed, Without Skin, Solids and Liquids									
1 cup, whole, without pits (258g)	214	0	0	0	55	4.1	0	1	28
Apricots, Canned, Heavy Syrup, Drained									
1 cup, whole (182g)	151	0	0	0	39	4.9	34	1	7
Apricots, Canned, Juice Packed, with Skin, Solids and Liquids									
1 apricot, half with liquid (36g)	17	0	0	0	4	0.6	4	0	1
Apricots, Canned, Light Syrup Packed, with Skin, Solids and Liquids									
1 apricot, half with liquid (40g)	25	0	0	0	7	0.6	6	0	2
Apricots, Canned, Water Packed, with Skin, Solids and Liquids									
1 apricot, half with liquid (36g)	10	0	0	0	2	0.6	2	0	1

Food Serving size	Cal.	(g) Total Fat	(g) Sat. Fat	(mg) Chol.	(g) Carb.	(g) Fiber	(g) Sug.	(g) Prot.	(mg) Sod.
Apricots, Canned, Water Packed, Without Skin, Solids and Liquids									
1 cup, whole, without pits (227g)	50	0	0	0	12	2.5	0	2	25
Apricots, Dehydrated (Low-moisture), Sulfured, Stewed									
1 cup (249g)	314	1	0	0	81	0	0	5	12
Apricots, Dehydrated (Low-moisture), Sulfured, Uncooked									
1 cup (119g)	381	1	0	0	99	0	0	6	15
Apricots, Dried, Sulfured, Stewed, with Sugar									
1 cup, halves (270g)	305	0	0	0	79	11.1	0	3	8
Apricots, Dried, Sulfured, Stewed, Without Sugar									
1 cup, halves (250g)	213	0	0	0	55	6.5	49	3	10
Apricots, Dried, Sulfured, Uncooked									
1 half (3.5g)	8	0	0	0	2	0.3	2	0	0
Apricots, Frozen, Sweetened									
1 cup (242g)	237	0	0	0	61	5.3	0	2	10
Avocados, Raw, All Commercial Varieties									
1 cup, pureed (230g)	368	34	5	0	20	15.4	2	5	16
Avocados, Raw, California									
1 fruit, without skin and seed (136g)	227	21	3	0	12	9.2	0	3	11
Balsam-Pear (Bitter Gourd), Leafy Tips, Raw									
.5 cup (24g)	7	0	0	0	1	0	0	1	3
Balsam-Pear (Bitter Gourd), Pods, Cooked, Boiled, Drained, Without Salt									
.5 cup, (1/2" pieces) (62g)	12	0	0	0	3	1.2	1	1	4
Balsam-Pear (Bitter Gourd), Pods, Raw									
1 balsam-pear (124g)	21	0	0	0	5	3.5	0	1	6
Bananas, Dehydrated, or Banana Powder									
1 tbsp (6.2g)	21	0	0	0	5	0.6	3	0	0
Bananas, Raw									
1 cup, sliced (150g)	134	0	0	0	34	3.9	18	2	2
Blackberries, Canned, Heavy Syrup, Solids and Liquids									
1 cup (256g)	236	0	0	0	59	8.7	50	3	8
Blackberries, Frozen, Unsweetened									
1 package (18 oz) (510g)	326	2	0	0	80	25.5	54	6	5
Blueberries, Canned, Heavy Syrup, Solids and Liquids									
1 cup (256g)	225	1	0	0	56	4.1	52	2	8

Food Serving size	Cal.	(g) Total Fat	(g) Sat. Fat	(mg) Chol.	(g) Carb.	(g) Fiber	(g) Sug.	(g) Prot.	(mg) Sod.
Blueberries, Canned, Light Syrup, Drained 1 cup (244g)	215	1	0	0	55	6.3	43	3	7
Blueberries, Frozen, Sweetened 1 package (10 oz) (284g)	241	0	0	0	62	6.2	56	1	3
Blueberries, Frozen, Unsweetened 1 package (20 oz) (567g)	289	4	0	0	69	15.3	48	2	6
Blueberries, Raw 50 berries (68g)	39	0	0	0	10	1.6	7	1	1
Blueberries, Wild, Canned, Heavy Syrup, Drained 1 cup (319g)	341	1	0	0	90	15.6	62	2	3
Blueberries, Wild, Frozen 1 cup, frozen (140g)	80	0	0	0	19	6.2	0	0	4
Boysenberries, Canned, Heavy Syrup 1 cup (256g)	225	0	0	0	57	6.7	0	3	8
Boysenberries, Frozen, Unsweetened 1 package (10 oz) (284g)	142	1	0	0	35	15.1	20	3	3
Carambola (Starfruit), Raw 1 cup, sliced (108g)	33	0	0	0	7	3	4	1	2
Chayote, Fruit, Cooked, Boiled, Drained, Without Salt 1 cup (1" pieces) (160g)	38	1	0	0	8	4.5	0	1	2
Cherries, Sour, Red, Canned, Extra Heavy Syrup Packed, Solids and Liquids 1 cup (261g)	298	0	0	0	76	2.1	0	2	18
Cherries, Sour, Red, Canned, Heavy Syrup Packed, Solids and Liquids 1 cup (256g)	233	0	0	0	60	2.8	57	2	18
Cherries, Sour, Red, Canned, Light Syrup Packed, Solids and Liquids 1 cup (252g)	189	0	0	0	49	2	0	2	18
Cherries, Sour, Red, Canned, Water Packed, Solids and Liquids (Including USDA Commodity) 1 cup (244g)	88	0	0	0	22	2.7	19	2	17
Cherries, Sour, Red, Frozen, Unsweetened 1 package (18 oz) (510g)	235	2	1	0	56	8.2	46	5	5
Cherries, Sweet, Canned, Extra Heavy Syrup Packed, Solids and Liquids 1 cup, pitted (261g)	266	0	0	0	68	3.9	0	2	8
Cherries, Sweet, Canned, Juice Packed, Solids and Liquids 1 cup, pitted (250g)	135	0	0	0	35	3.8	31	2	8

Food Serving size	Cal.	(g) Total Fat	(g) Sat. Fat	(mg) Chol.	(g) Carb.	(g) Fiber	(g) Sug.	(g) Prot.	(mg) Sod.
Cherries, Sweet, Canned, Light Syrup Packed, Solids and Liquids									
1 cup, pitted (252g)	169	0	0	0	44	3.8	40	2	8
Cherries, Sweet, Canned, Pitted, Heavy Syrup Packed, Solids and Liquids									
1 cup (253g)	210	0	0	0	54	3.5	41	2	8
Cherries, Sweet, Canned, Water Packed, Solids and Liquids									
1 cup, pitted (248g)	114	0	0	0	29	3.7	25	2	2
Cherries, Sweet, Frozen, Sweetened									
1 package (10 oz) (284g)	253	0	0	0	64	6	58	3	3
Cherries, Sweetened, Canned, Pitted, Heavy Syrup, Drained									
1 cup (179g)	149	0	0	0	38	4.1	29	1	5
Clementines, Raw									
1 fruit (74g)	35	0	0	0	9	1.3	7	1	1
Cranberries, Dried, Sweetened									
.33 cup (40g)	123	1	0	0	33	2.3	26	0	1
Cranberry Sauce, Canned, Sweetened									
1 slice (1/2" thick, approx 8 slices per can) (57g)	86	0	0	0	22	0.6	22	0	17
Currants, European Black, Raw									
1 cup (112g)	71	0	0	0	17	0	0	2	2
Currants, Red and White, Raw									
1 cup (112g)	63	0	0	0	15	4.8	8	2	1
Currants, Zante, Dried									
1 cup (144g)	408	0	0	0	107	9.8	97	6	12
Dates, Deglet Noor									
1 date, pitted (7.1g)	20	0	0	0	5	0.6	4	0	0
Dates, Medjool									
1 date, pitted (24g)	66	0	0	0	18	1.6	16	0	0
Durians, Raw or Frozen									
1 fruit (602g)	885	32	0	0	163	22.9	0	9	12
Elderberries, Raw									
1 cup (145g)	106	1	0	0	27	10.2	0	1	9
Figs, Canned, Extra Heavy Syrup Packed, Solids and Liquids									
1 cup (261g)	279	0	0	0	73	0	0	1	3
Figs, Canned, Heavy Syrup Packed, Solids and Liquids									
1 fig, with liquid (28g)	25	0	0	0	6	0.6	6	0	0

Food Serving size	Cal.	(g) Total Fat	(g) Sat. Fat	(mg) Chol.	(g) Carb.	(g) Fiber	(g) Sug.	(g) Prot.	(mg) Sod.
Figs, Canned, Light Syrup Packed, Solids and Liquids									
1 fig, with liquid (28g)	19	0	0	0	5	0.5	5	0	0
Figs, Canned, Water Packed, Solids and Liquids									
1 fig, with liquid (27g)	14	0	0	0	4	0.6	3	0	0
Figs, Dried, Stewed									
1 cup (259g)	277	1	0	0	71	10.9	60	4	10
Figs, Dried, Uncooked									
1 fig (8.4g)	21	0	0	0	5	0.8	4	0	1
Fruit Butters, Apple									
1 tbsp (17g)	29	0	0	0	7	0.3	6	0	3
Fruit Cocktail, Canned, Extra Heavy Syrup, Solids and Liquids									
1 cup (260g)	229	0	0	0	60	2.9	0	1	16
Fruit Cocktail, Canned, Extra Light Syrup, Solids and Liquids									
.5 cup (123g)	55	0	0	0	14	1.4	0	0	5
Fruit Cocktail, Canned, Heavy Syrup, Drained									
1 cup (214g)	150	0	0	0	40	3.6	37	1	13
Fruit Cocktail, Canned, Heavy Syrup, Solids and Liquids									
1 cup (248g)	181	0	0	0	47	2.5	44	1	15
Fruit Cocktail, Canned, Juice Packed, Solids and Liquids									
1 cup (237g)	109	0	0	0	28	2.4	26	1	9
Fruit Cocktail, Canned, Light Syrup, Solids and Liquids									
1 cup (242g)	138	0	0	0	36	2.4	34	1	15
Fruit Cocktail, Canned, Water Packed, Solids and Liquids									
1 cup (237g)	76	0	0	0	20	2.4	18	1	9
Fruit Leather, Pieces									
1 package (27g)	97	1	0	0	22	0	16	0	109
Fruit Leather, Rolls									
1 small (14g)	52	0	0	0	12	0	7	0	44
Fruit Salad, Canned, Extra Heavy Syrup, Solids and Liquids									
1 cup (259g)	228	0	0	0	59	2.6	0	1	13
Fruit Salad, Canned, Heavy Syrup, Solids and Liquids									
1 cup (255g)	186	0	0	0	49	2.6	46	1	15
Fruit Salad, Canned, Juice Packed, Solids and Liquids									
1 cup (249g)	125	0	0	0	32	2.5	0	1	12

Food Serving size	Cal.	(g) Total Fat	(g) Sat. Fat	(mg) Chol.	(g) Carb.	(g) Fiber	(g) Sug.	(g) Prot.	(mg) Sod.
Fruit Salad, Canned, Light Syrup, Solids and Liquids 1 cup (252g)	146	0	0	0	38	2.5	0	1	15
Fruit Salad, Canned, Water Packed, Solids and Liquids 1 cup (245g)	74	0	0	0	19	2.5	0	1	7.
Fruit Salad, Tropical, Canned, with Heavy Syrup, Solids and Liquids 1 cup (257g)	221	0	0	0	57	3.3	0	1	5
Fruit, Mixed (Peach and Pear and Pineapple), Canned, Heavy Syrup, Solids and Liquids 1 cup (255g)	184	0	0	0	48	2.6	0	1	10
Fruit, Mixed (Peach, Cherry-Sweetened and Sour, Raspberry, Grape, Boysenberry) Frozen, Sweetened 1 package (10 oz) (284g)	278	1	0	0	69	5.4	0	4	9
Fruit, Mixed (Prune and Apricot and Pear), Dried 1 package (11 oz) (293g)	712	1	0	0	188	22.9	0	7	53
Gooseberries, Canned, Light Syrup Packed, Solids and Liquids 1 cup (252g)	184	1	0	0	47	6	0	2	5
Grapefruit, Raw, Pink and Red and White, All Areas .5 large (approx 4-1/2″ dia) (166g)	53	0	0	0	13	1.8	12	1	0
Grapefruit, Raw, Pink and Red, All Areas .5 fruit (3-3/4″ dia) (123g)	52	0	0	0	13	2	8	1	0
Grapefruit, Raw, Pink and Red, California and Arizona .5 fruit (3-3/4″ dia) (123g)	46	0	0	0	12	0	0	1	1
Grapefruit, Raw, Pink and Red, Florida .5 fruit (3-3/4″ dia) (123g)	37	0	0	0	9	1.4	0	1	0
Grapefruit, Raw, White, All Areas .5 fruit (3-3/4″ dia) (118g)	39	0	0	0	10	1.3	9	1	0
Grapefruit, Raw, White, California .5 fruit (3-3/4″ dia) (118g)	44	0	0	0	11	0	0	1	0
Grapefruit, Raw, White, Florida .5 fruit (3-3/4″ dia) (118g)	38	0	0	0	10	0	0	1	0
Grapefruit, Sections, Canned, Juice Packed, Solids and Liquids 1 cup (249g)	92	0	0	0	23	1	22	2	17
Grapefruit, Sections, Canned, Light Syrup Packed, Solids and Liquids 1 cup (254g)	152	0	0	0	39	1	38	1	5

Food Serving size	Cal.	(g) Total Fat	(g) Sat. Fat	(mg) Chol.	(g) Carb.	(g) Fiber	(g) Sug.	(g) Prot.	(mg) Sod.
Grapefruit, Sections, Canned, Water Packed, Solids and Liquids									
1 cup (244g)	88	0	0	0	22	1	21	1	5
Grapes, American Type (Slip Skin), Raw									
1 grape (2.4g)	2	0	0	0	0	0	0	0	0
Grapes, Canned, Thompson Seedless, Heavy Syrup Packed, Solids and Liquids									
1 cup (256g)	195	0	0	0	50	1.5	49	1	13
Grapes, Canned, Thompson Seedless, Water Packed, Solids and Liquids									
1 cup (245g)	98	0	0	0	25	1.5	24	1	15
Grapes, Muscadine, Raw									
1 grape (6g)	3	0	0	0	1	0.2	0	0	0
Grapes, Red or Green (European Type, Such as Thompson Seedless), Raw									
10 grapes (49g)	34	0	0	0	9	0.4	8	0	1
Guava Nectar, Canned									
1 cup (251g)	158	0	0	0	41	2.5	33	0	15
Guavas, Common, Raw									
1 fruit, without refuse (55g)	37	1	0	0	8	3	5	1	1
Guavas, Strawberry, Raw									
1 fruit, without refuse (6g)	4	0	0	0	1	0.3	0	0	2
Jackfruit, Raw									
1 cup, 1″ pieces (151g)	143	1	0	0	35	2.3	29	3	3
Java-plum (Jambolan), Raw									
3 fruits (9g)	5	0	0	0	1	0	0	0	1
Kiwifruit, Gold, Raw									
1 fruit (86g)	52	0	0	0	12	1.7	9	1	3
Kiwifruit, Green, Raw									
1 fruit (2″ diameter) (69g)	42	0	0	0	10	2.1	6	1	2
Kumquats, Raw									
1 fruit, without refuse (19g)	13	0	0	0	3	1.2	2	0	2
Lemon Peel, Raw									
1 tsp (2g)	1	0	0	0	0	0.2	0	0	0
Lemons, Raw, Without Peel									
1 fruit (2-1/8″ diameter) (58g)	17	0	0	0	5	1.6	1	1	1
Litchis, Dried									
1 fruit (2.5g)	6	0	0	0	1	0.1	1	0	0

Food Serving size	Cal.	(g) Total Fat	(g) Sat. Fat	(mg) Chol.	(g) Carb.	(g) Fiber	(g) Sug.	(g) Prot.	(mg) Sod.
Litchis, Raw 1 fruit, without refuse (9.6g)	6	0	0	0	2	0.1	1	0	0
Loganberries, Frozen 1 cup, unthawed (147g)	81	0	0	0	19	7.8	11	2	1
Longans, Raw 1 fruit, without refuse (3.2g)	2	0	0	0	0	0	0	0	0
Loquats, Raw 1 large (20g)	9	0	0	0	2	0.3	0	0	0
Mammy-apple (Mamey), Raw 1 fruit, without refuse (846g)	431	4	1	0	106	25.4	0	4	127
Mango Nectar, Canned 1 cup (251g)	128	0	0	0	33	0.8	31	0	13
Mangos, Raw 1 fruit, without refuse (336g)	202	1	0	0	50	5.4	46	3	3
Mangosteen, Canned, Syrup Packed 1 cup (216g)	158	1	0	0	39	3.9	0	1	15
Maraschino Cherries, Canned, Drained 1 cherry (NLEA serving) (5g)	8	0	0	0	2	0.2	2	0	0
Melon Balls, Frozen 1 cup, unthawed (173g)	57	0	0	0	14	1.2	0	1	54
Melon, Cantaloupe, Raw 1 cup, cubes (160g)	54	0	0	0	13	1.4	13	1	26
Melon, Casaba, Raw 1 melon (1640g)	459	2	0	0	108	14.8	93	18	148
Melon, Honeydew, Raw 1 cup, balls (177g)	64	0	0	0	16	1.4	14	1	32
Mulberries, Raw 10 fruits (15g)	6	0	0	0	1	0.3	1	0	2
Nance, Frozen, Unsweetened 3 fruits, without pits thawed (9.8g)	7	0	0	0	2	0.7	1	0	0
Nectarines, Raw 1 small (2-1/3″ dia) (129g)	57	0	0	0	14	2.2	10	1	0
Orange Peel, Raw 1 tsp (2g)	2	0	0	0	1	0.2	0	0	0

Food Serving size	Cal.	(g) Total Fat	(g) Sat. Fat	(mg) Chol.	(g) Carb.	(g) Fiber	(g) Sug.	(g) Prot.	(mg) Sod.
Oranges, Raw, California, Valencia 1 fruit (2-5/8″ dia) (121g)	59	0	0	0	14	3	0	1	0
Oranges, Raw, All Commercial Varieties 1 large (3-1/16″ dia) (184g)	86	0	0	0	22	4.4	17	2	0
Oranges, Raw, Florida 1 fruit (2-5/8″ dia) (141g)	65	0	0	0	16	3.4	13	1	0
Oranges, Raw, Navels 1 fruit (2-7/8″ dia) (140g)	69	0	0	0	18	3.1	12	1	1
Oranges, Raw, with Peel 1 fruit, without seeds (159g)	100	0	0	0	25	7.2	0	2	3
Orange-strawberry-banana Juice 1 fl oz (29.2g)	15	0	0	0	4	0.1	0	0	1
Papaya Nectar, Canned 1 fl oz (31.2g)	18	0	0	0	5	0.2	4	0	2
Papaya, Canned, Heavy Syrup, Drained 1 piece (39g)	80	0	0	0	22	0.6	20	0	4
Passion-fruit (Granadilla), Purple, Raw 1 fruit, without refuse (18g)	17	0	0	0	4	1.9	2	0	5
Passion-fruit Juice, Purple, Raw 1 fl oz (30.9g)	16	0	0	0	4	0.1	4	0	2
Passion-fruit Juice, Yellow, Raw 1 fl oz (30.9g)	19	0	0	0	4	0.1	4	0	2
Peaches, Canned, Extra Heavy Syrup Pack, Solids and Liquids 1 cup, halves or slices (262g)	252	0	0	0	68	2.6	0	1	21
Peaches, Canned, Extra Light Syrup, Solids and Liquids 1 cup, halves or slices (247g)	104	0	0	0	27	2.5	0	1	12
Peaches, Canned, Heavy Syrup Pack, Solids and Liquids 1 half, with liquid (98g)	73	0	0	0	20	1.3	18	0	6
Peaches, Canned, Heavy Syrup, Drained 1 half (73g)	53	0	0	0	13	0.9	11	0	4
Peaches, Canned, Juice Packed, Solids and Liquids 1 cup, halves or slices (248g)	109	0	0	0	29	3.2	25	2	10
Peaches, Canned, Light Syrup Pack, Solids and Liquids 1 half, with liquid (98g)	53	0	0	0	14	1.3	13	0	5

Food Serving size	Cal.	(g) Total Fat	(g) Sat. Fat	(mg) Chol.	(g) Carb.	(g) Fiber	(g) Sug.	(g) Prot.	(mg) Sod.
Peaches, Canned, Water Packed, Solids and Liquids									
1 half, with liquid (98g)	24	0	0	0	6	1.3	5	0	3
Peaches, Dehydrated (Low-moisture), Sulfured, Stewed									
1 cup (242g)	322	1	0	0	83	0	0	5	10
Peaches, Dehydrated (Low-moisture), Sulfured, Uncooked									
1 cup (116g)	377	1	0	0	96	0	0	6	12
Peaches, Dried, Sulfured, Stewed, with Sugar									
1 cup (270g)	278	1	0	0	72	6.5	0	3	5
Peaches, Dried, Sulfured, Stewed, Without Sugar									
1 cup (258g)	199	1	0	0	51	7	44	3	5
Peaches, Dried, Sulfured, Uncooked									
1 half (13g)	31	0	0	0	8	1.1	5	0	1
Peaches, Frozen, Sliced, Sweetened									
10 slices (155g)	146	0	0	0	37	2.8	34	1	9
Peaches, Raw									
1 small (2-1/2″ dia) (130g)	51	0	0	0	12	2	11	1	0
Peaches, Spiced, Canned, Heavy Syrup Pack, Solids and Liquids									
1 cup, whole (242g)	182	0	0	0	49	3.1	45	1	10
Pears, Asian, Raw									
1 fruit, 3-3/8″ high x 3″ diameter (275g)	116	1	0	0	29	9.9	19	1	0
Pears, Canned, Extra Heavy Syrup Pack, Solids and Liquids									
1 half, with liquid (79g)	77	0	0	0	20	1.3	0	0	4
Pears, Canned, Extra Light Syrup Pack, Solids and Liquids									
1 half, with liquid (76g)	36	0	0	0	9	1.2	0	0	2
Pears, Canned, Heavy Syrup Pack, Solids and Liquids									
1 half, with liquid (76g)	56	0	0	0	15	1.2	12	0	4
Pears, Canned, Heavy Syrup, Drained									
1 half (48g)	36	0	0	0	9	1.3	8	0	2
Pears, Canned, Juice Packed, Solids and Liquids									
1 half, with liquid (76g)	38	0	0	0	10	1.2	7	0	3
Pears, Canned, Light Syrup Pack, Solids and Liquids									
1 half, with liquid (76g)	43	0	0	0	12	1.2	9	0	4
Pears, Canned, Water Packed, Solids and Liquids									
1 half, with liquid (76g)	22	0	0	0	6	1.2	5	0	2

Food Serving size	Cal.	(g) Total Fat	(g) Sat. Fat	(mg) Chol.	(g) Carb.	(g) Fiber	(g) Sug.	(g) Prot.	(mg) Sod.
Pears, Dried, Sulfured, Stewed, with Sugar									
1 cup, halves (280g)	392	1	0	0	104	16.2	0	2	8
Pears, Dried, Sulfured, Stewed, Without Sugar									
1 cup, halves (255g)	324	1	0	0	86	16.3	70	2	8
Pears, Dried, Sulfured, Uncooked									
1 half (18g)	47	0	0	0	13	1.4	11	0	1
Pears, Raw, Bartlett									
1 small (152g)	96	0	0	0	23	4.7	15	1	2
Pears, Raw, Bosc									
1 small (159g)	107	0	0	0	26	4.9	16	1	2
Pears, Raw, Green Anjou									
1 small (172g)	114	0	0	0	27	5.3	17	1	2
Pears, Raw, Red Anjou									
1 medium (157g)	97	0	0	0	23	4.7	15	1	2
Persimmons, Japanese, Dried									
1 fruit, without refuse (34g)	93	0	0	0	25	4.9	0	0	1
Persimmons, Japanese, Raw									
1 fruit (2-1/2″ dia) (168g)	118	0	0	0	31	6	21	1	2
Persimmons, Native, Raw									
1 fruit, without refuse (25g)	32	0	0	0	8	0	0	0	0
Pineapple, Canned, Extra Heavy Syrup Packed, Solids and Liquids									
1 cup, crushed, sliced, or chunks (260g)	216	0	0	0	56	2.1	0	1	3
Pineapple, Canned, Heavy Syrup Packed, Solids and Liquids									
1 slice, or ring (3″ dia) with liquid (49g)	38	0	0	0	10	0.4	8	0	0
Pineapple, Canned, Juice Packed, Drained									
1 cup, crushed (195g)	117	0	0	0	30	2.5	28	1	2
Pineapple, Canned, Juice Packed, Solids and Liquids									
1 slice, or ring (3″ dia) with liquid (47g)	28	0	0	0	7	0.4	7	0	0
Pineapple, Canned, Light Syrup Packed, Solids and Liquids									
1 slice, or ring (3″ dia) with liquid (48g)	25	0	0	0	6	0.4	6	0	0

Food Serving size	Cal.	(g) Total Fat	(g) Sat. Fat	(mg) Chol.	(g) Carb.	(g) Fiber	(g) Sug.	(g) Prot.	(mg) Sod.
Pineapple, Canned, Water Packed, Solids and Liquids 1 slice, or ring (3″ dia) with liquid (47g)	15	0	0	0	4	0.4	4	0	0
Pineapple, Frozen, Chunks, Sweetened 1 cup, chunks (245g)	211	0	0	0	54	2.7	52	1	5
Pineapple, Raw, All Varieties 1 fruit (905g)	453	1	0	0	119	12.7	89	5	9
Pineapple, Raw, Extra Sweet Variety 1 slice (4-2/3″ dia x 3/4″ thick) (166g)	85	0	0	0	22	2.3	17	1	2
Pineapple, Raw, Traditional Variety 1 slice (4-2/3″ dia x 3/4″ thick) (175g)	79	0	0	0	21	0	15	1	2
Pitanga, (Surinam-Cherry), Raw 1 fruit, without refuse (7g)	2	0	0	0	1	0	0	0	0
Plantains, Cooked 1 cup, slices (154g)	179	0	0	0	48	3.5	22	1	8
Plantains, Green, Fried 10 slices (1/4″ thick) (53g)	164	6	2	0	26	1.9	2	1	1
Plantains, Raw 1 medium (179g)	218	1	0	0	57	4.1	27	2	7
Plantains, Yellow, Fried, Latino Restaurant 1 cup (169g)	399	13	3	0	69	5.4	37	2	10
Plums, Canned, Heavy Syrup, Drained 1 cup, with pits yields (183g)	163	0	0	0	42	2.7	39	1	35
Plums, Canned, Purple, Extra Heavy Syrup Packed, Solids and Liquids 1 cup, pitted (261g)	264	0	0	0	69	2.6	0	1	50
Plums, Canned, Purple, Heavy Syrup Packed, Solids and Liquids 1 plum, with liquid (46g)	41	0	0	0	11	0.4	10	0	9
Plums, Canned, Purple, Juice Packed, Solids and Liquids 1 plum, with liquid (46g)	27	0	0	0	7	0.4	7	0	0
Plums, Canned, Purple, Light Syrup Packed, Solids and Liquids 1 plum, with liquid (46g)	29	0	0	0	7	0.4	7	0	9
Plums, Canned, Purple, Water Packed, Solids and Liquids 1 plum, with liquid (46g)	19	0	0	0	5	0.4	5	0	0

Food Serving size	Cal.	(g) Total Fat	(g) Sat. Fat	(mg) Chol.	(g) Carb.	(g) Fiber	(g) Sug.	(g) Prot.	(mg) Sod.
Plums, Dried (Prunes), Sweetened, with Added Sugar									
1 cup, pitted (248g)	308	1	0	0	82	9.4	0	3	5
Plums, Dried (Prunes), Sweetened, Without Added Sugar									
1 cup, pitted (248g)	265	0	0	0	70	7.7	62	2	2
Plums, Dried (Prunes), Uncooked									
1 prune, pitted (9.5g)	23	0	0	0	6	0.7	4	0	0
Pomegranates, Raw									
1 pomegranate, (4″ diameter) (282g)									
	234	3	0	0	53	11.3	39	5	8
Prickly Pears, Raw									
1 fruit, without refuse (103g)	42	1	0	0	10	3.7	0	1	5
Prunes, Canned, Heavy Syrup Packed, Solids and Liquids									
5 prunes, with liquid (86g)	90	0	0	0	24	3.3	0	1	3
Prunes, Dehydrated (Low-moisture), Sweetened									
1 cup (280g)	316	1	0	0	83	0	0	3	6
Prunes, Dehydrated (Low-moisture), Uncooked									
1 cup (132g)	447	1	0	0	118	0	0	5	7
Pummelo, Raw									
1 fruit, without refuse (609g)	231	0	0	0	59	6.1	0	5	6
Quinces, Raw									
1 fruit, without refuse (92g)	52	0	0	0	14	1.7	0	0	4
Raisins, Golden, Seedless									
1 cup (not packed) (145g)	438	1	0	0	115	5.8	86	5	17
Raisins, Seeded									
1 cup (not packed) (145g)	429	1	0	0	114	9.9	0	4	41
Raisins, Seedless									
1 cup (not packed) (145g)	434	1	0	0	115	5.4	86	4	16
Rambutan, Canned, Syrup Packed									
1 cup (214g)	175	0	0	0	45	1.9	0	1	24
Raspberries, Canned, Red, Heavy Syrup Packed, Solids and Liquids									
1 cup (256g)	233	0	0	0	60	8.4	51	2	8
Raspberries, Frozen, Red, Sweetened									
1 package (10 oz) (284g)	293	0	0	0	74	12.5	62	2	3

Food Serving size	Cal.	(g) Total Fat	(g) Sat. Fat	(mg) Chol.	(g) Carb.	(g) Fiber	(g) Sug.	(g) Prot.	(mg) Sod.
Raspberries, Raw 1 pint, as purchased, yields (312g)	162	2	0	0	37	20.3	14	4	3
Sapodilla, Raw 1 sapodilla (170g)	141	2	0	0	34	9	0	1	20
Sapote, Mamey, Raw 1 fruit, without refuse (558g)	692	3	1	0	179	30.1	112	8	39
Squash, Summer, All Varieties, Cooked, Boiled, Drained, with Salt 1 cup, slices (180g)	36	1	0	0	8	2.5	5	2	427
Squash, Summer, All Varieties, Cooked, Boiled, Drained, Without Salt 1 cup, sliced (180g)	36	1	0	0	8	2.5	5	2	2
Squash, Summer, All Varieties, Raw 1 large (323g)	52	1	0	0	11	3.6	7	4	6
Squash, Summer, Crookneck and Straightneck, Canned, Drained, Solid, Without Salt 1 cup, mashed (240g)	31	0	0	0	7	3.4	3	1	12
Squash, Summer, Crookneck and Straightneck, Cooked, Boiled, Drained, with Salt 1 cup, slices (180g)	34	1	0	0	7	2	4	2	427
Squash, Summer, Crookneck and Straightneck, Cooked, Boiled, Drained, Without Salt .5 cup, slices (90g)	21	0	0	0	3	1	2	1	1
Squash, Summer, Crookneck and Straightneck, Frozen, Cooked, Boiled, Drained, with Salt 1 cup, slices (192g)	48	0	0	0	11	2.7	4	2	465
Squash, Summer, Crookneck and Straightneck, Frozen, Cooked, Boiled, Drained, Without Salt 1 cup, slices (192g)	48	0	0	0	11	2.7	4	2	12
Squash, Summer, Crookneck and Straightneck, Frozen, Unprepared 1 cup, slices (130g)	26	0	0	0	6	1.6	0	1	7
Squash, Summer, Crookneck and Straightneck, Raw 1 cup, sliced (127g)	24	0	0	0	5	1.3	4	1	3
Squash, Summer, Scallop, Cooked, Boiled, Drained, with Salt .5 cup, mashed (120g)	19	0	0	0	4	2.3	2	1	284
Squash, Summer, Scallop, Cooked, Boiled, Drained, Without Salt 1 cup, sliced (180g)	29	0	0	0	6	3.4	3	2	2

Food Serving size	Cal.	(g) Total Fat	(g) Sat. Fat	(mg) Chol.	(g) Carb.	(g) Fiber	(g) Sug.	(g) Prot.	(mg) Sod.
Squash, Summer, Scallop, Raw									
1 cup, slices (130g)	23	0	0	0	5	0	0	2	1
Squash, Summer, Zucchini, Including Skin, Cooked, Boiled, Drained, with Salt									
.5 cup, mashed (120g)	18	0	0	0	3	1.2	2	1	287
Squash, Summer, Zucchini, Including Skin, Cooked, Boiled, Drained, Without Salt									
.5 cup, mashed (120g)	18	0	0	0	3	1.2	2	1	4
Squash, Summer, Zucchini, Including Skin, Frozen, Cooked, Boiled, Drained, with Salt									
1 cup (223g)	31	0	0	0	7	2.9	4	3	531
Squash, Summer, Zucchini, Including Skin, Frozen, Cooked, Boiled, Drained, Without Salt									
1 cup (223g)	38	0	0	0	8	2.9	4	3	4
Squash, Summer, Zucchini, Including Skin, Frozen, Unprepared									
1 package (3 lb) (1361g)	231	2	0	0	49	17.7	23	16	27
Squash, Summer, Zucchini, Including Skin, Raw									
1 cup, sliced (113g)	19	0	0	0	4	1.1	3	1	9
Squash, Summer, Zucchini, Italian Style, Canned									
1 cup (227g)	66	0	0	0	16	0	0	2	849
Squash, Winter, Acorn, Cooked, Baked, with Salt									
1 cup, cubes (205g)	115	0	0	0	30	9	0	2	492
Squash, Winter, Acorn, Cooked, Baked, Without Salt									
1 cup, cubes (205g)	115	0	0	0	30	9	0	2	8
Squash, Winter, Acorn, Cooked, Boiled, Mashed, with Salt									
1 cup, mashed (245g)	83	0	0	0	22	6.4	0	2	586
Squash, Winter, Acorn, Cooked, Boiled, Mashed, Without Salt									
1 cup, mashed (245g)	83	0	0	0	22	6.4	0	2	7
Squash, Winter, Acorn, Raw									
1 squash (4 inch dia) (431g)	172	0	0	0	45	6.5	0	3	13
Squash, Winter, All Varieties, Cooked, Baked, with Salt									
1 cup, cubes (205g)	80	1	0	0	18	5.7	7	2	486
Squash, Winter, All Varieties, Cooked, Baked, Without Salt									
1 cup, cubes (205g)	76	1	0	0	18	5.7	7	2	2
Squash, Winter, All Varieties, Raw									
1 cup, cubes (116g)	39	0	0	0	10	1.7	3	1	5

Food Serving size	Cal.	(g) Total Fat	(g) Sat. Fat	(mg) Chol.	(g) Carb.	(g) Fiber	(g) Sug.	(g) Prot.	(mg) Sod.
Squash, Winter, Butternut, Cooked, Baked, with Salt									
1 cup, cubes (205g)	82	0	0	0	22	6.6	4	2	492
Squash, Winter, Butternut, Cooked, Baked, Without Salt									
1 cup, cubes (205g)	82	0	0	0	22	6.6	4	2	8
Squash, Winter, Butternut, Frozen, Cooked, Boiled, with Salt									
1 cup, mashed (240g)	94	0	0	0	24	0	0	3	571
Squash, Winter, Butternut, Frozen, Cooked, Boiled, Without Salt									
1 cup, mashed (240g)	94	0	0	0	24	0	0	3	5
Squash, Winter, Butternut, Frozen, Unprepared									
1 package (4 lb) (1814g)	1034	2	0	0	261	23.6	51	32	36
Squash, Winter, Butternut, Raw									
1 cup, cubes (140g)	63	0	0	0	16	2.8	3	1	6
Squash, Winter, Hubbard, Cooked, Baked, with Salt									
1 cup, cubes (205g)	103	1	0	0	22	0	0	5	500
Squash, Winter, Hubbard, Cooked, Baked, Without Salt									
1 cup, cubes (205g)	103	1	0	0	22	10	10	5	16
Squash, Winter, Hubbard, Cooked, Boiled, Mashed, with Salt									
1 cup, mashed (236g)	71	1	0	0	15	6.8	7	3	569
Squash, Winter, Hubbard, Cooked, Boiled, Mashed, Without Salt									
1 cup, mashed (236g)	71	1	0	0	15	6.8	7	3	12
Squash, Winter, Hubbard, Raw									
1 cup, cubes (116g)	46	1	0	0	10	0	0	2	8
Squash, Winter, Spaghetti, Cooked, Boiled, Drained or Baked, with Salt									
1 cup (155g)	42	0	0	0	10	2.2	4	1	394
Squash, Winter, Spaghetti, Cooked, Boiled, Drained or Baked, Without Salt									
1 cup (155g)	42	0	0	0	10	2.2	4	1	28
Squash, Winter, Spaghetti, Raw									
1 cup, cubes (101g)	31	1	0	0	7	0	0	1	17
Squash, Zucchini, Baby, Raw									
1 medium (11g)	2	0	0	0	0	0.1	0	0	0
Strawberries, Canned, Heavy Syrup Packed, Solids and Liquids									
1 cup (254g)	234	1	0	0	60	4.3	55	1	10
Strawberries, Frozen, Sweetened, Sliced									
1 package (10 oz) (284g)	273	0	0	0	74	5.4	68	2	9

Food Serving size	Cal.	(g) Total Fat	(g) Sat. Fat	(mg) Chol.	(g) Carb.	(g) Fiber	(g) Sug.	(g) Prot.	(mg) Sod.
Strawberries, Frozen, Sweetened, Whole									
1 package (10 oz) (284g)	222	0	0	0	60	5.4	53	1	3
Strawberries, Frozen, Unsweetened									
1 cup, unthawed (149g)	52	0	0	0	14	3.1	7	1	3
Strawberries, Raw									
1 cup, pureed (232g)	74	1	0	0	18	4.6	11	2	2
Sugar-Apples, (Sweetsop), Raw									
1 fruit, (2-7/8″ diameter) (155g)	146	0	0	0	37	6.8	0	3	14
Tamarinds, Raw									
1 fruit (3″ x 1″) (2g)	5	0	0	0	1	0.1	1	0	1
Tangerines (Mandarin Oranges), Canned, Juice Packed									
1 cup (249g)	92	0	0	0	24	1.7	22	2	12
Tangerines (Mandarin Oranges), Canned, Juice Packed, Drained									
1 cup (189g)	72	0	0	0	18	2.3	16	1	9
Tangerines (Mandarin Oranges), Canned, Light Syrup Packed									
1 cup (252g)	154	0	0	0	41	1.8	39	1	15
Tangerines (Mandarin Oranges), Raw									
1 small (2-1/4″ dia) (76g)	40	0	0	0	10	1.4	8	1	2
Tomatillos, Raw									
.5 cup, chopped or diced (66g)	21	1	0	0	4	1.3	3	1	1
Watermelon, Raw									
1 cup, diced (152g)	46	0	0	0	11	0.6	9	1	2

Fruit Juice Drinks/Juice Cocktails

Food Serving size	Cal.	(g) Total Fat	(g) Sat. Fat	(mg) Chol.	(g) Carb.	(g) Fiber	(g) Sug.	(g) Prot.	(mg) Sod.
Apple Cider-flavored Drink, Powder, Low Calorie, with Vitamin C, Prepared									
1 fl oz (30g)	0	0	0	0	0	0	0	0	4
Apple Cider-flavored Drink, Powder, Vitamin C and Sugar									
1 packet (21g)	83	0	0	0	21	0	1	0	20
Apple Juice, Canned or Bottled, Unsweetened, with Added Vitamin C									
1 fl oz (31g)	14	0	0	0	4	0.1	3	0	1
Apple Juice, Canned or Bottled, Unsweetened, with Added Vitamin C, Calcium, and Potassium									
10 fl oz (295g)	142	1	0	0	34	0.9	28	0	15
Apple Juice, Canned or Bottled, Unsweetened, Without Added Vitamin C									
1 fl oz (31g)	14	0	0	0	4	0.1	3	0	1

Food Serving size	Cal.	(g) Total Fat	(g) Sat. Fat	(mg) Chol.	(g) Carb.	(g) Fiber	(g) Sug.	(g) Prot.	(mg) Sod.
Apple Juice, Frozen Concentrate, Unsweetened, Diluted with 3 Volumes Water, with Vitamin C									
1 fl oz (29.9g)	14	0	0	0	3	0	0	0	2
Apple Juice, Frozen Concentrate, Unsweetened, Diluted, with 3 Volumes Water, Without Vitamin C									
1 fl oz (29.9g)	14	0	0	0	3	0	3	0	2
Apple Juice, Frozen Concentrate, Unsweetened, Undiluted, with Vitamin C									
1 can (6 fl oz) (211g)	350	1	0	0	87	0	82	1	53
Apple Juice, Frozen Concentrate, Unsweetened, Undiluted, Without Vitamin C									
1 can (6 fl oz) (211g)	350	1	0	0	87	0.8	82	1	53
Apricot Nectar, Canned, with Vitamin C									
1 fl oz (31.4g)	18	0	0	0	5	0.2	0	0	1
Apricot Nectar, Canned, Without Vitamin C									
1 fl oz (31.4g)	18	0	0	0	5	0.2	4	0	1
Apricots, Canned, Water Packed, with Skin, Solids and Liquids									
1 apricot, half with liquid (36g)	10	0	0	0	2	0.6	2	0	1
Blackberry Juice, Canned									
1 cup (250g)	95	2	0	0	20	0.3	19	1	3
Citrus Fruit Juice Drink, Frozen Concentrate									
1 can (12 fl oz) (423g)	685	0	0	0	170	0.8	121	5	13
Citrus Fruit Juice Drink, Frozen Concentrate, Prepared with Water									
1 serving, 8 fl oz (237g)	111	0	0	0	28	0	23	0	9
Cranberry Juice Cocktail, Bottled									
1 cup (8 fl oz) (253g)	137	0	0	0	34	0	30	0	5
Cranberry Juice Cocktail, Bottled, Low Calorie, with Calcium, Saccharin and Corn Sweetener									
1 cup (8 fl oz) (237g)	45	0	0	0	11	0	11	0	7
Cranberry Juice Cocktail, Frozen Concentrate									
1 can (12 fl oz) (435g)	874	0	0	0	224	0.9	185	0	17
Cranberry Juice Cocktail, Frozen Concentrate, Prepared with Water									
1 fl oz (29.6g)	14	0	0	0	3	0	3	0	1
Cranberry Juice, Unsweetened									
1 fl oz (31.6g)	15	0	0	0	4	0	0	0	1
Cranberry-apple Juice Drink, Bottled									
1 cup (8 fl oz) (245g)	154	0	0	0	39	0	36	0	5

Food Serving size	Cal.	(g) Total Fat	(g) Sat. Fat	(mg) Chol.	(g) Carb.	(g) Fiber	(g) Sug.	(g) Prot.	(mg) Sod.
Cranberry-apple Juice Drink, Low Calorie, with Vitamin C									
1 fl oz (30g)	6	0	0	0	1	0	0	0	2
Cranberry-apricot Juice Drink, Bottled									
1 cup (8 fl oz) (245g)	157	0	0	0	40	0.2	0	0	5
Cranberry-grape Juice Drink, Bottled									
1 cup (8 fl oz) (245g)	137	0	0	0	34	0.2	0	0	7
Fruit Punch Drink, Frozen Concentrate									
1 can (12 fl oz) (418g)	677	0	0	0	173	1.7	0	1	33
Grape Juice Cocktail, Frozen Concentrate, Diluted with 3 Volumes Water with Added Vitamin C									
1 fl oz (31.2g)	16	0	0	0	4	0	4	0	1
Grape Juice Cocktail, Frozen Concentrate, Undiluted, with Added Vitamin C									
1 can (6 fl oz) (216g)	387	1	0	0	96	0.6	95	1	15
Grape Juice Drink, Canned									
1 fl oz (31.3g)	18	0	0	0	5	0	4	0	3
Grape Juice, Canned or Bottled, Unsweetened, with Added Vitamin C and Calcium									
1 fl oz (31.6g)	20	0	0	0	5	0.1	4	0	2
Grape Juice, Canned or Bottled, Unsweetened, Without Added Vitamin C									
1 fl oz (31.6g)	19	0	0	0	5	0.1	4	0	2
Grapefruit Juice, Pink, Raw									
1 fruit, yields (196g)	76	0	0	0	18	0	0	1	2
Grapefruit Juice, White, Canned, Sweetened									
1 fl oz (31.2g)	14	0	0	0	3	0	3	0	1
Grapefruit Juice, White, Canned, Unsweetened									
1 fl oz (30.9g)	12	0	0	0	3	0	3	0	0
Grapefruit Juice, White, Frozen Concentrate, Unsweetened, Diluted with 3 Volumes Water									
1 fl oz (30.9g)	13	0	0	0	3	0	3	0	0
Grapefruit Juice, White, Frozen Concentrate, Unsweetened, Undiluted									
1 can (6 fl oz) (207g)	302	1	0	0	72	0.8	71	4	6
Grapefruit Juice, White, Raw									
1 fl oz (30.9g)	12	0	0	0	3	0	3	0	0
Juice, Apple and Grape Blend, with Added Vitamin C									
8 fl oz (250g)	125	0	0	0	31	0	27	0	18

Food Serving size	Cal.	(g) Total Fat	(g) Sat. Fat	(mg) Chol.	(g) Carb.	(g) Fiber	(g) Sug.	(g) Prot.	(mg) Sod.
Juice, Apple, Grape, and Pear Blend, with Added Ascorbic Acid and Calcium									
8 fl oz (250g)	130	0	0	0	32	0.5	25	0	13
Lemon Juice, Canned or Bottled									
1 tbsp (15g)	3	0	0	0	1	0.1	0	0	3
Lemon Juice, Frozen, Unsweetened, Single Strength									
1 fl oz (30.5g)	7	0	0	0	2	0.1	1	0	0
Lemon Juice, Raw									
1 fl oz (30.5g)	7	0	0	0	2	0.1	1	0	0
Lemonade, Frozen Concentrate, Pink, Prepared with Water									
1 fl oz (30.9g)	13	0	0	0	3	0	3	0	1
Lemonade, Frozen Concentrate, White									
1 can (12 fl oz) (438g)	858	3	0	0	219	1.3	195	1	31
Lemonade, Frozen Concentrate, White, Prepared with Water									
1 fl oz (30.9g)	12	0	0	0	3	0	3	0	1
Lemonade, Low Calorie, with Aspartame, Powder									
1 serving (2g)	7	0	0	0	2	0	0	0	0
Lemonade, Low Calorie, with Aspartame, Powder, Prepared with Water									
1 fl oz (29.8g)	1	0	0	0	0	0	0	0	1
Lime Juice, Canned or Bottled, Unsweetened									
1 fl oz (30.8g)	6	0	0	0	2	0.1	0	0	5
Lime Juice, Raw									
1 fl oz (30.8g)	8	0	0	0	3	0.1	1	0	1
Limeade, Frozen Concentrate									
1 can (12 fl oz) (437g)	1079	0	0	0	272	0	262	0	0
Limeade, Frozen Concentrate, Prepared with Water									
1 serving, 1 cup 8 fl oz (247g)	128	0	0	0	34	0	33	0	7
Limes, Raw									
1 NLEA serving (67g)	20	0	0	0	7	1.9	1	0	1
Orange and Apricot Juice Drink, Canned									
1 cup, (8 fl oz) (250g)	128	0	0	0	32	0.3	30	1	5
Orange Breakfast Drink, Ready-to-drink									
1 fl oz (31.3g)	13	0	0	0	3	0.1	2	0	1
Orange Breakfast Drink, Ready-to-drink, with Added Nutrients									
1 cup (8 fl oz) (253g)	134	0	0	0	33	0.3	20	0	137

Food Serving size	Cal.	(g) Total Fat	(g) Sat. Fat	(mg) Chol.	(g) Carb.	(g) Fiber	(g) Sug.	(g) Prot.	(mg) Sod.
Orange Drink, Breakfast Type, with Juice and Pulp, Frozen Concentrate									
1 can (12 fl oz) (436g)	667	0	0	0	170	0.4	166	2	113
Orange Drink, Breakfast Type, with Juice and Pulp, Frozen Concentrate, Prepared with Water									
1 serving, 8 fl oz (250g)	113	0	0	0	28	0	28	0	25
Orange Drink, Canned, with Added Vitamin C									
1 cup (8 fl oz) (248g)	122	0	0	0	31	0	27	0	7
Orange Juice Drink									
1 fl oz (31.1g)	17	0	0	0	4	0.1	0	0	1
Orange Juice, Canned, Unsweetened									
1 fl oz (31.1g)	15	0	0	0	3	0.1	3	0	1
Orange Juice, Chilled, Including from Concentrate									
1 fl oz (31.1g)	15	0	0	0	4	0.1	3	0	1
Orange Juice, Chilled, Including from Concentrate, Fortified with Calcium									
1 fl oz (31.1g)	15	0	0	0	4	0.1	3	0	1
Orange Juice, Chilled, Including from Concentrate, Fortified with Calcium and Vitamin D									
1 fl oz (31.1g)	15	0	0	0	4	0.1	3	0	1
Orange Juice, Chilled, Including from Concentrate, with Added Calcium and Vitamins A, D, and E									
1 fl oz (31.1g)	15	0	0	0	4	0.1	3	0	1
Orange Juice, Frozen Concentrate, Unsweetened, Diluted with 3 Volumes of Water									
1 fl oz (31.1g)	12	0	0	0	3	0.1	2	0	1
Orange Juice, Frozen Concentrate, Unsweetened, Undiluted									
1 fl oz (33g)	49	0	0	0	12	0.3	10	1	2
Orange Juice, Frozen Concentrate, Unsweetened, Undiluted, with Added Calcium									
1 fl oz (33g)	49	0	0	0	11	0.3	10	1	2
Orange Juice, Raw									
1 fl oz (31g)	14	0	0	0	3	0.1	3	0	0
Orange-flavor Drink, Breakfast Type, Powder									
1 serving, 2 tbsp (26g)	100	0	0	0	26	0.1	24	0	4
Orange-flavor Drink, Breakfast Type, Powder, Prepared with Water									
1 serving, 6 fl oz (203g)	99	0	0	0	26	0.2	24	0	10
Orange-flavor Drink, Breakfast Type, with Pulp, Frozen Concentrate									
1 can (12 fl oz) (424g)	729	2	0	0	182	0.8	177	0	102

Food Serving size	Cal.	(g) Total Fat	(g) Sat. Fat	(mg) Chol.	(g) Carb.	(g) Fiber	(g) Sug.	(g) Prot.	(mg) Sod.
Orange-flavor Drink, Breakfast Type, with Pulp, Frozen Concentrate Prepared with Water									
1 serving, 8 fl oz (248g)	122	0	0	0	30	0	30	0	25
Orange-grapefruit Juice, Canned, Unsweetened									
1 fl oz (30.9g)	13	0	0	0	3	0	3	0	1
Peach Nectar, Canned with Vitamin C									
1 fl oz (31.1g)	17	0	0	0	4	0.2	0	0	2
Peach Nectar, Canned, Without Vitamin C									
1 fl oz (31.1g)	17	0	0	0	4	0.2	4	0	2
Pear Nectar, Canned, with Vitamin C									
1 fl oz (31.2g)	19	0	0	0	5	0.2	5	0	1
Pear Nectar, Canned, Without Vitamin C									
1 fl oz (31.2g)	19	0	0	0	5	0.2	5	0	1
Pineapple and Grapefruit Juice Drink, Canned									
1 cup (8 fl oz) (250g)	118	0	0	0	29	0.3	29	1	35
Pineapple and Orange Juice Drink, Canned									
1 cup (8 fl oz) (250g)	125	0	0	0	30	0.3	29	3	8
Pineapple Juice, Dole, Canned, Not from Concentrate, Unsweetened, with Added Vitamins A, C, and E									
1 fl oz (31.3g)	18	0	0	0	4	0.1	3	0	1
Pineapple Juice, Canned, Unsweetened, with Added Vitamin C									
1 fl oz (31.3g)	17	0	0	0	4	0.1	3	0	1
Pineapple Juice, Canned, Unsweetened, Without Vitamin C									
1 fl oz (31.3g)	17	0	0	0	4	0.1	3	0	1
Pineapple Juice, Frozen Concentrate, Unsweetened, Diluted with 3 Volumes Water									
1 fl oz (31.2g)	16	0	0	0	4	0.1	4	0	0
Pineapple Juice, Frozen Concentrate, Unsweetened, Undiluted									
1 can (6 fl oz) (216g)	387	0	0	0	96	1.5	94	3	6
Pomegranate Juice, Bottled									
1 fl oz (31.4g)	17	0	0	0	4	0	4	0	3
Prune Juice, Canned									
1 fl oz (32g)	23	0	0	0	6	0.3	5	0	1
Tangerine Juice, Canned, Sweetened									
1 fl oz (31.1g)	16	0	0	0	4	0.1	4	0	0

Food Serving size	Cal.	(g) Total Fat	(g) Sat. Fat	(mg) Chol.	(g) Carb.	(g) Fiber	(g) Sug.	(g) Prot.	(mg) Sod.
Tangerine Juice, Frozen Concentrate, Sweetened, Diluted with 3 Volumes Water									
1 fl oz (30.1g)	14	0	0	0	3	0	0	0	0
Tangerine Juice, Frozen Concentrate, Sweetened, Undiluted									
1 can (6 fl oz) (214g)	345	1	0	0	83	1.3	0	3	6
Tangerine Juice, Raw									
1 fl oz (30.9g)	13	0	0	0	3	0.1	3	0	0
Tomato and Vegetable Juice, Low Sodium									
1 fl oz (30.2g)	7	0	0	0	1	0.2	0	0	21
Tomato Juice, Canned, with Salt									
6 fl oz (182g)	31	0	0	0	8	0.7	6	1	490
Tomato Juice, Canned, Without Salt									
1 fl oz (30.4g)	5	0	0	0	1	0.1	1	0	3

Dairy

Why Eat Dairy?

Consuming dairy products provides health benefits, especially improved bone health. Intake of dairy products is also associated with a reduced risk of cardiovascular disease and type 2 diabetes, and with lower blood pressure in adults. Foods in the dairy group provide nutrients that are vital for health and maintenance of your body. These nutrients include calcium, potassium, vitamin D, and protein. Calcium is used for building bones and teeth and in maintaining bone mass. Diets rich in potassium may help to maintain healthy blood pressure. Vitamin D functions in the body to maintain proper levels of calcium and phosphorous, thereby helping to build and maintain bones. Vitamin D is also important for a healthy immune system.

Daily Goal

Three cups for an adult on a 2,000-calorie diet
One-cup equivalents:

1 cup milk	⅓ cup shredded cheese
1 cup yogurt	2 oz processed cheese
1½ oz hard cheese	2 cups cottage cheese

Shopping Tips

- Choose low-fat or fat-free dairy products.
- If you don't or can't consume milk, choose lactose-free products and soy, almond, or rice milk.
- Look for good sources of calcium: 10% DV or higher.
- Use fat-free or low-fat yogurt as a snack or to make dips or smoothies.

Shopping List Essentials

Milk, low-fat or fat-free	Soy milk, unsweetened and
Yogurt, low-fat or fat-free	calcium-fortified
Cottage cheese, low-fat or fat-free	Cheese, reduced-fat
Lactose-free milk, if needed	

Red Flags

The fat in dairy products is highly saturated, so the lower the fat content the better. Move from whole milk to reduced-fat, to low-fat, to fat-free (also referred to as skim) gradually to let your taste buds adjust. Fortified rice and almond milk, though sometimes used as a milk alternative do not contain appreciable amounts of protein. When choosing these milk alternatives make sure you consider other protein sources to insure you are consuming adequate amounts.

Preparation Pointer

Use plain yogurt as a substitution for mayonnaise and sour cream. Use yogurt and milk along with fruit in a blender to make smoothies for a nutritious snack or dessert.

Food Serving size	Cal.	(g) Total Fat	(g) Sat. Fat	(mg) Chol.	(g) Carb.	(g) Fiber	(g) Sug.	(g) Prot.	(mg) Sod.
Milk									
Milk, Chocolate Beverage, Hot Cocoa, Homemade									
1 fl oz (31.2g)	24	1	0	2	3	0.3	3	1	14
Milk, Chocolate, Fluid, Commercial, Lowfat, with Added Vitamins A and D									
1 quart (1000g)	710	10	6	30	126	5	99	32	610
Milk, Chocolate, Fluid, Commercial, Reduced Fat, with Added Calcium									
1 fl oz (31.2g)	24	1	0	2	4	0.2	3	1	21
Milk, Chocolate, Fluid, Commercial, Reduced Fat, with Added Vitamins A and D									
1 fl oz (31.2g)	24	1	0	2	4	0.2	3	1	21
Milk, Chocolate, Fluid, Commercial, Whole, with Added Vitamins A and D									
1 fl oz (31.2g)	26	1	1	4	3	0.2	3	1	19
Milk, Condensed, Evaporated, Nonfat, with Added Vitamins A and D									
1 cup (256g)	200	1	0	10	29	0	29	19	294
Milk, Condensed, Evaporated, with Added Vitamin D, No Added Vitamin A									
1 cup (252g)	338	19	12	73	25	0	25	17	267
Milk, Condensed, Evaporated, with Vitamin A									
.5 cup (126g)	169	10	6	37	13	0	0	9	134
Milk, Condensed, Evaporated, Without Added Vitamins A and D									
1 fl oz (31.5g)	43	2	1	9	3	0	3	2	33
Milk, Condensed, Sweetened									
1 cup (306g)	982	27	17	104	166	0	166	24	389
Milk, Dry, Nonfat, Calcium Reduced									
.25 lb (113g)	400	0	0	2	59	0	0	40	2576
Milk, Dry, Whole, with Added Vitamin D									
1 cup (128g)	635	34	21	124	49	0	49	34	475
Milk, Dry, Whole, Without Added Vitamin D									
.25 cup (32g)	434	1	1	24	62	0	62	43	642
Milk, Fluid, Nonfat, Calcium Fortified (Fat Free or Skim)									
1 fl oz (30.9g)	11	0	0	1	1	0	0	1	16
Milk, Human, Mature, Fluid									
1 cup (246g)	172	11	5	34	17	0	17	3	42
Milk, Lowfat, Fluid, 1% Milk Fat, Protein Fortified, with Added Vitamins A and D									
1 quart (984g)	472	12	7	39	54	0	0	39	571

Food Serving size	Cal.	(g) Total Fat	(g) Sat. Fat	(mg) Chol.	(g) Carb.	(g) Fiber	(g) Sug.	(g) Prot.	(mg) Sod.
Milk, Lowfat, Fluid, 1% Milk Fat, with Added Nonfat Milk Solids, with Vitamins A and D									
1 quart (980g)	421	10	6	39	49	0	0	34	510
Milk, Lowfat, Fluid, 1% Milk Fat, with Added Vitamins A and D									
1 fl oz (30.5g)	13	0	0	2	2	0	2	1	13
Milk, Fluid, 1% Fat, Without Added Vitamins A and D									
1 quart (976g)	410	9	6	49	49	0	51	33	429
Milk, Low Sodium, Fluid, Whole									
1 fl oz (30.6g)	19	1	1	4	1	0	1	1	1
Milk, Nonfat, Fluid, Protein Fortified, with Added Vitamins A and D (Fat Free or Skim)									
1 quart (984g)	403	2	2	20	55	0	0	39	581
Milk, Nonfat, Fluid, with Added Nonfat Milk Solids, Vitamins A and D									
1 fl oz (30.6g)	11	0	0	1	2	0	2	1	16
Milk, Nonfat, Fluid, with Added Vitamins A and D (Fat Free or Skim)									
1 fl oz (30.6g)	10	0	0	1	2	0	2	1	13
Milk, Nonfat, Fluid, Without Added Vitamins A and D (Fat Free or Skim)									
1 quart (980g)	333	1	0	20	49	0	50	33	412
Milk, Producer, Fluid, 3.7% Milk Fat									
1 quart (976g)	625	36	22	137	45	0	0	32	478
Milk, Reduced Fat, Fluid, 2% Milk Fat, Protein Fortified, with Added Vitamins A and D									
1 quart (984g)	551	19	12	79	54	0	52	39	581
Milk, Reduced Fat, Fluid, 2% Milk Fat, with Added Nonfat Milk Solids and Vitamins A and D									
1 quart (980g)	500	19	12	78	49	0	0	34	510
Milk, Reduced Fat, Fluid, 2% Milk Fat, with Added Vitamins A and D									
1 fl oz (30.5g)	15	1	0	2	1	0	2	1	14
Milk, Reduced Fat, Fluid, 2% Milk Fat, with Nonfat Milk Solids, Without Vitamin A									
1 quart (980g)	549	19	12	78	54	0	0	39	578
Milk, Reduced Fat, Fluid, 2% Milk Fat, without Added Vitamins A and D									
1 quart (984g)	492	19	12	79	47	0	50	32	462
Milk, Reduced Fat, Ready-to-drink, Flavored and Sweetened, with Calcium, Vitamins A and D									
1 cup (244g)	188	4	3	20	29	1	28	7	120

Food Serving size	Cal.	(g) Total Fat	(g) Sat. Fat	(mg) Chol.	(g) Carb.	(g) Fiber	(g) Sug.	(g) Prot.	(mg) Sod.
Milk, Whole, 3.25% Milk Fat, with Added Vitamin D									
1 fl oz (30.5g)	19	1	1	3	1	0	2	1	13
Milk, Whole, 3.25% Milk Fat, Without Added Vitamins A and D									
1 tbsp (15g)	9	0	0	2	1	0	1	0	6

Milk-based Desserts

Food Serving size	Cal.	Total Fat	Sat. Fat	Chol.	Carb.	Fiber	Sug.	Prot.	Sod.
Corn Pudding, Home Prepared									
.667 cup (#6 scoop) (167g)	219	8	4	120	28	2	11	7	471
Cream, Fluid, Heavy Whipping									
1 cup, fluid (yields 2 cups whipped) (238g)	821	88	55	326	7	0	7	5	90
Cream, Fluid, Light Whipping									
1 cup, fluid (yields 2 cups whipped) (239g)	698	74	46	265	7	0	7	5	81
Dessert Topping, Powder									
1 portion, amount to make 1 tbsp (1.3g)	8	1	0	0	1	0	1	0	2
Dessert Topping, Powder, 1.5 oz Prepared with 1/2 Cup Milk									
1 tbsp (4g)	8	1	0	0	1	0	1	0	3
Dessert Topping, Pressurized									
1 tbsp (4g)	11	1	1	0	1	0	1	0	2
Dessert Topping, Semi Solid, Frozen									
1 tbsp (4g)	13	1	1	0	1	0	1	0	1
Desserts, Mousse, Chocolate, Prepared from Recipe									
1 recipe, yields (808g)	1818	129	74	1131	130	4.8	120	33	307
Desserts, Pudding, Chocolate, Dry Mix, Regular									
1 portion, amount to make 1/2 cup (25g)	91	1	0	0	22	1.1	11	1	88
Desserts, Rennin, Chocolate, Dry Mix									
1 package (2 oz) (57g)	207	2	1	0	52	2.9	0	1	40
Desserts, Rennin, Tablets, Unsweetened									
1 package (0.35 oz) (9.9g)	8	0	0	0	2	0	0	0	2579
Desserts, Rennin, Vanilla, Dry Mix									
1 package (1.5 oz) (43g)	165	0	0	0	43	0	0	0	3

Food Serving size	Cal.	(g) Total Fat	(g) Sat. Fat	(mg) Chol.	(g) Carb.	(g) Fiber	(g) Sug.	(g) Prot.	(mg) Sod.
Egg Custard, Dry Mix 1 portion, amount to make 1/2 cup (21g)	86	1	0	54	17	0	0	1	59
Flan, Caramel Custard, Dry Mix 1 portion, amount to make 1/2 cup (21g)	73	0	0	0	19	0	0	0	91
Frozen Novelites, Ice Cream, Chocolate or Caramel Covered, with Nuts 1 bar (54g)	171	11	7	1	17	0.3	0	2	50
Frozen Novelites, Juice Type, Juice with Cream 2.5 oz (71g)	82	1	1	5	17	0.1	0	1	30
Frozen Novelties, Fat Free Fudgesicle Bars 1 serving, 1 pop (51g)	65	0	0	2	14	0.9	10	3	48
Ice Cream, Breyers, 98% Fat Free Chocolate 1 serving, 1/2 cup (68g)	92	1	1	5	21	3.9	14	3	51
Ice Cream, Breyers, 98% Fat Free Vanilla 1 serving, 1/2 cup (68g)	93	1	1	5	21	3.7	14	2	50
Ice Cream, Breyers, All Natural Light French Chocolate 1 serving, 1/2 cup (68g)	137	5	3	28	20	0.7	16	4	51
Ice Cream, Breyers, All Natural Light French Vanilla 1 serving, 1/2 cup (68g)	118	4	2	36	18	0.1	14	3	50
Ice Cream, Breyers, All Natural Light Mint Chocolate Chip 1 serving, 1/2 cup (68g)	133	5	3	10	19	0.4	17	3	46
Ice Cream, Breyers, All Natural Light Vanilla 1 serving, 1/2 cup (68g)	110	3	2	10	17	0.1	15	3	48
Ice Cream, Breyers, All Natural Light Vanilla/Chocolate/Strawberry 1 serving, 1/2 cup (68g)	109	3	2	10	18	0.3	15	3	47
Ice Cream, Breyers, No Sugar Added, Butter Pecan 1 serving, 1/2 cup (68g)	122	7	3	12	14	0.6	4	3	112
Ice Cream, Breyers, No Sugar Added, Chocolate Caramel 1 serving, 1/2 cup (71g)	107	4	3	11	18	0.7	4	3	55
Ice Cream, Breyers, No Sugar Added, French Vanilla 1 serving, 1/2 cup (68g)	105	5	3	36	14	0.3	5	3	59
Ice Cream, Breyers, No Sugar Added, Vanilla 1 serving, 1/2 cup (69g)	99	4	3	12	15	0.3	4	3	46

Food Serving size	Cal.	(g) Total Fat	(g) Sat. Fat	(mg) Chol.	(g) Carb.	(g) Fiber	(g) Sug.	(g) Prot.	(mg) Sod.
Ice Cream, Breyers, No Sugar Added, Vanilla Fudge Twirl									
1 serving, 1/2 cup (72g)	110	4	3	12	18	0.6	4	3	52
Ice Cream, Breyers, No Sugar Added, Vanilla/Chocolate/Strawberry									
1 serving, 1/2 cup (68g)	97	4	3	12	15	0.5	4	3	46
Ice Cream, Chocolate									
.5 cup (4 fl oz) (66g)	143	7	4	22	19	0.8	17	3	50
Ice Cream, Chocolate, Light									
1 unit (100g)	187	7	4	28	26	0.8	25	5	71
Ice Cream, Chocolate, Light, No Sugar Added									
1 serving, 1/2 cup (72g)	125	4	3	12	19	0.6	4	3	54
Ice Cream, Chocolate, Rich									
1 cubic inch (10.2g)	26	2	1	6	2	0.1	5	0	6
Ice Cream, French Vanilla, Soft-serve									
.5 cup (4 fl oz) (86g)	191	11	6	78	19	0.6	18	4	52
Ice Cream, Regular, Low Carbohydrate, Chocolate									
1 individual (3.5 fl oz) (58g)	137	7	4	20	16	2.8	4	2	44
Ice Cream, Regular, Low Carbohydrate, Vanilla									
.5 cup (4 fl oz) (66g)	143	8	4	21	15	3.2	4	2	32
Ice Cream, Strawberry									
.5 cup (4 fl oz) (66g)	127	6	3	19	18	0.6	0	2	40
Ice Cream, Vanilla									
1 serving, 1/2 cup (66g)	137	7	4	29	16	0.5	14	2	53
Ice Cream, Vanilla, Light									
1 serving, 1/2 cup (76g)	137	4	2	21	22	0.2	17	4	56
Ice Cream, Vanilla, Light, No Sugar Added									
1 serving, 1/2 cup (68g)	115	5	3	18	15	0	4	3	65
Ice Cream, Vanilla, Light, Soft-serve									
1 serving, 1/2 cup (88g)	111	2	1	11	19	0	16	4	62
Ice Cream, Vanilla, Rich									
.5 cup (107g)	266	17	11	98	24	0	22	4	65
Kraft Cheeze Whiz, Light Pasteurized Process Cheese Product									
2 tbsp (33g)	75	3	2	12	6	0.1	3	6	597
Kraft Free Singles American Nonfat Pasteurized Process Cheese Product									
2 tbsp (35g)	31	0	0	3	2	0	1	5	273

Food Serving size	Cal.	(g) Total Fat	(g) Sat. Fat	(mg) Chol.	(g) Carb.	(g) Fiber	(g) Sug.	(g) Prot.	(mg) Sod.
Kraft Velveeta Light Reduced Fat Pasteurized Process Cheese Product									
1 oz (28g)	62	3	2	12	3	0	2	5	444
Light Ice Cream, Soft-serve, Blended with Cookie Pieces									
12 fl oz, cup (337g)	570	19	9	51	86	0.3	0	13	253
Light Ice Cream, Soft-serve, Blended with Milk Chocolate Candies									
12 fl oz, cup (348g)	633	22	13	56	93	0.7	13	14	188
Milk Dessert, Frozen, Milk Fat Free, Chocolate									
1 cup (137g)	229	1	1	0	52	0	0	6	133
Milk Shakes, Thick Chocolate									
1 container (10.6 oz) (300g)	357	8	5	33	63	0.9	63	9	333
Milk Shakes, Thick Vanilla									
1 container (11 oz) (313g)	351	9	6	38	56	0	56	12	297
Puddings, All Flavors Except Chocolate, Low Calorie, Instant, Dry Mix									
1 package, 4 servings (32g)	112	0	0	0	27	0.3	0	0	1360
Puddings, Banana, Dry Mix, Instant									
1 portion, amount to make 1/2 cup (25g)	92	0	0	0	23	0	19	0	375
Puddings, Banana, Dry Mix, Instant, with Added Oil									
1 portion, amount to make 1/2 cup (25g)	97	1	0	0	22	0	0	0	375
Puddings, Banana, Dry Mix, Regular									
1 portion, amount to make 1/2 cup (22g)	81	0	0	0	20	0.1	16	0	173
Puddings, Banana, Dry Mix, Regular with Added Oil									
1 portion, amount to make 1/2 cup (22g)	85	1	0	0	19	0.1	0	0	173
Puddings, Chocolate Flavor, Low Calorie, Instant, Dry Mix									
1 package, 1.4 oz box, 4 servings (40g)	142	1	0	0	31	2.4	1	2	1135
Puddings, Chocolate Flavor, Low Calorie, Regular, Dry Mix									
1 package (40g)	146	1	1	0	30	4	5	4	1330
Puddings, Chocolate, Dry Mix, Instant									
1 portion, amount to make 1/2 cup (25g)	95	0	0	0	22	0.9	17	1	357

Food Serving size	Cal.	(g) Total Fat	(g) Sat. Fat	(mg) Chol.	(g) Carb.	(g) Fiber	(g) Sug.	(g) Prot.	(mg) Sod.
Puddings, Chocolate, Dry Mix, Instant, Prepared with Whole Milk 1 package, yields (2 cups) (570g)	684	18	10	51	112	4.6	68	18	559
Puddings, Chocolate, Dry Mix, Instant, Prepared with Whole Milk 1 package, yields (2 cups) (587g)	652	18	11	65	110	5.9	0	18	1667
Puddings, Chocolate, Ready-to-eat 1 container, refrigerated, 4 oz container (108g)	153	5	1	1	25	0	19	2	164
Puddings, Coconut Cream, Dry Mix, Instant 1 portion, amount to make 1/2 cup (25g)	97	1	1	0	23	1	16	0	260
Puddings, Coconut Cream, Dry Mix, Instant, Prepared with 2% Milk 1 package, yields (2 cups) (587g)	628	14	8	35	113	0.6	0	17	1444
Puddings, Coconut Cream, Dry Mix, Instant, Prepared with Whole Milk 1 package, yields (2 cups) (587g)	687	21	12	65	112	0.6	0	17	1444
Puddings, Coconut Cream, Dry Mix, Regular 1 portion, amount to make 1/2 cup (25g)	109	3	3	0	20	0.4	20	0	171
Puddings, Coconut Cream, Dry Mix, Regular, Prepared with 2% Milk 1 package, yields (2 cups) (559g)	581	14	10	39	100	1.1	0	17	911
Puddings, Coconut Cream, Dry Mix, Regular, Prepared with Whole Milk 1 package, yields (2 cups) (559g)	637	21	14	67	99	1.1	0	17	906
Puddings, Lemon, Dry Mix, Instant 1 portion, amount to make 1/2 cup (25g)	95	0	0	0	24	0	0	0	333
Puddings, Lemon, Dry Mix, Instant, Prepared with Whole Milk 1 package, yields (2 cups) (587g)	675	17	10	65	118	0	0	16	1567
Puddings, Lemon, Dry Mix, Regular 1 portion, amount to make 1/2 cup (21g)	76	0	0	0	19	0	0	0	106

Food Serving size	Cal.	(g) Total Fat	(g) Sat. Fat	(mg) Chol.	(g) Carb.	(g) Fiber	(g) Sug.	(g) Prot.	(mg) Sod.
Puddings, Lemon, Dry Mix, Regular with Added Oil, Phosphorus, and Sodium 1 portion, amount to make 1/2 cup (21g)									
	77	0	0	0	19	0	0	0	178
Puddings, Rice, Dry Mix 1 portion, amount to make 1/2 cup (27g)									
	102	0	0	0	25	0.2	0	1	99
Puddings, Rice, Ready-to-eat 1 serving, 4 oz refrigerated (113g)									
	133	3	2	20	22	1	16	4	139
Puddings, Tapioca, Dry Mix 1 portion, amount to make 1/2 cup (23g)									
	85	0	0	0	22	0	15	0	110
Puddings, Tapioca, Dry Mix, with No Added Salt 1 portion, amount to make 1/2 cup (23g)									
	85	0	0	0	22	0	0	0	2
Puddings, Tapioca, Ready-to-eat 1 container, refrigerated 4 oz (110g)									
	143	4	1	1	24	0	16	2	160
Puddings, Tapioca, Ready-to-eat, Fat Free 1 container, refrigerated 4 oz (112g)									
	105	0	0	1	24	0	16	2	209
Puddings, Vanilla, Dry Mix, Instant 1 portion, amount to make 1/2 cup (25g)									
	94	0	0	0	23	0	23	0	360
Puddings, Vanilla, Dry Mix, Instant, Prepared with Whole Milk 1 package, yields (2 cups) (569g)									
	649	17	10	63	112	0	103	15	1627
Puddings, Vanilla, Dry Mix, Regular 1 portion, amount to make 1/2 cup (22g)									
	83	0	0	0	21	0.1	17	0	140
Puddings, Vanilla, Dry Mix, Regular with Added Oil 1 portion, amount to make 1/2 cup (22g)									
	81	0	0	0	20	0	0	0	166
Puddings, Vanilla, Dry Mix, Regular, Prepared with Whole Milk 1 package, yields (2 cups) (559g)									
	632	16	9	50	106	0.6	96	16	872

Food Serving size	Cal.	(g) Total Fat	(g) Sat. Fat	(mg) Chol.	(g) Carb.	(g) Fiber	(g) Sug.	(g) Prot.	(mg) Sod.
Puddings, Vanilla, Ready-to-eat 1 container, refrigerated 4 oz (110g)	143	4	1	1	25	0	19	2	156
Puddings, Vanilla, Ready-to-eat, Fat Free 1 serving, 3.5 oz shelf stable (99g)	88	0	0	0	20	0	15	2	189
Sherbet, Orange 1 bar (2.75 fl oz) (66g)	95	1	1	1	20	0.9	16	1	30
Sour Cream, Imitation, Cultured 1 oz (28.35g)	59	6	5	0	2	0	2	1	29
Sour Cream, Reduced Fat 1 cup (230g)	416	32	20	81	16	0	1	16	161
Sour Cream, Light 1 cup (230g)	313	24	15	81	16	0	1	8	191
Sour Cream, Fat Free 1 cup (230g)	170	0	0	21	36	0	1	7	324
Sour Dressing, Non-butterfat, Cultured, Filled Cream-type 1 cup (235g)	418	39	31	12	11	0	11	8	113

Cheeses

Food Serving size	Cal.	(g) Total Fat	(g) Sat. Fat	(mg) Chol.	(g) Carb.	(g) Fiber	(g) Sug.	(g) Prot.	(mg) Sod.
Cheese, Pasteurized Process, American, Vitamin D Fortified 1 slice, 3/4 oz (21g)	65	5	3	16	2	0	1	4	274
Cheese Fondue .5 cup (108g)	247	15	9	49	4	0	0	15	143
Cheese Food, Cold Pack, American 1 package (8 oz) (227g)	751	56	35	145	19	0	0	45	2193
Cheese Food, Pasteurized Process, American, Without Added Vitamin D 1 oz (28.35g)	94	7	4	23	2	0	2	5	359
Cheese Food, Pasteurized Process, Swiss 1 package (8 oz) (227g)	733	55	35	186	10	0	0	50	3523
Cheese Product, Pasteurized Process, American, Reduced Fat, Fortified with Vitamin D 1 slice, 2/3 oz (19g)	46	3	2	10	2	0	2	3	228
Cheese Sauce, Prepared from Recipe 2 tbsp (30g)	59	4	2	11	2	0	0	3	148

Food Serving size	Cal.	(g) Total Fat	(g) Sat. Fat	(mg) Chol.	(g) Carb.	(g) Fiber	(g) Sug.	(g) Prot.	(mg) Sod.
Cheese Spread, Cream Cheese Base 1 oz (28.35g)	84	8	5	26	1	0	3	2	191
Cheese Spread, Pasteurized Process, American 1 jar (5 oz) (142g)	412	30	19	78	12	0	0	23	2308
Cheese Spread, Pasteurized Process, American 1 cup (244g)	708	52	33	134	21	0	18	40	3965
Cheese, American Cheddar, Imitation 1 cubic inch (18g)	43	3	2	6	2	0	0	3	242
Cheese, Blue 1 cubic inch (17g)	60	5	3	13	0	0	0	4	195
Cheese, Brick 1 cup, shredded (113g)	419	34	21	106	3	0	1	26	633
Cheese, Brie 1 cup, sliced (144g)	481	40	25	144	1	0	1	30	906
Cheese, Camembert 1 cup (246g)	738	60	38	177	1	0	1	49	2071
Cheese, Cheddar 1 cup, melted (244g)	991	83	47	249	3	0	1	59	1571
Cheese, Cheddar, Sharp, Sliced 1 slice, 3/4 oz slice (21g)	86	7	4	21	0	0	0	5	135
Cheese, Colby 1 cup, shredded (113g)	445	36	23	107	3	0	1	27	683
Cheese, Cottage, Creamed, Large or Small Curd 1 cup, large curd (not packed) (210g)	206	9	4	36	7	0	6	23	764
Cheese, Cottage, Creamed, with Fruit 1 cup, (not packed) (226g)	219	9	5	29	10	0.5	5	24	777
Cheese, Cottage, Lowfat, 1% Milk Fat 1 cup, (not packed) (226g)	81	1	1	5	3	0	3	14	459
Cheese, Cottage, Lowfat, 2% Milk Fat 1 cup, (not packed) (226g)	183	5	3	27	11	0	9	24	696
Cheese, Cottage, Nonfat, Uncreamed, Dry, Large or Small Curd 4 oz (113g)	81	0	0	8	8	0	2	12	420
Cheese, Cream 1 cup (232g)	793	79	45	255	9	0	7	14	847

Food Serving size	Cal.	(g) Total Fat	(g) Sat. Fat	(mg) Chol.	(g) Carb.	(g) Fiber	(g) Sug.	(g) Prot.	(mg) Sod.
Cheese, Cream, Lowfat 1 tbsp (15g)	30	2	1	8	1	0	1	1	71
Cheese, Edam 1 package (7 oz) (198g)	707	55	35	176	3	0	3	49	1608
Cheese, Feta 1 oz (28.35g)	75	6	4	25	1	0	1	4	260
Cheese, Fontina 1 cup, shredded (108g)	420	34	21	125	2	0	2	28	864
Cheese, Gjetost 1 package (8 oz) (227g)	1058	67	43	213	97	0	0	22	1362
Cheese, Goat, Hard Type 1 oz (28.35g)	127	10	7	29	1	0	1	9	118
Cheese, Goat, Semisoft Type 1 oz (28.35g)	102	8	6	22	0	0	0	6	116
Cheese, Goat, Soft Type 1 oz (28.35g)	74	6	4	13	0	0	0	5	129
Cheese, Gouda 1 package (7 oz) (198g)	705	54	35	226	4	0	4	49	1622
Cheese, Gruyere 1 slice (1oz) (28g)	116	9	5	31	0	0	0	8	200
Cheese, Limburger 1 oz (28.35g)	93	8	5	26	0	0	0	6	227
Cheese, Lowfat, Cheddar or Colby 1 cup, shredded (113g)	195	8	5	24	2	0	1	28	986
Cheese, Low Sodium, Cheddar or Colby 1 cup, shredded (113g)	450	37	23	113	2	0	1	28	24
Cheese, Mexican, Blend, Reduced Fat .25 cup (28g)	79	5	3	17	1	0	0	7	217
Cheese, Mexican, Queso Anejo 1 oz (28.35g)	106	8	5	30	1	0	1	6	321
Cheese, Mexican, Queso Asadero 1 cup, shredded (113g)	402	32	20	119	3	0	3	26	797
Cheese, Mexican, Queso Chihuahua 1 cup, shredded (113g)	423	34	21	119	6	0	6	24	697

Food Serving size	Cal.	(g) Total Fat	(g) Sat. Fat	(mg) Chol.	(g) Carb.	(g) Fiber	(g) Sug.	(g) Prot.	(mg) Sod.
Cheese, Monterey 1 cup, shredded (113g)	421	34	22	101	1	0	1	28	678
Cheese, Monterey, Lowfat 1 cup, shredded (113g)	350	24	16	73	1	0	0	32	637
Cheese, Mozzarella, Low Sodium 1 cup, shredded (113g)	316	19	12	61	4	0	0	31	18
Cheese, Mozzarella, Nonfat 1 cup, shredded (113g)	159	0	0	20	4	2	4	36	840
Cheese, Mozzarella, Part Skim Milk, Low Moisture 1 cup, shredded (113g)	340	22	13	73	7	0	3	28	771
Cheese, Mozzarella, Whole Milk 1 oz (28.35g)	85	6	4	22	1	0	0	6	178
Cheese, Mozzarella, Whole Milk, Low Moisture 1 cubic inch (18g)	57	4	3	16	0	0	0	4	75
Cheese, Muenster 1 cup, shredded (113g)	416	34	22	108	1	0	1	26	710
Cheese, Muenster, Lowfat 1 cubic inch (18g)	49	3	2	11	1	0	0	4	108
Cheese, Neufchatel 1 package (3 oz) (85g)	215	19	11	63	3	0	3	8	284
Cheese, Parmesan, Dry Grated, Reduced Fat 1 tbsp (5g)	13	1	1	4	0	0	0	1	76
Cheese, Parmesan, Grated 1 tbsp (5g)	21	1	1	4	1	0	0	1	90
Cheese, Parmesan, Hard 1 cubic inch (10.3g)	40	3	2	7	0	0	0	4	165
Cheese, Parmesan, Low Sodium 1 tbsp (5g)	23	1	1	4	0	0	0	2	3
Cheese, Parmesan, Shredded 1 tbsp (5g)	21	1	1	4	0	0	0	2	85
Cheese, Pasteurized Process, American 1 cup, melted (244g)	915	76	48	229	4	0	1	54	3060
Cheese, Pasteurized Process, American 1 cubic inch (18g)	68	6	4	17	0	0	0	4	117

Food Serving size	Cal.	(g) Total Fat	(g) Sat. Fat	(mg) Chol.	(g) Carb.	(g) Fiber	(g) Sug.	(g) Prot.	(mg) Sod.
Cheese, Pasteurized Process, American, Lowfat									
1 cup, shredded (113g)	203	8	5	40	4	0	0	28	1616
Cheese, Pasteurized Process, Cheddar or American, Fat Free									
1 slice (3/4 oz) (21g)	31	0	0	2	3	0	0	5	321
Cheese, Pasteurized Process, Cheddar or American, Low Sodium									
1 cup, shredded (113g)	425	35	22	106	2	0	0	25	8
Cheese, Pasteurized Process, Pimiento									
1 cup, melted (244g)	915	76	48	229	4	0.2	2	54	2233
Cheese, Pasteurized Process, Swiss									
1 cubic inch (18g)	60	5	3	15	0	0	0	4	123
Cheese, Pasteurized Process, Swiss									
1 cup, shredded (113g)	377	28	18	96	2	0	1	28	1548
Cheese, Pasteurized Process, Swiss, Lowfat									
1 cup, shredded (113g)	186	6	4	40	5	0	3	29	1616
Cheese, Port de Salut									
1 cup, shredded (113g)	398	32	19	139	1	0	1	27	603
Cheese, Provolone									
1 oz (28.35g)	100	8	5	20	1	0	0	7	248
Cheese, Provolone, Reduced Fat									
1 oz (28.35g)	78	5	3	16	1	0	0	7	174
Cheese, Ricotta, Part Skim Milk									
1 oz (28.35g)	39	2	1	9	1	0	0	3	28
Cheese, Ricotta, Whole Milk									
1 cup (246g)	428	32	20	125	7	0	1	28	207
Cheese, Romano									
1 package (5 oz) (142g)	550	38	24	148	5	0	1	45	2035
Cheese, Roquefort									
1 package (3 oz) (85g)	314	26	16	77	2	0	0	18	1538
Cheese Spread, American or Cheddar Cheese Base, Reduced Fat									
1 package (566g)	996	50	32	215	61	0	40	76	6237
Cheese, Substitute, Mozzarella									
1 oz (28.35g)	70	3	1	0	7	0	7	3	194
Cheese, Swiss									
1 cup, melted (244g)	927	68	43	224	13	0	3	66	171

Food Serving size	Cal.	(g) Total Fat	(g) Sat. Fat	(mg) Chol.	(g) Carb.	(g) Fiber	(g) Sug.	(g) Prot.	(mg) Sod.
Cheese, Swiss, Lowfat 1 cup, shredded (108g)	187	6	4	38	4	0	0	31	281
Cheese, Swiss, Low Sodium 1 cup, shredded (108g)	404	30	19	99	4	0	1	31	15
Cheese, Tilsit 1 package (6 oz) (170g)	578	44	29	173	3	0	0	41	1280
Imitation Cheese, American or Cheddar, Low Cholesterol 1 cubic inch (18g)	70	6	1	3	0	0	0	5	121
Kraft Velveeta Pasteurized Process Cheese Spread 1 slice (21g)	64	5	3	17	2	0	2	3	315
Whey, Acid, Fluid 1 quart (984g)	236	1	1	10	50	0	50	7	472
Whey, Acid, Dried 1 tbsp (2.9g)	10	0	0	0	2	0	2	0	28
Whey, Sweet, Fluid 1 quart (984g)	266	4	2	20	51	0	51	8	531
Whey, Sweet, Dried 1 tbsp (7.5g)	26	0	0	0	6	0	6	1	81

Yogurt

Food Serving size	Cal.	(g) Total Fat	(g) Sat. Fat	(mg) Chol.	(g) Carb.	(g) Fiber	(g) Sug.	(g) Prot.	(mg) Sod.
Kraft Breyers Light n' Lively Lowfat Strawberry Yogurt (1% Milk Fat) 1 container (8 oz) (227g)	245	2	1	20	50	0.5	44	7	102
Kraft Breyers Light Nonfat Strawberry Yogurt (with Aspartame and Fructose Sweetener) 1 container (8 oz) (227g)	125	0	0	11	22	0	17	8	102
Kraft Breyers Lowfat Strawberry Yogurt (1% Milk Fat) 2 tbsp (32g)	31	0	0	3	6	0.1	6	1	17
Kraft Breyers Smooth and Creamy Lowfat Strawberry Yogurt (1% Milk Fat) 1 container (4.4 oz) (125g)	128	1	1	11	25	0.4	22	5	69

Dairy Alternatives

Food Serving size	Cal.	(g) Total Fat	(g) Sat. Fat	(mg) Chol.	(g) Carb.	(g) Fiber	(g) Sug.	(g) Prot.	(mg) Sod.
Beverages, Almond Milk, Chocolate, Rtd. 1 cup (240g)	120	3	0	0	23	1	21	2	170
Beverages, Almond Milk, Sweetened, Vanilla Flavor Rtd. 1 cup (240g)	91	2	0	0	16	1	15	1	151

Food Serving size	Cal.	(g) Total Fat	(g) Sat. Fat	(mg) Chol.	(g) Carb.	(g) Fiber	(g) Sug.	(g) Prot.	(mg) Sod.
Cream Substitute, Fluid with Hydrogenated Vegetable Oils and Soy Protein									
1 fl oz (30g)	41	3	1	0	3	0	3	0	20
Cream Substitute, Liquid, Light									
1 fl oz (30g)	21	1	0	0	3	0	0	0	18
Cream Substitute, with Lauric Acid Oil									
.5 cup (120g)	163	12	11	0	14	0	0	1	95
Cream, Fluid, Half and Half									
1 tbsp (15g)	20	2	1	6	1	0	1	0	6
Cream, Fluid, Light Coffee or Table									
1 tbsp (15g)	29	3	2	10	1	0	1	0	6
Cream, Half and Half, Fat Free									
1 pint (484g)	286	7	4	24	44	0	24	13	484
Cream, Sour, Cultured									
1 cup (230g)	478	45	41	0	15	0	15	6	235
Cream, Sour, Reduced Fat, Cultured									
1 cup (242g)	327	29	18	94	10	0	0	7	215
Cream, Substitute, Powder									
1 tsp (2g)	11	1	1	0	1	0	1	0	2
Cream, Whipped, Cream Topping, Pressurized									
1 tbsp (3g)	8	1	0	2	0	0	0	0	4
Dairy Drink Mix, Chocolate, Reduced Calorie, with Aspartame, Powder, Prepared with Water and Ice									
1 serving (243g)	70	1	0	5	11	1.9	7	5	148
Dairy Drink Mix, Chocolate, Reduced Calorie, with Low-calorie Sweeteners, Powder									
1 packet (.75 oz) (21g)	69	1	0	5	11	2	7	5	138
Frozen Novelties, Fruit and Juice Bars									
1 bar (3 fl oz) (92g)	80	0	0	0	19	0.9	16	1	4
Frozen Novelties, Ice Type, Fruit, No Sugar Added									
1 bar (51g)	12	0	0	0	3	0	0	0	3
Frozen Novelties, Ice Type, Italian, Restaurant Prepared									
.5 cup (116g)	61	0	0	0	16	0	0	0	5
Frozen Novelties, Ice Type, Lime									
.5 cup (4 fl oz) (99g)	127	0	0	0	32	0	32	0	22

Food Serving size	Cal.	(g) Total Fat	(g) Sat. Fat	(mg) Chol.	(g) Carb.	(g) Fiber	(g) Sug.	(g) Prot.	(mg) Sod.
Frozen Novelties, Ice Type, Pineapple-coconut .5 cup (4 fl oz) (99g)	112	3	2	0	24	0.7	0	0	35
Frozen Novelties, Ice Type, Pop 1 serving, 1.75 fl oz pop (52g)	41	0	0	0	10	0	7	0	4
Frozen Novelties, Ice Type, Pop, with Low Calorie Sweetener 1 serving, 1.75 fl oz pop (55g)	13	0	0	0	3	0	0	0	6
Frozen Novelties, Ice Type, Sugar Free, Orange, Cherry, and Grape Popsicle 1 serving, 1.75 fl oz pop (55g)	12	0	0	0	3	0	1	0	6
Frozen Novelties, Juice Type, Orange 1 fl oz (29.8g)	28	0	0	0	7	0	0	0	2
Frozen Novelties, Juice Type, Popsicle Scribblers 1 serving, 1.2 fl oz pop (33g)	27	0	0	0	6	0	5	0	4
Frozen Novelties, Klondike, Slim-a-Bear Chocolate Cone 1 serving, 1 cone (79g)	177	3	1	2	36	3.4	19	3	126
Frozen Novelties, Klondike, Slim-a-Bear Chocolate Sandwich 1 serving, 1 sandwich (64g)	136	2	1	3	28	3.1	14	4	120
Frozen Novelties, Klondike, Slim-a-Bear Fudge Brownie, 98% Fat Free, No Sugar Added 1 serving, 3.5 fl oz bar (74g)	92	1	1	5	22	4.4	5	3	89
Frozen Novelties, Klondike, Slim-a-Bear Mint Sandwich 1 serving, 1 sandwich (64g)	134	1	0	3	28	2.8	14	4	122
Frozen Novelties, Klondike, Slim-a-Bear Vanilla Cone 1 serving, 1 cone (79g)	175	3	1	2	35	3	20	3	126
Frozen Novelties, Klondike, Slim-a-Bear Vanilla Sandwich 1 serving, 1 sandwich (64g)	135	1	0	3	28	2.8	14	4	122
Frozen Novelties, No Sugar Added, Creamsicle Pops 1 serving, 1 pop (44g)	25	0	0	1	6	0.1	1	1	18
Frozen Novelties, No Sugar Added, Fudgesicle Pops 1 serving (84g)	88	1	0	2	19	1.3	3	3	86
Frozen Novelties, Sugar Free, Creamsicle Pops 1 serving, 2 pops (80g)	39	2	2	0	10	6	0	1	5
Frozen Yogurt, Chocolate 1 cup (174g)	221	6	4	23	38	4	0	5	110
Frozen Yogurt, Chocolate, Soft-serve .5 cup (4 fl oz) (72g)	115	4	3	4	18	1.6	0	3	71

Food Serving size	Cal.	(g) Total Fat	(g) Sat. Fat	(mg) Chol.	(g) Carb.	(g) Fiber	(g) Sug.	(g) Prot.	(mg) Sod.
Frozen Yogurt, Flavors Other than Chocolate									
1 cup (174g)	221	6	4	23	38	0	0	5	110
Frozen Yogurt, Vanilla, Soft-serve									
.5 cup (72g)	114	4	2	1	17	0	17	3	63
Kraft Breakstone's Fat-free Sour Cream									
2 tbsp (31g)	29	0	0	3	5	0	2	2	23
Milk Substitute, Fluid, with Lauric Acid Oil									
1 quart (976g)	595	33	30	0	60	0	0	17	761
Milk, Buttermilk, Dried									
1 cup (120g)	464	7	4	83	59	0	59	41	620
Milk, Buttermilk, Fluid, Cultured, Lowfat									
1 fl oz (30.6g)	12	0	0	1	1	0	1	1	58
Milk, Buttermilk, Fluid, Cultured, Reduced Fat									
1 fl oz (30.6g)	17	1	0	2	2	0	0	1	26
Milk, Dry, Nonfat, Instant, with Added Vitamins A and D									
1 envelope (1-1/3 cup) (91g)	326	1	0	16	47	0	47	32	500
Milk, Dry, Nonfat, Instant, Without Added Vitamins A and D									
1 envelope (1-1/3 cup) (91g)	326	1	0	16	47	0	47	32	50
Milk, Dry, Nonfat, Regular, with Added Vitamins A and D									
1 cup (120g)	434	1	1	24	62	0	62	43	642
Milk, Dry, Nonfat, Regular, Without Added Vitamins A and D									
.25 cup (30g)	109	0	0	6	16	0	16	11	161
Milk, Filled, Fluid, with Blend of Hydrogenated Vegetable Oils									
1 quart (976g)	615	34	7	20	46	0	0	33	556
Milk, Filled, Fluid, with Lauric Acid Oil									
1 fl oz (30.5g)	19	1	1	1	1	0	1	1	17
Milk, Goat, Fluid, with Added Vitamin D									
1 cup (244g)	168	10	7	27	11	0	11	9	122
Milk, Imitation, Non-soy									
1 fl oz (30.5g)	14	1	0	0	2	0	0	0	17
Milk, Indian Buffalo, Fluid									
1 quart (976g)	947	67	45	185	51	0	0	37	508
Milk, Sheep, Fluid									
1 quart (980g)	1058	69	45	265	53	0	0	59	431

Food Serving size	Cal.	(g) Total Fat	(g) Sat. Fat	(mg) Chol.	(g) Carb.	(g) Fiber	(g) Sug.	(g) Prot.	(mg) Sod.
Silk Banana-strawberry Soy Yogurt									
1 container (170g)	150	2	0	0	29	1	18	4	26
Silk Black Cherry Soy Yogurt									
1 container (170g)	150	2	0	0	29	1	20	4	20
Silk Blueberry Soy Yogurt									
1 container (170g)	150	2	0	0	29	1	21	4	26
Silk Chai, Soy Milk									
1 cup (243g)	129	3	1	0	19	0	14	6	100
Silk Chocolate, Soy Milk									
1 cup (243g)	141	3	1	0	23	1.9	19	5	100
Silk Coffee, Soy Milk									
1 cup (243g)	151	3	1	0	25	0	23	5	100
Silk French Vanilla Creamer									
1 tbsp (15g)	20	1	0	0	3	0	3	0	10
Silk Hazelnut Creamer									
1 tbsp (15g)	20	1	0	0	3	0	3	0	10
Silk Key Lime Soy Yogurt									
1 container (170g)	150	2	0	0	30	1	21	4	26
Silk Light Chocolate, Soy Milk									
1 cup (243g)	119	2	0	0	22	1.9	19	5	100
Silk Light Plain, Soy Milk									
1 cup (243g)	70	2	0	0	8	1	6	6	119
Silk Light Vanilla, Soy Milk									
1 cup (243g)	80	2	0	0	10	1	7	6	95
Silk Mocha, Soy Milk									
1 cup (243g)	141	3	1	0	22	0	18	5	100
Silk Nog, Soy Milk									
.5 cup (122g)	90	2	0	0	15	0	12	3	74
Silk Original Creamer									
1 tbsp (15g)	15	1	0	0	1	0	0	0	10
Silk Peach, Soy Yogurt									
1 container (170g)	160	2	0	0	32	1	25	4	26
Silk Plain, Soy Milk									
1 cup (243g)	100	4	1	0	8	1	6	7	119

Food Serving size	Cal.	(g) Total Fat	(g) Sat. Fat	(mg) Chol.	(g) Carb.	(g) Fiber	(g) Sug.	(g) Prot.	(mg) Sod.
Silk Plain, Soy Yogurt 1 container (227g)	150	4	0	0	22	0.9	12	6	30
Silk Plus Fiber, Soy Milk 1 cup (243g)	100	3	1	0	14	5.1	7	6	95
Silk Plus for Bone Health, Soy Milk 1 cup (243g)	100	3	1	0	11	1.9	7	6	95
Silk Plus Omega-3 DHA, Soy Milk 1 cup (243g)	109	5	1	0	8	1	6	7	119
Silk Raspberry, Soy Yogurt 1 container (170g)	150	2	0	0	30	1	22	4	26
Silk Strawberry, Soy Yogurt 1 container (170g)	160	2	0	0	31	1	22	4	26
Silk Unsweetened, Soy Milk 1 cup (243g)	80	4	1	0	4	1	1	7	85
Silk Vanilla, Soy Milk 1 cup (243g)	100	3	1	0	10	1	7	6	95
Silk Vanilla, Soy Yogurt (Family Size) 1 container (227g)	179	4	0	0	31	0.9	24	6	30
Silk Vanilla, Soy Yogurt (Single Serving Size) 1 container (170g)	150	3	0	0	25	1	18	5	20
Silk Very Vanilla, Soy Milk 1 cup (243g)	129	4	1	0	19	1	16	6	141
Soy Milk (All Flavors), Enhanced 1 cup (243g)	109	5	1	0	8	1	6	7	122
Soy Milk (All Flavors), Lowfat, with Added Calcium and Vitamins A and D 1 cup (243g)	104	2	0	0	17	1.9	9	4	90
Soy Milk (All Flavors), Nonfat, with Added Calcium and Vitamins A and D 1 cup (243g)	68	0	0	0	10	0.5	9	6	139
Soy Milk (All Flavors), Unsweetened, with Added Calcium with Added Vitamins A and D 1 cup (243g)	80	4	1	0	4	1.2	1	7	90
Soy Milk, Chocolate and Other Flavors, Light with Added Calcium and Vitamins A and D 1 cup (243g)	114	2	0	0	20	1.7	17	5	112

Food Serving size	Cal.	(g) Total Fat	(g) Sat. Fat	(mg) Chol.	(g) Carb.	(g) Fiber	(g) Sug.	(g) Prot.	(mg) Sod.
Soy Milk, Chocolate, Nonfat, with Added Calcium and Vitamins A and D									
1 cup (243g)	107	0	0	0	21	0.5	9	6	139
Soy Milk, Chocolate, Unfortified									
1 fl oz (30.6g)	19	0	0	0	3	0.1	2	1	16
Soy Milk, Chocolate, with Added Calcium and Vitamins A and D									
1 fl oz (30.6g)	19	0	0	0	3	0.1	2	1	16
Soy Milk, Original and Vanilla, Light with Added Calcium and Vitamins A and D									
1 cup (243g)	73	2	0	0	9	0.7	6	6	117
Soy Milk, Original and Vanilla, Light, Unsweetened, with Added Calcium and Vitamins A and D									
1 cup (243g)	83	2	0	0	9	1.5	1	6	153
Soy Milk, Original and Vanilla, Unfortified									
1 fl oz (30.6g)	17	1	0	0	2	0.2	1	1	16
Soy Milk, Original and Vanilla, with Added Calcium and Vitamins A and D									
1 fl oz (30.6g)	13	0	0	0	2	0.1	1	1	14
Tofu Yogurt									
1 cup (262g)	246	5	1	0	42	0.5	6	9	92
Reddi Whip Fat Free Whipped Topping									
1 cup (75g)	112	4	2	12	19	0.3	12	2	54
Whipped Cream Substitute, Dietetic, Made from Powder Mix									
1 cup (80g)	80	5	3	0	8	0	4	1	85
Whipped Topping, Frozen, Lowfat									
1 cup (75g)	168	10	8	2	18	0	0	2	54
Yogurt Parfait, Lowfat, with Fruit and Granola									
1 item (149g)	125	2	1	4	24	1.6	0	5	73
Yogurt, Frozen, Chocolate, Nonfat Milk, with Low Calorie Sweetener									
1 cup (186g)	199	1	1	7	37	3.7	0	8	151
Yogurt, Fruit Variety, Nonfat, Fortified with Vitamin D									
1 container (4.4 oz) (125g)	119	0	0	3	24	0	24	6	73
Yogurt, Fruit, Lowfat, 10 Grams Protein per 8 oz									
1 cup (8 fl oz) (245g)	250	3	2	10	47	0	47	11	142
Yogurt, Fruit, Lowfat, 10 Grams Protein per 8 oz, Fortified with Vitamin D									
1 cup (8 fl oz) (245g)	173	2	1	7	32	0	32	7	99
Yogurt, Fruit, Lowfat, 11 Grams Protein per 8 oz									
.5 container (4 oz) (113g)	119	2	1	7	21	0	0	5	73

Food Serving size	Cal.	(g) Total Fat	(g) Sat. Fat	(mg) Chol.	(g) Carb.	(g) Fiber	(g) Sug.	(g) Prot.	(mg) Sod.
Yogurt, Fruit, Lowfat, 9 Grams Protein per 8 oz									
1 container (4.4 oz) (125g)	124	1	1	6	23	0	23	5	66
Yogurt, Fruit, Lowfat, 9 Grams Protein per 8 oz, Fortified with Vitamin D									
1 container (4.4 oz) (125g)	124	1	1	6	23	0	23	5	66
Yogurt, Fruit, Lowfat, with Low Calorie Sweetener									
1 cup (8 fl oz) (245g)	257	3	2	15	46	0	7	12	142
Yogurt, Fruit, Lowfat, with Low Calorie Sweetener, Fortified with Vitamin D									
1 cup (8 fl oz) (245g)	257	3	2	15	46	0	7	12	142
Yogurt, Fruit, Variety, Nonfat									
1 container (4.4 oz) (125g)	119	0	0	3	24	0	1	6	73
Yogurt, Plain, Lowfat, 12 Grams Protein per 8 oz									
1 container (8 oz) (227g)	143	4	2	14	16	0	16	12	159
Yogurt, Plain, Skim Milk, 13 Grams Protein per 8 oz									
1 container (8 oz) (227g)	127	0	0	5	17	0	17	13	175
Yogurt, Plain, Whole Milk, 8 Grams Protein per 8 oz									
1 container (8 oz) (227g)	138	7	5	30	11	0	11	8	104
Yogurt, Vanilla, Lowfat, 11 Grams Protein per 8 oz									
1 container (8 oz) (227g)	193	3	2	11	31	0	31	11	150
Yogurt, Vanilla, Lowfat, 11 Grams Protein per 8 oz, Fortified with Vitamin D									
1 container (8 oz) (227g)	193	3	2	11	31	0	31	11	150

Protein Foods

ChooseMyPlate.gov

Why Eat Proteins?

Protein foods include meat, poultry, fish, eggs, nuts, and seeds. They provide nutrients that are vital for health and maintenance of your body. These include protein, B vitamins (niacin, thiamin, riboflavin, B_{12}, and B_6), vitamin E, iron, zinc, and magnesium. Proteins function as building blocks for bones, muscles, cartilage, skin, and blood. Proteins are responsible for growth and repair of the body. B vitamins help the body release energy from food, play a vital role in the function of the nervous system, aid in the formation of red blood cells, and help build tissues. Iron is used to carry oxygen in the blood. Fish contains a range of nutrients essential for optimal health, notably the omega-3 fatty acids, EPA, and DHA. Eating about 8–12 ounces per week of a variety of fish and seafood contributes to the prevention of heart disease. The omega-3 content of animal proteins like eggs and beef is higher in grass-fed, free-range animals making them better choices than conventionally raised animals when available.

Daily Goal

5½ ounces for an adult on a 2,000-calorie diet
8 ounces of fish per week
One-ounce equivalents:

1 ounce lean meat, poultry, or fish
1 egg
½ ounce nuts or seeds
1 tablespoon peanut butter or
    almond butter

¼ cup cooked dried beans, lentils,
    or peas
¼ cup tofu/roasted soybeans

Shopping Tips

- Choose low-fat or lean cuts of meat.
- Use low-fat cooking methods—bake, broil, or grill.
- Vary your meals with more fish, beans, peas, lentils, nuts, and seeds.
- Select fish rich in omega-3 fats: salmon, trout, or herring.
- Trim visible fat and skin from meat before cooking.

Shopping List Essentials

| Lean beef | Turkey | Eggs | Beans | Lentils |
| Chicken | Fish | Almonds | Walnuts | Edamame |

161

Red Flags

Choosing proteins that are high in saturated fat and cholesterol may increase your risk for coronary heart disease. These include fatty cuts of beef, pork, and lamb; regular (75% to 85% lean) ground beef; regular sausages, hot dogs, and bacon; some luncheon meats, such as regular bologna and salami; and some poultry, such as duck. Avoid or limit processed meats, which often contain known carcinogens (nitrates and nitrites) and high levels of sodium. Caution should be used when choosing fish, especially by pregnant and nursing women and young children, since some types of fish are high in mercury. High-mercury fish include tuna, swordfish, shark, king mackerel, and tilefish.

Preparation Pointer

Of all the animal proteins, fish may be the fastest cooking and yet many home cooks avoid fish. Baked, grilled, or cooked on the stove, use the 10-minute rule. Measure the fish at the thickest point and cook it 10 minutes per inch, turning it halfway through. If it measures less than an inch, it does not need to be turned over. If purchasing fresh fish, check with the fish purveyor that it is fresh. If using frozen, defrost in the refrigerator or in a shallow dish of warm water, turning the package and changing the water as needed until defrosted. Canned fish (like salmon) is useful in soups, stews, and fish cakes/burgers. Lemon, garlic, and dill are commonly used to add flavor to fish. Orange, lime, mustard, and other herbs create many tasty fish dishes as well.

Food Serving size	Cal.	(g) Total Fat	(g) Sat. Fat	(mg) Chol.	(g) Carb.	(g) Fiber	(g) Sug.	(g) Prot.	(mg) Sod.
Meats									
Bacon Bits, Meatless 1 tbsp (7g)	33	2	0	0	2	0.7	0	2	124
Bacon, Meatless 1 oz, cooked yield (16g)	50	5	1	0	1	0.4	0	2	234
Bacon, Pre-Sliced, Reduced/Low Sodium, Unprepared 1 package (446g)	1815	175	0	0	4	0	4	56	2096
Beef Jerky, Chopped and Formed 1 piece, large (20g)	82	5	2	10	2	0.4	2	7	416
Beef, Bologna, Reduced Sodium 1 slice, medium (28g)	87	8	3	16	1	0	0	3	191
Beef, Bottom Sirloin, Tri-tip Roast, Lean and Fat, 0" Fat, Choice, Cooked, Roasted 1 roast (yield from 714 g raw meat) (591g)	1306	73	27	502	0	0	0	152	296
Beef, Bottom Sirloin, Tri-tip Roast, Lean and Fat, 0" Fat, Select, Cooked, Roasted 1 roast (yield from 666 g raw meat) (547g)	1099	53	20	443	0	0	0	145	306
Beef, Bottom Sirloin, Tri-tip Steak, Lean, 0" fat, All Grades, Cooked, Broiled 1 lb (453.6g)	1134	60	22	485	0	0	0	139	331
Beef, Brisket, Flat Half, Lean and Fat, 0" Fat, All Grades, Cooked, Braised 1 steak (yield from 418 g raw meat) (270g)	575	22	9	248	0	0	0	89	146
Beef, Brisket, Flat Half, Lean and Fat, 0" Fat, All Grades, Cooked, Braised 3 oz (85g)	174	6	2	85	0	0	0	28	46
Beef, Brisket, Flat Half, Lean and Fat, 0" Fat, Select, Cooked, Braised 1 steak (247g)	489	15	6	252	0	0	0	84	138
Beef, Brisket, Flat Half, Lean and Fat, 0" Fat, Select, Cooked, Braised 1 steak (yield from 388 g raw meat) (247g)	506	17	7	230	0	0	0	83	141
Beef, Brisket, Flat Half, Lean and Fat, 1/8" Fat, All Grades, Cooked, Braised 1 steak (yield from raw steak weighing 550 g) (380g)	1098	70	28	403	0	0	0	110	182
Beef, Brisket, Flat Half, Lean and Fat, 1/8" Fat, Choice, Cooked, Braised 1 steak (yield from 593 g raw meat) (409g)	1219	80	34	438	0	0	0	117	188

Food Serving size	Cal.	(g) Total Fat	(g) Sat. Fat	(mg) Chol.	(g) Carb.	(g) Fiber	(g) Sug.	(g) Prot.	(mg) Sod.
Beef, Brisket, Flat Half, Lean and Fat, 1/8" Fat, Select, Cooked, Braised									
1 steak (350g)	980	61	24	375	0	0	0	101	172
Beef, Brisket, Flat Half, Lean, 1/8" Fat, All Grades, Cooked, Braised									
1 lb (453.6g)	889	27	10	440	0	0	0	150	245
Beef, Brisket, Flat Half, Lean, 1/8" Fat, Choice, Cooked, Braised									
1 lb (453.6g)	921	31	12	440	0	0	0	150	240
Beef, Brisket, Point Half, Lean and Fat, 1/8" Fat, All Grades, Cooked, Braised									
1 piece, cooked excluding refuse (yield from 1 lb raw meat with refuse) (332g)	1159	90	35	305	0	0	0	81	229
Beef, Brisket, Whole, Lean and Fat, 1/8" Fat, All Grades, Cooked, Braised									
1 piece, cooked, excluding refuse (yield from 1 lb raw meat with refuse) (329g)	1089	81	31	306	0	0	0	85	211
Beef, Chuck Eye Country-style Ribs, Boneless, Lean, 0" Fat, All Grades, Cooked, Braised									
1 piece (227g)	672	47	20	218	0	0	0	63	148
Beef, Chuck Eye Country-style Ribs, Boneless, Lean, 0" Fat, Choice, Cooked									
1 piece (224g)	679	48	21	215	0	0	0	61	146
Beef, Chuck Eye Country-style Ribs, Boneless, Lean, 0" Fat, Select, Cooked, Braised									
1 piece (231g)	658	44	19	219	0	0	0	66	152
Beef, Chuck Eye Roast, Boneless, America's Beef Roast, Lean, 0" Fat, All Grades, Cooked									
1 roast (609g)	1114	52	21	512	0	0	0	162	487
Beef, Chuck Eye Roast, Boneless, America's Beef Roast, Lean, 0" Fat, Choice, Cooked									
1 roast (586g)	1113	55	22	498	0	0	0	155	463
Beef, Chuck Eye Roast, Boneless, America's Beef Roast, Lean, 0" Fat, Select, Cooked									
1 roast (645g)	1109	46	19	522	0	0	0	174	522
Beef, Chuck Eye Steak, Boneless, Lean, 0" Fat, All Grades, Cooked, Grilled									
1 steak (308g)	644	33	15	271	0	0	17	86	231
Beef, Chuck Eye Steak, Boneless, Lean, 0" Fat, Choice, Cooked, Grilled									
1 steak (307g)	660	35	15	267	0	0	15	86	230
Beef, Chuck Eye Steak, Boneless, Lean, 0" Fat, Select, Cooked, Grilled									
1 steak (309g)	615	30	15	281	0	0	16	86	229

Food Serving size	Cal.	(g) Total Fat	(g) Sat. Fat	(mg) Chol.	(g) Carb.	(g) Fiber	(g) Sug.	(g) Prot.	(mg) Sod.
Beef, Chuck for Stew, Lean and Fat, All Grades, Cooked, Braised									
1 lb (453.6g)	866	31	13	449	0	0	0	147	304
Beef, Chuck for Stew, Lean and Fat, Choice, Cooked, Braised									
1 lb (453.6g)	165	6	2	82	0	0	0	28	55
Beef, Chuck for Stew, Lean and Fat, Select, Cooked, Braised									
1 lb (453.6g)	158	5	2	87	0	0	0	27	58
Beef, Chuck, Arm Pot Roast, Lean and Fat, 0" Fat, All Grades, Cooked, Braised									
1 roast (yield from 1601 g raw meat) (1166g)	3463	224	88	1353	0	0	0	337	548
Beef, Chuck, Arm Pot Roast, Lean and Fat, 0" Fat, Select, Cooked, Braised									
1 roast (yield from 1675 g raw meat) (1236g)	3498	217	85	1421	0	0	0	361	593
Beef, Chuck, Arm Pot Roast, Lean and Fat, 1/8" Fat, All Grades, Cooked, Braised									
1 piece, cooked, excluding refuse (yield from 1 lb raw meat with refuse) (258g)	779	50	20	310	0	0	0	78	129
Beef, Chuck, Arm Pot Roast, Lean and Fat, 1/8" Fat, Choice, Cooked, Braised									
1 piece, cooked, excluding refuse (yield from 1 lb raw meat with refuse) (yield 258g)	797	51	20	312	0	0	0	78	126
Beef, Chuck, Arm Pot Roast, Lean and Fat, 1/8" Fat, Select, Cooked, Braised									
1 piece, cooked, excluding refuse (yield from 1 lb raw meat with refuse) (yield 257g)	758	48	19	306	0	0	0	77	129
Beef, Chuck, Arm Pot Roast, Lean, 0" Fat, Choice, Cooked, Braised									
1 roast (yield from 1528 g raw meat) (1095g)	2321	84	32	1095	0	0	0	365	591
Beef, Chuck, Arm Pot Roast, Lean, 0" Fat, Select, Cooked, Braised									
1 roast (yield from 1675 g raw meat) (1236g)	2410	72	27	1211	0	0	0	412	680
Beef, Chuck, Arm Pot Roast, Lean, 1/8" Fat, All Grades, Cooked, Braised									
1 lb (453.6g)	971	33	13	472	0	0	0	157	254
Beef, Chuck, Arm Pot Roast, Lean, 1/8" Fat, Choice, Cooked, Braised									
1 lb (453.6g)	1016	38	14	481	0	0	0	157	254
Beef, Chuck, Blade Roast, Lean and Fat, 1/8" Fat, All Grades, Cooked, Braised									
1 piece, cooked, excluding refuse (yield from 1 lb raw meat with refuse) (247g)	842	62	25	257	0	0	0	66	161

Food Serving size	Cal.	(g) Total Fat	(g) Sat. Fat	(mg) Chol.	(g) Carb.	(g) Fiber	(g) Sug.	(g) Prot.	(mg) Sod.
Beef, Chuck, Blade Roast, Lean and Fat, 1/8" Fat, Choice, Cooked, Braised									
1 piece, cooked, excluding refuse (yield from 1 lb raw meat with refuse) (247g)									
	887	67	27	254	0	0	0	65	158
Beef, Chuck, Blade Roast, Lean and Fat, 1/8" Fat, Select, Cooked, Braised									
1 piece, cooked, excluding refuse (yield from 1 lb raw meat with refuse) (247g)									
	785	55	22	257	0	0	0	68	163
Beef, Chuck, Clod Roast, Lean and Fat, 0" Fat, All Grades, Cooked, Roasted									
1 lb (453.6g)	939	49	18	313	0	0	6	117	322
Beef, Chuck, Clod Roast, Lean Only, to 1/4" Fat, All Grades, Cooked, Roasted									
1 lb (453.6g)	785	31	10	322	0	0	0	120	322
Beef, Chuck, Clod Roast, Lean, 0" Fat, All Grades, Cooked, Roasted									
1 lb (453.6g)	780	29	9	304	0	0	0	122	336
Beef, Chuck, Clod Roast, Lean and Fat, 0" Fat, Choice, Cooked, Roasted									
1 lb (453.6g)	980	56	19	304	0	0	0	112	322
Beef, Chuck, Clod Roast, Lean and Fat, 0" Fat, Select, Cooked, Roasted									
1 lb (453.6g)	889	40	15	331	0	0	0	124	327
Beef, Chuck, Clod Steak, Lean Only, to 1/4" Fat, All Grades, Cooked, Braised									
1 lb (453.6g)	857	32	10	426	0	0	4	133	272
Beef, Chuck, Clod, Shoulder Tender, Medium, Lean and Fat, 0" Fat, All Grades, Cooked, Grilled									
1 serving (3 oz) (85g)	150	6	2	66	0	0	0	22	50
Beef, Chuck, Clod, Shoulder Tender, Medium, Lean and Fat, 0" Fat, Choice, Cooked, Grilled									
1 serving (3 oz) (85g)	154	7	2	65	0	0	0	22	51
Beef, Chuck, Clod, Shoulder Tender, Medium, Lean and Fat, 0" Fat, Select, Cooked, Grilled									
1 serving (3 oz) (85g)	146	5	1	68	0	0	0	22	49
Beef, Chuck, Clod, Shoulder Top and Center Steak, Lean and Fat, 0", All Grades, Grilled									
1 serving (3 oz) (85g)	155	7	2	65	0	0	8	22	51
Beef, Chuck, Clod, Top and Center, Steak, Lean and Fat, 0" Fat, Select, Cooked, Grilled									
1 serving (3 oz) (85g)	150	6	2	65	0	0	8	23	53
Beef, Chuck, Clod, Top Blade, Steak, Lean and Fat, 0" Fat, All Grades, Cooked, Grilled									
1 serving (3 oz) (85g)	189	11	4	71	0	0	15	21	65

Food Serving size	Cal.	(g) Total Fat	(g) Sat. Fat	(mg) Chol.	(g) Carb.	(g) Fiber	(g) Sug.	(g) Prot.	(mg) Sod.
Beef, Chuck, Clod, Top Blade, Steak, Lean and Fat, 0" Fat, Choice, Cooked, Grilled									
1 serving (3 oz) (85g)	194	12	5	71	0	0	17	21	66
Beef, Chuck, Clod, Top Blade, Steak, Lean and Fat, 0" Fat, Select, Cooked, Grilled									
1 serving (3 oz) (85g)	180	10	4	71	0	0	11	21	65
Beef, Chuck, Eye Country-style Ribs, Boneless, Lean and Fat, 0" Fat, All Grades, Cooked									
1 piece (227g)	672	47	20	218	0	0	0	63	148
Beef, Chuck, Eye Country-style Ribs, Boneless, Lean and Fat, 0" Fat, Choice, Cooked									
1 piece (224g)	679	48	21	215	0	0	0	61	146
Beef, Chuck, Eye Country-style Ribs, Boneless, Lean and Fat, 0" Fat, Select, Cooked									
1 piece (231g)	658	44	20	222	0	0	0	66	152
Beef, Chuck, Eye Roast, Boneless, America's Beef Roast, Lean and Fat, 0", All Grades, Cooked, Roasted									
1 roast (609g)	1437	93	39	505	0	0	0	150	463
Beef, Chuck, Eye Roast, Boneless, America's Beef Roast, Lean and Fat, 0", Choice, Cooked, Roasted									
1 roast (586g)	1412	93	38	498	0	0	0	143	440
Beef, Chuck, Eye Roast, Boneless, America's Beef Roast, Lean and Fat, 0" Fat, Select, Cooked, Roasted									
1 roast (645g)	1477	93	40	522	0	0	0	160	490
Beef, Chuck, Eye Steak, Boneless, Lean and Fat, 0" Fat, All Grades, Cooked, Grilled									
1 steak (308g)	853	60	27	268	0	0	16	77	219
Beef, Chuck, Eye Steak, Boneless, Lean and Fat, 0" Fat, Choice, Cooked, Grilled									
1 steak (307g)	869	62	27	264	0	0	0	77	218
Beef, Chuck, Eye Steak, Boneless, Lean and Fat, 0" Fat, Select, Cooked, Grilled									
1 steak (309g)	825	57	27	275	0	0	15	77	216
Beef, Chuck, Mock Tender Steak, Boneless, Lean and Fat, 0" Fat, All Grades, Cooked									
1 steak (198g)	253	9	4	135	0	0	0	42	158
Beef, Chuck, Mock Tender Steak, Boneless, Lean and Fat, 0" Fat, All Grades, Cooked									
1 steak (141g)	310	14	5	159	0	0	0	45	94

Food Serving size	Cal.	(g) Total Fat	(g) Sat. Fat	(mg) Chol.	(g) Carb.	(g) Fiber	(g) Sug.	(g) Prot.	(mg) Sod.
Beef, Chuck, Mock Tender Steak, Boneless, Lean and Fat, 0" Fat, Choice, Cooked									
1 steak (141g)	317	15	5	155	0	0	0	45	93
Beef, Chuck, Mock Tender Steak, Boneless, Lean and Fat, 0" Fat, Select, Cooked									
1 steak (141g)	298	13	5	165	0	0	0	45	97
Beef, Chuck, Mock Tender Steak, Boneless, Lean, 0" Fat, All Grades, Cooked, Braised									
1 steak (141g)	268	9	4	161	0	0	15	47	96
Beef, Chuck, Mock Tender Steak, Boneless, Lean, 0" Fat, Choice, Cooked, Braised									
1 steak (141g)	278	10	4	157	0	0	0	47	94
Beef, Chuck, Mock Tender Steak, Boneless, Lean, 0" Fat, Select, Cooked, Braised									
1 steak (141g)	255	8	3	166	0	0	4	46	99
Beef, Chuck, Mock Tender Steak, Lean and Fat, 0" Fat, All Grades, Cooked, Broiled									
1 lb (453.6g)	726	25	8	286	0	0	10	117	322
Beef, Chuck, Mock Tender Steak, Lean and Fat, 0" Fat, USDA Choice, Cooked, Broiled									
1 lb (453.6g)	730	26	8	295	0	0	0	117	331
Beef, Chuck, Mock Tender Steak, Lean and Fat, 0" Fat, USDA Select, Cooked, Broiled									
1 lb (453.6g)	721	24	9	272	0	0	0	118	308
Beef, Chuck, Mock Tender Steak, Lean, 0" Fat, All Grades, Cooked, Broiled									
1 lb (453.6g)	721	25	8	286	0	0	12	117	322
Beef, Chuck, Mock Tender Steak, Lean, 0" Fat, Choice, Cooked, Broiled									
3 oz (1 serving) (85g)	137	5	1	80	0	0	0	22	62
Beef, Chuck, Mock Tender Steak, Lean, 0" Fat, Select, Cooked, Broiled									
3 oz (1 serving) (85g)	133	4	2	84	0	0	0	22	58
Beef, Chuck, Pot Roast, Lean, 1/8" Fat, Select, Cooked, Braised									
1 lb (453.6g)	930	29	11	467	0	0	0	157	259
Beef, Chuck, Short Ribs, Boneless, 0" Fat, Choice, Cooked, Broiled									
1 piece (272g)	680	41	19	277	0	0	0	78	204
Beef, Chuck, Short Ribs, Boneless, Lean and Fat, 0" Fat, All Grades, Cooked, Braised									
1 piece (289g)	881	65	29	289	0	0	14	74	202

Food Serving size	Cal.	(g) Total Fat	(g) Sat. Fat	(mg) Chol.	(g) Carb.	(g) Fiber	(g) Sug.	(g) Prot.	(mg) Sod.
Beef, Chuck, Short Ribs, Boneless, Lean and Fat, 0" Fat, Choice, Cooked, Braised									
1 piece (272g)	862	65	29	267	0	0	32	69	190
Beef, Chuck, Short Ribs, Boneless, Lean and Fat, 0" Fat, Select, Cooked, Braised									
1 piece (315g)	904	64	29	324	0	0	0	81	224
Beef, Chuck, Short Ribs, Boneless, Lean, 0" Fat, All Grades, Cooked, Braised									
1 piece (289g)	694	40	19	303	0	0	0	83	217
Beef, Chuck, Short Ribs, Boneless, Lean, 0" Fat, Select, Cooked, Braised									
1 piece (315g)	706	38	18	340	0	0	0	91	236
Beef, Chuck, Shoulder Clod, Top and Center, Steak, Lean and Fat, 0" Fat, Choice, Cooked, Grilled									
1 serving (3 oz) (85g)	156	7	3	63	0	0	2	22	50
Beef, Chuck, Top Blade, Lean and Fat, 0" Fat, All Grades, Cooked, Broiled									
1 lb (453.6g)	980	53	18	277	0	0	16	117	304
Beef, Chuck, Top Blade, Lean and Fat, 0" Fat, Choice, Cooked, Broiled									
1 lb (453.6g)	1030	59	19	263	0	0	8	117	308
Beef, Chuck, Top Blade, Lean and Fat, 0" Fat, Select, Cooked, Broiled									
1 lb (453.6g)	907	45	16	304	0	0	17	116	304
Beef, Chuck, Top Blade, Lean Only, to 0" Fat, All Grades, Cooked, Broiled									
1 lb (453.6g)	921	46	15	272	0	0	14	119	308
Beef, Chuck, Top Blade, Lean, 0" Fat, Choice, Cooked, Broiled									
3 oz (1 serving) (85g)	184	10	3	79	0	0	0	22	58
Beef, Chuck, Top Blade, Lean, 0" Fat, Select, Cooked, Broiled									
3 oz (1 serving) (85g)	156	7	2	80	0	0	0	22	58
Beef, Chuck, Under Blade Center Steak, Boneless, Denver Cut, Lean and Fat, All Grades, Cooked									
1 steak (353g)	801	48	20	332	1	0	0	92	258
Beef, Chuck, Under Blade Center Steak, Boneless, Denver Cut, Lean, 0" Fat									
1 steak (356g)	812	48	20	328	1	0	0	94	260
Beef, Chuck, Under Blade Center Steak, Boneless, Denver Cut, Lean, 0" Fat									
1 steak (353g)	777	45	19	332	0	0	0	94	258
Beef, Chuck, Under Blade Center Steak, Boneless, Denver Cut, Lean, 0" Fat, Select, Cooked									
1 steak (349g)	729	40	17	335	0	0	0	93	258

Food Serving size	Cal.	(g) Total Fat	(g) Sat. Fat	(mg) Chol.	(g) Carb.	(g) Fiber	(g) Sug.	(g) Prot.	(mg) Sod.
Beef, Chuck, Under Blade Pot Roast, Boneless, Lean and Fat, 0" Fat, Choice, Cooked, Braised									
1 roast (658g)	2013	141	56	658	0	0	0	174	401
Beef, Chuck, Under Blade Pot Roast, Boneless, Lean and Fat, 0" Fat, Select, Cooked, Braised									
1 roast (629g)	1812	120	49	616	0	0	0	171	403
Beef, Chuck, Under Blade Pot Roast, Boneless, Lean, 0" Fat, All Grades, Cooked									
1 roast (647g)	1398	68	26	673	0	0	0	198	421
Beef, Chuck, Under Blade Pot Roast, Boneless, Lean, 0" Fat, All Grades, Cooked, Braised									
1 roast (960g)	1344	58	26	634	3	0	0	203	778
Beef, Chuck, Under Blade Pot Roast, Boneless, Lean, 0" Fat, Choice, Cooked, Braised									
1 roast (658g)	1520	73	29	691	0	0	0	200	415
Beef, Chuck, Under Blade Pot Roast, Boneless, Lean, 0" Fat, Select, Cooked, Braised									
1 roast (629g)	1359	59	22	642	0	0	0	193	421
Beef, Chuck, Under Blade Steak, Boneless, Lean and Fat, 0" Fat, All Grades									
1 steak (449g)	1235	81	33	431	0	0	0	127	292
Beef, Chuck, Under Blade Steak, Boneless, Lean and Fat, 0" Fat, Choice, Cooked									
1 steak (445g)	1264	86	34	436	0	0	0	123	285
Beef, Chuck, Under Blade Steak, Boneless, Lean and Fat, 0" Fat, Select, Cooked									
1 steak (454g)	1185	73	30	427	0	0	0	132	300
Beef, Chuck, Under Blade Steak, Boneless, Lean, 0" Fat, All Grades, Cooked, Braised									
1 steak (449g)	983	47	18	480	0	0	0	141	292
Beef, Chuck, Under Blade Steak, Boneless, Lean, 0" Fat, Choice, Cooked, Braised									
1 steak (445g)	988	49	19	472	0	0	0	138	289
Beef, Chuck, Under Blade Steak, Boneless, Lean, 0" Fat, Select, Cooked, Braised									
1 steak (454g)	976	44	16	490	0	0	0	145	300
Beef, Chuck, Under Blade, Pot Roast, Boneless, Lean and Fat, 0" Fat, All Grades, Cooked, Broiled									
1 roast (647g)	1883	133	53	641	0	0	0	173	401

Food Serving size	Cal.	(g) Total Fat	(g) Sat. Fat	(mg) Chol.	(g) Carb.	(g) Fiber	(g) Sug.	(g) Prot.	(mg) Sod.
Beef, Composite of Retail Cuts, Lean and Fat, 0" Fat, All Grades, Cooked									
1 piece, cooked, excluding refuse (yield from 1 lb raw meat with refuse) (279g)									
	762	48	19	243	0	0	0	76	173
Beef, Composite of Retail Cuts, Lean and Fat, 0" Fat, Choice, Cooked									
1 piece, cooked, excluding refuse (yield from 1 lb raw meat with refuse) (240g)									
	790	52	20	243	0	0	0	76	173
Beef, Composite of Retail Cuts, Lean and Fat, 0" Fat, Select, Cooked									
1 piece, cooked, excluding refuse (yield from 1 lb raw meat with refuse) (244g)									
	728	44	17	240	0	0	0	77	176
Beef, Composite of Retail Cuts, Lean and Fat, 1/8" Fat, All Grades, Cooked									
1 piece, cooked, excluding refuse (yield from 1 lb raw meat with refuse) (285g)									
	829	56	22	248	0	0	0	75	180
Beef, Composite of Retail Cuts, Lean and Fat, 1/8" Fat, Choice, Cooked									
1 piece, cooked, excluding refuse (yield from 1 lb raw meat with refuse) (285g)									
	858	60	23	248	0	0	0	75	177
Beef, Composite of Retail Cuts, Lean and Fat, 1/8" Fat, Prime, Cooked									
1 piece, cooked, excluding refuse (yield from 1 lb raw meat with refuse) (296g)									
	885	61	25	246	0	0	0	78	186
Beef, Composite of Retail Cuts, Lean and Fat, 1/8" Fat, Select, Cooked									
1 piece, cooked, excluding refuse (yield from 1 lb raw meat with refuse) (286g)									
	795	52	21	246	0	0	0	76	180
Beef, Composite of Retail Cuts, Lean, 0" Fat, All Grades, Cooked									
1 piece, cooked, excluding refuse (yield from 1 lb raw meat with refuse) (242g)									
	511	22	9	208	0	0	0	72	160
Beef, Composite of Retail Cuts, Lean, 0" Fat, Choice, Cooked									
1 piece, cooked, excluding refuse (yield from 1 lb raw meat with refuse) (240g)									
	526	24	9	206	0	0	0	72	158
Beef, Composite of Retail Cuts, Lean, 0" Fat, Select, Cooked									
1 piece, cooked, excluding refuse (yield from 1 lb raw meat with refuse) (244g)									
	490	20	8	210	0	0	0	73	161
Beef, Cured, Breakfast Strips, Cooked									
1 package, cooked (yield from 12 oz raw product) (170g)									
	763	58	24	202	2	0	0	53	3830
Beef, Cured, Corned Beef, Brisket, Cooked									
1 piece, cooked, excluding refuse (yield from 1 lb raw meat with refuse) (320g)									
	803	61	20	314	2	0	0	58	3114

Food Serving size	Cal.	(g) Total Fat	(g) Sat. Fat	(mg) Chol.	(g) Carb.	(g) Fiber	(g) Sug.	(g) Prot.	(mg) Sod.
Beef, Cured, Corned beef, Canned 1 slice (3/4 oz) (21g)	53	3	1	18	0	0	0	6	211
Beef, Cured, Dried 10 slices (28g)	43	1	0	22	1	0	1	9	781
Beef, Cured, Luncheon Meat, Jellied 1 slice (1 oz) (4" x 4" x 3/32" thick) (28g)	31	1	0	10	0	0	0	5	370
Beef, Cured, Pastrami 1 slice (1 oz) (28g)	41	2	1	19	0	0	0	6	248
Beef, Cured, Sausage, Cooked, Smoked 1 oz (28.35g)	88	8	3	19	1	0	0	4	321
Beef, Cured, Smoked, Chopped Beef 1 slice (1 oz) (28g)	37	1	1	13	1	0	0	6	352
Beef, Cured, Thin-sliced Beef 5 slices (21g)	37	1	0	9	1	0	0	6	302
Beef, Flank, Steak, Lean and Fat, 0" Fat, All Grades, Cooked, Broiled 1 steak (yield from 475 g raw meat) (383g)	735	32	13	303	0	0	0	106	214
Beef, Flank, Steak, Lean and Fat, 0" Fat, Choice, Cooked, Braised 1 piece, cooked, excluding refuse (yield from 1 lb raw meat with refuse) (262 grams)	689	43	18	189	0	0	0	71	183
Beef, Flank, Steak, Lean and Fat, 0" Fat, Choice, Cooked, Broiled 1 steak (yield from 483 g raw meat) (387g)	782	36	15	313	0	0	0	107	205
Beef, Flank, Steak, Lean and Fat, 0" Fat, Select, Cooked, Broiled 1 steak (yield from 467 g raw meat) (379g)	694	27	11	296	0	0	0	105	220
Beef, Flank, Steak, Lean, 0" Fat, Choice, Cooked, Braised 1 piece, cooked, excluding refuse (yield from 1 lb raw meat with refuse) (262 grams)	583	32	14	175	0	0	0	69	177
Beef, Flank, Steak, Lean, 0" Fat, Choice, Cooked, Broiled 1 steak (387 grams)	751	32	13	310	0	0	0	108	217
Beef, Ground, 70% Lean Meat/30% Fat, Crumbles, Cooked, Pan-browned 1 portion (yield from 1/2 lb raw meat) (139g)	366	25	10	124	0	0	0	36	133

Food Serving size	Cal.	(g) Total Fat	(g) Sat. Fat	(mg) Chol.	(g) Carb.	(g) Fiber	(g) Sug.	(g) Prot.	(mg) Sod.
Beef, Ground, 70% Lean Meat/30% Fat, Loaf, Cooked, Baked									
1 loaf (yield from 1 lb raw meat) (284g)									
	684	44	17	250	0	0	0	68	207
Beef, Ground, 70% Lean Meat/30% Fat, Patty, Cooked, Broiled									
1 patty (70g)	194	13	5	62	0	0	0	18	57
Beef, Ground, 70% Lean Meat/30% Fat, Patty, Cooked, Pan-broiled									
1 patty (77g)	183	12	5	65	0	0	0	18	71
Beef, Ground, 75% Lean Meat, 25% Fat, Crumbles, Cooked, Pan-browned									
1 portion (yield from 1/2 lb raw meat) (139g)									
	385	25	10	124	0	0	8	37	129
Beef, Ground, 75% Lean Meat, 25% Fat, Loaf, Cooked, Baked									
1 loaf (yield from 1 lb raw meat) (284g)									
	721	47	18	233	0	0	19	70	199
Beef, Ground, 75% Lean Meat, 25% Fat, Patty, Cooked, Broiled									
1 patty (yield from 1/4 lb raw meat) (70g)									
	195	13	5	62	0	0	1	18	55
Beef, Ground, 75% Lean Meat, 25% Fat, Patty, Cooked, Pan-broiled									
1 patty (yield from 1/4 lb raw meat) (77g)									
	191	13	5	64	0	0	4	18	67
Beef, Ground, 80% Lean Meat, 20% Fat, Crumbles, Cooked, Pan-browned									
1 portion (yield from 1/2 lb raw meat) (149g)									
	405	26	10	133	0	0	7	40	136
Beef, Ground, 80% Lean Meat, 20% Fat, Loaf, Cooked, Baked									
1 loaf (yield from 1 lb raw meat) (309g)									
	785	50	19	278	0	0	11	78	207
Beef, Ground, 80% Lean Meat, 20% Fat, Patty, Cooked, Broiled									
1 patty (yield from 1/4 lb raw meat) (77g)									
	209	14	5	70	0	0	2	20	58
Beef, Ground, 80% Lean Meat, 20% Fat, Patty, Cooked, Pan-broiled									
1 patty (yield from 1/4 lb raw meat) (83g)									
	204	13	5	71	0	0	4	20	69
Beef, Ground, 85% Lean Meat, 15% Fat, Crumbles, Cooked, Pan-browned									
1 portion (yield from 1/2 lb raw meat) (149g)									
	381	23	9	134	0	0	4	41	133
Beef, Ground, 85% Lean Meat, 15% Fat, Loaf, Cooked, Baked									
1 loaf (yield from 1 lb raw meat) (309g)									
	742	44	17	281	0	0	21	80	198

Food Serving size	Cal.	(g) Total Fat	(g) Sat. Fat	(mg) Chol.	(g) Carb.	(g) Fiber	(g) Sug.	(g) Prot.	(mg) Sod.
Beef, Ground, 85% Lean Meat, 15% Fat, Patty, Cooked, Broiled 1 patty (yield from 1/4 lb raw meat) (77g)									
	193	12	5	69	0	0	2	20	55
Beef, Ground, 85% Lean Meat, 15% Fat, Patty, Cooked, Pan-broiled 1 patty (yield from 1/4 lb raw meat) (83g)									
	193	12	4	71	0	0	4	20	66
Beef, Ground, 90% Lean Meat, 10% Fat, Crumbles, Cooked, Pan-browne 1 portion (yield from 1/2 lb raw meat) (154g)									
	354	19	7	137	0	0	5	44	134
Beef, Ground, 90% Lean Meat, 10% Fat, Loaf, Cooked, Baked 1 loaf (yield from 1 lb raw meat) (323g)									
	691	36	14	278	0	0	10	86	197
Beef, Ground, 90% Lean Meat, 10% Fat, Patty, Cooked, Broiled 1 patty (yield from 1/4 lb raw meat) (82g)									
	178	10	4	70	0	0	4	21	56
Beef, Ground, 90% Lean Meat, 10% Fat, Patty, Cooked, Pan-broiled 1 patty (yield from 1/4 lb raw meat) (86g)									
	175	9	4	71	0	0	4	22	65
Beef, Ground, 95% Lean Meat, 5% Fat, Crumbles, Cooked, Pan-browned 1 portion (yield from 1/2 lb raw meat) (154g)									
	297	12	5	137	0	0	8	45	131
Beef, Ground, 95% Lean Meat, 5% Fat, Loaf, Cooked, Baked 1 loaf (yield from 1 lb raw meat) (323g)									
	562	21	9	236	0	0	14	88	187
Beef, Ground, 95% Lean Meat, 5% Fat, Patty, Cooked, Broiled 1 patty (yield from 1/4 lb raw meat) (82g)									
	140	5	2	62	0	0	1	22	53
Beef, Ground, 95% Lean Meat, 5% Fat, Patty, Cooked, Pan-broiled 1 patty (yield from 1/4 lb raw meat) (86g)									
	141	5	2	65	0	0	5	22	61
Beef, Ground, Patties, Frozen, Cooked, Broiled 3 oz (85g)	251	19	7	71	0	0	0	20	65
Beef, Loin, Bottom Sirloin Butt, Tri-tip, Lean, 0" Fat, All Grades, Cooked, Roasted 1 roast (569g)	1036	47	18	444	0	0	0	152	313
Beef, Loin, Porterhouse Steak, Lean and Fat, 0" Fat, USDA Choice, Cooked, Broiled 1 lb (453.6g)	1284	91	34	313	0	0	0	107	295

Food Serving size	Cal.	(g) Total Fat	(g) Sat. Fat	(mg) Chol.	(g) Carb.	(g) Fiber	(g) Sug.	(g) Prot.	(mg) Sod.
Beef, Loin, T-bone Steak, Lean & Fat, 0" Fat, USDA Choice, Cooked, Broiled									
1 lb (453.6g)	1170	78	29	277	0	0	0	109	304
Beef, Plate, Inside Skirt Steak, Lean, 0" Fat, All Grades, Cooked, Broiled									
3 oz (1 serving) (85g)	174	9	3	72	0	0	0	23	65
Beef, Plate, Outside Skirt Steak, Lean and Fat, 0" Fat, All Grades, Cooked Broiled									
1 lb (453.6g)	1157	78	32	268	0	0	22	107	417
Beef, Plate, Outside Skirt Steak, Lean, 0" Fat, All Grades, Cooked, Broiled									
3 oz (1 serving) (85g)	198	12	5	77	0	0	0	21	80
Beef, Plate, Skirt Steak, Lean and Fat, 0" Fat, All Grades, Cooked, Broiled									
1 lb (453.6g)	998	55	21	272	0	0	0	119	340
Beef, Retail Cuts, Fat, Cooked									
3 oz (85g)	578	60	24	81	0	0	0	9	20
Beef, Rib Eye, Small End (Ribs 10-12) Lean, 0" Fat, Select, Cooked, Broiled									
1 steak (231g)	420	14	5	219	0	0	0	69	146
Beef, Rib Eye, Small End (Ribs 10-12), Lean and Fat, 0" Fat, All Grades, Cooked, Broiled									
1 steak (yield from 295 g raw meat) (233g)	580	34	13	207	0	0	0	64	130
Beef, Rib Eye, Small End (Ribs 10-12), Lean and Fat, 0" Fat, Choice, Cooked, Broiled									
1 steak (yield from 297 g raw meat) (236g)	625	40	15	208	0	0	0	63	125
Beef, Rib Eye, Small End (Ribs 10-12), Lean and Fat, 0" Fat, Select, Cooked, Broiled									
1 steak (yield from 294 g raw meat) (231g)	541	29	11	213	0	0	0	65	136
Beef, Rib Eye, Small End (Ribs 10-12), Lean, 0" Fat, Choice, Cooked, Broiled									
3 oz (85g)	174	8	3	77	0	0	0	25	51
Beef, Rib, Large End (Ribs 6-9), Lean and Fat, 0" Fat, Choice, Cooked, Roasted									
1 piece, cooked, excluding refuse (yield from 1 lb raw meat with refuse) (290g)	1079	88	36	247	0	0	0	66	186
Beef, Rib, Large End (Ribs 6-9), Lean and Fat, 0" Fat, Select, Cooked, Roasted									
1 piece, cooked, excluding refuse (yield from 1 lb raw meat with refuse) (286g)	947	73	29	240	0	0	0	67	186

Food Serving size	Cal.	(g) Total Fat	(g) Sat. Fat	(mg) Chol.	(g) Carb.	(g) Fiber	(g) Sug.	(g) Prot.	(mg) Sod.
Beef, Rib, Large End (Ribs 6-9), Lean and Fat, 1/8" Fat, All Grades, Cooked, Broiled									
1 piece, cooked, excluding refuse (yield from 1 lb raw meat with refuse) (267g)									
	902	73	30	214	0	0	0	58	171
Beef, Rib, Large End (Ribs 6-9), Lean and Fat, 1/8" Fat, All Grades, Cooked, Roasted									
1 piece, cooked, excluding refuse (yield from 1 lb raw meat with refuse) (292g)									
	1037	83	34	248	0	0	0	67	187
Beef, Rib, Large End (Ribs 6-9), Lean and Fat, 1/8" Fat, Choice, Cooked, Broiled									
1 piece, cooked, excluding refuse (yield from 1 lb raw meat with refuse) (267g)									
	988	83	34	216	0	0	0	56	168
Beef, Rib, Large End (Ribs 6-9), Lean and Fat, 1/8" Fat, Choice, Cooked, Roasted									
1 piece, cooked, excluding refuse (yield from 1 lb raw meat with refuse) (296g)									
	1119	93	37	252	0	0	0	67	186
Beef, Rib, Large End (Ribs 6-9), Lean and Fat, 1/8" Fat, Prime, Cooked, Broiled									
1 piece, cooked, excluding refuse (yield from 1 lb raw meat with refuse) (278g)									
	1123	97	40	239	0	0	0	57	172
Beef, Rib, Large End (Ribs 6-9), Lean and Fat, 1/8" Fat, Prime, Cooked, Roasted									
1 piece, cooked, ecluding refuse (yield from 1 lb raw meat with refuse) (281g)									
	1104	92	38	239	0	0	0	64	180
Beef, Rib, Large End (Ribs 6-9), Lean and Fat, 1/8" Fat, Select, Cooked, Broiled									
1 piece, cooked, excluding refuse (yield from 1 lb raw meat with refuse) (267g)									
	865	69	28	214	0	0	0	58	171
Beef, Rib, Large End (Ribs 6-9), Lean and Fat, 1/8" Fat, Select, Cooked, Roasted									
1 piece, cooked, excluding refuse (yield from 1 lb raw meat with refuse) (292g)									
	972	75	30	245	0	0	0	68	190
Beef, Rib, Large End (Ribs 6-9), Lean, 0" Fat, All Grades, Cooked, Roasted									
1 piece, cooked, excluding refuse (yield from 1lb raw meat with refuse) (214g)									
	509	29	11	173	0	0	0	59	156
Beef, Rib, Large End (Ribs 6-9), Lean, 0" Fat, Choice, Cooked, Roasted									
1 piece, cooked, excluding refuse (yield from 1 lb raw meat with refuse) (290g)									
	524	31	12	168	0	0	0	57	151
Beef, Rib, Large End (Ribs 6-9), Lean, 0" Fat, Select, Cooked, Roasted									
1 piece, cooked, excluding refuse (yield from 1 lb raw meat with refuse) (217g)									
	477	25	10	176	0	0	0	60	158

Food Serving size	Cal.	(g) Total Fat	(g) Sat. Fat	(mg) Chol.	(g) Carb.	(g) Fiber	(g) Sug.	(g) Prot.	(mg) Sod.
Beef, Rib, Short Ribs, Lean and Fat, Choice, Cooked, Braised									
1 piece, cooked, excluding refuse (yield from 1 lb raw meat with refuse) (225g)									
	1060	94	40	212	0	0	0	49	113
Beef, Rib, Short Ribs, Lean, Choice, Cooked, Braised									
3 oz (85g)	251	15	7	79	0	0	0	26	49
Beef, Rib, Small End (Ribs 10-12), Lean and Fat, 0" Fat, All Grades, Cooked, Broiled									
1 steak (yield from 233 g raw meat) (233g)									
	580	34	13	207	0	0	0	64	130
Beef, Rib, Small End (Ribs 10-12), Lean and Fat, 0" Fat, Choice, Cooked, Broiled									
1 piece, cooked, excluding refuse (yield from 1 lb raw meat with refuse) (272g)									
	849	62	25	226	0	0	0	67	174
Beef, Rib, Small End (Ribs 10-12), Lean and Fat, 0" Fat, Select, Cooked, Broiled									
1 piece, cooked, excluding refuse (yield from 1 lb raw meat with refuse) (265g)									
	755	52	21	220	0	0	0	66	170
Beef, Rib, Small End (Ribs 10-12), Lean and Fat, 1/8" Fat, All Grades, Cooked, Broiled									
1 piece, cooked, excluding refuse (yield from 1 lb raw meat with refuse) (268g)									
	780	54	21	260	0	0	0	69	142
Beef, Rib, Small End (Ribs 10-12), Lean and Fat, 1/8" Fat, All Grades, Cooked, Roasted									
1 piece, cooked, excluding refuse (yield from 1 lb raw meat with refuse) (282g)									
	962	77	31	234	0	0	0	64	178
Beef, Rib, Small End (Ribs 10-12), Lean and Fat, 1/8" Fat, Choice, Cooked, Broiled									
1 steak (yield from 320 g raw meat) (256g)									
	778	57	22	241	0	0	0	63	125
Beef, Rib, Small End (Ribs 10-12), Lean and Fat, 1/8" Fat, Choice, Cooked, Roasted									
1 piece, cooked, excluding refuse (yield from 1 lb raw meat with refuse) (278g)									
	998	81	33	231	0	0	0	62	175
Beef, Rib, Small End (Ribs 10-12), Lean and Fat, 1/8" Fat, Prime, Cooked, Broiled									
1 piece, cooked, excluding refuse (yield from 1 lb raw meat with refuse) (268g)									
	949	75	31	222	0	0	0	65	169

Food Serving size	Cal.	(g) Total Fat	(g) Sat. Fat	(mg) Chol.	(g) Carb.	(g) Fiber	(g) Sug.	(g) Prot.	(mg) Sod.
Beef, Rib, Small End (Ribs 10-12), Lean and Fat, 1/8" Fat, Prime, Cooked, Roasted 1 piece, cooked, excluding refuse (yield from 1 lb raw meat with refuse) (276g)	1134	97	40	232	0	0	0	61	179
Beef, Rib, Small End (Ribs 10-12), Lean and Fat, 1/8" Fat, Select, Cooked, Broiled 1 steak (yield from 1 raw steak weighing 321g)	681	44	17	252	0	0	0	67	142
Beef, Rib, Small End (Ribs 10-12), Lean and Fat, 1/8" Fat, Select, Cooked, Roasted 1 piece, cooked, excluding refuse (yield from 1 lb raw meat with refuse) (285g)	921	71	29	237	0	0	0	65	182
Beef, Rib, Small End (Ribs 10-12), Lean, 0" Fat, All Grades, Cooked, Broiled 1 steak (yield from 296 g raw meat) (233g)	450	18	7	212	0	0	0	69	142
Beef, Rib, Small End (Ribs 10-12), Lean, 0" Fat, Choice, Cooked, Broiled 1 piece, cooked, excluding refuse (yield from 1 lb raw meat with refuse) (220g)	495	26	10	176	0	0	0	62	152
Beef, Rib, Small End (Ribs 10-12), Lean, 0" Fat, Select, Cooked, Broiled 1 piece, cooked, excluding refuse (yield from 1 lb raw meat with refuse) (220g)	436	19	8	176	0	0	0	62	152
Beef, Rib, Small End (Ribs 10-12), Lean, 1/8" Fat, All Grades, Cooked, Broiled 1 lb (453.6g)	885	35	13	395	0	0	0	134	281
Beef, Rib, Small End (Ribs 10-12), Lean, 1/8" Fat, Choice, Cooked, Broiled 1 lb (453.6g)	916	41	16	399	0	0	0	128	263
Beef, Rib, Small End (Ribs 10-12), Lean, 1/8" Fat, Select, Cooked, Broiled 1 lb (453.6g)	853	28	11	445	0	0	25	140	299
Beef, Rib, Whole (Ribs 6-12), Lean and Fat, 1/8" Fat, All Grades, Cooked, Broiled 1 piece, cooked, excluding refuse (yield from 1 lb raw meat with refuse) (267g)	900	71	29	219	0	0	0	60	168
Beef, Rib, Whole (Ribs 6-12), Lean and Fat, 1/8" Fat, All Grades, Cooked, Roasted 1 piece, cooked, excluding refuse (yield from 1 lb raw meat with refuse) (289g)	1014	81	33	243	0	0	0	66	185
Beef, Rib, Whole (Ribs 6-12), Lean and Fat, 1/8" Fat, Choice, Cooked, Broiled 1 piece, cooked, excluding refuse (yield from 1 lb raw meat with refuse) (267g)	940	76	31	219	0	0	0	59	168

Food Serving size	Cal.	(g) Total Fat	(g) Sat. Fat	(mg) Chol.	(g) Carb.	(g) Fiber	(g) Sug.	(g) Prot.	(mg) Sod.
Beef, Rib, Whole (Ribs 6-12), Lean and Fat, 1/8" Fat, Choice, Cooked, Roasted									
1 piece, cooked, excluding refuse (yield from 1 lb raw meat with refuse) (289g)									
	1055	86	35	243	0	0	0	65	185
Beef, Rib, Whole (Ribs 6-12), Lean and Fat, 1/8" Fat, Prime, Cooked, Broiled									
1 piece, cooked, excluding refuse (yield from 1 lb raw meat with refuse) (274g)									
	1058	89	37	233	0	0	0	60	170
Beef, Rib, Whole (Ribs 6-12), Lean and Fat, 1/8" Fat, Prime, Cooked, Roasted									
1 piece, cooked, excluding refuse (yield from 1 lb raw meat with refuse) (278g)									
	1112	94	39	236	0	0	0	63	181
Beef, Rib, Whole (Ribs 6-12), Lean and Fat, 1/8" Fat, Select, Cooked, Broiled									
1 piece, cooked, excluding refuse (yield from 1 lb raw meat with refuse) (264g)									
	832	64	26	214	0	0	0	60	169
Beef, Rib, Whole (Ribs 6-12), Lean and Fat, 1/8" Fat, Select, Cooked, Roasted									
1 piece, cooked, excluding refuse (yield from 1 lb raw meat with refuse) (289g)									
	954	74	30	243	0	0	0	67	188
Beef, Round, Bottom Round Roast, Lean, 0" Fat, Select, Cooked, Roasted									
1 roast (yield from 572 g raw meat) (464g)									
	784	25	9	353	0	0	0	131	176
Beef, Round, Bottom Round Roast, Lean, 1/8" Fat, Select, Cooked, Roasted									
1 lb (453.6g)	744	21	7	336	0	0	19	129	172
Beef, Round, Bottom Round, Roast, Lean and Fat, 0" Fat, All Grades, Cooked, Roasted									
1 roast (yield from 600 g raw meat) (489g)									
	914	38	14	386	0	0	0	134	176
Beef, Round, Bottom Round, Roast, Lean and Fat, 0" Fat, Choice, Cooked, Roasted									
1 roast (yield from 627 g raw meat) (515g)									
	1025	48	17	417	0	0	0	138	180
Beef, Round, Bottom Round, Roast, Lean and Fat, 0" Fat, Select, Cooked, Roasted									
1 roast (yield from 572 g raw meat) (464g)									
	812	28	10	357	0	0	0	130	172
Beef, Round, Bottom Round, Roast, Lean and Fat, 1/8" Fat, All Grades, Cooked, Roasted									
1 piece, cooked, excluding refuse (yield from 1 lb raw meat with refuse) (338g)									
	737	39	15	287	0	0	0	89	118

Food Serving size	Cal.	(g) Total Fat	(g) Sat. Fat	(mg) Chol.	(g) Carb.	(g) Fiber	(g) Sug.	(g) Prot.	(mg) Sod.
Beef, Round, Bottom Round, Roast, Lean and Fat, 1/8" Fat, Choice, Cooked, Roasted 1 piece, cooked, excluding refuse (yield from 1 lb raw meat with refuse) (338g)	754	42	16	291	0	0	0	88	115
Beef, Round, Bottom Round, Roast, Lean and Fat, 1/8" Fat, Select, Cooked, Roasted 1 piece, cooked, excluding refuse (yield from 1 lb raw meat with refuse) (338g)	717	37	14	284	0	0	0	90	118
Beef, Round, Bottom Round, Roast, Lean, 0" Fat, All Grades, Cooked, Roasted 1 roast (yield from 600 g raw meat) (489g)	866	32	11	377	0	0	0	136	176
Beef, Round, Bottom Round, Roast, Lean, 1/8" Fat, All Grades, Cooked 1 oz (28.35g)	46	2	1	22	0	0	0	8	10
Beef, Round, Bottom Round, Roast, Lean, 1/8" Fat, Choice, Cooked, Roasted 1 lb (453.6g)	812	31	11	349	0	0	0	125	163
Beef, Round, Bottom Round, Steak, Lean and Fat, 0" Fat, All Grades, Cooked, Braised 1 steak (yield from 290 g raw meat) (185g)	413	16	6	176	0	0	0	62	81
Beef, Round, Bottom Round, Steak, Lean and Fat, 0" Fat, Choice, Cooked, Braised 1 steak (yield from 299 g raw meat) (191g)	426	17	6	181	0	0	0	63	82
Beef, Round, Bottom Round, Steak, Lean and Fat, 0" Fat, Select, Cooked, Braised 1 steak (yield from 281 g raw meat) (179g)	369	11	4	163	0	0	0	62	82
Beef, Round, Bottom Round, Steak, Lean and Fat, 1/8" Fat, All Grades, Cooked, Braised 1 piece, cooked, excluding refuse (yield from 1 lb raw meat with refuse) (281g)	694	33	13	281	0	0	0	92	121
Beef, Round, Bottom Round, Steak, Lean and Fat, 1/8" Fat, Choice, Cooked, Braised 1 steak (yield from 341 g raw meat) (227g)	577	29	11	229	0	0	0	75	95

Food Serving size	Cal.	(g) Total Fat	(g) Sat. Fat	(mg) Chol.	(g) Carb.	(g) Fiber	(g) Sug.	(g) Prot.	(mg) Sod.
Beef, Round, Bottom Round, Steak, Lean and Fat, 1/8" Fat, Select, Cooked, Braised									
1 steak (yield from raw steak weighing 340 g) (226g)									
	542	25	10	221	0	0	0	74	97
Beef, Round, Bottom Round, Steak, Lean, 0" Fat, All Grades, Cooked, Braised									
1 steak (yield from 290 g raw meat) (185g)									
	396	14	5	172	0	0	0	63	81
Beef, Round, Bottom Round, Steak, Lean, 0" Fat, Choice, Cooked, Braised									
3 oz (85g)	190	8	3	81	0	0	0	28	37
Beef, Round, Bottom Round, Steak, Lean, 0" Fat, Select, Cooked, Braised									
3 oz (85g)	175	5	2	77	0	0	0	30	39
Beef, Round, Bottom Round, Steak, Lean, 1/8" Fat, All Grades, Cooked, Braised									
1 lb (453.6g)	980	35	12	426	0	0	0	156	204
Beef, Round, Bottom Round, Steak, Lean, 1/8" Fat, Choice, Cooked, Braised									
1 lb (453.6g)	1034	41	14	440	0	0	0	155	204
Beef, Round, Bottom Round, Steak, Lean, 1/8" Fat, Select, Cooked, Braised									
1 lb (453.6g)	930	29	10	417	0	0	0	156	209
Beef, Round, Eye of Round, Roast, Lean and Fat, 0" Fat, All Grades, Cooked, Roasted									
1 roast (yield from 436 g raw meat) (346g)									
	578	15	6	263	0	0	0	103	232
Beef, Round, Eye of Round, Roast, Lean and Fat, 0" Fat, Choice, Cooked, Roasted									
1 roast (yield from 445 g raw meat) (355g)									
	589	17	6	266	0	0	0	101	131
Beef, Round, Eye of Round, Roast, Lean and Fat, 0" Fat, Select, Cooked, Roasted									
1 roast (yield from 426 g raw meat) (337g)									
	570	16	6	256	0	0	0	100	131
Beef, Round, Eye of Round, Roast, Lean and Fat, 1/8" Fat, All Grades, Cooked, Roasted									
1 piece, cooked, excluding refuse (yield from 1 lb raw meat with refuse) (333g)									
	693	32	12	280	0	0	0	94	123
Beef, Round, Eye of Round, Roast, Lean and Fat, 1/8" Fat, Choice, Cooked, Roasted									
1 piece, cooked, excluding refuse (yield from 1 lb raw meat with refuse) (333g)									
	706	33	13	286	0	0	0	95	123

Food Serving size	Cal.	(g) Total Fat	(g) Sat. Fat	(mg) Chol.	(g) Carb.	(g) Fiber	(g) Sug.	(g) Prot.	(mg) Sod.
Beef, Round, Eye of Round, Roast, Lean and Fat, 1/8" Fat, Select, Cooked, Roasted 1 roast (yield from 530 g raw meat) (417g)	851	39	15	346	0	0	0	117	154
Beef, Round, Eye of Round, Roast, Lean, 0" Fat, All Grades, Cooked, Roasted 1 roast (yield from 436 g raw meat) (346g)	564	13	5	263	0	0	0	103	232
Beef, Round, Eye of Round, Roast, Lean, 0" Fat, Choice, Cooked, Roasted 1 roast (yield from 445 g raw meat) (355g)	589	15	5	263	0	0	0	106	234
Beef, Round, Eye of Round, Roast, Lean, 0" Fat, Select, Cooked, Roasted 1 roast (yield from 426 g raw meat) (337g)	529	12	4	266	0	0	0	99	212
Beef, Round, Eye of Round, Roast, Lean, 1/8" Fat, All Grades, Cooked, Roasted 1 lb (453.6g)	767	21	7	345	0	0	0	135	172
Beef, Round, Eye of Round, Roast, Lean, 1/8" Fat, Choice, Cooked, Roasted 1 lb (453.6g)	794	24	8	354	0	0	0	135	177
Beef, Round, Eye of Round, Roast, Lean, 1/8" Fat, Select, Cooked, Roasted 1 lb (453.6g)	739	19	6	340	0	0	15	134	177
Beef, Round, Full Cut, Lean and Fat, 1/8" Fat, Choice, Cooked, Broiled 3 oz (85g)	200	11	4	67	0	0	0	23	53
Beef, Round, Full Cut, Lean and Fat, 1/8" Fat, Select, Cooked, Broiled 1 piece, cooked, excluding refuse (yield from 1 lb raw meat with refuse) (313g)	682	35	13	247	0	0	0	86	194
Beef, Round, Full Cut, Lean, 1/4" Fat, Choice, Cooked, Broiled 1 piece, cooked, excluding refuse (yield from 1 lb raw meat with refuse) (313g)	736	41	15	247	0	0	0	86	194
Beef, Round, Full Cut, Lean, 1/4" Fat, Select, Cooked, Broiled 1 piece, cooked, excluding refuse (yield from 1 lb raw meat with refuse) (285g)	485	15	5	220	0	0	0	82	180
Beef, Round, Knuckle, Tip Center, Steak, Lean and Fat, 0" Fat, All Grades, Cooked, Grilled 1 steak (150g)	266	10	4	116	0	0	6	41	78
Beef, Round, Knuckle, Tip Center, Steak, Lean and Fat, 0" Fat, Choice, Cooked, Grilled 1 steak (156g)	293	13	4	117	0	0	2	42	80

Food Serving size	Cal.	(g) Total Fat	(g) Sat. Fat	(mg) Chol.	(g) Carb.	(g) Fiber	(g) Sug.	(g) Prot.	(mg) Sod.
Beef, Round, Knuckle, Tip Center, Steak, Lean and Fat, 0" Fat, Select, Cooked, Grilled 1 steak (160g)	259	9	3	118	0	0	3	43	85
Beef, Round, Knuckle, Tip Side, Steak, Lean and Fat, 0" Fat, All Grades, Cooked, Grilled 1 serving (3 oz) (85g)	143	4	2	68	0	0	3	25	46
Beef, Round, Knuckle, Tip Side, Steak, Lean and Fat, 0" Fat, Choice, Cooked, Grilled 1 serving (3 oz) (85g)	148	5	2	70	0	0	3	24	47
Beef, Round, Knuckle, Tip Side, Steak, Lean and Fat, 0" Fat, Select, Cooked, Grilled 1 serving (3 oz) (85g)	136	3	1	66	0	0	4	25	44
Beef, Round, Out Round, Bottom Round, Steak, Lean and Fat, 0" Fat, All Grades, Cooked, Grilled 1 serving (3 oz) (85g)	155	6	2	65	0	0	0	23	49
Beef, Round, Out Round, Bottom Round, Steak, Lean and Fat, 0" Fat, Choice, Cooked, Grilled 1 serving (3 oz) (85g)	162	7	3	66	0	0	2	23	48
Beef, Round, Out Round, Bottom Round, Steak, Lean and Fat, 0" Fat, Select, Cooked, Grilled 1 serving (3 oz) (85g)	141	4	1	64	0	0	11	24	51
Beef, Round, Tip Round, Roast, Lean and Fat, 0" Fat, All Grades, Cooked, Roasted 1 piece, cooked, excluding refuse (yield from 1 lb raw meat with refuse) (330g)	620	27	10	257	0	0	0	88	116
Beef, Round, Tip Round, Roast, Lean and Fat, 0" Fat, Choice, Cooked, Roasted 1 roast (yield from 1405 g raw meat) (1138g)	2230	101	37	910	0	0	0	307	398
Beef, Round, Tip Round, Roast, Lean and Fat, 0" Fat, Select, Cooked, Roasted 1 roast (yield from 1388 g raw meat) (1141g)	2065	86	31	867	0	0	0	303	399
Beef, Round, Tip Round, Roast, Lean and Fat, 1/8" Fat, All Grades, Cooked, Roasted 1 piece, cooked, excluding refuse (yield from 1 lb raw meat with refuse) (326g)	714	37	14	267	0	0	0	89	263
Beef, Round, Tip Round, Roast, Lean and Fat, 1/8" Fat, Choice, Cooked, Roasted 1 piece, cooked, excluding refuse (yield from 1 lb raw meat with refuse) (325g)	741	40	15	267	0	0	0	89	205

Food Serving size	Cal.	(g) Total Fat	(g) Sat. Fat	(mg) Chol.	(g) Carb.	(g) Fiber	(g) Sug.	(g) Prot.	(mg) Sod.
Beef, Round, Tip Round, Roast, Lean and Fat, 1/8" Fat, Select, Cooked, Roasted 1 piece, cooked, excluding refuse (yield from 1 lb raw meat with refuse) (327g)	687	33	12	268	0	0	0	90	209
Beef, Round, Tip Round, Roast, Lean, 0" Fat, All Grades, Cooked, Roasted 1 piece, cooked, excluding refuse (yield from 1 lb raw meat with refuse) (320g)	557	20	7	237	0	0	0	88	115
Beef, Round, Tip Round, Roast, Lean, 0" Fat, Choice, Cooked, Roasted 1 roast (yield from 1405 g raw meat) (1138g)	2003	73	26	865	0	0	0	315	410
Beef, Round, Tip Round, Roast, Lean, 0" Fat, Select, Cooked, Roasted 1 roast (yield from 1388 g raw meat) (1141g)	1700	50	18	810	0	0	0	312	411
Beef, Round, Top Round, Lean and Fat, 0" Fat, All Grades, Cooked, Braised 1 piece, cooked, excluding refuse (yield from 1 lb raw meat with refuse) (267g)	558	17	6	240	0	0	0	95	120
Beef, Round, Top Round, Lean and Fat, 0" Fat, Choice, Cooked, Braised 1 piece, cooked, excluding refuse (yield from 1 lb raw meat with refuse) (267g)	577	19	7	240	0	0	0	95	120
Beef, Round, Top Round, Lean and Fat, 0" Fat, Select, Cooked, Braised 1 piece, cooked, excluding refuse (yield from 1 lb raw meat with refuse) (267g)	534	14	5	240	0	0	0	95	120
Beef, Round, Top Round, Lean and Fat, 1/8" Fat, All Grades, Cooked, Braised 1 piece, cooked, excluding refuse (yield from 1 lb raw meat) (286g)	681	29	11	257	0	0	0	98	129
Beef, Round, Top Round, Lean and Fat, 1/8" Fat, Choice, Cooked, Braised 1 piece, cooked, excluding refuse (yield from 1 lb raw meat with refuse) (289g)	723	34	13	260	0	0	0	99	130
Beef, Round, Top Round, Lean and Fat, 1/8" Fat, Choice, Cooked, Pan-fried 1 piece, cooked, excluding refuse (yield from 1 lb raw meat with refuse) (283g)	753	39	13	275	0	0	0	93	192
Beef, Round, Top Round, Lean and Fat, 1/8" Fat, Select, Cooked, Braised 1 piece, cooked, excluding refuse (yield from 1 lb raw meat with refuse) (286g)	644	24	9	257	0	0	0	99	129
Beef, Round, Top Round, Lean, 0" Fat, Choice, Cooked, Braised 1 piece, cooked, excluding refuse (yield from 1 lb raw meat with refuse) (261g)	540	15	5	235	0	0	0	94	117

Food Serving size	Cal.	(g) Total Fat	(g) Sat. Fat	(mg) Chol.	(g) Carb.	(g) Fiber	(g) Sug.	(g) Prot.	(mg) Sod.
Beef, Round, Top Round, Lean, 0" Fat, Select, Cooked, Braised 1 piece, cooked, excluding refuse (yield from 1 lb raw meat with refuse) (261g)									
	496	10	4	235	0	0	0	94	117
Beef, Round, Top Round, Lean, 1/8" Fat, Choice, Cooked, Pan-fried 1 piece, cooked, excluding refuse (yield from 1 lb raw meat with refuse) (283g)									
	645	24	7	289	6	0	0	96	184
Beef, Round, Top Round, Steak, Lean and Fat, 0" Fat, All Grades, Cooked, Broiled 1 steak (yield from 381 g raw meat) (277g)									
	521	16	6	235	0	0	0	88	114
Beef, Round, Top Round, Steak, Lean and Fat, 0" Fat, Choice, Cooked, Broiled 1 steak (yield from 396 g raw meat) (284g)									
	568	20	7	253	0	0	0	90	119
Beef, Round, Top Round, Steak, Lean and Fat, 0" Fat, Select, Cooked, Broiled 1 steak (yield from 368 g meat) (269g)									
	476	12	4	215	0	0	0	85	113
Beef, Round, Top Round, Steak, Lean and Fat, 1/8" Fat, All Grades, Cooked, Broiled 1 piece, cooked, excluding refuse (yield from 1 lb raw meat with refuse) (326g)									
	665	29	11	293	0	0	0	100	134
Beef, Round, Top Round, Steak, Lean and Fat, 1/8" Fat, Choice, Cooked, Broiled 1 steak (yield from raw steak weighing 492 g) (347g)									
	777	36	14	319	0	0	0	107	139
Beef, Round, Top Round, Steak, Lean and Fat, 1/8" Fat, Prime, Cooked, Broiled 1 piece, cooked, excluding refuse (yield from 1 lb raw meat with refuse) (332g)									
	747	34	12	279	0	0	0	104	203
Beef, Round, Top Round, Steak, Lean and Fat, 1/8" Fat, Select, Cooked, Broiled 1 steak (yield from raw steak weighing 491 g) (359g)									
	722	28	11	312	0	0	0	110	147
Beef, Round, Top Round, Steak, Lean, 0" Fat, All Grades, Cooked, Broiled 1 steak (277g)									
	515	16	5	233	0	0	0	88	116
Beef, Round, Top Round, Steak, Lean, 0" Fat, Choice, Cooked, Broiled 1 steak (284g)									
	559	19	7	250	0	0	0	90	122
Beef, Round, Top Round, Steak, Lean, 0" Fat, Select, Cooked, Broiled 1 steak (269g)									
	473	12	4	215	0	0	0	85	113
Beef, Round, Top Round, Steak, Lean, 1/8" Fat, All Grades, Cooked, Broiled 1 lb (453.6g)									
	839	25	9	381	0	0	0	144	191

Food Serving size	Cal.	(g) Total Fat	(g) Sat. Fat	(mg) Chol.	(g) Carb.	(g) Fiber	(g) Sug.	(g) Prot.	(mg) Sod.
Beef, Round, Top Round, Steak, Lean, 1/8" Fat, Choice, Cooked, Broiled									
1 lb (453.6g)	875	28	10	390	0	0	0	145	191
Beef, Round, Top Round, Steak, Lean, 1/8" Fat, Select, Cooked, Broiled									
1 lb (453.6g)	803	21	7	372	0	0	0	143	195
Beef, Shank Crosscuts, Lean, 1/4" Fat, Choice, Cooked, Simmered									
1 piece, cooked, excluding refuse (yield from 1 lb raw meat with refuse) (170g)									
	342	11	4	133	0	0	0	57	109
Beef, Short Loin, Porterhouse Steak, Lean and Fat, 0" Fat, All Grades, Cooked, Broiled									
1 lb (453.6g)	1252	87	33	304	0	0	0	109	295
Beef, Short Loin, Porterhouse Steak, Lean and Fat, 0" Fat, USDA Select, Cooked, Broiled									
1 lb (453.6g)	1211	82	32	290	0	0	0	111	295
Beef, Short Loin, Porterhouse Steak, Lean and Fat, 1/8" Fat, All Grades, Cooked, Broiled									
3 oz (85g)	252	19	7	60	0	0	3	20	54
Beef, Short Loin, Porterhouse Steak, Lean and Fat, 1/8" Fat, Choice, Cooked, Broiled									
3 oz (85g)	254	19	7	63	0	0	0	20	54
Beef, Short Loin, Porterhouse Steak, Lean and Fat, 1/8" Fat, Select, Cooked, Broiled									
3 oz (85g)	250	18	7	55	0	0	3	20	54
Beef, Short Loin, Porterhouse Steak, Lean, 0" Fat, All Grades, Cooked, Broiled									
1 lb (453.6g)	962	51	18	281	0	0	0	118	313
Beef, Short Loin, Porterhouse Steak, Lean, 0" Fat, Choice, Cooked, Broiled									
1 serving (85g)	190	11	4	77	0	0	0	22	59
Beef, Short Loin, Porterhouse Steak, Lean, 0" Fat, Select, Cooked, Broiled									
1 serving (85g)	165	7	3	71	0	0	0	23	59
Beef, Short Loin, T-bone Steak, Lean and Fat, 0" Fat, All Grades, Cooked, Broiled									
1 lb (453.6g)	1120	72	28	272	0	0	0	110	304
Beef, Short Loin, T-bone Steak, Lean and Fat, 0" Fat, USDA Select, Cooked, Broiled									
1 lb (453.6g)	1043	64	25	268	0	0	0	111	308
Beef, Short Loin, T-bone Steak, Lean and Fat, 1/8" Fat, All Grades, Cooked, Broiled									
3 oz (85g)	238	17	6	53	0	0	6	21	56

Food Serving size	Cal.	(g) Total Fat	(g) Sat. Fat	(mg) Chol.	(g) Carb.	(g) Fiber	(g) Sug.	(g) Prot.	(mg) Sod.
Beef, Short Loin, T-bone Steak, Lean and Fat, 1/8" Fat, Choice, Cooked, Broiled									
3 oz (85g)	243	17	7	55	0	0	0	20	56
Beef, Short Loin, T-bone Steak, Lean and Fat, 1/8" Fat, Select, Cooked, Broiled									
3 oz (85g)	225	15	6	48	0	0	3	21	56
Beef, Short Loin, T-bone Steak, Lean, 0" Fat, All Grades, Cooked, Broiled									
1 lb (453.6g)	857	39	14	249	0	0	0	118	322
Beef, Short Loin, T-bone Steak, Lean, 0" Fat, Choice, Cooked, Broiled									
1 serving (85g)	168	8	3	71	0	0	0	22	60
Beef, Short Loin, T-bone Steak, Lean, 0" Fat, Select, Cooked, Broiled									
1 serving (85g)	150	6	2	68	0	0	0	22	60
Beef, Short Loin, T-bone Steak, Lean, 1/4" Fat, All Grades, Cooked, Broiled									
1 lb (453.6g)	916	44	16	259	0	0	0	123	340
Beef, Short Loin, Top Loin, Lean and Fat, 1/8" Fat, Prime, Cooked, Broiled									
1 steak, excluding refuse (yield from 1 raw steak, with refuse, weighing 242 g) (167g)	518	37	15	132	0	0	0	43	107
Beef, Short Loin, Top Loin, Steak, Lean and Fat, 0" Fat, All Grades, Cooked, Broiled									
1 steak, excluding refuse (yield from 1 raw steak, with refuse, weighing 223 g) (155g)	299	12	5	126	0	0	0	45	91
Beef, Short Loin, Top Loin, Steak, Lean and Fat, 0" Fat, Choice, Cooked, Broiled									
3 oz (85g)	174	8	3	71	0	0	0	24	48
Beef, Short Loin, Top Loin, Steak, Lean and Fat, 0" Fat, Select, Cooked, Broiled									
1 steak (yield from 186 g raw meat) (150g)	270	9	4	119	0	0	0	44	92
Beef, Short Loin, Top Loin, Steak, Lean and Fat, 1/8" Fat, All Grades, Cooked, Broiled									
1 steak, excluding refuse (yield from 1 raw steak, with refuse, weighing 242 g) (165g)	436	28	11	158	0	0	0	44	89
Beef, Short Loin, Top Loin, Steak, Lean and Fat, 1/8" Fat, Choice, Cooked, Broiled									
3 oz (1 serving) (85g)	236	16	6	85	0	0	0	22	44
Beef, Short Loin, Top Loin, Steak, Lean and Fat, 1/8" Fat, Select, Cooked, Broiled									
3 oz (85g)	213	13	5	79	0	0	0	23	48
Beef, Short Loin, Top Loin, Steak, Lean, 0" Fat, All Grades, Cooked, Broiled									
3 oz (85g)	155	5	2	67	0	0	0	25	51

Food Serving size	Cal.	(g) Total Fat	(g) Sat. Fat	(mg) Chol.	(g) Carb.	(g) Fiber	(g) Sug.	(g) Prot.	(mg) Sod.
Beef, Short Loin, Top Loin, Steak, Lean, 0" Fat, Choice, Cooked, Broiled									
3 oz (85g)	163	6	2	69	0	0	0	25	50
Beef, Short Loin, Top Loin, Steak, Lean, 0" Fat, Select, Cooked, Broiled									
3 oz (85g)	146	4	2	65	0	0	0	25	53
Beef, Short Loin, Top Loin, Steak, Lean, 1/8" Fat, All Grades, Cooked, Broiled									
1 lb (453.6g)	857	32	12	367	0	0	0	133	277
Beef, Short Loin, Top Loin, Steak, Lean, 1/8" Fat, Choice, Cooked, Broiled									
1 lb (453.6g)	912	38	15	381	0	0	0	132	272
Beef, Short Loin, Top Loin, Steak, Lean, 1/8" Fat, Select, Cooked, Broiled									
1 lb (453.6g)	803	26	10	354	0	0	40	134	281
Beef, Shoulder Pot Roast, Boneless, Lean and Fat, 0" Fat, All Grades, Cooked, Braised									
1 roast (787g)	1605	70	24	763	0	0	0	244	480
Beef, Shoulder Pot Roast, Boneless, Lean and Fat, 0" Fat, Choice, Cooked, Braised									
1 roast (793g)	1642	73	26	769	0	0	0	245	476
Beef, Shoulder Pot Roast, Boneless, Lean and Fat, 0" Fat, Select, Cooked, Braised									
1 roast (779g)	1558	66	22	763	0	0	0	243	483
Beef, Shoulder Pot Roast, Boneless, Lean, 0" Fat, All Grades, Cooked, Braised									
1 roast (787g)	1543	61	20	771	0	0	167	248	480
Beef, Shoulder Pot Roast, Boneless, Lean, 0" Fat, Choice, Cooked, Braised									
1 roast (793g)	1586	66	22	769	0	0	24	248	476
Beef, Shoulder Pot Roast, Boneless, Lean, 0" Fat, Select, Cooked, Braised									
1 roast (779g)	1480	55	17	771	0	0	190	247	491
Beef, Shoulder Steak, Boneless, Lean and Fat, 0" Fat, All Grades, Cooked, Grilled									
1 steak (287g)	522	20	8	232	0	0	4	81	192
Beef, Shoulder Steak, Boneless, Lean and Fat, 0" Fat, Choice, Cooked, Grilled									
1 steak (280g)	521	20	9	227	0	0	12	79	188
Beef, Shoulder Steak, Boneless, Lean and Fat, 0" Fat, Select, Cooked, Grilled									
1 steak (297g)	526	18	8	244	0	0	0	84	199
Beef, Shoulder Steak, Boneless, Lean Only, 0" Fat, Choice, Cooked, Grilled									
3 oz (1 serving) (85g)	151	5	2	67	0	0	0	24	58
Beef, Shoulder Steak, Boneless, Lean, 0" Fat, All Grades, Cooked, Grilled									
3 oz (1 serving) (85g)	149	5	2	69	0	0	6	24	58

Food Serving size	Cal.	(g) Total Fat	(g) Sat. Fat	(mg) Chol.	(g) Carb.	(g) Fiber	(g) Sug.	(g) Prot.	(mg) Sod.
Beef, Shoulder Steak, Boneless, Lean, 0" Fat, Select, Cooked, Grilled									
3 oz (1 serving) (85g)	144	4	2	70	0	0	0	24	58
Beef, Shoulder Top Blade Steak, Boneless, Lean and Fat, 0" Fat, All Grades, Cooked, Grilled									
1 steak (186g)	391	21	8	177	0	0	0	51	158
Beef, Shoulder Top Blade Steak, Boneless, Lean and Fat, 0" Fat, Choice, Cooked, Grilled									
1 steak (177g)	389	22	9	163	0	0	0	49	149
Beef, Shoulder Top Blade Steak, Boneless, Lean and Fat, 0" Fat, Select, Cooked, Grilled									
1 steak (199g)	386	18	8	195	0	0	0	55	175
Beef, Shoulder Top Blade Steak, Boneless, Lean, 0" Fat, All Grades, Cooked, Grilled									
1 steak (186g)	365	17	7	177	0	0	0	52	162
Beef, Shoulder Top Blade Steak, Boneless, Lean, 0" Fat, Choice, Cooked, Grilled									
1 steak (177g)	358	17	7	165	0	0	0	50	150
Beef, Shoulder Top Blade Steak, Boneless, Lean, 0" Fat, Select, Cooked, Grilled									
1 steak (199g)	372	17	7	195	0	0	0	56	177
Beef, Sirloin, Tri-tip Steak, Lean and Fat, 0" Fat, All Grades, Cooked, Broiled									
1 lb (453.6g)	1202	69	26	308	0	0	0	136	327
Beef, Tenderloin, Lean and Fat, 0" Fat, Select, Cooked, Broiled									
1 steak (yield from 136 g raw meat) (108g)	221	11	4	90	0	0	0	29	63
Beef, Tenderloin, Lean and Fat, 1/8" Fat, All Grades, Cooked, Roasted									
3 oz (85g)	275	21	8	72	0	0	0	20	48
Beef, Tenderloin, Lean and Fat, 1/8" Fat, Choice, Cooked, Roasted									
3 oz (85g)	281	22	9	72	0	0	0	20	55
Beef, Tenderloin, Lean and Fat, 1/8" Fat, Prime, Cooked, Roasted									
3 oz (85g)	292	23	9	75	0	0	0	20	47
Beef, Tenderloin, Lean and Fat, 1/8" Fat, Select, Cooked, Roasted									
3 oz (85g)	269	20	8	72	0	0	0	20	48
Beef, Tenderloin, Steak, Lean and Fat, 0" Fat, All Grades, Cooked, Broiled									
1 steak, excluding refuse (yield from 1 raw steak, with refuse, weighing 135 g) (93g)	203	10	4	80	0	0	0	26	52

Food Serving size	Cal.	(g) Total Fat	(g) Sat. Fat	(mg) Chol.	(g) Carb.	(g) Fiber	(g) Sug.	(g) Prot.	(mg) Sod.
Beef, Tenderloin, Steak, Lean and Fat, 0" Fat, Choice, Cooked, Broiled 1 steak (yield from 161 g raw meat) (126g)									
	291	16	6	113	0	0	0	35	69
Beef, Tenderloin, Steak, Lean and Fat, 1/8" Fat, All Grades, Cooked, Broiled 1 steak, excluding refuse (yield from 1 raw steak, with refuse, weighing 154 g) (104g)									
	278	18	7	101	0	0	0	28	56
Beef, Tenderloin, Steak, Lean and Fat, 1/8" Fat, Choice, Cooked, Broiled 3 oz (85g)									
	232	15	6	84	0	0	0	22	44
Beef, Tenderloin, Steak, Lean and Fat, 1/8" Fat, Prime, Cooked, Broiled 1 steak, excluding refuse (yield from 1 raw steak, with refuse, weighing 154 g) (106g)									
	326	24	9	91	0	0	0	27	63
Beef, Tenderloin, Steak, Lean and Fat, 1/8" Fat, Select, Cooked, Broiled 3 oz (85g)									
	223	14	6	82	0	0	0	23	48
Beef, Tenderloin, Steak, Lean, 0" Fat, All Grades, Cooked, Broiled 3 oz (85g)									
	164	7	3	69	0	0	0	24	50
Beef, Tenderloin, Steak, Lean, 0" Fat, Choice, Cooked, Broiled 3 oz (85g)									
	175	8	3	72	0	0	0	25	50
Beef, Tenderloin, Steak, Lean, 0" Fat, Select, Cooked, Broiled 3 oz (85g)									
	152	6	2	65	0	0	0	24	50
Beef, Tenderloin, Steak, Lean, 1/8" Fat, All Grades, Cooked, Broiled 1 lb (453.6g)									
	907	38	14	372	0	0	0	132	272
Beef, Tenderloin, Steak, Lean, 1/8" Fat, Choice, Cooked, Broiled 1 lb (453.6g)									
	934	41	16	386	0	0	0	132	268
Beef, Tenderloin, Steak, Lean, 1/8" Fat, Select, Cooked, Broiled 1 lb (453.6g)									
	880	35	13	376	0	0	35	132	281
Beef, Top Sirloin, Steak, Lean and Fat, 0" Fat, All Grades, Cooked, Broiled 1 steak (yield from 518 g raw meat) (384g)									
	814	37	14	338	0	0	0	113	234
Beef, Top Sirloin, Steak, Lean and Fat, 0" Fat, Choice, Cooked, Broiled 1 steak (yield from 532 g raw meat) (393g)									
	861	41	16	350	0	0	0	114	228
Beef, Top Sirloin, Steak, Lean and Fat, 0" Fat, Select, Cooked, Broiled 1 steak (yield from 505 g raw meat) (375g)									
	773	33	13	326	0	0	0	111	236

Food Serving size	Cal.	(g) Total Fat	(g) Sat. Fat	(mg) Chol.	(g) Carb.	(g) Fiber	(g) Sug.	(g) Prot.	(mg) Sod.
Beef, Top Sirloin, Steak, Lean and Fat, 1/8" Fat, All Grades, Cooked, Broiled									
1 piece, cooked, excluding refuse (yield from 1 lb raw meat with refuse) (306g)									
	744	44	17	282	0	0	0	82	171
Beef, Top Sirloin, Steak, Lean and Fat, 1/8" Fat, Choice, Cooked, Broiled									
1 piece, cooked, excluding refuse (yield from 1 lb raw meat with refuse) (306g)									
	786	48	19	294	0	0	0	82	165
Beef, Top Sirloin, Steak, Lean and Fat, 1/8" Fat, Choice, Cooked, Pan-fried									
1 piece, cooked, excluding refuse (yield from 1 lb raw meat with refuse) (307g)									
	961	65	25	301	0	0	0	88	218
Beef, Top Sirloin, Steak, Lean and Fat, 1/8" Fat, Select, Cooked, Broiled									
1 steak (yield from 1 raw steak weighing 624 g) (485g)									
	1116	62	24	432	0	0	0	132	276
Beef, Top Sirloin, Steak, Lean, 0" Fat, All Grades, Cooked, Broiled									
1 piece, cooked, excluding refuse (yield from 1 lb raw meat with refuse) (292g)									
	534	17	6	239	0	0	0	89	187
Beef, Top Sirloin, Steak, Lean, 0" Fat, Choice, Cooked, Broiled									
1 steak (yield from 532 g raw meat) (393g)									
	739	26	10	326	0	0	0	119	248
Beef, Top Sirloin, Steak, Lean, 0" Fat, Select, Cooked, Broiled									
1 steak (yield from 505 g raw meat) (375g)									
	664	19	7	304	0	0	0	116	248
Beef, Top Sirloin, Steak, Lean, 1/8" Fat, All Grades, Cooked, Broiled									
1 lb (453.6g)	807	26	10	358	0	0	0	133	277
Beef, Top Sirloin, Steak, Lean, 1/8" Fat, Choice, Cooked, Broiled									
1 lb (453.6g)	848	30	12	367	0	0	0	134	277
Beef, Top Sirloin, Steak, Lean, 1/8" Fat, Select, Cooked, Broiled									
1 lb (453.6g)	771	22	9	349	0	0	0	133	281
Beef, Variety Meats and By-products, Brain, Cooked, Pan-fried									
1 piece, cooked, excluding refuse (yield from 1 lb raw meat with refuse) (351g)									
	688	56	13	7002	0	0	0	44	555
Beef, Variety Meats and By-products, Brain, Cooked, Simmered									
1 piece, cooked, excluding refuse (391g)									
	590	41	9	12121	6	0	0	46	422
Beef, Variety Meats and By-products, Heart, Cooked, Simmered									
3 oz (85g)	140	4	1	180	0	0	0	24	50
Beef, Variety Meats and By-products, Kidneys, Cooked, Simmered									
3 oz (85g)	134	4	1	609	0	0	0	23	80

Food Serving size	Cal.	(g) Total Fat	(g) Sat. Fat	(mg) Chol.	(g) Carb.	(g) Fiber	(g) Sug.	(g) Prot.	(mg) Sod.
Beef, Variety Meats and By-products, Liver, Cooked, Braised									
1 slice (68g)	130	4	1	269	3	0	0	20	54
Beef, Variety Meats and By-products, Liver, Cooked, Pan-fried									
1 slice (82g)	144	4	1	312	4	0	0	22	63
Beef, Variety Meats and By-products, Lungs, Cooked, Braised									
3 oz (85g)	102	3	1	235	0	0	0	17	86
Beef, Variety Meats and By-products, Pancreas, Cooked, Braised									
3 oz (85g)	230	15	5	223	0	0	0	23	51
Beef, Variety Meats and By-products, Spleen, Cooked, Braised									
3 oz (85g)	123	4	1	295	0	0	0	21	48
Beef, Variety Meats and By-products, Thymus, Cooked, Braised									
1 piece, cooked, excluding refuse (yield from 1 lb raw meat with refuse) (381g)									
	1215	95	33	1120	0	0	0	83	442
Beef, Variety Meats and By-products, Tongue, Cooked, Simmered									
3 oz (85g)	241	19	7	112	0	0	0	16	55
Bison, Ground, Grass-fed, Cooked									
3 oz (85g)	152	7	3	60	0	0	0	22	65
Canadian Bacon, Cooked, Pan-Fried									
NA	19	0	0	9	0	0	0	4	133
Carl Buddig, Cooked Corned Beef, Chopped, Pressed									
1 serving, 2 oz (57g)	81	4	2	37	1	0	0	11	765
Carl Buddig, Cooked, Smoked, Beef Pastrami, Chopped, Pressed									
1 package (71g)	100	5	2	46	1	0	0	14	750
Carl Buddig, Smoked Sliced Beef									
1 package (71g)	99	5	2	48	0	0	0	14	1016
Carl Buddig, Smoked Sliced Chicken, Light and Dark Meat									
1 package (71g)	117	7	2	38	0	0	0	13	677
Carl Buddig, Smoked Sliced Ham									
1 package (71g)	116	7	2	39	1	0	0	13	981
Carl Buddig, Smoked Sliced Turkey, Light and Dark Meat									
1 package (71g)	114	6	2	40	1	0	0	12	778
Game Meat, Antelope, Cooked, Roasted									
1 piece, cooked (yield from 1 lb raw meat, boneless) (340g)									
	510	9	3	428	0	0	0	100	184

Food Serving size	Cal.	(g) Total Fat	(g) Sat. Fat	(mg) Chol.	(g) Carb.	(g) Fiber	(g) Sug.	(g) Prot.	(mg) Sod.
Game Meat, Bear, Cooked, Simmered									
1 piece, cooked (yield from 1 lb raw meat, boneless) (277g)									
	717	37	10	271	0	0	0	90	197
Game Meat, Beaver, Cooked, Roasted									
1 piece, cooked (yield from 1 lb raw meat, boneless) (313g)									
	664	22	6	366	0	0	0	109	185
Game Meat, Beefalo, Composite of Cuts, Cooked, Roasted									
1 piece, cooked (yield from 1 lb raw meat, boneless) (340g)									
	639	21	9	197	0	0	0	104	279
Game Meat, Bison, Chuck, Shoulder Clod, Lean, 3-5 lb. Roasted, Cooked, Braised									
1 roast (yield from 1247 g raw meat) (774g)									
	1494	42	18	859	0	0	0	261	441
Game Meat, Bison, Ground, Cooked, Pan-broiled									
1 serving (3 oz) (85g)	202	13	0	71	0	0	0	20	62
Game Meat, Bison, Lean, Cooked, Roasted									
3 oz (85g)	122	2	1	70	0	0	0	24	48
Game Meat, Bison, Rib Eye, Lean, 1" Steak, Cooked, Broiled									
1 steak (yield from 232.8 g raw meat)									
	317	10	4	141	0	0	0	53	93
Game Meat, Bison, Top Round, Lean, 1" Steak, Cooked, Broiled									
1 steak (180g)	313	9	4	153	0	0	0	54	74
Game Meat, Bison, Top Sirloin, Lean, 1" Steak, Cooked, Broiled									
1 steak (yield from 309.7 g raw meat) (194g)									
	332	11	5	167	0	0	0	54	103
Game Meat, Boar, Wild, Cooked, Roasted									
1 piece, cooked (yield from 1 lb raw meat, boneless) (340g)									
	544	15	4	262	0	0	0	96	204
Game Meat, Buffalo, Water, Cooked, Roasted									
1 piece, cooked (yield from 1 lb raw meat, boneless) (340g)									
	445	6	2	207	0	0	0	91	190
Game Meat, Caribou, Cooked, Roasted									
1 piece, cooked (yield from 1 lb raw meat, boneless) (340g)									
	568	15	6	371	0	0	0	101	204
Game Meat, Deer, Cooked, Roasted									
1 piece, cooked (yield from 1 lb raw meat, boneless) (340g)									
	537	11	4	381	0	0	0	103	184

Food Serving size	Cal.	(g) Total Fat	(g) Sat. Fat	(mg) Chol.	(g) Carb.	(g) Fiber	(g) Sug.	(g) Prot.	(mg) Sod.
Game Meat, Deer, Ground, Cooked, Pan-broiled									
1 serving (3 oz) (85g)	159	7	3	83	0	0	0	22	66
Game Meat, Deer, Loin, Lean, 1" Steak, Cooked, Broiled									
1 serving (3 oz) (85g)	128	2	1	67	0	0	0	26	48
Game Meat, Deer, Shoulder Clod, Lean, 3-5 lb. Roasted, Cooked, Braised									
1 roast (293g)	560	12	7	331	0	0	0	106	152
Game Meat, Deer, Tenderloin, Lean, 0.5-1 lb. Roasted, Cooked, Broiled									
1 roast, (yield from 271.8 g raw meat)	301	5	2	178	0	0	0	60	115
Game Meat, Deer, Top Round, Lean, 1" Steak, Cooked, Broiled									
1 serving (3 oz) (85g)	129	2	1	72	0	0	0	27	38
Game Meat, Elk, Cooked, Roasted									
1 piece, cooked (yield from 1 lb raw meat, boneless) (340g)	496	6	2	248	0	0	0	103	207
Game Meat, Elk, Ground, Cooked, Pan-broiled									
1 serving (3 oz) (85g)	164	7	3	66	0	0	0	23	72
Game Meat, Elk, Loin, Lean, Cooked, Broiled									
1 serving (3 oz) (85g)	142	3	1	64	0	0	0	26	46
Game Meat, Elk, Round, Lean, Cooked, Broiled									
1 serving (3 oz) (85g)	133	2	1	66	0	0	0	26	43
Game Meat, Elk, Tenderloin, Lean, Cooked, Broiled									
1 serving (3 oz) (85g)	138	3	1	61	0	0	0	26	43
Game Meat, Goat, Cooked, Roasted									
1 piece, cooked (yield from 1 lb raw meat, boneless) (340g)	486	10	3	255	0	0	0	92	292
Game Meat, Horse, Cooked, Roasted									
1 piece, cooked (yield from 1 lb raw meat, boneless) (340g)	595	21	6	231	0	0	0	96	187
Game Meat, Moose, Cooked, Roasted									
1 piece, cooked (yield from 1 lb raw meat, boneless) (340g)	456	3	1	265	0	0	0	100	235
Game Meat, Muskrat, Cooked, Roasted									
1 piece, cooked (yield from 1 lb raw meat, boneless) (313g)	732	37	0	379	0	0	0	94	297

Food Serving size	Cal.	(g) Total Fat	(g) Sat. Fat	(mg) Chol.	(g) Carb.	(g) Fiber	(g) Sug.	(g) Prot.	(mg) Sod.
Game Meat, Rabbit, Domesticated, Composite of Cuts, Cooked, Roasted									
1 piece, cooked (yield from 1 lb raw meat, boneless) (313g)									
	617	25	8	257	0	0	0	91	147
Game Meat, Rabbit, Domesticated, Composite of Cuts, Cooked, Stewed									
1 piece, cooked (yield from 1 lb raw meat, boneless) (299g)									
	517	10	3	368	0	0	0	99	135
Game Meat, Rabbit, Wild, Cooked, Stewed									
1 piece, cooked (yield from 1 lb raw meat, boneless) (299g)									
	147	3	1	105	0	0	0	28	38
Game Meat, Raccoon, Cooked, Roasted									
1 piece, cooked (yield from 1 lb raw meat, boneless) (399g)									
	1017	58	16	387	0	0	0	117	315
Game Meat, Squirrel, Cooked, Roasted									
1 piece, cooked (yield from 1 lb raw meat, boneless) (313g)									
	541	15	2	379	0	0	0	96	372
Goose, Domesticated, Meat and Skin, Cooked, Roasted									
1 unit (yield from 1 lb ready-to-cook goose) (188g)									
	573	41	13	171	0	0	0	47	132
Goose, Domesticated, Meat Only, Cooked, Roasted									
.5 goose (591g)	1407	75	27	567	0	0	0	171	449
Lamb, Australian, Imported, Fresh, Composite of Retail Cuts, Lean and Fat, 1/8" Fat, Cooked									
1 piece, cooked, excluding refuse (yield from 1 lb raw meat with refuse) (270g)									
	691	45	21	235	0	0	0	66	205
Lamb, Australian, Imported, Fresh, Composite of Retail Cuts, Lean, 1/8" Fat, Cooked									
1 piece, cooked, excluding refuse (yield from 1 lb raw meat with refuse) (236g)									
	474	23	10	205	0	0	0	63	189
Lamb, Australian, Imported, Fresh, Fat, Cooked									
1 piece, cooked, excluding refuse (yield from 1 lb raw meat with refuse) (248g)									
	1585	165	86	206	0	0	0	23	126
Lamb, Australian, Imported, Fresh, Foreshank, Lean and Fat, 1/8" Fat, Cooked, Braised									
1 piece, cooked, excluding refuse (yield from 1 lb raw meat with refuse) (211g)									
	498	30	14	192	0	0	0	52	196

Food Serving size	Cal.	(g) Total Fat	(g) Sat. Fat	(mg) Chol.	(g) Carb.	(g) Fiber	(g) Sug.	(g) Prot.	(mg) Sod.
Lamb, Australian, Imported, Fresh, Foreshank, Lean, 1/8" Fat, Cooked, Braised 1 piece, cooked, excluding refuse (yield from 1 lb raw meat with refuse) (180g)	297	9	3	166	0	0	0	50	180
Lamb, Australian, Imported, Fresh, Leg, Center Slice, Bone-in, Lean and Fat, 1/8" Fat, Cooked, Broiled 3 oz (85g)	183	10	5	72	0	0	0	22	55
Lamb, Australian, Imported, Fresh, Leg, Center Slice, Bone-in, Lean, 1/8" Fat, Cooked, Broiled 3 oz (85g)	156	7	3	72	0	0	0	23	56
Lamb, Australian, Imported, Fresh, Leg, Shank Half, Lean and Fat, 1/8" Fat, Cooked, Roasted 1 piece, cooked, excluding refuse (yield from 1 lb raw meat with refuse) (277g)	640	38	18	230	0	0	0	70	186
Lamb, Australian, Imported, Fresh, Leg, Shank Half, Lean, 1/8" Fat, Cooked, Roasted 1 piece, cooked, excluding refuse (yield from 1 lb raw meat with refuse) (246g)	448	18	7	204	0	0	0	67	170
Lamb, Australian, Imported, Fresh, Leg, Sirloin Chops, Boneless, Lean and Fat, 1/8" Fat, Cooked, Broiled 3 oz (85g)	200	12	5	72	0	0	0	22	54
Lamb, Australian, Imported, Fresh, Leg, Sirloin Chops, Boneless, Lean, 1/8" Fat, Cooked, Broiled 3 oz (85g)	160	7	3	72	0	0	0	23	56
Lamb, Australian, Imported, Fresh, Leg, Sirloin Half, Boneless, Lean and Fat, 1/8" Fat, Cooked, Roasted 1 piece, cooked, excluding refuse (yield from 1 lb raw meat with refuse) (306g)	860	59	28	312	0	0	0	76	239
Lamb, Australian, Imported, Fresh, Leg, Sirloin Half, Boneless, Lean, 1/8" Fat, Cooked, Roasted 1 piece, cooked, excluding refuse (yield from 1 lb raw meat with refuse) (259g)	557	28	12	272	0	0	0	72	215
Lamb, Australian, Imported, Fresh, Leg, Whole (Shank and Sirloin), Lean and Fat, 1/8" Fat, Cooked, Roasted 1 piece, cooked, excluding refuse (yield from 1 lb raw meat with refuse) (284g)	693	43	20	250	0	0	0	71	199

Food Serving size	Cal.	(g) Total Fat	(g) Sat. Fat	(mg) Chol.	(g) Carb.	(g) Fiber	(g) Sug.	(g) Prot.	(mg) Sod.
Lamb, Australian, Imported, Fresh, Leg, Whole (Shank and Sirloin), Lean, 1/8" Fat, Cooked, Roasted									
1 piece, cooked, excluding refuse (yield from 1 lb raw meat with refuse) (251g)									
	477	20	8	223	0	0	0	69	181
Lamb, Australian, Imported, Fresh, Loin, Lean and Fat, 1/8" Fat, Cooked, Broiled									
3 oz (85g)	186	10	5	70	0	0	0	22	66
Lamb, Australian, Imported, Fresh, Loin, Lean, 1/8" Fat, Cooked, Broiled									
3 oz (85g)	163	7	3	69	0	0	0	23	68
Lamb, Australian, Imported, Fresh, Rib, Lean and Fat, 1/8" Fat, Cooked, Roasted									
1 piece, cooked, excluding refuse (yield from 1 lb raw meat with refuse) (286g)									
	792	58	28	229	0	0	0	64	220
Lamb, Australian, Imported, Fresh, Rib, Lean, 1/8" Fat, Cooked, Roasted									
1 piece, cooked, excluding refuse (yield from 1 lb raw meat with refuse) (241g)									
	506	28	12	193	0	0	0	59	198
Lamb, Australian, Imported, Fresh, Shoulder, Arm, Lean and Fat, 1/8" Fat, Cooked, Braised									
3 oz (85g)	264	17	8	90	0	0	0	25	62
Lamb, Australian, Imported, Fresh, Shoulder, Arm, Lean, 1/8" Fat, Cooked, Braised									
3 oz (85g)	202	9	4	94	0	0	0	29	66
Lamb, Australian, Imported, Fresh, Shoulder, Blade, Lean and Fat, 1/8" Fat, Cooked, Broiled									
1 piece, cooked, excluding refuse (yield from 1 lb raw meat with refuse) (273g)									
	794	60	29	229	0	0	0	59	240
Lamb, Australian, Imported, Fresh, Shoulder, Blade, Lean, 1/8" Fat, Cooked, Broiled									
1 piece, cooked, excluding refuse (yield from 1 lb raw meat with refuse) (233g)									
	538	34	15	198	0	0	0	56	219
Lamb, Australian, Imported, Fresh, Shoulder, Whole (Arm and Blade), Lean and Fat, 1/8" Fat, Cooked									
1 piece, cooked, excluding refuse (yield from 1 lb raw meat with refuse) (262g)									
	776	57	27	233	0	0	0	62	223
Lamb, Australian, Imported, Fresh, Shoulder, Whole (Arm and Blade), Lean, 1/8" Fat, Cooked									
1 piece, cooked, excluding refuse (yield from 1 lb raw meat with refuse) (222g)									
	517	30	13	202	0	0	0	58	202

Food Serving size	Cal.	(g) Total Fat	(g) Sat. Fat	(mg) Chol.	(g) Carb.	(g) Fiber	(g) Sug.	(g) Prot.	(mg) Sod.
Lamb, Domestic, Composite of Retail Cuts, Fat, 1/4" Fat, Choice, Cooked 1 piece, cooked, excluding refuse (yield from 1 lb raw meat with refuse) (187g)	385	18	6	172	0	0	0	53	142
Lamb, Domestic, Composite of Retail Cuts, Lean and Fat, 1/4" Fat, Choice, Cooked 1 piece, cooked, excluding refuse (yield from 1 lb raw meat with refuse) (242g)	711	51	21	235	0	0	0	59	174
Lamb, Domestic, Composite of Retail Cuts, Lean and Fat, 1/8" Fat, Choice, Cooked 1 piece, cooked, excluding refuse (yield from 1 lb raw meat with refuse) (250g)	678	45	19	240	0	0	0	64	180
Lamb, Domestic, Composite of Retail Cuts, Lean, 1/4" Fat, Choice, Cooked 1 unit, cooked (yield from 1 lb raw meat) (286g)	676	169	77	326	0	0	0	35	166
Lamb, Domestic, Cubed for Stew (Leg and Shoulder), Lean, 1/4" Fat, Cooked, Braised 1 unit, cooked (yield from 1 lb raw meat) (272g)	607	24	9	294	0	0	0	92	190
Lamb, Domestic, Cubed for Stew (Leg and Shoulder), Lean, 1/4" Fat, Cooked, Broiled 1 unit, cooked (yield from 1 lb raw meat) (327g)	608	24	9	294	0	0	0	92	249
Lamb, Domestic, Foreshank, Lean and Fat, 1/4" Fat, Choice, Cooked, Braised 3 oz (85g)	207	11	5	90	0	0	0	24	61
Lamb, Domestic, Foreshank, Lean and Fat, 1/8" Fat, Cooked, Braised 3 oz (85g)	207	11	5	90	0	0	0	24	61
Lamb, Domestic, Foreshank, Lean, 1/4" Fat, Choice, Cooked, Braised 3 oz (85g)	159	5	2	88	0	0	0	26	63
Lamb, Domestic, Leg, Shank Half, Lean and Fat, 1/4" Fat, Choice, Cooked, Roasted 1 piece, cooked, excluding refuse (yield from 1 lb raw meat with refuse) (269g)	605	33	14	242	0	0	0	71	175
Lamb, Domestic, Leg, Shank Half, Lean and Fat, 1/8" Fat, Choice, Cooked, Roasted 1 piece, cooked, excluding refuse (yield from 1 lb raw meat with refuse) (267g)	579	30	12	240	0	0	0	71	174

Food Serving size	Cal.	(g) Total Fat	(g) Sat. Fat	(mg) Chol.	(g) Carb.	(g) Fiber	(g) Sug.	(g) Prot.	(mg) Sod.
Lamb, Domestic, Leg, Shank Half, Lean, 1/4" Fat, Choice, Cooked, Roasted									
1 piece, cooked, excluding refuse (yield from 1 lb raw meat with refuse) (238g)									
	428	16	6	207	0	0	0	67	157
Lamb, Domestic, Leg, Sirloin Half, Lean and Fat, 1/4" Fat, Choice, Cooked, Roasted									
1 piece, cooked, excluding refuse (yield from 1 lb raw meat with refuse) (262 g)									
	765	54	23	254	0	0	0	65	178
Lamb, Domestic, Leg, Sirloin Half, Lean and Fat, 1/8" Fat, Choice, Cooked, Roasted									
1 piece, cooked, excluding refuse (yield from 1 lb raw meat with refuse) (260g)									
	738	51	21	250	0	0	0	65	177
Lamb, Domestic, Leg, Sirloin Half, Lean, 1/4" Fat, Choice, Cooked, Roasted									
1 piece, cooked, excluding refuse (yield from 1 lb raw meat with refuse) (238g)									
	428	16	6	207	0	0	0	67	157
Lamb, Domestic, Leg, Whole (Shank and Sirloin), Lean and Fat, 1/4" Fat, Choice, Cooked, Roasted									
1 piece, cooked, excluding refuse (yield from 1 lb raw meat with refuse) (265g)									
	684	44	18	246	0	0	0	68	175
Lamb, Domestic, Leg, Whole (Shank and Sirloin), Lean and Fat, 1/8" Fat, Choice, Cooked, Roasted									
1 piece, cooked, excluding refuse (yield from 1 lb raw meat with refuse) (260g)									
	629	37	15	239	0	0	0	68	174
Lamb, Domestic, Leg, Whole (Shank and Sirloin), Lean, 1/4" Fat, Choice, Cooked, Roasted									
1 piece, cooked, excluding refuse (yield from 1 lb raw meat with refuse) (218g)									
	416	17	6	194	0	0	0	62	148
Lamb, Domestic, Loin, Lean and Fat, 1/4" Fat, Choice, Cooked, Broiled									
1 chop, excluding refuse (yield from 1 raw chop, with refuse, weighing 120g) (64g)									
	202	15	6	64	0	0	0	16	49
Lamb, Domestic, Loin, Lean and Fat, 1/4" Fat, Choice, Cooked, Roasted									
1 piece, cooked, excluding refuse (yield from 1 raw chop with refuse, weighing 120g) (65g)									
	831	63	28	256	0	0	0	61	172
Lamb, Domestic, Loin, Lean and Fat, 1/8" Fat, Choice, Cooked, Broiled									
1 steak, excluding refuse (yield from 1 raw steak, with refuse, weighing 102 g) (53g)									
	157	11	5	52	0	0	0	14	41
Lamb, Domestic, Loin, Lean and Fat, 1/8" Fat, Choice, Cooked, Roasted									
1 piece, cooked, excluding refuse (yield from 1 lb raw meat with refuse) (265g)									
	769	56	24	246	0	0	0	62	170

Food Serving size	Cal.	(g) Total Fat	(g) Sat. Fat	(mg) Chol.	(g) Carb.	(g) Fiber	(g) Sug.	(g) Prot.	(mg) Sod.
Lamb, Domestic, Loin, Lean, 1/4" Fat, Choice, Cooked, Broiled 1 chop, excluding refuse (yield from 1 raw chop, with refuse, weighing 120 g) (46g)									
	99	4	2	44	0	0	0	14	39
Lamb, Domestic, Loin, Lean, 1/4" Fat, Choice, Cooked, Roasted 1 piece, cooked, excluding refuse (yield from 1 lb raw meat with refuse) (193g)									
	390	19	7	168	0	0	0	51	127
Lamb, Domestic, Rib, Lean and Fat, 1/4" Fat, Choice, Cooked, Broiled 1 piece, cooked, excluding refuse (yield from 1 lb raw meat with refuse) (229g)									
	827	68	29	227	0	0	0	51	174
Lamb, Domestic, Rib, Lean and Fat, 1/4" Fat, Choice, Cooked, Roasted 3 oz (85g)									
	305	25	11	82	0	0	0	18	62
Lamb, Domestic, Rib, Lean and Fat, 1/8" Fat, Choice, Cooked, Broiled 1 piece, cooked, excluding refuse (yield from 1 lb raw meat with refuse) (222g)									
	755	60	25	218	0	0	0	51	171
Lamb, Domestic, Rib, Lean and Fat, 1/8" Fat, Choice, Cooked, Roasted 1 piece, cooked, excluding refuse (yield from 1 lb raw meat with refuse) (248g)									
	846	68	29	238	0	0	0	54	184
Lamb, Domestic, Rib, Lean, 1/4" Fat, Choice, Cooked, Broiled 3 oz (85g)									
	200	11	4	77	0	0	0	24	72
Lamb, Domestic, Rib, Lean, 1/4" Fat, Choice, Cooked, Roasted 1 piece, cooked, excluding refuse (yield from 1 lb raw meat with refuse) (159g)									
	369	21	8	140	0	0	0	42	129
Lamb, Domestic, Shoulder, Arm, Lean and Fat, 1/4" Fat, Choice, Cooked, Braised 1 chop, excluding refuse (yield from 1 raw chop, with refuse, weighing 160 g) (70g)									
	242	17	7	84	0	0	0	21	50
Lamb, Domestic, Shoulder, Arm, Lean and Fat, 1/4" Fat, Choice, Cooked, Broiled 1 chop, excluding refuse (yield from 1 raw chop, with refuse, weighing 160 g) (93g)									
	261	18	8	89	0	0	0	23	72
Lamb, Domestic, Shoulder, Arm, Lean and Fat, 1/4" Fat, Choice, Cooked, Roasted 1 piece, cooked, excluding refuse (yield from 1 lb raw meat with refuse) (286g)									
	798	58	25	263	0	0	0	64	186
Lamb, Domestic, Shoulder, Arm, Lean and Fat, 1/8" Fat, Choice, Cooked, Braised 1 steak, excluding refuse (yield from 1 raw steak, with refuse, weighing 102 g) (45g)									
	152	10	4	54	0	0	0	14	32

Food Serving size	Cal.	(g) Total Fat	(g) Sat. Fat	(mg) Chol.	(g) Carb.	(g) Fiber	(g) Sug.	(g) Prot.	(mg) Sod.
Lamb, Domestic, Shoulder, Arm, Lean and Fat, 1/8" Fat, Choice, Roasted									
1 piece, cooked, excluding refuse (yield from 1 lb raw meat with refuse) (284g)									
	758	53	23	258	0	0	0	65	185
Lamb, Domestic, Shoulder, Arm, Lean and Fat, 1/8" Fat, Cooked, Broiled									
1 steak, excluding refuse (yield from 1 raw steak, with refuse, weighing 102 g) (59g)									
	159	11	5	57	0	0	0	15	46
Lamb, Domestic, Shoulder, Arm, Lean, 1/4" Fat, Choice, Cooked, Braised									
1 chop, excluding refuse (yield from 1 raw chop, with refuse, weighing 160 g) (55g)									
	153	8	3	67	0	0	0	20	42
Lamb, Domestic, Shoulder, Arm, Lean, 1/4" Fat, Choice, Cooked, Broiled									
1 chop, excluding refuse (yield from 1 raw chop, with refuse, weighing 160 g) (74g)									
	148	7	3	68	0	0	0	21	61
Lamb, Domestic, Shoulder, Arm, Lean, 1/4" Fat, Choice, Cooked, Roasted									
3 oz (85g)	163	8	3	73	0	0	0	22	57
Lamb, Domestic, Shoulder, Blade, Lean and Fat, 1/4" Fat, Choice, Cooked, Braised									
1 piece, cooked, excluding refuse (yield from 1 lb raw meat with refuse) (209g)									
	721	52	22	242	0	0	0	60	157
Lamb, Domestic, Shoulder, Blade, Lean and Fat, 1/4" Fat, Choice, Cooked, Broiled									
1 piece, cooked, excluding refuse (yield from 1 lb raw meat with refuse) (252g)									
	701	50	21	239	0	0	0	58	207
Lamb, Domestic, Shoulder, Blade, Lean and Fat, 1/4" Fat, Choice, Cooked, Roasted									
1 piece, cooked, excluding refuse (yield from 1 lb raw meat with refuse) (258g)									
	725	53	22	237	0	0	0	57	170
Lamb, Domestic, Shoulder, Blade, Lean and Fat, 1/8" Fat, Choice, Cooked, Braised									
1 piece, cooked, excluding refuse (yield from 1 lb raw meat with refuse) (207g)									
	702	49	20	240	0	0	0	60	155
Lamb, Domestic, Shoulder, Blade, Lean and Fat, 1/8" Fat, Choice, Cooked, Broiled									
1 piece, cooked, excluding refuse (yield from 1 lb raw meat with refuse) (250g)									
	668	46	19	238	0	0	0	59	208
Lamb, Domestic, Shoulder, Blade, Lean and Fat, 1/8" Fat, Choice, Cooked, Roasted									
1 piece, cooked, excluding refuse (yield from 1 lb raw meat with refuse) (256g)									
	691	49	20	236	0	0	0	58	172

Food Serving size	Cal.	(g) Total Fat	(g) Sat. Fat	(mg) Chol.	(g) Carb.	(g) Fiber	(g) Sug.	(g) Prot.	(mg) Sod.
Lamb, Domestic, Shoulder, Blade, Lean, 1/4" Fat, Choice, Cooked, Braised									
1 piece, cooked, excluding refuse (yield from 1 lb raw meat with refuse) (168g)	484	28	11	197	0	0	0	54	133
Lamb, Domestic, Shoulder, Blade, Lean, 1/4" Fat, Choice, Cooked, Broiled									
1 piece, cooked, excluding refuse (yield from 1 lb raw meat with refuse) (207g)	437	23	8	188	0	0	0	53	182
Lamb, Domestic, Shoulder, Blade, Lean, 1/4" Fat, Choice, Cooked, Roasted									
1 piece, cooked, excluding refuse (yield from 1 lb raw meat with refuse) (210g)	439	24	9	183	0	0	0	52	143
Lamb, Domestic, Shoulder, Whole (Arm and Blade), Lean and Fat, 1/4" Fat, Choice, Cooked, Braised									
1 piece, cooked, excluding refuse (yield from 1 lb raw meat) (218g)	750	54	23	253	0	0	0	63	164
Lamb, Domestic, Shoulder, Whole (Arm and Blade), Lean and Fat, 1/4" Fat, Choice, Cooked, Broiled									
1 piece, cooked, excluding refuse (yield from 1 lb raw meat with refuse) (248g)	689	48	20	241	0	0	0	61	193
Lamb, Domestic, Shoulder, Whole (Arm and Blade), Lean and Fat, 1/4" Fat, Choice, Cooked, Roasted									
1 piece, cooked, excluding refuse (yield from 1 lb raw meat with refuse) (269g)	742	54	23	247	0	0	0	61	178
Lamb, Domestic, Shoulder, Whole (Arm and Blade), Lean and Fat, 1/8" Fat, Choice, Cooked, Braised									
1 piece, cooked, excluding refuse (yield from 1 lb raw meat with refuse) (213g)	720	50	21	249	0	0	0	63	158
Lamb, Domestic, Shoulder, Whole (Arm and Blade), Lean and Fat, 1/8" Fat, Choice, Cooked, Broiled									
1 piece, cooked, excluding refuse (yield from 1 lb raw meat with refuse) (242g)	649	45	18	230	0	0	0	58	198
Lamb, Domestic, Shoulder, Whole (Arm and Blade), Lean and Fat, 1/8" Fat, Choice, Cooked, Roasted									
1 piece, cooked, excluding refuse (yield from 1 lb raw meat with refuse) (263g)	707	50	21	239	0	0	0	60	174
Lamb, Domestic, Shoulder, Whole (Arm and Blade), Lean, 1/4" Fat, Choice, Cooked, Braised									
1 piece, cooked, excluding refuse (yield from 1 lb raw meat with refuse) (174g)	492	28	11	204	0	0	0	57	137

Food Serving size	Cal.	(g) Total Fat	(g) Sat. Fat	(mg) Chol.	(g) Carb.	(g) Fiber	(g) Sug.	(g) Prot.	(mg) Sod.
Lamb, Domestic, Shoulder, Whole (Arm and Blade), Lean, 1/4" Fat, Choice, Cooked, Broiled 1 piece, cooked, excluding refuse (yield from 1 lb raw meat with refuse) (202g)									
	424	21	8	188	0	0	0	55	168
Lamb, Domestic, Shoulder, Whole (Arm and Blade), Lean, 1/4" Fat, Choice, Cooked, Roasted 1 piece, cooked, excluding refuse (yield from 1 lb raw meat with refuse) (217g)									
	443	23	9	189	0	0	0	54	148
Lamb, Ground, Cooked, Broiled 1 unit, cooked (yield from 1 lb raw meat) (313g)									
	886	62	25	304	0	0	0	77	254
Lamb, New Zealand, Imported, Frozen, Composite of Retail Cuts, Fat, Cooked 1 unit, cooked (yield from 1 lb raw meat with refuse) (286g)									
	1676	173	90	312	0	0	0	28	100
Lamb, New Zealand, Imported, Frozen, Composite of Retail Cuts, Lean and Fat, 1/8" Fat, Cooked 1 piece, cooked, excluding refuse (yield from 1 lb raw meat with refuse) (242g)									
	653	44	21	257	0	0	0	61	111
Lamb, New Zealand, Imported, Frozen, Composite of Retail Cuts, Lean and Fat, Cooked 1 piece, cooked, excluding refuse (yield from 1 lb raw meat with refuse) (222g)									
	677	49	25	242	0	0	0	54	102
Lamb, New Zealand, Imported, Frozen, Composite of Retail Cuts, Lean, Cooked 1 piece, cooked, excluding refuse (yield from 1 lb raw meat with refuse) (164g)									
	338	15	6	179	0	0	0	49	82
Lamb, New Zealand, Imported, Frozen, Foreshank, Lean and Fat, 1/8" Fat, Cooked, Braised 1 piece, cooked, excluding refuse (yield from 1 lb raw meat with refuse) (168g)									
	433	27	13	171	0	0	0	45	79
Lamb, New Zealand, Imported, Frozen, Leg, Whole (Shank and Sirloin), Lean and Fat, 1/8" Fat, Cooked, Roasted 1 piece, cooked, excluding refuse (yield from 1 lb raw meat with refuse) (253g)									
	592	35	17	256	0	0	0	64	111
Lamb, New Zealand, Imported, Frozen, Leg, Whole (Shank and Sirloin), Lean and Fat, Cooked, Roasted 1 piece, cooked, excluding refuse (yield from 1 lb raw meat with refuse) (258g)									
	635	40	20	261	0	0	0	64	111

Food Serving size	Cal.	(g) Total Fat	(g) Sat. Fat	(mg) Chol.	(g) Carb.	(g) Fiber	(g) Sug.	(g) Prot.	(mg) Sod.
Lamb, New Zealand, Imported, Frozen, Leg, Whole (Shank and Sirloin), Lean, Cooked, Roasted 1 piece, cooked, excluding refuse (yield from 1 lb raw meat with refuse) (218g)	395	15	7	218	0	0	0	60	98
Lamb, New Zealand, Imported, Frozen, Loin, Lean and Fat, 1/8" Fat, Cooked, Broiled 1 chop, excluding refuse (yield from 1 raw chop, with refuse, weighing 85 g) (42g)	124	9	4	47	0	0	0	10	21
Lamb, New Zealand, Imported, Frozen, Loin, Lean and Fat, Cooked, Broiled 1 chop, excluding refuse (yield from 1 raw chop, with refuse, weighing 85 g) (43g)	135	10	5	48	0	0	0	10	21
Lamb, New Zealand, Imported, Frozen, Loin, Lean, Cooked, Broiled 1 chop, excluding refuse (yield from 1 raw chop, with refuse, weighing 85 g) (30g)	60	2	1	34	0	0	0	9	17
Lamb, New Zealand, Imported, Frozen, Rib, Lean and Fat, 1/8" Fat, Cooked, Roasted 1 piece, cooked, excluding refuse (yield from 1 lb raw meat with refuse) (233g)	739	60	30	231	0	0	0	46	103
Lamb, New Zealand, Imported, Frozen, Rib, Lean and Fat, Cooked, Roasted 3 oz (85g)	289	24	12	85	0	0	0	16	37
Lamb, New Zealand, Imported, Frozen, Rib, Lean, Cooked, Roasted 3 oz (85g)	167	9	4	80	0	0	0	21	41
Lamb, New Zealand, Imported, Frozen, Shoulder, Whole (Arm and Blade), Lean and Fat, 1/8" Fat, Cooked, Braised 1 piece, cooked, excluding refuse (yield from 1 lb raw meat with refuse) (233g)	797	56	27	287	0	0	0	69	121
Lamb, New Zealand, Imported, Frozen, Shoulder, Whole (Arm and Blade), Lean and Fat, Cooked, Braised 1 piece, cooked, excluding refuse (yield from 1 lb raw meat with refuse) (206g)	735	54	26	253	0	0	0	58	105
Lamb, New Zealand, Imported, Frozen, Shoulder, Whole (Arm and Blade), Lean, Cooked, Braised 1 piece, cooked, excluding refuse (yield from 1 lb raw meat with refuse) (157g)	447	24	11	199	0	0	0	53	88
Lamb, Variety Meats and By-products, Brain, Cooked, Braised 1 unit, cooked (yield from 1 lb raw meat) (347g)	503	35	9	7089	0	0	0	44	465

Food Serving size	Cal.	(g) Total Fat	(g) Sat. Fat	(mg) Chol.	(g) Carb.	(g) Fiber	(g) Sug.	(g) Prot.	(mg) Sod.
Lamb, Variety Meats and By-products, Brain, Cooked, Pan-fried 1 unit, cooked (yield from 1 lb raw meat) (240g)	655	53	14	6010	0	0	0	41	377
Lamb, Variety Meats and By-products, Heart, Cooked, Braised 1 unit, cooked (yield from 1 lb raw meat) (191g)	353	15	6	476	4	0	0	48	120
Lamb, Variety Meats and By-products, Kidneys, Cooked, Braised 1 unit, cooked (yield from 1 lb raw meat) (255g)	349	9	3	1441	3	0	0	60	385
Lamb, Variety Meats and By-products, Liver, Cooked, Braised 1 unit, cooked (yield from 1 lb raw meat) (336g)	739	30	11	1683	9	0	0	103	188
Lamb, Variety Meats and By-products, Liver, Cooked, Pan-fried 1 unit, cooked (yield from 1 lb raw meat) (322g)	766	41	16	1587	12	0	0	82	399
Lamb, Variety Meats and By-products, Lungs, Cooked, Braised 1 unit, cooked (yield from 1 lb raw meat) (381g)	431	12	4	1082	0	0	0	76	320
Lamb, Variety Meats and By-products, Pancreas, Cooked, Braised 1 unit, cooked (yield from 1 lb raw meat) (231g)	541	35	16	924	0	0	0	53	120
Lamb, Variety Meats and By-products, Spleen, Cooked, Braised 1 unit, cooked (yield from 1 lb raw meat) (295g)	460	14	5	1136	0	0	0	78	171
Lamb, Variety Meats and By-products, Tongue, Cooked, Braised 1 unit, cooked (yield from 1 lb raw meat) (255g)	701	52	20	482	0	0	0	55	171
Lamb, Domestic, Shoulder, Blade, Lean and Fat, 1/8" Fat, Choice, Cooked, Roasted 3 oz (85g)	230	16	7	78	0	0	0	19	57
Lambs, Quarters, Cooked, Boiled, Drained, with Salt 1 cup, chopped (180g)	58	1	0	0	9	3.8	1	6	477
Loma Linda Redi-burger, Canned, Unprepared 1 slice, 5/8" (85g)	124	2	0	0	7	3.7	1	19	432
Loma Linda Swiss Steak with Gravy, Canned, Unprepared 1 piece (92g)	127	6	1	1	10	2.9	1	9	433

Food Serving size	Cal.	(g) Total Fat	(g) Sat. Fat	(mg) Chol.	(g) Carb.	(g) Fiber	(g) Sug.	(g) Prot.	(mg) Sod.
Loma Linda Tender Bits, Canned, Unprepared									
6 pieces (85g)	115	4	1	0	7	3.7	1	13	521
Loma Linda Tender Rounds with Gravy, Canned, Unprepared									
6 pieces (80g)	116	4	1	1	6	2.8	1	13	354
Pastrami, Beef, 98% Fat Free									
1 serving, 6 slices (57g)	54	1	0	27	1	0	0	11	576
Pork Skins, Barbecue Flavor									
.5 oz (14.2g)	76	5	2	16	0	0	0	8	379
Pork Skins, Plain									
.5 oz (14.2g)	77	4	2	13	0	0	0	9	258
Pork, Cured, Bacon, Cooked, Baked									
1 slice, cooked (8.1g)	44	3	1	9	0	0	0	3	175
Pork, Cured, Bacon, Cooked, Broiled, Pan-fried or Roasted									
1 slice, cooked (8g)	43	3	1	9	0	0	0	3	185
Pork, Cured, Bacon, Cooked, Broiled, Pan-fried or Roasted, Reduced Sodium									
1 slice, cooked (8g)	43	3	1	9	0	0	0	3	82
Pork, Cured, Bacon, Cooked, Microwaved									
1 slice, raw (28g)	133	10	3	31	0	0	0	11	499
Pork, Cured, Bacon, Cooked, Pan-fried									
1 slice, cooked (7.9g)	51	4	1	11	0	0	0	4	185
Pork, Cured, Breakfast Strips, Cooked									
3 slices, cooked (raw product packed 15 per 12-oz bag) (34g)	156	12	4	36	0	0	0	10	714
Pork, Cured, Canadian-style Bacon, Grilled									
2 slices (6 per 6-oz pkg.) (47g)	87	4	1	27	1	0	0	11	727
Pork, Cured, Canadian-style Bacon, Unheated									
2 slices (6 per 6-oz pkg.) (57g)	89	4	1	29	1	0	0	12	803
Pork, Cured, Fat (from Ham and Arm Picnic), Roasted									
3 oz (85g)	502	53	19	73	0	0	0	6	530
Pork, Cured, Feet, Pickled									
1 lb (453.6g)	635	45	13	376	0	0	0	53	4291
Pork, Cured, Ham, Extra Lean and Regular, Canned, Roasted									
3 oz (85g)	142	7	2	35	0	0	0	18	908
Pork, Cured, Ham–Water Added, Rump, Bone-in, Lean and Fat, Heated, Roasted									
1 serving (3 oz) (85g)	137	7	2	54	1	0	1	17	936

Food Serving size	Cal.	(g) Total Fat	(g) Sat. Fat	(mg) Chol.	(g) Carb.	(g) Fiber	(g) Sug.	(g) Prot.	(mg) Sod.
Pork, Cured, Ham–Water Added, Rump, Bone-in, Lean and Fat, Unheated									
1 lb (453.6g)	780	57	19	245	4	0	3	63	4849
Pork, Cured, Ham–Water Added, Rump, Bone-in, Lean, Heated, Roasted									
1 roast, rump (2970g)	3594	106	37	1841	26	0	25	636	34155
Pork, Cured, Ham–Water Added, Shank, Bone-in, Lean and Fat, Heated, Roasted									
1 roast, shank (3054g)	6108	408	133	2016	41	0	24	569	30174
Pork, Cured, Ham–Water Added, Shank, Bone-in, Lean and Fat, Unheated									
1 lb (453.6g)	758	50	16	236	1	0	3	76	4373
Pork, Cured, Ham–Water Added, Shank, Bone-in, Lean, Heated, Roasted									
1 roast, shank (3054g)	3909	135	43	1985	37	0	28	639	32372
Pork, Cured, Ham–Water Added, Slice, Bone-in, Lean and Fat, Heated, Pan-broiled									
1 serving (3 oz) (85g)	141	7	2	56	1	0	1	18	1113
Pork, Cured, Ham–Water Added, Slice, Bone-in, Lean and Fat, Unheated									
1 lb (453.6g)	744	49	16	249	5	0	5	71	4586
Pork, Cured, Ham–Water Added, Slice, Bone-in, Lean, Heated, Pan-broiled									
1 slice (436g)	724	38	13	288	7	0	7	91	5707
Pork, Cured, Ham–Water Added, Slice, Boneless, Lean and Fat, Heated, Pan-broiled									
1 serving (3 oz) (85g)	106	4	1	46	1	0	1	16	1030
Pork, Cured, Ham–Water Added, Slice, Boneless, Lean, Heated, Pan-broiled									
1 slice (189g)	236	10	3	102	3	0	3	35	2291
Pork, Cured, Ham–Water Added, Whole, Boneless, Lean and Fat, Heated, Roasted									
1 roast (1867g)	2352	102	33	1008	29	0	29	332	22049
Pork, Cured, Ham–Water Added, Whole, Boneless, Lean and Fat, Unheated									
1 lb, whole (453.6g)	549	24	9	227	6	0	6	77	5108
Pork, Cured, Ham–Water Added, Whole, Boneless, Lean, Heated, Roasted									
1 roast, whole (1867g)	2184	82	27	990	26	0	29	336	22273
Pork, Cured, Ham and Water Product, Rump, Bone-in, Lean and Fat, Heated, Roasted									
1 roast, rump (2533g)	4711	291	96	1697	29	0	26	493	29915
Pork, Cured, Ham and Water Product, Rump, Bone-in, Lean and Fat, Unheated									
1 lb (453.6g)	780	57	19	245	4	0	3	63	4849

Food Serving size	Cal.	(g) Total Fat	(g) Sat. Fat	(mg) Chol.	(g) Carb.	(g) Fiber	(g) Sug.	(g) Prot.	(mg) Sod.
Pork, Cured, Ham and Water Product, Rump, Bone-in, Lean, Heated, Roasted									
1 serving (3 oz) (85g)	111	4	1	56	1	0	1	18	1077
Pork, Cured, Ham and Water Product, Rump, Bone-in, Lean, Unheated									
1 lb (453.6g)	485	15	5	263	6	0	4	81	4854
Pork, Cured, Ham and Water Product, Shank, Bone-in, Lean and Fat, Heated, Roasted									
1 roast, shank (3204g)	7497	554	183	2307	45	0	32	582	30278
Pork, Cured, Ham and Water Product, Shank, Bone-in, Lean and Fat, Unheated									
1 lb (453.6g)	758	50	16	236	3	0	3	76	4373
Pork, Cured, Ham and Water Product, Shank, Bone-in, Lean, Heated, Roasted									
1 serving (3 oz) (85g)	112	4	1	61	1	0	1	18	888
Pork, Cured, Ham and Water Product, Slice, Bone-in, Lean and Fat, Heated, Pan-broiled									
1 slice (446g)	691	35	12	285	6	0	5	89	5298
Pork, Cured, Ham and Water Product, Slice, Bone-in, Lean and Fat, Unheated									
1 lb (453.6g)	676	42	14	227	12	0	4	62	4985
Pork, Cured, Ham and Water Product, Slice, Bone-in, Lean, Heated, Pan-broiled									
1 slice (446g)	544	16	5	285	6	0	5	93	5517
Pork, Cured, Ham and Water Product, Slice, Boneless, Lean and Fat, Heated, Pan-broiled									
1 serving (3 oz) (85g)	105	4	1	38	4	0	4	13	1181
Pork, Cured, Ham and Water Product, Slice, Boneless, Lean, Heated, Pan-broiled									
1 serving (3 oz) (85g)	105	4	1	38	4	0	4	13	1182
Pork, Cured, Ham and Water Product, Whole, Boneless, Lean and Fat, Heated, Roasted									
1 roast (1995g)	2454	109	37	858	92	0	92	277	26633
Pork, Cured, Ham and Water Product, Whole, Boneless, Lean and Fat, Unheated									
1 lb, whole (453.6g)	531	23	7	195	19	0	19	64	5933
Pork, Cured, Ham and Water Product, Whole, Boneless, Lean, Heated, Roasted									
1 roast (1995g)	2454	109	37	858	92	0	92	277	26633
Pork, Cured, Ham with Natural Juices, Rump, Bone-in, Lean and Fat, Heated, Roasted									
1 roast, rump (2673g)	4731	251	83	1925	16	0	12	601	22480
Pork, Cured, Ham with Natural Juices, Slice, Bone-in, Lean, Heated, Pan-broiled									
1 slice (445g)	668	19	5	356	0	0	0	123	3716

Food Serving size	Cal.	(g) Total Fat	(g) Sat. Fat	(mg) Chol.	(g) Carb.	(g) Fiber	(g) Sug.	(g) Prot.	(mg) Sod.
Pork, Cured, Ham with Natural Juices, Slice, Bone-in, Lean, Unheated									
1 slice (430g)	529	12	3	271	0	0	0	105	3702
Pork, Cured, Ham with Natural Juices, Slice, Boneless, Lean and Fat, Heated, Pan-broiled									
1 serving (3 oz) (85g)	100	3	1	49	1	0	1	18	986
Pork, Cured, Ham with Natural Juices, Slice, Boneless, Lean, Heated, Pan-broiled									
1 slice (277g)	327	9	3	161	3	0	3	58	3213
Pork, Cured, Ham with Natural Juices, Spiral Sliced, Boneless, Lean and Fat, Heated, Roasted									
1 roast (920g)	1279	47	4	589	10	0	10	204	8988
Pork, Cured, Ham with Natural Juices, Spiral Sliced, Boneless, Lean and Fat, Unheated									
1 lb, spiral slice (453.6g)	585	26	8	259	5	0	5	85	3996
Pork, Cured, Ham with Natural Juices, Spiral Sliced, Boneless, Lean, Unheated									
1 lb, spiral slice (453.6g)	494	15	5	259	6	0	6	87	4060
Pork, Cured, Ham with Natural Juices, Spiral Sliced, Meat Only, Boneless, Lean, Heated, Roasted									
1 roast (920g)	1159	35	5	580	10	0	10	208	9071
Pork, Cured, Ham with Natural Juices, Whole, Boneless, Lean and Fat, Heated, Roasted									
1 roast (1497g)	1707	47	16	838	13	0	12	307	17650
Pork, Cured, Ham with Natural Juices, Whole, Boneless, Lean and Fat, Unheated									
1 lb, whole (453.6g)	508	16	5	240	5	0	5	88	4971
Pork, Cured, Ham with Natural Juices, Whole, Boneless, Lean, Heated, Roasted									
1 roast (1497g)	1692	45	16	838	13	0	12	308	17665
Pork, Cured, Ham with Natural Juices, Whole, Boneless, Lean, Unheated									
1 lb (453.6g)	499	15	4	240	5	0	5	88	4981
Pork, Cured, Ham, Boneless, Extra Lean (Approximately 5% Fat), Roasted									
3 oz (85g)	123	5	2	45	1	0	0	18	1023
Pork, Cured, Ham, Boneless, Extra Lean and Regular, Roasted									
3 oz (85g)	140	7	2	48	0	0	0	19	1177
Pork, Cured, Ham, Boneless, Low Sodium, Extra Lean and Regular, Roasted									
1 oz, boneless (28.35g)	47	2	1	16	0	0	0	6	275
Pork, Cured, Ham, Boneless, Regular (Approximately 11% Fat), roasted									
3 oz (85g)	151	8	3	50	0	0	0	19	1275

Food Serving size	Cal.	(g) Total Fat	(g) Sat. Fat	(mg) Chol.	(g) Carb.	(g) Fiber	(g) Sug.	(g) Prot.	(mg) Sod.
Pork, Cured, Ham, Center Slice, Lean and Fat, Unheated									
4 oz (113g)	229	15	5	61	0	0	0	23	1566
Pork, Cured, Ham, Extra Lean (Approximately 4% Fat), Canned, Roasted									
3 oz (85g)	116	4	1	26	0	0	0	18	965
Pork, Cured, Ham, Extra Lean (Approximately 4% Fat), Canned, Unheated									
1 oz (28.35g)	34	1	0	11	0	0	0	5	356
Pork, Cured, Ham, Extra Lean and Regular, Canned, Roasted									
3 oz (85g)	142	7	2	35	0	0	0	18	908
Pork, Cured, Ham, Low Sodium, Lean and Fat, Cooked									
1 oz, boneless (28.35g)	49	2	1	16	0	0	0	6	275
Pork, Cured, Ham, Patties, Grilled									
1 unit, cooked (yield from 1 lb raw meat) (413g)	1412	127	46	297	7	0	0	55	4390
Pork, Cured, Ham, Regular (Approximately 13% Fat), Canned, Roasted									
3 oz (85g)	192	13	4	53	0	0	0	17	800
Pork, Cured, Ham, Regular (Approximately 13% Fat), Canned, Unheated									
1 oz (28.35g)	54	4	1	11	0	0	0	5	352
Pork, Cured, Ham, Rump, Bone-in, Lean and Fat, Heated, Roasted									
1 roast, rump (2874g)	5087	255	82	2041	20	0	20	748	24314
Pork, Cured, Ham, Rump, Bone-in, Lean, Heated, Roasted									
1 roast, rump (2874g)	3794	88	26	2041	20	0	20	748	24314
Pork, Cured, Ham, Slice, Bone-in, Lean and Fat, Heated, Pan-broiled									
1 serving (3 oz) (85g)	153	7	1	62	0	0	1	22	724
Pork, Cured, Ham, Slice, Bone-in, Lean, Heated, Pan-broiled									
1 slice (366g)	659	31	6	267	3	0	3	93	3118
Pork, Cured, Ham, Whole, Lean and Fat, Roasted									
3 oz (85g)	207	14	5	53	0	0	0	18	1009
Pork, Cured, Ham, Whole, Lean, Roasted									
3 oz (85g)	133	5	2	47	0	0	0	21	1128
Pork, Cured, Shoulder, Arm Picnic, Lean and Fat, Roasted									
3 oz (85g)	238	18	7	49	0	0	0	17	911
Pork, Cured, Shoulder, Arm Picnic, Lean, Roasted									
3 oz (85g)	145	6	2	41	0	0	0	21	1046
Pork, Cured, Shoulder, Blade Roll, Lean and Fat, Roasted									
1 piece, cooked (yield from 1 lb unheated product) (376g)	1079	88	32	252	1	0	0	65	3658

Food Serving size	Cal.	(g) Total Fat	(g) Sat. Fat	(mg) Chol.	(g) Carb.	(g) Fiber	(g) Sug.	(g) Prot.	(mg) Sod.
Pork, Fresh, Backribs, Lean and Fat, Cooked, Roasted 1 ribs (yield from 1 lb raw meat with refuse) (878g)									
	248	18	7	71	0	0	0	20	80
Pork, Fresh, Composite (Leg, Loin, Shoulder and Spareribs), Lean and Fat, Cooked 3 oz (85g)									
	588	34	12	217	0	0	0	65	141
Pork, Fresh, Composite of Retail Cuts (Leg, Loin, and Shoulder), Lean, Cooked 3 oz (85g)	464	21	7	194	0	0	0	64	127
Pork, Fresh, Composite of Retail Cuts (Loin and Shoulder Blade), Lean and Fat, Cooked 1 piece, cooked, excluding refuse (yield from 1 lb raw meat with refuse) (261g)									
	613	36	12	217	0	0	0	68	144
Pork, Fresh, Composite of Retail Cuts (Loin and Shoulder Blade), Lean, Cooked 1 piece, cooked, excluding refuse (yield from 1 lb raw meat with refuse) (236g)									
	498	22	8	201	0	0	0	70	135
Pork, Fresh, Enhanced, Loin, Tenderloin, Lean and Fat, Cooked, Roasted 1 roast (508g)	615	19	6	290	2	0	0	109	1168
Pork, Fresh, Enhanced, Shoulder (Boston Butt), Blade (Steaks), Lean and Fat, Braised 1 steak (264g)	694	45	17	256	0	0	0	68	399
Pork, Fresh, Fat, Cooked 4 oz (113g)	707	75	27	89	0	0	0	8	63
Pork, Fresh, Ground, Cooked 3 oz (85g)	252	18	7	80	0	0	0	22	62
Pork, Fresh, Leg (Ham), Rump Half, Lean and Fat, Cooked, Roasted 3 oz (85g)	178	9	3	72	0	0	0	23	65
Pork, Fresh, Leg (Ham), Rump Half, Lean, Cooked, Roasted 1 roast (3027g)	4995	140	44	2603	0	0	0	874	2422
Pork, Fresh, Leg (Ham), Shank Half, Lean and Fat, Cooked, Roasted 1 roast (2900g)	6728	389	134	2639	0	0	0	753	2349
Pork, Fresh, Leg (Ham), Shank Half, Lean, Cooked, Roasted 1 roast (2900g)	5075	169	53	2697	0	0	0	832	2436
Pork, Fresh, Leg (Ham), Whole, Lean and Fat, Cooked, Roasted 3 oz (85g)	232	15	5	80	0	0	0	23	51

Food Serving size	Cal.	(g) Total Fat	(g) Sat. Fat	(mg) Chol.	(g) Carb.	(g) Fiber	(g) Sug.	(g) Prot.	(mg) Sod.
Pork, Fresh, Leg (Ham), Whole, Lean, Cooked, Roasted 3 oz (85g)	179	8	3	80	0	0	0	25	54
Pork, Fresh, Loin, Blade (Chops), Bone-in, Lean, Cooked, Braised 1 chop (206g)	457	23	5	179	0	0	0	58	144
Pork, Fresh, Loin, Blade (Chops), Bone-in, Lean, Cooked, Broiled 1 chop (219g)	423	21	5	171	0	0	0	55	166
Pork, Fresh, Loin, Blade (Chops), Bone-in, Lean and Fat, Cooked, Braised 1 chop (206g)	525	32	9	177	0	0	0	55	142
Pork, Fresh, Loin, Blade (Chops), Bone-in, Lean and Fat, Cooked, Broiled 1 chop (219g)	506	31	10	171	0	0	0	52	162
Pork, Fresh, Loin, Blade (Chops), Bone-in, Lean, Cooked, Braised 1 chop (206g)	457	23	5	179	0	0	0	58	144
Pork, Fresh, Loin, Blade (Chops), Bone-in, Lean, Cooked, Broiled 1 chop (219g)	423	21	5	171	0	0	0	55	166
Pork, Fresh, Loin, Blade (Chops), Bone-in, Lean, Cooked, Pan-fried 1 chop (215g)	550	36	9	176	0	0	0	54	183
Pork, Fresh, Loin, Blade (Roasts), Bone-in, Lean and Fat, Cooked, Roasted 1 roast (830g)	2108	139	49	689	0	0	0	202	631
Pork, Fresh, Loin, Blade (Roasts), Bone-in, Lean, Cooked, Roasted 1 roast (830g)	1801	99	33	689	0	0	0	213	647
Pork, Fresh, Loin, Blade (Roasts), Boneless, Lean and Fat, Cooked, Roasted 1 roast (848g)	1688	88	31	644	0	0	0	225	568
Pork, Fresh, Loin, Center Loin (Chops), Bone-in, Lean and Fat, Cooked, Braised 1 chop (187g)	453	25	9	151	0	0	0	53	137
Pork, Fresh, Loin, Center Loin (Chops), Bone-in, Lean, Cooked, Braised 1 chop (187g)	374	15	5	151	0	0	0	56	140
Pork, Fresh, Loin, Center Loin (Chops), Bone-in, Lean, Cooked, Broiled 3 oz (85g)	153	6	2	71	0	0	0	23	48
Pork, Fresh, Loin, Center Loin (Chops), Bone-in, Lean, Cooked, Pan-fried 1 chop (172g)	335	13	4	134	0	0	0	51	170
Pork, Fresh, Loin, Center Loin (Roasts), Bone-in, Lean and Fat, Cooked, Roasted 1 roast (900g)	2079	115	44	684	0	0	0	243	747
Pork, Fresh, Loin, Center Loin (Roasts), Bone-in, Lean, Cooked, Roasted 1 roast (900g)	1746	72	26	675	0	0	0	257	774

Food Serving size	Cal.	(g) Total Fat	(g) Sat. Fat	(mg) Chol.	(g) Carb.	(g) Fiber	(g) Sug.	(g) Prot.	(mg) Sod.
Pork, Fresh, Loin, Center Loin (Chops), Bone-in, Lean and Fat, Cooked, Pan-fried									
1 chop (172g)	409	23	8	136	0	0	0	48	162
Pork, Fresh, Loin, Center Rib (Chops), Bone-in, Lean, Cooked, Broiled									
1 chop, excluding refuse (yield from 1 raw chop, with refuse, weighing 151 g) (67g)									
	125	6	2	44	0	0	0	17	38
Pork, Fresh, Loin, Center Rib (Chops), Bone-in, Lean and Fat, Cooked, Braised									
1 chop (187g)	389	17	5	148	0	0	0	54	135
Pork, Fresh, Loin, Center Rib (Chops), Bone-in, Lean and Fat, Cooked, Broiled									
3 oz (85g)	189	11	4	57	0	0	0	21	47
Pork, Fresh, Loin, Center Rib (Chops), Bone-in, Lean, Cooked, Broiled									
1 chop, excluding refuse (yield from 1 raw chop, with refuse, weighing 151 g) (67g)									
	125	6	2	44	0	0	0	17	38
Pork, Fresh, Loin, Center Rib (Chops), Bone-in, Lean, Cooked, Pan-fried									
1 chop (172g)	335	13	4	134	0	0	0	51	170
Pork, Fresh, Loin, Center Rib (Chops), Boneless, Lean and Fat, Cooked, Braised									
1 chop, excluding refuse (yield from 1 raw chop, with refuse, weighing 113 g) (81g)									
	207	13	5	59	0	0	0	21	32
Pork, Fresh, Loin, Center Rib (Chops), Boneless, Lean and Fat, Cooked, Broiled									
1 chop, excluding refuse (yield from 1 raw chop, with refuse, weighing 113 g) (80g)									
	208	13	5	66	0	0	0	22	50
Pork, Fresh, Loin, Center Rib (Chops), Boneless, Lean and Fat, Cooked, Pan-fried									
1 chop, excluding refuse (yield from 1 raw chop, with refuse, weighing 113 g) (75g)									
	205	14	5	55	0	0	0	19	38
Pork, Fresh, Loin, Center Rib (Chops), Boneless, Lean, Cooked, Braised									
1 chop, excluding refuse (yield from 1 raw chop, with refuse, weighing 113 g) (72g)									
	152	7	3	51	0	0	0	20	30
Pork, Fresh, Loin, Center Rib (Chops), Boneless, Lean, Cooked, Broiled									
1 chop, excluding refuse (yield from 1 raw chop, with refuse, weighing 113 g) (71g)									
	153	7	3	58	0	0	0	21	46
Pork, Fresh, Loin, Center Rib (Chops), Boneless, Lean, Cooked, Pan-fried									
1 chop, excluding refuse (yield from 1 raw chop, with refuse, weighing 113 g) (66g)									
	148	8	3	46	0	0	0	18	34
Pork, Fresh, Loin, Center Rib (Roasts), Bone-in, Lean and Fat, Cooked, Roasted									
1 roast (783g)	1942	115	43	611	0	0	0	211	713
Pork, Fresh, Loin, Center Rib (Roasts), Bone-in, Lean, Cooked, Roasted									
1 roast (783g)	1613	72	25	611	0	0	0	226	744

Food Serving size	Cal.	(g) Total Fat	(g) Sat. Fat	(mg) Chol.	(g) Carb.	(g) Fiber	(g) Sug.	(g) Prot.	(mg) Sod.
Pork, Fresh, Loin, Center Rib (Roasts), Boneless, Lean and Fat, Cooked, Roasted 1 piece, cooked, excluding refuse (yield from 1 lb raw meat with refuse) (317g)	799	48	17	257	0	0	0	86	152
Pork, Fresh, Loin, Center Rib (Roasts), Boneless, Lean, Cooked, Roasted 1 piece, cooked, excluding refuse (yield from 1 lb raw meat with refuse) (283g)	606	29	10	235	0	0	0	82	142
Pork, Fresh, Loin, Sirloin (Chops), Bone-in, Lean and Fat, Cooked, Braised 1 chop (180g)	421	22	8	157	0	0	0	52	104
Pork, Fresh, Loin, Sirloin (Chops), Bone-in, Lean and Fat, Cooked, Broiled 1 chop (195g)	433	23	8	170	0	0	0	53	168
Pork, Fresh, Loin, Sirloin (Chops), Bone-in, Lean, Cooked, Braised 1 chop (180g)	351	12	4	158	0	0	0	56	104
Pork, Fresh, Loin, Sirloin (Chops), Bone-in, Lean, Cooked, Broiled 1 chop (195g)	339	11	3	172	0	0	0	57	174
Pork, Fresh, Loin, Sirloin (Chops), Boneless, Lean and Fat, Cooked, Braised 1 chop, excluding refuse (yield from 1 raw chop, with refuse, weighing 113 g) (82g)	140	4	2	66	0	0	0	23	46
Pork, Fresh, Loin, Sirloin (Chops), Boneless, Lean and Fat, Cooked, Broiled 1 chop (159g)	270	9	3	121	0	0	0	45	103
Pork, Fresh, Loin, Sirloin (Roasts), Bone-in, Lean and Fat, Cooked, Roasted 1 roast, without refuse (yield from 1 cooked roast, with refuse, weighing 1515 g) (1046g)	2406	135	43	931	0	0	0	279	596
Pork, Fresh, Loin, Sirloin (Roasts), Bone-in, Lean, Cooked, Roasted 1 roast, without refuse (985g)	2009	93	28	877	0	0	0	274	581
Pork, Fresh, Loin, Sirloin (Roasts), Boneless, Lean and Fat, Cooked, Roasted 1 roast (638g)	1225	47	16	536	0	0	0	189	421
Pork, Fresh, Loin, Sirloin (Roasts), Boneless, Lean, Cooked, Roasted 1 roast (638g)	1136	34	11	536	0	0	0	194	421
Pork, Fresh, Loin, Tenderloin, Lean and Fat, Cooked, Broiled 1 chop, excluding refuse (yield from 1 raw chop, with refuse, weighing 113 g) (76g)	153	6	2	71	0	0	0	23	49
Pork, Fresh, Loin, Tenderloin, Lean and Fat, Cooked, Roasted 1 roast (402g)	591	16	5	293	0	0	0	105	229
Pork, Fresh, Loin, Tenderloin, Lean, Cooked, Broiled 1 chop, excluding refuse (yield from 1 raw chop, with refuse, weighing 113 g) (73g)	137	5	2	69	0	0	0	22	47

Food Serving size	Cal.	(g) Total Fat	(g) Sat. Fat	(mg) Chol.	(g) Carb.	(g) Fiber	(g) Sug.	(g) Prot.	(mg) Sod.
Pork, Fresh, Loin, Tenderloin, Lean, Cooked, Roasted 1 piece, cooked, excluding refuse (yield from 1 lb raw meat with refuse) (333g)									
	476	12	4	243	0	0	0	87	190
Pork, Fresh, Loin, Top Loin (Chops), Boneless, Lean and Fat, Cooked, Braised 1 chop (135g)	270	11	4	97	0	0	0	39	89
Pork, Fresh, Loin, Top Loin (Chops), Boneless, Lean and Fat, Cooked, Broiled 3 oz (85g)	167	8	3	62	0	0	0	23	37
Pork, Fresh, Loin, Top Loin (Chops), Boneless, Lean and Fat, Cooked, Pan-fried 1 chop (142g)	278	11	4	99	0	0	0	42	122
Pork, Fresh, Loin, Top Loin (Chops), Boneless, Lean, Cooked, Braised 1 chop (135g)	230	6	2	96	0	0	0	41	90
Pork, Fresh, Loin, Top Loin (Chops), Boneless, Lean, Cooked, Broiled 1 chop (145g)	251	9	3	104	0	0	0	40	65
Pork, Fresh, Loin, Top Loin (Chops), Boneless, Lean, Cooked, Pan-fried 3 oz (85g)	146	4	2	59	0	0	0	26	74
Pork, Fresh, Loin, Top Loin (Roasts), Boneless, Lean and Fat, Cooked, Roasted 1 roast (848g)	1628	75	24	678	0	0	0	224	390
Pork, Fresh, Loin, Top Loin (Roasts), Boneless, Lean, Cooked, Roasted 3 oz (85g)	147	5	2	67	0	0	0	23	40
Pork, Fresh, Loin, Whole, Lean and Fat, Cooked, Braised 1 chop, excluding refuse (yield from 1 raw chop, with refuse, weighing 151 g) (89g)									
	213	12	5	71	0	0	0	24	43
Pork, Fresh, Loin, Whole, Lean and Fat, Cooked, Broiled 1 chop, excluding refuse (yield from 1 raw chop, with refuse, weighing 151 g) (87g)									
	211	12	5	70	0	0	0	24	54
Pork, Fresh, Loin, Whole, Lean and Fat, Cooked, Roasted 1 chop, excluding refuse (yield from 1 raw chop, with refuse, weighing 151 g) (89g)									
	221	13	5	73	0	0	0	24	53
Pork, Fresh, Loin, Whole, Lean, Cooked, Braised 1 chop, excluding refuse (yield from 1 raw chop, with refuse, weighing 151 g) (80g)									
	163	7	3	63	0	0	0	23	40
Pork, Fresh, Loin, Whole, Lean, Cooked, Broiled 1 chop, excluding refuse (yield from 1 raw chop, with refuse, weighing 151 g) (79g)									
	166	8	3	62	0	0	0	23	51

Food Serving size	Cal.	(g) Total Fat	(g) Sat. Fat	(mg) Chol.	(g) Carb.	(g) Fiber	(g) Sug.	(g) Prot.	(mg) Sod.
Pork, Fresh, Loin, Whole, Lean, Cooked, Roasted 1 chop, excluding refuse (yield from 1 raw chop, with refuse, weighing 151 g) (81g)									
	169	8	3	66	0	0	0	23	47
Pork, Fresh, Shoulder (Boston Butt), Blade (Steaks), Lean and Fat, Cooked, Braised 1 steak, without refuse (yield from 1 cooked steak, with refuse, weighing 249 g) (185g)									
	494	33	12	181	0	0	0	46	107
Pork, Fresh, Shoulder (Boston Butt), Blade (Steaks), Lean, Cooked, Braised 1 steak (249g)									
	580	33	13	249	0	0	0	66	149
Pork, Fresh, Shoulder, Arm Picnic, Lean and Fat, Cooked, Braised 1 roast (2252g)									
	5292	323	109	1937	0	0	0	560	2162
Pork, Fresh, Shoulder, Arm Picnic, Lean and Fat, Cooked, Roasted 1 piece, cooked, excluding refuse (yield from 1 lb raw meat with refuse) (191g)									
	435	24	8	181	0	0	0	51	153
Pork, Fresh, Shoulder, Arm Picnic, Lean, Cooked, Braised 1 roast (2252g)									
	4369	200	64	1959	0	0	0	603	2252
Pork, Fresh, Shoulder, Arm Picnic, Lean, Cooked, Roasted 3 oz (85g)									
	269	20	7	80	0	0	0	20	60
Pork, Fresh, Shoulder, Blade, Boston (Roasts), Lean and Fat, Cooked, Roasted 1 piece, cooked, excluding refuse (yield from 1 lb raw meat with refuse) (262g)									
	705	49	18	225	0	0	0	61	176
Pork, Fresh, Shoulder, Blade, Boston (Roasts), Lean, Cooked, Roasted 1 piece, cooked, excluding refuse (yield from 1 lb raw meat with refuse) (238g)									
	552	34	12	202	0	0	0	58	209
Pork, Fresh, Shoulder, Blade, Boston (Steaks), Lean and Fat, Cooked, Broiled 1 steak, excluding refuse (yield from 1 raw steak, with refuse, weighing 300 g) (169g)									
	438	28	10	161	0	0	0	43	117
Pork, Fresh, Shoulder, Blade, Boston (Steaks), Lean, Cooked, Broiled 1 steak, excluding refuse (yield from 1 raw steak, with refuse, weighing 300 g) (147g)									
	334	18	7	138	0	0	0	39	109
Pork, Fresh, Shoulder, Whole, Lean and Fat, Cooked, Roasted 3 oz (85g)									
	248	18	7	77	0	0	0	20	58
Pork, Fresh, Shoulder, Whole, Lean, Cooked, Roasted 3 oz (85g)									
	196	12	4	77	0	0	0	22	64

Food Serving size	Cal.	(g) Total Fat	(g) Sat. Fat	(mg) Chol.	(g) Carb.	(g) Fiber	(g) Sug.	(g) Prot.	(mg) Sod.
Pork, Fresh, Top Loin (Chops), Boneless, Enhanced, Lean and Fat, Cooked, Pan-broiled									
1 chop, boneless (yield from 189 g raw meat) (150g)									
	285	11	4	113	0	0	0	43	308
Pork, Fresh, Variety Meats and By-products, Brain, Cooked, Braised									
3 oz (85g)	117	8	2	2169	0	0	0	10	77
Pork, Fresh, Variety Meats and By-products, Chitterlings, Cooked, Simmered									
3 oz (85g)	198	17	8	235	0	0	0	11	15
Pork, Fresh, Variety Meats and By-products, Liver, Cooked, Braised									
3 oz (85g)	140	4	1	302	3	0	0	22	42
Pork, Fresh, Variety Meats and By-products, Lungs, Cooked, Braised									
3 oz (85g)	84	3	1	329	0	0	0	14	69
Pork, Leg Sirloin Tip Roast, Boneless, Lean and Fat, Cooked, Braised									
1 piece (609g)	950	16	5	512	0	0	0	189	262
Pork, Loin, Leg Cap Steak, Boneless, Lean and Fat, Cooked, Broiled									
1 piece (194g)	307	9	3	157	0	0	0	53	147
Pork, Oriental Style, Dehydrated									
1 cup (22g)	135	14	5	15	0	0	0	3	151
Pork, Shoulder Breast, Boneless, Lean and Fat, Cooked, Broiled									
1 piece (373g)	604	17	5	291	0	0	0	106	201
Pork, Shoulder, Petite Tender, Boneless, Lean and Fat, Cooked, Broiled									
1 piece (92g)	143	4	1	75	0	0	0	25	49
Pork Loin, Fresh, Backribs, Bone-in, Cooked-Roasted, Lean									
1 ribs (878g)	2239	155	55	738	0	0	0	212	860
Salami Pork Beef, Less Sodium									
3.527 oz (100g)	396	31	11	90	15	0.2	6	15	623
Salami, Cooked, Beef									
1 oz (28.35g)	74	6	3	20	1	0	0	4	323
Salami, Dry or Hard, Pork									
1 slice (3-1/8" dia x 1/16" thick) (10g)									
	41	3	1	8	0	0	0	2	226
Salami, Dry or Hard, Pork, Beef									
1 oz (28g)	106	9	3	30	0	0	0	6	492
Salami, Italian Pork									
1 oz (28g)	119	10	4	22	0	0	0	6	529

Food Serving size	Cal.	(g) Total Fat	(g) Sat. Fat	(mg) Chol.	(g) Carb.	(g) Fiber	(g) Sug.	(g) Prot.	(mg) Sod.
Salami, Italian, Pork and Beef, Dry, Sliced, 50% Less Sodium									
1 serving, 5 slices (28g)	98	7	3	25	2	0	0	6	262
Scrapple, Pork									
1 oz, cooked (25g)	53	3	1	12	4	0.1	0	2	121
Sheepshead, Cooked, Dry Heat									
3 oz (85g)	107	1	0	54	0	0	0	22	62
Veal, Breast, Fat, Cooked									
1 oz (28.35g)	146	15	6	27	0	0	0	3	14
Veal, Breast, Plate Half, Boneless, Lean and Fat, Cooked, Braised									
1 piece, cooked, excluding refuse (yield from 1 lb raw meat with refuse) (291g)	821	55	22	326	0	0	0	75	186
Veal, Breast, Point Half, Boneless, Lean and Fat, Cooked, Braised									
1 piece, cooked, excluding refuse (yield from 1 lb raw meat with refuse) (274g)	680	39	15	312	0	0	0	77	181
Veal, Breast, Whole, Boneless, Lean and Fat, Cooked, Braised									
1 piece, cooked, excluding refuse (yield from 1 lb raw meat with refuse) (283g)	753	47	19	320	0	0	0	76	184
Veal, Breast, Whole, Boneless, Lean, Cooked, Braised									
1 piece, cooked, excluding refuse (yield from 1 lb raw meat with refuse) (237g)	517	23	9	275	0	0	0	72	161
Veal, Composite of Retail Cuts, Fat, Cooked									
1 unit, cooked (yield from 1 lb raw meat) (290g)	1862	194	94	212	0	0	0	27	165
Veal, Composite of Retail Cuts, Lean and Fat, Cooked									
1 piece, cooked, excluding refuse (yield from 1 lb raw meat with refuse) (209g)	483	24	9	238	0	0	0	63	182
Veal, Composite of Retail Cuts, Lean, Cooked									
1 piece, cooked, excluding refuse (yield from 1 lb raw meat with refuse) (192g)	376	13	4	227	0	0	0	61	171
Veal, Cubed for Stew (Leg and Shoulder), Lean, Cooked, Braised									
1 unit, cooked (yield from 1 lb raw meat) (263g)	494	11	3	381	0	0	0	92	245
Veal, Ground, Cooked, Broiled									
1 unit, cooked (yield from 1 lb raw meat) (299g)	514	23	9	308	0	0	0	73	248

Food Serving size	Cal.	(g) Total Fat	(g) Sat. Fat	(mg) Chol.	(g) Carb.	(g) Fiber	(g) Sug.	(g) Prot.	(mg) Sod.
Veal, Leg (Top Round), Lean and Fat, Cooked, Braised 1 unit, cooked (yield from 1 lb raw meat) (272g)									
	574	17	7	364	0	0	0	98	182
Veal, Leg (Top Round), Lean and Fat, Cooked, Pan-fried, Breaded 1 unit, cooked (yield from 1 lb raw meat) (295g)									
	702	27	9	330	29	0.9	2	81	1339
Veal, Leg (Top Round), Lean and Fat, Cooked, Pan-fried, Not Breaded 3 oz (85g)									
	179	7	3	89	0	0	0	27	65
Veal, Leg (Top Round), Lean and Fat, Cooked, Roasted 1 unit, cooked (yield from 1 lb raw meat) (358g)									
	573	17	7	369	0	0	0	99	243
Veal, Leg (Top Round), Lean, Cooked, Braised 1 piece, cooked, excluding refuse (yield from 1 lb raw meat with refuse) (267g)									
	542	14	5	360	0	0	0	98	179
Veal, Leg (Top Round), Lean, Cooked, Pan-fried, Breaded 1 unit, cooked (yield from 1 lb raw meat) (295g)									
	637	18	5	333	29	0.6	2	84	1342
Veal, Leg (Top Round), Lean, Cooked, Pan-fried, Not Breaded 1 piece, cooked, excluding refuse (yield from 1 lb raw meat with refuse) (289g)									
	529	13	4	309	0	0	0	96	223
Veal, Leg (Top Round), Lean, Cooked, Roasted 1 piece, cooked, excluding refuse (yield from 1 lb raw meat with refuse) (351g)									
	527	12	4	362	0	0	0	99	239
Veal, Loin, Lean and Fat, Cooked, Braised 1 chop, excluding refuse (yield from 1 raw chop, with refuse, weighing 195g) (80g)									
	227	14	5	94	0	0	0	24	64
Veal, Loin, Lean and Fat, Cooked, Roasted 1 piece, cooked, excluding refuse (yield from 1 lb raw meat with refuse) (229g)									
	497	28	12	236	0	0	0	57	213
Veal, Loin, Lean, Cooked, Braised 1 chop, excluding refuse (yield from 1 raw chop, with refuse, weighing 195g) (69g)									
	156	6	2	86	0	0	0	23	58
Veal, Loin, Lean, Cooked, Roasted 1 piece, cooked, excluding refuse (yield from 1 lb raw meat with refuse) (208g)									
	364	14	5	220	0	0	0	55	200

Food Serving size	Cal.	(g) Total Fat	(g) Sat. Fat	(mg) Chol.	(g) Carb.	(g) Fiber	(g) Sug.	(g) Prot.	(mg) Sod.
Veal, Rib, Lean and Fat, Cooked, Braised 1 piece, cooked, excluding refuse (yield from 1 lb raw meat with refuse) (163g)									
	355	13	4	235	0	0	0	56	161
Veal, Rib, Lean and Fat, Cooked, Roasted 1 piece, cooked, excluding refuse (yield from 1 lb raw meat with refuse) (215g)									
	381	16	4	247	0	0	0	55	209
Veal, Rib, Lean, Cooked, Braised 3 oz (85g)									
	185	7	2	122	0	0	0	29	84
Veal, Rib, Lean, Cooked, Roasted 3 oz (85g)									
	150	6	2	98	0	0	0	22	82
Veal, Shank (Fore and Hind), Lean and Fat, Cooked, Braised 1 piece, cooked, excluding refuse (yield from 1 lb raw meat with refuse) (194g)									
	371	12	4	241	0	0	0	61	180
Veal, Shank (Fore and Hind), Lean, Cooked, Braised 1 piece, cooked, excluding refuse (yield from 1 lb raw meat with refuse) (223g)									
	395	10	3	281	0	0	0	72	210
Veal, Shoulder, Arm, Lean and Fat, Cooked, Braised 1 steak, excluding refuse (yield from 1 raw steak, with refuse, weighing 385 g) (173g)									
	408	18	7	256	0	0	0	58	151
Veal, Shoulder, Arm, Lean and Fat, Cooked, Roasted 1 piece, cooked, excluding refuse (yield from 1 lb raw meat with refuse) (283g)									
	518	23	10	306	0	0	0	72	255
Veal, Shoulder, Arm, Lean, Cooked, Braised 1 steak, excluding refuse (yield from 1 raw steak, with refuse, weighing 385 g) (160g)									
	322	9	2	248	0	0	0	57	144
Veal, Shoulder, Arm, Lean, Cooked, Roasted 1 piece, cooked, excluding refuse (yield from 1 lb raw meat with refuse) (272g)									
	446	16	6	296	0	0	0	71	248
Veal, Shoulder, Blade, Lean and Fat, Cooked, Braised 1 piece, cooked, excluding refuse (yield from 1 lb raw meat with refuse) (186g)									
	419	19	7	285	0	0	0	58	182
Veal, Shoulder, Blade, Lean and Fat, Cooked, Roasted 1 piece, cooked, excluding refuse (yield from 1 lb raw meat with refuse) (244g)									
	454	21	8	285	0	0	0	61	244
Veal, Shoulder, Blade, Lean, Cooked, Braised 1 piece, cooked, excluding refuse (yield from 1 lb raw meat with refuse) (174g)									
	345	11	3	275	0	0	0	57	176

Food Serving size	Cal.	(g) Total Fat	(g) Sat. Fat	(mg) Chol.	(g) Carb.	(g) Fiber	(g) Sug.	(g) Prot.	(mg) Sod.
Veal, Shoulder, Blade, Lean, Cooked, Roasted									
1 piece, cooked, excluding refuse (yield from 1 lb raw meat with refuse) (236g)									
	404	16	6	281	0	0	0	61	241
Veal, Shoulder, Whole (Arm and Blade), Lean and Fat, Cooked, Braised									
1 piece, cooked, excluding refuse (yield from 1 lb raw meat with refuse) (191g)									
	435	19	7	241	0	0	0	61	181
Veal, Shoulder, Whole (Arm and Blade), Lean and Fat, Cooked, Roasted									
1 piece, cooked, excluding refuse (yield from 1 lb raw meat with refuse) (258g)									
	475	22	9	292	0	0	0	65	248
Veal, Shoulder, Whole (Arm and Blade), Lean, Cooked, Braised									
1 piece, cooked, excluding refuse (yield from 1 lb raw meat with refuse) (182g)									
	362	11	3	237	0	0	0	61	177
Veal, Shoulder, Whole (Arm and Blade), Lean, Cooked, Roasted									
1 piece, cooked, excluding refuse (yield from 1 lb raw meat with refuse) (251g)									
	427	17	6	286	0	0	0	65	243
Veal, Sirloin, Lean and Fat, Cooked, Braised									
1 piece, cooked, excluding refuse (yield from 1 lb raw meat with refuse) (205g)									
	517	27	11	221	0	0	0	64	162
Veal, Sirloin, Lean and Fat, Cooked, Roasted									
1 piece, cooked, excluding refuse (yield from 1 lb raw meat with refuse) (269g)									
	543	28	12	274	0	0	0	68	223
Veal, Sirloin, Lean, Cooked, Braised									
1 piece, cooked, excluding refuse (yield from 1 lb raw meat with refuse) (183g)									
	373	12	3	207	0	0	0	62	148
Veal, Sirloin, Lean, Cooked, Roasted									
1 piece, cooked, excluding refuse (yield from 1 lb raw meat with refuse) (251g)									
	422	16	6	261	0	0	0	66	213
Veal, Variety Meats and By-products, Brain, Cooked, Braised									
1 unit, cooked (yield from 1 lb raw meat) (339g)									
	461	33	7	10509	0	0	0	39	529
Veal, Variety Meats and By-products, Brain, Cooked, Pan-fried									
1 unit, cooked (yield from 1 lb raw meat) (330g)									
	703	55	13	6996	0	0	0	48	581
Veal, Variety Meats and By-products, Heart, Cooked, Braised									
1 unit, cooked (yield from 1 lb raw meat) (198g)									
	368	13	4	348	0	0	0	58	115

Food Serving size	Cal.	(g) Total Fat	(g) Sat. Fat	(mg) Chol.	(g) Carb.	(g) Fiber	(g) Sug.	(g) Prot.	(mg) Sod.
Veal, Variety Meats and By-products, Kidneys, Cooked, Braised									
1 unit, cooked (yield from 1 lb raw meat) (184g)	300	10	3	1455	0	0	0	48	202
Veal, Variety Meats and By-products, Liver, Cooked, Braised									
1 slice (80g)	154	5	2	409	3	0	0	23	62
Veal, Variety Meats and By-products, Liver, Cooked, Pan-fried									
1 slice (67g)	129	4	1	325	3	0	0	18	57
Veal, Variety Meats and By-products, Lungs, Cooked, Braised									
1 unit, cooked (yield from 1 lb raw meat) (300g)	312	8	3	789	0	0	0	56	168
Veal, Variety Meats and By-products, Pancreas, Cooked, Braised									
1 unit, cooked (yield from 1 lb raw meat) (240g)	614	35	12	0	0	0	0	70	163
Veal, Variety Meats and By-products, Spleen, Cooked, Braised									
1 unit, cooked (yield from 1 lb raw meat) (345g)	445	10	3	1542	0	0	0	83	200
Veal, Variety Meats and By-products, Thymus, Cooked, Braised									
3 oz (85g)	106	3	1	298	0	0	0	19	50
Veal, Variety Meats and By-products, Tongue, Cooked, Braised									
1 unit, cooked (yield from 1 lb raw meat) (255g)	701	52	20	482	0	0	0	55	171
Worthington Choplets, Canned, Unprepared									
2 slices (92g)	95	1	0	0	4	2.6	0	18	420
Worthington Diced Chicken, Canned, Unprepared									
.25 cup (55g)	44	0	0	1	2	0.8	0	8	189

Poultry

Food Serving size	Cal.	(g) Total Fat	(g) Sat. Fat	(mg) Chol.	(g) Carb.	(g) Fiber	(g) Sug.	(g) Prot.	(mg) Sod.
Chicken Breast, Fat Free, Mesquite Flavor, Sliced									
1 serving, 2 slices (42g)	34	0	0	15	1	0	0	7	437
Chicken Breast, Oven-roasted, Fat Free, Sliced									
1 serving, 2 slices (42g)	33	0	0	15	1	0	0	7	457
Chicken Breast Tenders, Breaded, Cooked, Microwaved									
4 pieces (62g)	156	8	2	28	11	0	0	10	277
Chicken, Broiler, Rotisserie, BBQ, Breast Meat Only									
1 breast (384g)	553	14	3	330	0	0	0	108	1260

Food Serving size	Cal.	(g) Total Fat	(g) Sat. Fat	(mg) Chol.	(g) Carb.	(g) Fiber	(g) Sug.	(g) Prot.	(mg) Sod.
Chicken, Broiler, Rotisserie, BBQ, Breast Meat and Skin									
1 breast (384g)	672	29	8	346	0	0	0	101	1263
Chicken, Broilers or Fryers, Back, Meat and Skin, Cooked, Fried, Batter									
.5 back, bone removed (120g)	397	26	7	106	12	0	0	26	380
Chicken, Broilers or Fryers, Back, Meat and Skin, Cooked, Fried, Flour									
:5 back, bone removed (72g)	238	15	4	64	5	0	0	20	65
Chicken, Broilers or Fryers, Back, Meat and Skin, Cooked, Roasted									
.5 back, bone removed (53g)	159	11	3	47	0	0	0	14	46
Chicken, Broilers or Fryers, Back, Meat and Skin, Cooked, Rotisserie, Original									
1 serving (3 oz) (85g)	221	16	4	109	0	0	0	20	496
Chicken, Broilers or Fryers, Back, Meat and Skin, Cooked, Stewed									
1 unit (yield from 1 lb ready-to-cook chicken) (36g)	93	7	2	28	0	0	0	8	23
Chicken, Broilers or Fryers, Back, Meat Only, Cooked, Fried									
.5 back, bone and skin removed (58g)	167	9	2	54	3	0	0	17	57
Chicken, Broilers or Fryers, Back, Meat Only, Cooked, Roasted									
.5 back, bone and skin removed (40g)	96	5	1	36	0	0	0	11	38
Chicken, Broilers or Fryers, Back, Meat Only, Cooked, Rotisserie, Original									
1 serving (3 oz) (85g)	174	10	3	105	0	0	0	22	562
Chicken, Broilers or Fryers, Back, Meat Only, Cooked, Stewed									
.5 back, bone and skin removed (42g)	88	5	1	36	0	0	0	11	28
Chicken, Broilers or Fryers, Breast, Meat and Skin, Cooked, Fried, Batter									
.5 breast, bone removed (140g)	364	18	5	119	13	0.4	0	35	385
Chicken, Broilers or Fryers, Breast, Meat and Skin, Cooked, Fried, Flour									
.5 breast, bone removed (98g)	218	9	2	87	2	0.1	0	31	74
Chicken, Broilers or Fryers, Breast, Meat and Skin, Cooked, Roasted									
1 unit (yield from 1 lb ready-to-cook chicken) (58g)	114	5	1	49	0	0	0	17	41
Chicken, Broilers or Fryers, Breast, Meat and Skin, Cooked, Rotisserie, Original									
1 oz (28.35g)	52	2	1	27	0	0	0	8	98
Chicken, Broilers or Fryers, Breast, Meat and Skin, Cooked, Stewed									
1 unit (yield from 1 lb ready-to-cook chicken) (66g)	121	5	1	50	0	0	0	18	41

Food Serving size	Cal.	(g) Total Fat	(g) Sat. Fat	(mg) Chol.	(g) Carb.	(g) Fiber	(g) Sug.	(g) Prot.	(mg) Sod.
Chicken, Broilers or Fryers, Breast, Meat Only, Cooked, Fried .5 breast, bone and skin removed (86g)									
	161	4	1	78	0	0	0	29	68
Chicken, Broilers or Fryers, Breast, Meat Only, Cooked, Rotisserie, Original 3 oz (85g)	116	2	1	73	0	0	0	24	266
Chicken, Broilers or Fryers, Breast, Skinless, Boneless, Meat Only, Cooked, Braised 1 piece (181g)	284	6	2	210	0	0	0	58	85
Chicken, Broilers or Fryers, Breast, Skinless, Boneless, Meat Only, Cooked, Grilled 1 piece (196g)	296	6	2	204	0	0	0	60	102
Chicken, Broilers or Fryers, Breast, Skinless, Boneless, Meat Only, Enhanced, Braised 1 piece (195g)	283	7	2	193	0	0	0	55	335
Chicken, Broilers or Fryers, Breast, Skinless, Boneless, Meat Only, Enhanced, Grilled 1 piece (192g)	284	7	2	204	0	0	0	57	413
Chicken, Broilers or Fryers, Breast, Skinless, Boneless, Meat Only, Enhanced, Raw 1 piece (263g)	284	8	1	168	0	0	0	53	455
Chicken, Broilers or Fryers, Breast, Skinless, Boneless, Meat Only, Raw 1 piece (272g)	326	7	2	199	0	0	0	61	122
Chicken, Broilers or Fryers, Breast, Meat Only, Cooked, Roasted 1 unit (yield from 1 lb ready-to-cook chicken) (52g)									
	86	2	1	44	0	0	0	16	38
Chicken, Broilers or Fryers, Breast, Meat Only, Cooked, Stewed 1 unit (yield from 1 lb ready-to-cook chicken) (57g)									
	86	2	0	44	0	0	0	17	36
Chicken, Broilers or Fryers, Dark Meat, Drumstick, Meat and Skin, Cooked, Braised 1 drumstick, with skin (105g)	196	11	3	139	0	0	0	24	117
Chicken, Broilers or Fryers, Dark Meat, Drumstick, Meat Only, Cooked, Braised 1 drumstick, with skin (105g)	156	6	2	139	0	0	0	25	123
Chicken, Broilers or Fryers, Dark Meat, Drumstick, Meat Only, Cooked, Roasted 1 drumstick, with skin (105g)	163	6	2	137	0	0	0	25	134

Food Serving size	Cal.	(g) Total Fat	(g) Sat. Fat	(mg) Chol.	(g) Carb.	(g) Fiber	(g) Sug.	(g) Prot.	(mg) Sod.
Chicken, Broilers or Fryers, Dark Meat, Drumstick, Meat Only, Raw									
1 drumstick, without skin (122g)	142	5	1	109	0	0	0	24	139
Chicken, Broilers or Fryers, Dark Meat, Meat and Skin, Cooked, Fried, Batter									
.5 chicken, bone removed (278g)	498	31	8	149	16	0	0	36	493
Chicken, Broilers or Fryers, Dark Meat, Meat and Skin, Cooked, Fried, Flour									
.5 chicken, bone removed (184g)	524	31	8	169	8	0	0	50	164
Chicken, Broilers or Fryers, Dark Meat, Meat and Skin, Cooked, Roasted									
.5 chicken, bone removed (167g)	423	26	7	152	0	0	0	43	145
Chicken, Broilers or Fryers, Dark Meat, Meat and Skin, Cooked, Stewed									
.5 chicken, bone removed (184g)	429	27	7	151	0	0	0	43	129
Chicken, Broilers or Fryers, Dark Meat, Meat Only, Cooked, Fried									
1 unit (yield from 1 lb ready-to-cook chicken) (91g)	217	11	3	87	2	0	0	26	88
Chicken, Broilers or Fryers, Dark Meat, Meat Only, Cooked, Roasted									
1 unit (yield from 1 lb ready-to-cook chicken) (81g)	166	8	2	75	0	0	0	22	75
Chicken, Broilers or Fryers, Dark Meat, Meat Only, Cooked, Stewed									
1 unit (yield from 1 lb ready-to-cook chicken) (86g)	165	8	2	76	0	0	0	22	64
Chicken, Broilers or Fryers, Dark Meat, Thigh, Meat and Skin, Cooked, Braised									
1 thigh, with skin (129g)	295	20	5	179	0	0	0	29	98
Chicken, Broilers or Fryers, Dark Meat, Thigh, Meat Only, Cooked, Braised									
1 thigh, with skin (129g)	227	11	3	182	0	0	0	32	99
Chicken, Broilers or Fryers, Drumstick, Meat and Skin, Cooked, Fried, Batter									
1 drumstick, bone removed (72g)	193	11	3	62	6	0.2	0	16	194
Chicken, Broilers or Fryers, Drumstick, Meat and Skin, Cooked, Fried, Flour									
1 drumstick, bone removed (49g)	120	7	2	44	1	0	0	13	44
Chicken, Broilers or Fryers, Drumstick, Meat and Skin, Cooked, Roasted									
1 drumstick, without skin (96g)	183	10	3	125	0	0	0	22	118
Chicken, Broilers or Fryers, Drumstick, Meat and Skin, Cooked, Rotisserie, Original									
1 serving (3 oz) (85g)	183	10	3	133	0	0	0	23	349
Chicken, Broilers or Fryers, Drumstick, Meat and Skin, Cooked, Stewed									
1 unit (yield from 1 lb ready-to-cook chicken) (34g)	69	4	1	28	0	0	0	9	26

Food Serving size	Cal.	(g) Total Fat	(g) Sat. Fat	(mg) Chol.	(g) Carb.	(g) Fiber	(g) Sug.	(g) Prot.	(mg) Sod.
Chicken, Broilers or Fryers, Drumstick, Meat Only, Cooked, Fried 1 drumstick, bone and skin removed (42g)	82	3	1	39	0	0	0	12	40
Chicken, Broilers or Fryers, Drumstick, Meat Only, Cooked, Roasted 1 unit (yield from 1 lb ready-to-cook chicken) (26g)	45	1	0	24	0	0	0	7	25
Chicken, Broilers or Fryers, Drumstick, Meat Only, Cooked, Rotisserie, Original 1 serving (3oz) (85g)	150	6	1	136	0	0	0	24	354
Chicken, Broilers or Fryers, Drumstick, Meat Only, Cooked, Stewed 1 drumstick, bone and skin removed (46g)	78	3	1	40	0	0	0	13	37
Chicken, Broilers or Fryers, Giblets, Cooked, Fried 1 unit (yield from 1 lb ready-to-cook chicken) (13g)	36	2	0	58	1	0	0	4	15
Chicken, Broilers or Fryers, Giblets, Cooked, Simmered 1 cup, chopped or dice (145g)	228	7	2	641	0	0	0	39	97
Chicken, Broilers or Fryers, Leg, Meat and Skin, Cooked, Fried, Batter 1 leg, bone removed (158g)	431	26	7	142	14	0.5	0	34	441
Chicken, Broilers or Fryers, Leg, Meat and Skin, Cooked, Fried, Flour 1 leg, bone removed (112g)	284	16	4	105	3	0.1	0	30	99
Chicken, Broilers or Fryers, Leg, Meat and Skin, Cooked, Roasted 1 unit (yield from 1 lb ready-to-cook chicken) (69g)	475	23	6	328	0	0	0	62	253
Chicken, Broilers or Fryers, Leg, Meat and Skin, Cooked, Stewed 1 unit (yield from 1 lb ready-to-cook chicken) (75g)	165	10	3	63	0	0	0	18	55
Chicken, Broilers or Fryers, Leg, Meat Only, Cooked, Fried 1 leg, bone and skin removed (94g)	196	9	2	93	1	0	0	27	90
Chicken, Broilers or Fryers, Leg, Meat Only, Cooked, Roasted 1 leg, bone and skin (sum of drumstick+thigh+back meat only) (199g)	346	16	4	255	0	0	0	48	197
Chicken, Broilers or Fryers, Leg, Meat Only, Cooked, Stewed 1 cup, chopped or diced (160g)	296	13	4	142	0	0	0	42	125
Chicken, Broilers or Fryers, Light Meat, Meat and Skin, Cooked, Fried, Batter .5 chicken, bone removed (188g)	521	29	8	158	18	0	0	44	540

Food Serving size	Cal.	(g) Total Fat	(g) Sat. Fat	(mg) Chol.	(g) Carb.	(g) Fiber	(g) Sug.	(g) Prot.	(mg) Sod.
Chicken, Broilers or Fryers, Light Meat, Meat and Skin, Cooked, Fried, Flour									
.5 chicken, bone removed (130g)	320	16	4	113	2	0.1	0	40	100
Chicken, Broilers or Fryers, Light Meat, Meat and Skin, Cooked, Roasted									
.5 chicken, bone removed (132g)	293	14	4	111	0	0	0	38	99
Chicken, Broilers or Fryers, Light Meat, Meat and Skin, Cooked, Stewed									
.5 chicken, bone removed (150g)	302	15	4	111	0	0	0	39	95
Chicken, Broilers or Fryers, Light Meat, Meat Only, Cooked, Fried									
1 unit (yield from 1 lb ready-to-cook chicken) (64g)	123	4	1	58	0	0	0	21	52
Chicken, Broilers or Fryers, Light Meat, Meat Only, Cooked, Roasted									
1 unit (yield from 1 lb ready-to-cook chicken) (64g)	111	3	1	54	0	0	0	20	49
Chicken, Broilers or Fryers, Light Meat, Meat Only, Cooked, Stewed									
1 unit (yield from 1 lb ready-to-cook chicken) (71g)	113	3	1	55	0	0	0	21	46
Chicken, Broilers or Fryers, Meat and Skin and Giblets and Neck, Fried, Batter									
1 unit (yield from 1 lb ready-to-cook chicken) (308g)	896	54	14	317	28	0	0	70	875
Chicken, Broilers or Fryers, Meat and Skin and Giblets and Neck, Fried, Flour									
1 unit (yield from 1 lb ready-to-cook chicken) (212g)	577	32	9	237	7	0	0	61	182
Chicken, Broilers or Fryers, Meat and Skin and Giblets and Neck, Raw									
1 chicken (1046g)	2228	155	44	941	1	0	0	192	732
Chicken, Broilers or Fryers, Meat and Skin and Giblets and Neck, Roasted									
1 unit (yield from 1 lb ready-to-cook chicken) (205g)	480	27	8	219	0	0	0	55	162
Chicken, Broilers or Fryers, Meat and Skin and Giblets and Neck, Stewed									
1 unit (yield from 1 lb ready-to-cook chicken) (225g)	486	28	8	218	0	0	0	55	149
Chicken, Broilers or Fryers, Meat and Skin, Cooked, Fried, Batter									
.5 chicken, bone removed (466g)	809	49	13	244	26	0.8	0	63	818
Chicken, Broilers or Fryers, Meat and Skin, Cooked, Fried, Flour									
.5 chicken, bone removed (314g)	506	28	8	169	6	0.2	0	54	158
Chicken, Broilers or Fryers, Meat and Skin, Cooked, Roasted									
1 unit (yield from 1 lb ready-to-cook chicken) (178g)	425	24	7	157	0	0	0	49	146

Food Serving size	Cal.	(g) Total Fat	(g) Sat. Fat	(mg) Chol.	(g) Carb.	(g) Fiber	(g) Sug.	(g) Prot.	(mg) Sod.
Chicken, Broilers or Fryers, Meat and Skin, Cooked, Stewed 1 unit (yield from 1 lb ready-to-cook chicken) (200g)	438	25	7	156	0	0	0	49	134
Chicken, Broilers or Fryers, Meat Only, Cooked, Fried 1 unit (yield from 1 lb ready-to-cook chicken) (155g)	339	14	4	146	3	0.2	0	47	141
Chicken, Broilers or Fryers, Meat Only, Roasted 1 tbsp (8.7g)	17	1	0	8	0	0	0	3	7
Chicken, Broilers or Fryers, Meat Only, Stewed 1 tbsp (8.7g)	15	1	0	7	0	0	0	2	6
Chicken, Broilers or Fryers, Neck, Meat and Skin, Cooked, Fried, Batter 1 neck, bone removed (52g)	172	12	3	47	5	0	0	10	144
Chicken, Broilers or Fryers, Neck, Meat and Skin, Cooked, Fried, Flour 1 neck, bone removed (36g)	120	8	2	34	2	0	0	9	30
Chicken, Broilers or Fryers, Neck, Meat and Skin, Cooked, Simmered 1 neck, bone removed (38g)	94	7	2	27	0	0	0	7	20
Chicken, Broilers or Fryers, Neck, Meat Only, Cooked, Fried 1 neck, bone and skin removed (22g)	50	3	1	23	0	0	0	6	22
Chicken, Broilers or Fryers, Neck, Meat Only, Cooked, Simmered 1 neck, bone and skin removed (18g)	32	1	0	14	0	0	0	4	12
Chicken, Broilers or Fryers, Skin Only, Cooked, Fried, Batter .5 chicken, skin only (190g)	749	55	14	141	44	0	0	20	1104
Chicken, Broilers or Fryers, Skin Only, Cooked, Fried, Flour .5 chicken, skin only (56g)	281	24	7	41	5	0	0	11	30
Chicken, Broilers or Fryers, Skin Only, Cooked, Roasted .5 chicken, skin only (56g)	254	23	6	46	0	0	0	11	36
Chicken, Broilers or Fryers, Skin Only, Cooked, Stewed .5 chicken, skin only (72g)	261	24	7	45	0	0	0	11	40
Chicken, Broilers or Fryers, Thigh, Meat and Skin, Cooked, Fried, Batter 1 thigh, bone removed (86g)	238	14	4	80	8	0.3	0	19	248
Chicken, Broilers or Fryers, Thigh, Meat and Skin, Cooked, Fried, Flour 1 thigh, bone removed (62g)	162	9	3	60	2	0.1	0	17	55

Food Serving size	Cal.	(g) Total Fat	(g) Sat. Fat	(mg) Chol.	(g) Carb.	(g) Fiber	(g) Sug.	(g) Prot.	(mg) Sod.
Chicken, Broilers or Fryers, Thigh, Meat and Skin, Cooked, Roasted									
1 thigh, without skin (116g)	269	17	5	154	0	0	0	27	118
Chicken, Broilers or Fryers, Thigh, Meat and Skin, Cooked, Rotisserie, Original									
1 serving (85g)	198	13	4	112	0	0	0	19	293
Chicken, Broilers or Fryers, Thigh, Meat and Skin, Cooked, Stewed									
1 thigh, bone removed (68g)	158	10	3	57	0	0	0	16	48
Chicken, Broilers or Fryers, Thigh, Meat Only, Cooked, Fried									
1 thigh, bone and skin removed (52g)	113	5	1	53	1	0	0	15	49
Chicken, Broilers or Fryers, Thigh, Meat Only, Cooked, Roasted									
1 thigh, with skin (137g)	245	11	3	182	0	0	0	34	145
Chicken, Broilers or Fryers, Thigh, Meat Only, Cooked, Rotisserie, Original									
1 serving (3 oz) (85g)	167	9	2	111	0	0	0	20	286
Chicken, Broilers or Fryers, Thigh, Meat Only, Cooked, Stewed									
1 unit (yield from 1 lb ready-to-cook chicken) (33g)	64	3	1	30	0	0	0	8	25
Chicken, Broilers or Fryers, Wing, Meat and Skin, Cooked, Fried, Batter									
1 wing, bone removed (49g)	159	11	3	39	5	0.1	0	10	157
Chicken, Broilers or Fryers, Wing, Meat and Skin, Cooked, Fried, Flour									
1 wing, bone removed (32g)	103	7	2	26	1	0	0	8	25
Chicken, Broilers or Fryers, Wing, Meat and Skin, Cooked, Rotisserie, Original									
1 serving (3 oz) (85g)	226	16	4	119	0	0	0	21	519
Chicken, Broilers or Fryers, Wing, Meat and Skin, Cooked, Stewed									
1 unit (yield from 1 lb ready-to-cook chicken) (24g)	60	4	1	17	0	0	0	5	16
Chicken, Broilers or Fryers, Wing, Meat Only, Cooked, Fried									
1 wing, bone and skin removed (20g)	42	2	1	17	0	0	0	6	18
Chicken, Broilers or Fryers, Wing, Meat Only, Cooked, Roasted									
1 wing, bone and skin removed (21g)	43	2	0	18	0	0	0	6	19
Chicken, Broilers or Fryers, Wing, Meat Only, Cooked, Rotisserie, Original									
1 serving (3 oz) (85g)	167	8	2	119	0	0	0	24	616
Chicken, Broilers or Fryers, Wing, Meat Only, Cooked, Stewed									
1 unit (yield from 1 lb ready-to-cook chicken) (14g)	25	1	0	10	0	0	0	4	10

Food Serving size	Cal.	(g) Total Fat	(g) Sat. Fat	(mg) Chol.	(g) Carb.	(g) Fiber	(g) Sug.	(g) Prot.	(mg) Sod.
Chicken, Canned, Meat Only, with Broth									
1 can (5 oz) (142g)	234	11	3	88	0	0	0	31	714
Chicken, Capons, Giblets, Cooked, Simmered									
1 unit (yield from 1 lb ready-to cook capon) (11g)									
	18	1	0	48	0	0	0	3	6
Chicken, Capons, Meat and Skin and Giblets and Neck, Cooked, Roasted									
1 capon (1418g)	3205	165	47	1461	1	0	0	402	709
Chicken, Capons, Meat and Skin, Cooked, Roasted									
1 unit (yield from 1 lb ready-to cook capon) (196g)									
	449	23	6	169	0	0	0	57	96
Chicken, Cornish Game Hens, Meat and Skin, Cooked, Roasted									
.5 bird (129g)	334	23	7	169	0	0	0	29	83
Chicken, Cornish Game Hens, Meat Only, Cooked, Roasted									
.5 bird (110g)	147	4	1	117	0	0	0	26	69
Chicken, Dark Meat, Drumstick, Meat and Skin, Enhanced, Braised									
1 drumstick, without skin (95g)	174	10	3	126	0	0	0	20	157
Chicken, Dark Meat, Drumstick, Meat and Skin, Enhanced, Cooked, Roasted									
1 drumstick, without skin (91g)	164	8	2	116	0	0	0	22	169
Chicken, Dark Meat, Drumstick, Meat Only, Enhanced, Cooked, Braised									
1 drumstick, with skin (106g)	158	7	2	143	0	0	0	24	179
Chicken, Dark Meat, Drumstick, Meat Only, Enhanced, Cooked, Roasted									
1 drumstick, with skin (129g)	188	6	2	160	0	0	0	33	245
Chicken, Dark Meat, Thigh, Meat and Skin, Enhanced, Cooked, Braised									
1 thigh, without skin (132g)	284	19	5	165	0	0	0	27	244
Chicken, Dark Meat, Thigh, Meat and Skin, Enhanced, Cooked, Roasted									
1 thigh, without skin (112g)	240	15	5	143	0	0	0	26	195
Chicken, Dark Meat, Thigh, Meat Only, Enhanced, Cooked, Braised									
1 thigh, without skin (132g)	216	11	3	166	0	0	0	30	260
Chicken, Dark Meat, Thigh, Meat Only, Enhanced, Cooked, Roasted									
1 thigh, without skin (112g)	184	9	3	137	0	0	0	27	198
Chicken, Ground, Crumbles, Cooked, Pan-browned									
3 oz, crumbled (85g)	161	9	3	91	0	0	0	20	64
Chicken, Roasting, Dark Meat, Meat Only, Cooked, Roasted									
1 unit (yield from 1 lb ready-to-cook chicken) (94g)									
	167	8	2	71	0	0	0	22	89

Food Serving size	Cal.	(g) Total Fat	(g) Sat. Fat	(mg) Chol.	(g) Carb.	(g) Fiber	(g) Sug.	(g) Prot.	(mg) Sod.
Chicken, Roasting, Giblets, Cooked, Simmered									
1 unit (yield from 1 lb ready-to-cook chicken) (15g)	25	1	0	54	0	0	0	4	9
Chicken, Roasting, Light Meat, Meat Only, Cooked, Roasted									
1 unit (yield from 1 lb ready-to-cook chicken) (78g)	119	3	1	59	0	0	0	21	40
Chicken, Roasting, Meat and Skin and Giblets and Neck, Cooked, Roasted									
1 unit (yield from 1 lb ready-to-cook chicken) (235g)	517	31	9	221	0	0	0	56	167
Chicken, Roasting, Meat and Skin, Cooked, Roasted									
1 unit (yield from 1 lb ready-to-cook chicken) (210g)	468	28	8	160	0	0	0	50	153
Chicken, Roasting, Meat Only, Cooked, Roasted									
1 unit (yield from 1 lb ready-to-cook chicken) (171g)	286	11	3	128	0	0	0	43	128
Chicken, Skin (Drumsticks and Thighs), Cooked, Braised									
1 lb (453g)	2007	194	54	589	0	0	0	66	340
Chicken, Skin (Drumsticks and Thighs), Cooked, Roasted									
1 lb (453g)	2093	199	55	598	0	0	0	75	385
Chicken, Stewing, Dark Meat, Meat Only, Cooked, Stewed									
1 unit (yield from 1 lb ready-to-cook chicken) (73g)	188	11	3	69	0	0	0	21	69
Chicken, Stewing, Giblets, Cooked, Simmered									
1 unit (yield from 1 lb ready-to-cook chicken) (17g)	33	2	0	60	0	0	0	4	10
Chicken, Stewing, Light Meat, Meat Only, Cooked, Stewed									
1 unit (yield from 1 lb ready-to-cook chicken) (64g)	136	5	1	45	0	0	0	21	37
Chicken, Stewing, Meat and Skin, Cooked, Stewed									
1 unit (yield from 1 lb ready-to-cook chicken) (178g)	507	34	9	141	0	0	0	48	130
Chicken, Stewing, Meat Only, Cooked, Stewed									
1 unit (yield from 1 lb ready-to-cook chicken) (137g)	325	16	4	114	0	0	0	42	107
Chicken, Wing, Frozen, Glazed, Barbecue Flavor									
1 serving (86g)	181	11	3	108	3	0.5	2	17	529

Food Serving size	Cal.	(g) Total Fat	(g) Sat. Fat	(mg) Chol.	(g) Carb.	(g) Fiber	(g) Sug.	(g) Prot.	(mg) Sod.
Chicken, Wing, Frozen, Glazed, Barbecue Flavor, Heated (Conventional Oven)									
1 serving (96g)	232	14	4	131	3	0.5	2	21	537
Chicken, Wing, Frozen, Glazed, Barbecue Flavor, Heated (Microwave)									
1 serving (74g)	184	10	3	115	3	0.7	2	19	619
Dove, Cooked (Including Squab)									
1 cup, chopped or diced (140g)	298	18	5	162	0	0	0	33	80
Duck, Domesticated, Meat and Skin, Cooked, Roasted									
1 unit (yield from 1 lb ready-to-cook duck) (173g)	583	49	17	145	0	0	0	33	102
Duck, Domesticated, Meat Only, Cooked, Roasted									
1 unit (yield from 1 lb ready-to-cook duck) (100g)	201	11	4	89	0	0	0	23	65
Emu, Fan Fillet, Cooked, Broiled									
1 steak (394g)	607	9	2	323	0	0	0	123	209
Emu, Full Rump, Cooked, Broiled									
1 full rump, cooked (yield from 695 g raw meat) (496g)	833	13	4	640	0	0	0	167	546
Emu, Ground, Cooked, Pan-Broiled									
1 serving (3 oz) (85g)	139	4	1	74	0	0	0	24	55
Emu, Inside Drums, Cooked, Broiled									
1 inside drum, cooked (yield from 572 g raw meat) (416g)	649	8	3	379	0	0	0	135	491
Emu, Top Loin, Cooked, Broiled									
1 steak (244g)	371	8	2	215	0	0	0	71	142
Ground Turkey, 85% Lean, 15% Fat, Pan-broiled Crumbles									
3 oz (85g)	219	15	4	90	0	0	0	21	72
Ground Turkey, 85% Lean, 15% Fat, Patties, Broiled									
3 oz (85g)	212	14	4	89	0	0	0	22	69
Ground Turkey, 85% Lean, 15% Fat, Raw									
1 oz (28.35g)	51	4	1	22	0	0	0	5	15
Ground Turkey, 93% Lean, 7% Fat, Pan-broiled Crumbles									
3 oz (85g)	181	10	3	88	0	0	0	23	77
Ground Turkey, 93% Lean, 7% Fat, Patties, Broiled									
3 oz (85g)	176	10	3	90	0	0	0	22	77

Food Serving size	Cal.	(g) Total Fat	(g) Sat. Fat	(mg) Chol.	(g) Carb.	(g) Fiber	(g) Sug.	(g) Prot.	(mg) Sod.
Ground Turkey, 93% Lean, 7% Fat, Raw 1 lb (453g)	680	38	10	335	0	0	0	85	313
Ground Turkey, Fat Free, Pan-broiled Crumbles 3 oz (85g)	128	2	1	60	0	0	0	27	52
Ground Turkey, Fat Free, Patties, Broiled 1 oz (28.35g)	39	1	0	18	0	0	0	8	17
Ostrich, Ground, Cooked, Pan-Broiled 1 serving (3 oz) (85g)	149	6	2	71	0	0	0	22	68
Pastrami, Turkey 1 package (8 oz) (227g)	316	14	3	154	8	0.2	8	37	2549
Turkey and Gravy, Frozen 1 package (net weight, 5 oz) (142g)	95	4	1	26	7	0	0	8	787
Turkey Bacon, Cooked 1 oz (28g)	107	8	2	27	1	0	0	8	640
Turkey Bacon, Microwaved 1 raw per g (15g)	55	4	1	23	1	0	1	4	303
Turkey Breast Meat 1 slice (3-1/2" square; 8 per 6 oz package) (21g)	22	0	0	9	1	0.1	1	4	213
Turkey Breast, Low Salt, Prepackaged or Deli, Luncheon Meat 1 slice, NFS (28g)	32	0	0	12	1	0.1	1	6	216
Turkey Breast, Pre-basted, Meat and Skin, Cooked, Roasted .5 breast, bone removed (864g)	1089	30	8	363	0	0	0	191	3430
Turkey Breast, Sliced, Oven Roasted, Luncheon Meat 1 slice, (3-1/2" square; 8 per g oz package) (21g)	22	0	0	9	1	0.1	1	4	195
Turkey Ham, Cured Turkey Thigh Meat 1 serving (28g)	35	1	0	20	1	0.1	0	5	348
Turkey Ham, Sliced Especially Lean, Prepackaged or Deli-sliced 1 cubic inch (20g)	25	1	0	13	1	0	0	4	208
Turkey Patties, Breaded, Battered, Fried 1 thick, slice (approx 3" x 2" x 3/8") (42g)	119	8	2	32	7	0.2	0	6	336

Food Serving size	Cal.	(g) Total Fat	(g) Sat. Fat	(mg) Chol.	(g) Carb.	(g) Fiber	(g) Sug.	(g) Prot.	(mg) Sod.
Turkey Roast, Boneless, Frozen, Seasoned, Light and Dark Meat, Raw									
1 box (net weight, 2.5 lb) (1134g)	1361	25	8	601	73	0	0	200	7689
Turkey Roast, Boneless, Frozen, Seasoned, Light and Dark Meat, Roasted									
1 box (net weight, 1.72 lb) (782g)	1212	45	15	414	24	0	0	167	5318
Turkey Roll, Light and Dark Meat									
2 slices (57g)	85	4	1	31	1	0	0	10	272
Turkey Roll, Light Meat									
1 slice, rectangle (29g)	28	0	0	10	1	0	0	4	302
Turkey Sausage, Reduced Fat, Brown and Serve, Cooked									
1 cup (128g)	261	13	4	74	14	0.4	0	22	923
Turkey Sticks, Breaded, Battered, Fried									
1 stick (2.25 oz) (64g)	179	11	3	41	11	0	0	9	536
Turkey Thigh, Pre-basted, Meat and Skin, Cooked, Roasted									
1 thigh, bone removed (314g)	493	27	8	195	0	0	0	59	1372
Turkey, All Classes, Back, Meat and Skin, Cooked, Roasted									
.5 back, bone removed (262g)	639	38	11	238	0	0	0	70	191
Turkey, All Classes, Breast, Meat and Skin, Cooked, Roasted									
.5 breast, bone removed (864g)	1633	64	18	639	0	0	0	248	544
Turkey, All Classes, Dark Meat, Cooked, Roasted									
1 unit (yield from 1 lb ready-to-cook turkey) (91g)	171	7	2	77	0	0	0	26	72
Turkey, All Classes, Dark Meat, Meat and Skin, Cooked, Roasted									
1 unit (yield from 1 lb ready-to-cook turkey) (104g)	230	12	4	93	0	0	0	29	79
Turkey, All Classes, Giblets, Cooked, Simmered, Some Giblet Fat									
1 unit (yield from 1 lb ready-to-cook turkey) (10g)	20	1	0	29	0	0	0	2	6
Turkey, All Classes, Leg, Meat and Skin, Cooked, Roasted									
1 leg, bone removed (546g)	1136	54	17	464	1	0	0	152	420
Turkey, All Classes, Light Meat, Meat and Skin, Cooked, Roasted									
1 unit (yield from 1 lb ready-to-cook turkey) (136g)	268	11	3	103	0	0	0	39	86
Turkey, All Classes, Meat and Skin and Giblets and Neck, Cooked, Roasted									
1 turkey (4023g)	8247	380	111	3822	3	0	0	1126	2695

Food Serving size	Cal.	(g) Total Fat	(g) Sat. Fat	(mg) Chol.	(g) Carb.	(g) Fiber	(g) Sug.	(g) Prot.	(mg) Sod.
Turkey, All Classes, Meat and Skin, Cooked, Roasted									
1 unit (yield from 1 lb ready-to-cook turkey) (240g)									
	499	23	7	197	0	0	0	67	163
Turkey, All Classes, Meat Only, Cooked, Roasted									
1 unit (yield from 1 lb ready-to-cook turkey) (208g)									
	354	10	3	158	0	0	0	61	146
Turkey, All Classes, Neck, Meat Only, Cooked, Simmered									
1 neck, bone and skin removed (152g)									
	274	11	3	185	0	0	0	41	85
Turkey, All Classes, Skin Only, Cooked, Roasted									
.5 turkey, skin only (248g)	1099	98	26	280	1	0	0	49	131
Turkey, All Classes, Wing, Meat and Skin, Cooked, Roasted									
1 wing, bone removed (186g)	426	23	6	151	0	0	0	51	113
Turkey, Back, from Whole Bird, Enhanced, Meat and Skin, Roasted									
1 back (949g)	1945	108	30	826	0	0	0	245	2249
Turkey, Back, from Whole Bird, Enhanced, Meat Only, Roasted									
1 back (949g)	1205	20	6	655	0	0	0	256	2259
Turkey, Back, from Whole Bird, Non-Enhanced, Meat Only, Roasted									
1 back (911g)	1576	55	16	1166	0	0	0	252	947
Turkey, Breast, from Whole Bird, Enhanced, Meat Only, Roasted									
1 breast (1654g)	2101	34	10	1141	0	0	0	446	3937
Turkey, Breast, Smoked, Lemon Pepper Flavor, 97% Fat Free									
1 slice (28g)	27	0	0	13	0	0	0	6	325
Turkey, Diced, Light and Dark Meat, Seasoned									
.5 lb (227g)	313	14	4	125	2	0	0	42	1930
Turkey, Drumstick, from Whole Bird, Enhanced, Meat Only, Roasted									
1 drumstick (217g)	343	13	4	228	0	0	0	57	436
Turkey, Drumstick, from Whole Bird, Meat Only, Roasted									
1 drumstick (206g)	286	4	1	165	0	0	0	62	204
Turkey, Drumstick, Smoked, Cooked, with Skin and Bone Removed									
1 oz, with bone, cooked (yield after bone removed) (21g)									
	42	2	1	18	0	0	0	6	209
Turkey, From Whole, Enhanced, Light Meat, Meat Only, Cooked, Roasted									
1 lb (453g)	711	26	7	344	0	0	0	120	1074

Food Serving size	Cal.	(g) Total Fat	(g) Sat. Fat	(mg) Chol.	(g) Carb.	(g) Fiber	(g) Sug.	(g) Prot.	(mg) Sod.
Turkey, Fryer-roasters, Back, Meat and Skin, Cooked, Roasted 1 unit (yield from 1 lb ready-to-cook turkey) (37g)									
	75	4	1	40	0	0	0	10	26
Turkey, Fryer-roasters, Back, Meat Only, Cooked, Roasted .5 back, bone and skin removed (99g)									
	168	6	2	94	0	0	0	28	72
Turkey, Fryer-roasters, Breast, Meat and Skin, Cooked, Roasted .5 breast, bone removed (344g)	526	11	3	310	0	0	0	100	182
Turkey, Fryer-roasters, Breast, Meat Only, Cooked, Roasted .5 breast, bone and skin removed (306g)									
	413	2	1	254	0	0	0	92	159
Turkey, Fryer-roasters, Dark Meat, Meat and Skin, Cooked, Roasted .5 turkey, bone removed (374g)	681	26	8	438	0	0	0	104	284
Turkey, Fryer-roasters, Dark Meat, Meat Only, Cooked, Roasted 1 unit (yield from 1 lb ready-to-cook turkey) (91g)									
	147	4	1	102	0	0	0	26	72
Turkey, Fryer-roasters, Leg, Meat and Skin, Cooked, Roasted 1 leg, bone removed (245g)	417	13	4	172	0	0	0	70	196
Turkey, Fryer-roasters, Leg, Meat Only, Cooked, Roasted 1 leg, bone and skin removed (224g)									
	356	8	3	267	0	0	0	65	181
Turkey, Fryer-roasters, Light Meat, Meat and Skin, Cooked, Roasted .5 turkey, bone removed (433g)	710	20	5	411	0	0	0	125	247
Turkey, Fryer-roasters, Light Meat, Meat Only, Cooked, Roasted 1 unit (yield from 1 lb ready-to-cook turkey) (104g)									
	146	1	0	89	0	0	0	31	58
Turkey, Fryer-roasters, Meat and Skin and Giblets and Neck, Cooked, Roasted 1 turkey (1772g)	3030	100	29	2091	1	0	0	498	1152
Turkey, Fryer-roasters, Meat and Skin, Cooked, Roasted .5 turkey, bone removed (808g)									
	1390	46	13	848	0	0	0	228	533
Turkey, Fryer-roasters, Meat Only, Cooked, Roasted 1 unit (yield from 1 lb ready-to-cook turkey) (195g)									
	293	5	2	191	0	0	0	58	131
Turkey, Fryer-roasters, Skin Only, Cooked, Roasted .5 turkey, skin only (121g)	362	28	7	174	0	0	0	25	74

Food Serving size	Cal.	(g) Total Fat	(g) Sat. Fat	(mg) Chol.	(g) Carb.	(g) Fiber	(g) Sug.	(g) Prot.	(mg) Sod.
Turkey, Fryer-roasters, Wing, Meat and Skin, Cooked, Roasted									
1 wing, bone removed (90g)	186	9	2	104	0	0	0	25	66
Turkey, Fryer-roasters, Wing, Meat Only, Cooked, Roasted									
1 wing, bone and skin removed (60g)									
	98	2	1	61	0	0	0	19	47
Turkey, Light or Dark Meat, Smoked, Cooked, with Skin and Bone Removed									
1 oz, boneless (28.35g)	57	3	1	23	0	0	1	8	282
Turkey, Retail Parts, Breast, Meat and Skin, Cooked, Roasted									
1 breast (863g)	1415	46	14	682	0	0	0	250	984
Turkey, Retail Parts, Drumstick, Meat and Skin, Cooked, Roasted									
1 drumstick (275g)	542	26	7	330	0	0	0	78	308
Turkey, Retail Parts, Drumstick, Meat Only, Cooked, Roasted									
1 drumstick (275g)	476	18	5	325	0	0	0	79	308
Turkey, Retail Parts, Breast, Meat Only, Cooked, Roasted									
3 oz (85g)	116	2	1	60	0	0	0	25	97
Turkey, Retail Parts, Thigh, Meat and Skin, Cooked, Roasted									
1 thigh (348g)	637	33	10	404	1	0	0	83	351
Turkey, Retail Parts, Thigh, Meat Only, Cooked, Roasted									
1 thigh (348g)	553	22	7	404	2	0	0	87	362
Turkey, Retail Parts, Wing, Meat and Skin, Cooked, Roasted									
1 wing (375g)	881	50	14	431	0	0	0	108	398
Turkey, Retail Parts, Wing, Meat Only, Cooked, Roasted									
1 wing (375g)	638	21	5	364	0	0	0	113	386
Turkey, Retail Parts, Enhanced, Breast, Meat Only, Cooked, Roasted									
1 breast (852g)	1108	18	4	630	0	0	0	238	1568
Turkey, Thigh, from Whole Bird, Enhanced, Meat Only, Roasted									
1 thigh (327g)	517	20	6	343	0	0	0	85	657
Turkey, Thigh, from Whole Bird, Meat Only, Roasted									
1 thigh (319g)	526	19	6	408	0	0	0	88	332
Turkey, Whole, Enhanced, Meat and Skin, Roasted									
1 bird (4147g)	7299	332	95	3774	0	0	0	1082	9289
Turkey, Whole, Enhanced, Meat Only, Roasted									
1 bird (4147g)	5806	153	45	3483	0	0	0	1104	9248
Turkey, Whole, Meat and Skin, Cooked, Roasted									
1 bird (3812g)	7205	282	82	4155	2	0	0	1088	3926

Food Serving size	Cal.	(g) Total Fat	(g) Sat. Fat	(mg) Chol.	(g) Carb.	(g) Fiber	(g) Sug.	(g) Prot.	(mg) Sod.
Turkey, Whole, Meat Only, Cooked, Roasted									
1 bird (3812g)	6061	146	43	3850	0	0	0	1108	3850
Turkey, Wing, from Whole Bird, Enhanced, Meat Only, Roasted									
1 wing (219g)	278	5	1	151	0	0	0	59	521
Turkey, Wing, from Whole Bird, Non-Enhanced, Meat Only, Roasted									
1 wing (213g)	313	4	1	170	0	0	0	64	211
Turkey, Wing, Smoked, Cooked, with Skin and Bone Removed									
1 oz, with bone, cooked (yield after bone removed) (19g)	42	2	1	15	0	0	0	5	189
Turkey, Young Hen, Back, Meat and Skin, Cooked, Roasted									
1 unit (yield from 1 lb ready-to-cook turkey) (35g)	89	5	2	30	0	0	0	9	24
Turkey, Young Hen, Breast, Meat and Skin, Cooked, Roasted									
.5 breast, bone removed (686g)	1331	54	15	494	0	0	0	198	398
Turkey, Young Hen, Light Meat, Meat Only, Cooked, Roasted									
1 unit (yield from 1 lb ready-to-cook turkey) (119g)	192	4	1	81	0	0	0	36	71
Turkey, Young Hen, Meat and Skin and Giblets and Neck, Cooked, Roasted									
1 turkey (3300g)	7095	348	102	3102	2	0	0	924	2079
Turkey, Young Hen, Meat and Skin, Cooked, Roasted									
.5 turkey, bone removed (1524g)	3322	166	48	1189	0	0	0	428	975
Turkey, Young Hen, Meat Only, Cooked, Roasted									
1 unit (yield from 1 lb ready-to-cook turkey) (212g)	371	12	4	155	0	0	0	62	142
Turkey, Young Hen, Skin Only, Cooked, Roasted									
.5 turkey, skin only (196g)	945	87	23	208	0	0	0	37	86
Turkey, Young Hen, Wing, Meat and Skin, Cooked, Roasted									
1 wing, bone removed (174g)	414	23	6	134	0	0	0	48	97
Turkey, Young Tom, Back, Meat and Skin, Cooked, Roasted									
1 unit (yield from 1 lb ready-to-cook turkey) (33g)	79	5	1	31	0	0	0	9	25
Turkey, Young Tom, Breast, Meat and Skin, Cooked, Roasted									
.5 breast, bone removed (1329g)	2512	98	28	997	0	0	0	380	890
Turkey, Young Tom, Dark Meat, Meat and Skin, Cooked, Roasted									
.5 turkey, bone removed (1184g)	2557	128	39	1077	0	0	0	327	947

Food Serving size	Cal.	(g) Total Fat	(g) Sat. Fat	(mg) Chol.	(g) Carb.	(g) Fiber	(g) Sug.	(g) Prot.	(mg) Sod.
Turkey, Young Tom, Meats and Skin and Giblets and Neck, Cooked, Roasted									
1 turkey (5957g)	11854	525	154	5719	6	0	0	1666	4289
Turkey, Young Tom, Skin Only, Cooked, Roasted									
.5 turkey, skin only (374g)	1578	139	36	438	0	0	0	75	224
Turkey, Young Tom, Wing, Meat and Skin, Cooked, Roasted									
1 wing, bone removed (237g)	524	27	7	192	0	0	0	65	156

Sausages and Luncheon Meats

Food Serving size	Cal.	(g) Total Fat	(g) Sat. Fat	(mg) Chol.	(g) Carb.	(g) Fiber	(g) Sug.	(g) Prot.	(mg) Sod.
Bacon and Beef Sticks									
1 oz (28g)	145	12	4	29	0	0	0	8	398
Barbecue Loaf, Pork, Beef									
1 slice (5-7/8" x 3-1/2" x 1/16") (23g)	40	2	1	9	1	0	0	4	307
Beerwurst, Beer Salami, Pork									
1 slice (2-3/4" dia x 1/16") (6g)	14	1	0	4	0	0	0	1	74
Beerwurst, Beer Salami, Pork and Beef									
2 oz (56g)	155	13	5	35	2	0.5	0	8	410
Beerwurst, Pork and Beef									
1 serving, 2 oz (56g)	155	13	5	35	2	0.5	0	8	410
Blood Sausage									
4 slices (100g)	379	35	13	120	1	0	1	15	680
Bologna, Beef									
1 slice (28g)	84	7	3	16	1	0	1	3	284
Bologna, Chicken, Pork									
1 slice (28g)	94	9	3	24	1	0	0	3	347
Bologna, Chicken, Pork, Beef									
1 slice (28g)	76	6	2	23	2	0	0	3	314
Bologna, Chicken, Turkey, Pork									
1 slice (28g)	83	7	2	22	2	0	0	3	258
Bologna, Pork									
1 slice (4" dia x 1/8" thick) (23g)	57	5	2	14	0	0	0	4	209
Bologna, Pork and Turkey Lite									
1 serving, 2 oz (56g)	118	9	3	44	2	0	0	7	401
Bologna, Pork, Turkey and Beef									
1 oz (28.35g)	94	8	3	21	2	0	0	3	295

Food Serving size	Cal.	(g) Total Fat	(g) Sat. Fat	(mg) Chol.	(g) Carb.	(g) Fiber	(g) Sug.	(g) Prot.	(mg) Sod.
Bologna, Turkey 1 serving (28g)	59	4	1	21	1	0.1	1	3	300
Bratwurst, Beef and Pork, Smoked 1 serving, 2.33 oz (66g)	196	17	4	51	1	0	0	8	560
Bratwurst, Chicken, Cooked 1 serving, 2.96 oz (84g)	148	9	0	60	0	0	0	16	60
Bratwurst, Pork, Beef and Turkey, Lite, Smoked 1 serving, 2.33 oz (66g)	123	9	0	37	1	0	1	10	648
Bratwurst, Pork, Beef, Link 1 link (70g)	226	19	7	44	2	0	2	10	778
Bratwurst, Pork, Cooked 1 link, cooked (85g)	283	25	8	63	2	0	0	12	719
Bratwurst, Veal, Cooked 1 serving, 2.96 oz (84g)	286	27	13	66	0	0	0	12	50
Braunschweiger (a Liver Sausage), Pork 1 slice (2-1/2" dia x 1/4" thick) (18g)	59	5	2	32	1	0	0	3	176
Butcher Boy Meats, Inc., Turkey Franks 1 serving (56g)	134	10	3	58	3	0.1	1	8	651
Cheesefurter, Cheese Smoky, Pork, Beef 2.33 links (100g)	328	29	10	68	2	0	2	14	1082
Chicken Roll, Light Meat 1 package (170g)	187	5	1	77	8	0	1	28	1800
Chicken Spread 1 serving (56g)	88	10	2	31	2	0.2	0	10	404
Chorizo, Pork and Beef 1 link (4" long) (60g)	273	23	9	53	1	0	0	14	741
Corned Beef Loaf, Jellied 2 slices (57g)	87	3	1	27	0	0	0	13	543
Dutch Brand Loaf, Chicken, Pork and Beef 1 slice (38g)	104	9	3	23	1	0.1	0	5	299
Frankfurter Meat 1 serving (1 hot dog) (52g)	151	13	0	40	2	0	0	5	567
Frankfurter Meat, Heated 1 serving (1 hot dog) (52g)	145	13	0	38	3	0	0	5	527

Food Serving size	Cal.	(g) Total Fat	(g) Sat. Fat	(mg) Chol.	(g) Carb.	(g) Fiber	(g) Sug.	(g) Prot.	(mg) Sod.
Frankfurter, Beef 1 frankfurter (5 in long x 7/8 in dia, 8 per lb) (57g)									
	188	17	7	30	2	0	2	6	650
Frankfurter, Beef and Pork 1 frankfurter (45g)	137	12	5	23	1	0	0	5	369
Frankfurter, Beef and Pork, Lowfat 1 frankfurter (57g)	87	6	2	25	3	0	0	6	716
Frankfurter, Beef, Lowfat 1 frankfurter (57g)	131	11	5	23	1	0	0	7	593
Frankfurter, Beef, Pork and Turkey, Fat Free 1 frankfurter, 1 NLEA serving (57g)	62	1	0	23	6	0	0	7	502
Frankfurter, Pork 1 link (76g)	204	18	7	50	0	0.1	0	10	620
Frankfurter, Turkey 1 frankfurter (45g)	100	8	2	35	2	0	1	6	410
Frankfurter, Low Sodium 1 frankfurter (57g)	178	16	7	35	1	0	0	7	177
Ham and Cheese Loaf or Roll 2 slices (57g)	137	11	4	33	2	0	0	8	570
Ham and Cheese Spread 1 oz (28.35g)	69	5	2	17	1	0	0	5	339
Ham Salad Spread 1 oz (28.35g)	61	4	1	10	3	0	0	2	305
Ham, Chopped, Canned 1 slice (4-1/4" x 4-1/4" x 1/16") (21g)									
	50	4	1	10	0	0	0	3	269
Ham, Chopped, Not Canned 1 slice (4-1/4" x 4-1/4" x 1/16") (21g)									
	38	2	1	12	1	0	0	3	218
Ham, Honey Smoked, Cooked 1.94 oz (1 serving) (55g)	67	1	0	12	4	0	0	10	495
Ham, Minced 1 slice (4-1/4" x 4-1/4" x 1/16") (21g)									
	55	4	2	15	0	0	0	3	261
Ham, Sliced, Extra Lean 1 slice, rectangle (24g)	26	1	0	11	0	0	0	5	254

Food Serving size	Cal.	(g) Total Fat	(g) Sat. Fat	(mg) Chol.	(g) Carb.	(g) Fiber	(g) Sug.	(g) Prot.	(mg) Sod.
Ham, Sliced, Regular (Approximately 11% Fat) 1 slice (28g)	46	2	1	16	1	0.4	0	5	320
Headcheese, Pork 45g (45g)	71	5	2	31	0	0	0	6	423
Honey Loaf, Pork, Beef 1 slice (28g)	35	1	0	10	3	0.2	0	3	370
Honey Roll Sausage, Beef 1 oz (28.35g)	52	3	1	14	1	0	0	5	375
Hormel, Always Tender, Boneless Pork Loin, Fresh Pork 1 serving (112g)	162	8	3	55	1	0	0	21	401
Hormel, Always Tender, Center Cut Chops, Fresh Pork 1 serving (112g)	187	11	4	58	1	0	0	21	423
Hormel, Canadian Style Bacon 1 serving (56g)	68	3	1	27	1	0	1	9	569
Hormel, Cure 81 Ham 1 serving (84g)	89	3	1	43	0	0	0	15	872
Hormel, Pillow Pack, Sliced Turkey Pepperoni 1 serving (30g)	73	3	1	37	1	0	0	9	557
Hormel, Spam, Light Lunch Meat, Pork and Chicken, Minced, Canned, Vitamin C Added 1 oz (28g)	53	4	1	21	0	0	0	4	289
Hormel, Spam, Luncheon Meat, Pork with Ham, Minced, Canned 1 serving, 2 oz (56g)	174	15	6	39	2	0	0	7	767
Hormel, Wrangler Beef Franks 1 frankfurter (56g)	162	14	6	38	1	0	1	7	557
Kielbasa, Fully Cooked, Grilled 1 link (367g)	1237	109	36	268	18	0	9	46	3898
Kielbasa, Fully Cooked, Unheated 1 link (397g)	1290	118	38	242	15	0	8	43	3684
Kielbasa, Kolbassy, Pork, Beef, Nonfat Dry Milk 1 ring (467g)	1443	127	43	308	13	0	7	57	3115
Kielbasa, Polish, Turkey and Beef, Smoked 1 serving, 2 oz (56g)	127	10	3	39	2	0	0	7	672
Knackwurst, Knockwurst, Pork, Beef 1 oz (28.35g)	87	8	3	17	1	0	0	3	264

Food Serving size	Cal.	(g) Total Fat	(g) Sat. Fat	(mg) Chol.	(g) Carb.	(g) Fiber	(g) Sug.	(g) Prot.	(mg) Sod.
Lebanon, Bologna, Beef									
1 oz (28.35g)	49	3	1	16	0	0	0	5	390
Liver Cheese, Pork									
1 slice (38g)	116	10	3	66	1	0	0	6	466
Liver Sausage, Liverwurst, Pork									
1 oz (28.35g)	92	8	3	45	1	0	0	4	244
Liverwurst Spread									
.25 cup (55g)	168	14	5	65	3	1.4	1	7	385
Loma Linda Big Franks, Canned Unprepared									
1 link (51g)	111	6	1	0	3	1.8	2	11	217
Loma Linda Linketts, Canned, Unprepared									
1 link (35g)	73	4	1	0	2	1.1	0	7	140
Loma Linda Little Links, Canned, Unprepared									
2 links (46g)	102	6	1	0	3	1.9	0	9	217
Loma Linda Low Fat Big Franks, Canned, Unprepared									
1 link (51g)	79	2	0	0	2	2.1	0	12	245
Loma Linda Vege-burger, Canned, Unprepared									
.25 cup (55g)	63	1	0	0	2	1.4	0	12	122
Louis Rich, Franks (Turkey and Chicken)									
1 serving (45g)	85	6	2	41	2	0	1	5	511
Louis Rich, Turkey (Honey Roasted, Fat Free)									
1 serving (56g)	57	0	0	22	3	0	2	11	661
Louis Rich, Turkey Bacon									
1 serving (14g)	35	3	1	13	0	0	0	2	170
Louis Rich, Turkey Bologna									
1 serving (28g)	52	4	1	19	1	0	0	3	302
Louis Rich, Turkey Breast (Oven Roasted, Fat Free)									
1 serving (28g)	24	0	0	9	1	0	0	4	334
Louis Rich, Turkey Breast (Oven Roasted, Portion Fat Free)									
1 serving (56g)	50	0	0	22	1	0	0	11	659
Louis Rich, Turkey Breast (Smoked, Carving Board)									
1 slice (22g)	21	0	0	9	0	0	0	4	264
Louis Rich, Turkey Breast (Smoked, Portion Fat Free)									
1 serving (56g)	52	0	0	23	1	0	0	11	721

Food Serving size	Cal.	(g) Total Fat	(g) Sat. Fat	(mg) Chol.	(g) Carb.	(g) Fiber	(g) Sug.	(g) Prot.	(mg) Sod.
Louis Rich, Turkey Breast and White Turkey (Oven Roasted)									
1 serving (28g)	28	1	0	11	1	0	0	5	270
Louis Rich, Turkey Breast and White Turkey (Smoked Sliced)									
1 serving (28g)	28	1	0	12	1	0	0	5	257
Louis Rich, Turkey Ham (10% Water)									
1 serving (28g)	32	1	0	19	0	0	0	5	316
Louis Rich, Turkey Nuggets/Sticks (Breaded)									
1 serving (85g)	235	15	3	34	13	0.4	0	12	577
Louis Rich, Turkey Salami									
1 serving (28g)	41	3	1	21	0	0	0	4	281
Louis Rich, Turkey Salami Cotto									
1 serving (28g)	42	3	1	22	0	0	0	4	285
Louis Rich, Turkey Smoked Sausage									
1 serving (56g)	90	6	1	37	2	0	2	8	530
Luncheon Meat, Beef, Loaved									
2 slices (57g)	176	15	6	36	2	0	0	8	641
Luncheon Meat, Beef, Thin Sliced									
1 slice, rectangle (13.8g)	16	0	0	7	0	0	0	2	154
Luncheon Meat, Pork and Chicken, Minced, Canned, Including Spam Lite									
2 oz (1 serving) (56g)	110	8	3	42	1	0	1	9	578
Luncheon Meat, Pork, Beef									
1 slice (4" x 4" x 3/32" thick) (57g)	201	18	7	31	1	0	0	7	737
Luncheon Slices, Meatless									
1 slice, thin (14g)	26	2	0	0	1	0	0	2	100
Luxury Loaf, Pork									
2 slices (57g)	80	3	1	21	3	0	0	10	698
Macaroni and Cheese Loaf, Chicken, Pork and Beef									
1 slice (38g)	87	6	2	17	4	0	0	4	1
Meatballs, Frozen, Italian Style									
3 pieces (56g)	160	12	4	37	5	1.3	2	8	373
Meatballs, Meatless									
1 cup (144g)	284	13	2	0	12	6.6	0	30	792
Mortadella, Beef, Pork									
1 slice (15 per 8 oz package) (15g)	47	4	1	8	0	0	0	2	187

Food Serving size	Cal.	(g) Total Fat	(g) Sat. Fat	(mg) Chol.	(g) Carb.	(g) Fiber	(g) Sug.	(g) Prot.	(mg) Sod.
Mother's Loaf, Pork									
1 slice, (4-1/4" x 4-1/4" x 1/16") (21g)	59	5	2	9	2	0	0	3	237
New England Brand, Sausage, Pork, Beef									
1 oz (28.35g)	46	2	1	14	1	0	0	5	346
Olive Loaf, Pork									
2 slices (57g)	134	9	3	22	5	0	0	7	549
Oscar Mayer, Bologna (Beef)									
1 serving (1 slice) (28g)	88	8	4	18	1	0	0	3	330
Oscar Mayer, Bologna Light (Pork, Chicken, Beef)									
1 serving (1 slice) (28g)	57	4	2	16	2	0	1	3	313
Oscar Mayer, Braunschweiger Liver Sausage (Saren Tube)									
1 serving (56g)	191	17	6	90	1	0.1	0	8	626
Oscar Mayer, Braunschweiger Liver Sausage (Sliced)									
1 serving (1 slice) (28g)	93	8	3	50	1	0.1	0	4	325
Oscar Mayer, Chicken Breast (Honey Glazed)									
1 serving (4 slices) (52g)	57	1	0	28	2	0	2	10	748
Oscar Mayer, Chicken Breast (Oven Roasted, Fat Free)									
1 slice (13g)	11	0	0	6	0	0	0	2	161
Oscar Mayer, Ham (40% Ham/Water Product, Smoked, Fat Free)									
1 slice (16g)	12	0	0	6	0	0	0	2	173
Oscar Mayer, Ham (Chopped with Natural Juice)									
1 serving (1 slice) (28g)	50	3	1	17	1	0	1	5	350
Oscar Mayer, Ham (Water Added, Baked, Cooked, 96% Fat Free)									
1 serving (3 slices) (63g)	66	2	1	30	1	0	1	10	782
Oscar Mayer, Ham (Water, Boiled)									
1 slice (21g)	22	1	0	10	0	0	0	3	283
Oscar Mayer, Ham (Water, Honey)									
1 slice (21g)	23	1	0	9	1	0	1	4	262
Oscar Mayer, Ham (Water, Smoked, Cooked)									
1 slice (21g)	21	1	0	10	0	0	0	3	255
Oscar Mayer, Ham and Cheese Loaf									
1 serving (28g)	66	5	2	17	1	0	1	4	327
Oscar Mayer, Head Cheese									
1 serving (28g)	52	4	1	25	0	0	0	4	300

Food Serving size	Cal.	(g) Total Fat	(g) Sat. Fat	(mg) Chol.	(g) Carb.	(g) Fiber	(g) Sug.	(g) Prot.	(mg) Sod.
Oscar Mayer, Liver Cheese, Pork Fat Wrapped									
1 slice (38g)	119	10	4	80	1	0	0	6	420
Oscar Mayer, Luncheon Loaf (Spiced)									
1 serving (28g)	66	5	2	19	2	0	1	4	343
Oscar Mayer, Old Fashioned Loaf									
1 serving (28g)	65	5	2	17	2	0	1	4	332
Oscar Mayer, Olive Loaf (Chicken, Pork, Turkey)									
1 serving (28g)	74	6	2	20	2	0	1	3	369
Oscar Mayer, Pickle, Pimento Loaf (with Chicken)									
1 serving (28g)	75	6	2	22	3	0	2	3	357
Oscar Mayer, Pork Sausage Links (Cooked)									
1 link (24g)	82	7	3	18	0	0	0	4	201
Oscar Mayer, Salami, Beef Cotto									
1 slice (23g)	47*	4	2	19	0	0	0	3	301
Oscar Mayer, Salami (for Beer)									
1 slice (23g)	52	4	1	16	0	0	0	3	283
Oscar Mayer, Salami (Genoa)									
1 slice (9g)	35	3	1	9	0	0	0	2	164
Oscar Mayer, Salami (Hard)									
1 slice (9g)	33	3	1	9	0	0	0	2	178
Oscar Mayer, Salami Cotto (Beef, Pork, Chicken)									
1 slice (23g)	56	5	2	18	1	0	0	3	252
Oscar Mayer, Sandwich Spread (Pork, Chicken, Beef)									
1 serving (30g)	71	5	2	14	5	0.1	2	2	246
Oscar Mayer, Simmer Sausage, Beef Thuringer Cervalat									
1 slice (23g)	71	6	3	18	0	0	0	3	328
Oscar Mayer, Simmer Sausage, Thuringer Cervalat									
1 slice (23g)	70	6	2	19	0	0	0	3	329
Oscar Mayer, Smokies (Beef)									
1 serving (1 link) (43g)	127	11	5	27	1	0	1	5	416
Oscar Mayer, Smokies (Cheese)									
1 serving (43g)	130	12	4	30	1	0	1	6	450
Oscar Mayer, Smokies Links Sausage									
1 serving (43g)	130	12	4	27	1	0	1	5	433

Food Serving size	Cal.	(g) Total Fat	(g) Sat. Fat	(mg) Chol.	(g) Carb.	(g) Fiber	(g) Sug.	(g) Prot.	(mg) Sod.
Oscar Mayer, Smokies Sausage Little (Pork, Turkey)									
1 serving (57g)	172	15	5	36	1	0	1	7	583
Oscar Mayer, Smokies Sausage Little Cheese (Pork, Turkey)									
1 serving (57g)	180	16	6	38	1	0	0	8	591
Oscar Mayer, Turkey Breast (Smoked, Fat Free)									
1 slice (13g)	10	0	0	4	0	0	0	2	142
Oscar Mayer, Wieners (Beef Franks Bun Length)									
1 serving (1 link) (57g)	185	17	7	34	2	0	1	6	584
Oscar Mayer, Wieners (Beef Franks)									
1 serving (45g)	147	14	6	25	1	0	1	5	461
Oscar Mayer, Wieners (Fat Free Hot Dogs)									
1 serving (50g)	37	0	0	15	2	0	1	6	487
Oscar Mayer, Wieners (Light Pork, Turkey, Beef)									
1 serving (57g)	111	8	3	35	2	0	1	7	591
Oscar Mayer, Wieners (Pork, Turkey)									
1 serving (1 link) (45g)	147	13	4	32	1	0	1	5	445
Oscar Mayer, Wieners Little (Pork, Turkey)									
1 serving (57g)	177	16	6	31	1	0	1	6	592
Oven Roasted, Chicken Breast Roll									
1 serving, 2 oz (56g)	75	4	1	22	1	0	0	8	494
Pate de Foie Gras, Canned (Goose Liver Pate), Smoked									
1 oz (28.35g)	131	12	4	43	1	0	0	3	198
Pate, Chicken Liver, Canned									
1 oz (28.35g)	57	4	1	111	2	0	0	4	109
Pate, Goose Liver, Smoked, Canned									
1 oz (28.35g)	131	12	4	43	1	0	0	3	198
Pate, Liver, Not Specified, Canned									
1 oz (28.35g)	90	8	3	72	0	0	0	4	198
Pate, Truffle Flavor									
1 serving, 2 oz (56g)	183	16	6	59	4	0	0	6	452
Peppered Loaf, Pork, Beef									
3.52 slices (100g)	149	6	2	46	5	0	5	17	732
Pepperoni, Pork, Beef									
1 oz (28g)	138	12	4	29	0	0	0	6	493

Food Serving size	Cal.	(g) Total Fat	(g) Sat. Fat	(mg) Chol.	(g) Carb.	(g) Fiber	(g) Sug.	(g) Prot.	(mg) Sod.
Pickle and Pimento Loaf, Pork 2 slices (57g)	128	9	3	33	5	0.9	5	6	593
Picnic Loaf, Pork, Beef 2 slices (57g)	132	9	3	22	3	0	0	9	663
Pork and Beef Sausage, Fresh, Cooked 1 patty, cooked (raw dimensions: 3-7/8" dia x 1/4" thick) (27g)	107	10	3	19	1	0	0	4	251
Pork, Sausage Rice Links, Brown and Serve, Cooked 3 links, 1 NLEA serving (60g)	244	23	4	40	1	0	0	8	413
Pork Sausage, Link/Patty, Cooked, Pan-Fried 1 package (343g)	916	70	21	281	1	0	0	72	2394
Pork Sausage, Link/Patty, Fully Cooked, Microwaved 1 link (21g)	92	9	3	17	0	0	0	3	208
Pork Sausage, Link/Patty, Fully Cooked, Unheated 1 patty (37g)	145	14	4	27	0	0	0	5	300
Pork Sausage, Link/Patty, Reduced Fat, Unprepared 1 package (343g)	744	57	15	230	1	0	0	57	1993
Roast Beef, Deli Style, Prepackaged, Sliced 1 slice, rectangle (13.8g)	16	1	0	7	0	0	0	3	118
Sandwiches and Burgers, Roast Beef Sandwich with Cheese 1 sandwich (176g)	473	18	9	77	45	0	0	32	1633
Sandwiches and Burgers, Steak Sandwich 1 sandwich (204g)	459	14	4	73	52	0	0	30	798
Sausage Berliner Pork, Beef 1 oz (28.35g)	65	5	2	13	1	0	1	4	368
Sausage Italian Sweet Links 1 link, 3 oz (84g)	125	7	3	25	2	0	0	14	479
Sausage Simmered Pork and Beef Sticks with Cheddar Cheese 1 oz (28.35g)	119	11	3	25	1	0.1	0	5	415
Sausage Turkey Breakfast Links, Mild 2 oz, 2 links (56g)	132	10	2	90	1	0	0	9	358
Sausage, Chicken and Beef, Smoked 1 cubic inch (18g)	53	4	1	13	0	0	0	3	184

Food Serving size	Cal.	(g) Total Fat	(g) Sat. Fat	(mg) Chol.	(g) Carb.	(g) Fiber	(g) Sug.	(g) Prot.	(mg) Sod.
Sausage, Chicken, Beef, Pork, Skinless, Smoked									
1 link (84g)	181	12	4	101	7	0	2	11	869
Sausage, Italian Turkey, Smoked									
1 serving, 2 oz (56g)	88	5	2	30	3	0.5	2	8	520
Sausage, Italian, Pork, Cooked									
1 link, 5/lb (67g)	230	18	6	38	3	0.1	1	13	809
Sausage, Meatless									
1 patty (38g)	98	7	1	0	4	1.1	0	7	337
Sausage, Polish Pork and Beef, Smoked									
1 serving, 2.67 oz (76g)	229	20	7	54	2	0	0	9	644
Sausage, Polish, Beef with Chicken, Hot									
5 pieces (55g)	142	11	4	36	2	0	0	10	847
Sausage, Pork and Beef with Cheddar Cheese, Smoked									
12 oz, serving 2.7 oz (77g)	228	20	7	49	2	0	0	10	653
Sausage, Turkey, Hot, Smoked									
2 oz (56g)	88	5	2	30	3	0.5	2	8	670
Sausage, Vienna, Canned, Chicken, Beef, Pork									
7 sausages (drained contents from can, net wt 4 oz) (113g)	260	22	8	98	3	0	0	12	993
Smoked Link Sausage, Pork									
1 link, little (2" long x 3/4" dia) (16g)	49	5	1	10	0	0	0	2	132
Smoked Link Sausage, Pork and Beef, Flavor and Nonfat Dry Milk									
2 oz (57g)	153	12	4	37	2	0	2	8	725
Smoked Link Sausage, Pork and Beef, Nonfat Dry Milk									
1 link, little (2" long x 3/4" dia) (16g)	50	4	2	10	0	0	0	2	188
Swiss Wurst Pork and Beef with Swiss Cheese, Smoked									
1 serving, 2.7 oz (77g)	236	21	0	47	1	0	0	10	637
Thuringer, Cervalat, Simmer Sausage, Beef, Pork									
2 oz, 1 serving (56g)	203	17	6	41	2	0	0	10	728
Turkey and Pork Sausage, Fresh Bulk, Patty or Link, Cooked									
1 oz (28g)	86	6	2	24	0	0	0	6	246
Turkey, Pork and Beef Sausage, Low Fat, Smoked									
1 lb, 16 oz (453.6g)	458	11	4	95	52	2.7	0	36	3611

Food Serving size	Cal.	(g) Total Fat	(g) Sat. Fat	(mg) Chol.	(g) Carb.	(g) Fiber	(g) Sug.	(g) Prot.	(mg) Sod.
Turkey, Pork and Beef, Sausage, Reduced Fat, Smoked									
1 cubic inch (14g)	34	2	1	9	0	0	0	3	134
Turkey, White, Rotisserie, Deli Cut									
1.69 oz (1 serving) (48g)	54	1	0	26	4	0.2	2	6	576
Yachtwurst, with Pistachio Nuts, Cooked									
1 serving, 2 oz (56g)	150	13	4	36	1	0	0	8	524

Dry Beans and Peas

Food Serving size	Cal.	(g) Total Fat	(g) Sat. Fat	(mg) Chol.	(g) Carb.	(g) Fiber	(g) Sug.	(g) Prot.	(mg) Sod.
Chickpeas (Garbanzo Beans, Bengal Grams), Mature Seeds, Canned									
1 cup (240g)	286	3	0	0	54	10.6	0	12	718
Chickpeas (Garbanzo Beans, Bengal Grams), Mature Seeds, Raw									
1 tbsp (12.5g)	47	1	0	0	8	1.5	1	3	3
Chickpeas, Mature Seeds, Cooked, Boiled, with Salt									
1 cup (164g)	269	4	0	0	45	12.5	8	15	399
Chickpeas, Mature Seeds, Cooked, Boiled, Without Salt									
1 cup (164g)	269	4	0	0	45	12.5	8	15	11
Cowpeas (Blackeyes), Immature Seeds, Cooked, Boiled, Drained, with Salt									
1 cup (165g)	160	1	0	0	34	8.3	5	5	7
Cowpeas (Blackeyes), Immature Seeds, Frozen, Cooked, Boiled, Drained, Without Salt									
1 cup (170g)	224	1	0	0	40	10.9	8	14	9
Cowpeas (Blackeyes), Immature Seeds, Frozen, Unprepared									
1 package (10 oz) (284g)	395	2	1	0	71	14.2	0	26	17
Cowpeas, Cat Jang, Mature Seeds, Cooked, Boiled, with Salt									
1 cup (171g)	200	1	0	0	35	6.2	0	14	436
Cowpeas, Cat Jang, Mature Seeds, Cooked, Boiled, Without Salt									
1 cup (171g)	200	1	0	0	35	6.2	0	14	32
Cowpeas, Common (Blackeyes, Crowder, Southern), Mature Seeds, Raw									
1 tbsp (10.5g)	35	0	0	0	6	1.1	1	2	2
Cowpeas, Common (Blackeyes, Crowder, Southern), Mature, Cooked, Boiled, Without Salt									
1 cup (171g)	198	1	0	0	35	11.1	6	13	7
Cowpeas, Common, Mature Seeds, Canned with Pork									
1 cup (240g)	199	4	1	17	40	7.9	0	7	840

Food Serving size	Cal.	(g) Total Fat	(g) Sat. Fat	(mg) Chol.	(g) Carb.	(g) Fiber	(g) Sug.	(g) Prot.	(mg) Sod.
Cowpeas, Common, Mature Seeds, Canned, Plain									
1 cup (240g)	185	1	0	0	33	7.9	0	11	718
Cowpeas, Common, Mature Seeds, Cooked, Boiled, with Salt									
1 cup (171g)	198	1	0	0	35	11.1	6	13	410
Cowpeas, Leafy Tips, Cooked, Boiled, Drained, Without Salt									
1 cup, chopped (53g)	12	0	0	0	1	0	0	2	3
Cowpeas, Young Pods with Seeds, Cooked, Boiled, Drained, Without Salt									
1 cup (95g)	32	0	0	0	7	0	0	2	3
Frijoles Rojos Volteados (Refried Beans, Red, Canned)									
1 tbsp (15g)	22	1	0	0	2	0.7	0	1	56
Hummus, Commercial									
1 tbsp (15g)	25	1	0	0	2	0.9	0	1	57
Hummus, Home Prepared									
1 cup (246g)	435	21	3	0	49	9.8	1	12	595
Hyacinth Beans, Immature Seeds, Cooked, Boiled, Drained, with Salt									
1 cup (87g)	44	0	0	0	8	0	0	3	207
Hyacinth Beans, Immature Seeds, Cooked, Boiled, Drained, Without Salt									
1 cup (87g)	44	0	0	0	8	0	0	3	2
Hyacinth Beans, Immature Seeds, Raw									
1 cup (80g)	37	0	0	0	7	2.6	3	2	2
Hyacinth Beans, Mature Seeds, Cooked, Boiled, with Salt									
1 cup (194g)	227	1	0	0	40	0	0	16	471
Hyacinth Beans, Mature Seeds, Cooked, Boiled, Without Salt									
1 cup (194g)	227	1	0	0	40	0	0	16	14
Hyacinth Beans, Mature Seeds, Raw									
1 cup (210g)	722	4	1	0	128	0	0	50	44
Lupins, Mature Seeds, Cooked, Boiled, with Salt									
1 cup (166g)	193	5	1	0	15	4.6	0	26	398
Mothbeans, Mature Seeds, Cooked, Boiled, with Salt									
1 cup (177g)	207	1	0	0	37	0	0	14	435
Mung Beans, Mature Seeds, Cooked, Boiled, with Salt									
1 cup (202g)	212	1	0	0	39	15.4	4	14	481
Mung Beans, Mature Seeds, Cooked, Boiled, Without Salt									
1 cup (202g)	212	1	0	0	39	15.4	4	14	4

Food Serving size	Cal.	(g) Total Fat	(g) Sat. Fat	(mg) Chol.	(g) Carb.	(g) Fiber	(g) Sug.	(g) Prot.	(mg) Sod.
Mung Beans, Mature Seeds, Sprouted, Cooked, Boiled, Drained, with Salt									
1 cup (124g)	24	0	0	0	4	1	4	3	305
Mung Beans, Mature Seeds, Sprouted, Cooked, Boiled, Drained, Without Salt									
1 cup (124g)	26	0	0	0	5	1	4	3	12
Mung Beans, Mature Seeds, Sprouted, Cooked, Stir-fried									
1 cup (124g)	62	0	0	0	13	2.4	0	5	11
Mungo Beans, Mature Seeds, Cooked, Boiled, with Salt									
1 cup (180g)	189	1	0	0	33	11.5	4	14	437
Mungo Beans, Mature Seeds, Cooked, Boiled, Without Salt									
1 oz, dry, yield after cooking (69g)	72	0	0	0	13	4.4	1	5	5
Pigeon Peas (Reduced Grams), Mature Seeds, Cooked, Boiled, with Salt									
1 cup (168g)	203	1	0	0	39	11.3	0	11	405
Pigeon Peas (Reduced Grams), Mature Seeds, Cooked, Boiled, Without Salt									
1 cup (168g)	203	1	0	0	39	11.3	0	11	8
Pigeon Peas (Reduced Grams), Mature Seeds, Raw									
1 cup (205g)	703	3	1	0	129	30.8	0	44	35
Winged Beans, Mature Seeds, Cooked, Boiled, with Salt									
1 cup (172g)	253	10	1	0	26	0	0	18	428
Winged Beans, Mature Seeds, Cooked, Boiled, Without Salt									
1 cup (172g)	253	10	1	0	26	0	0	18	22

Nuts and Seeds

Food Serving size	Cal.	(g) Total Fat	(g) Sat. Fat	(mg) Chol.	(g) Carb.	(g) Fiber	(g) Sug.	(g) Prot.	(mg) Sod.
Acorns, Dried									
1 oz (28.35g)	144	9	1	0	15	0	0	2	0
Almond Butter, Plain, with Salt									
1 tbsp (16g)	98	9	1	0	3	1.6	1	3	34
Almond Butter, Plain, Without Salt									
1 tbsp (16g)	98	9	1	0	3	1.6	1	3	1
Almond Paste									
1 oz (28.35g)	130	8	1	0	14	1.4	10	3	3
Almonds									
1 cup, sliced (92g)	529	45	3	0	20	11.2	4	20	1
Almonds, Blanched									
1 tbsp (9.1g)	54	5	0	0	2	0.9	0	2	2

Food Serving size	Cal.	(g) Total Fat	(g) Sat. Fat	(mg) Chol.	(g) Carb.	(g) Fiber	(g) Sug.	(g) Prot.	(mg) Sod.
Almonds, Dry Roasted, with Salt 1 oz (22 whole kernels) (28.35g)	169	15	1	0	6	3.1	1	6	96
Almonds, Dry Roasted, Without Salt 1 oz (22 whole kernels) (28.35g)	169	15	1	0	6	3.1	1	6	1
Almonds, Honey Roasted, Unblanched 1 oz (28.35g)	168	14	1	0	8	3.9	0	5	37
Almonds, Oil Roasted, with Salt 1 oz (22 whole kernels) (28.35g)	172	16	1	0	5	3	1	6	96
Almonds, Oil Roasted, Without Salt 1 oz (22 whole kernels) (28.35g)	172	16	1	0	5	3	1	6	0
Beechnuts, Dried 1 oz (28.35g)	163	14	2	0	9	0	0	2	11
Brazil Nuts, Dried, Unblanched 1 kernel (5g)	33	3	1	0	1	0.4	0	1	0
Breadfruit Seeds, Boiled 1 oz (28.35g)	48	1	0	0	9	1.4	0	2	7
Breadfruit Seeds, Raw 1 oz (28.35g)	54	2	0	0	8	1.5	0	2	7
Breadfruit Seeds, Roasted 1 oz (28.35g)	59	1	0	0	11	1.7	0	2	8
Breadfruit, Raw .25 fruit, small (96g)	99	0	0	0	26	4.7	11	1	2
Broadbeans (Fava Beans), Mature Seeds, Canned 1 cup (256g)	182	1	0	0	32	9.5	0	14	1160
Broadbeans (Fava Beans), Mature Seeds, Cooked, Boiled, with Salt 1 cup (170g)	187	1	0	0	33	9.2	3	13	410
Broadbeans (Fava Beans), Mature Seeds, Cooked, Boiled, Without Salt 1 cup (170g)	187	1	0	0	33	9.2	3	13	9
Broadbeans (Fava Beans), Mature Seeds, Raw 1 tbsp (9.4g)	32	0	0	0	5	2.4	1	2	1
Broadbeans, Immature Seeds, Raw 1 broadbean (8g)	6	0	0	0	1	0.3	0	0	4

Food Serving size	Cal.	(g) Total Fat	(g) Sat. Fat	(mg) Chol.	(g) Carb.	(g) Fiber	(g) Sug.	(g) Prot.	(mg) Sod.
Butternuts, Dried 1 oz (28.35g)	174	16	0	0	3	1.3	0	7	0
Caraway Seeds 1 tsp (2.1g)	7	0	0	0	1	0.8	0	0	0
Cashew Butter, Plain, with Salt 1 oz (28.35g)	166	14	3	0	8	0.6	1	5	174
Cashew Butter, Plain, Without Salt 1 oz (28.35g)	166	14	3	0	8	0.6	0	5	4
Cashew Nuts, Dry Roasted, with Salt 1 oz (28.35g)	163	13	3	0	9	0.9	1	4	181
Cashew Nuts, Dry Roasted, Without Salt 1 tbsp (8.6g)	49	4	1	0	3	0.3	0	1	1
Cashew Nuts, Oil Roasted, with Salt 1 cup, halves and pieces (129g)	749	62	11	0	39	4.3	6	22	397
Cashew Nuts, Oil Roasted, Without Salt 1 cup, halves and pieces (129g)	748	62	11	0	39	4.3	6	22	17
Chestnuts, Chinese, Boiled and Steamed 1 oz (28.35g)	43	0	0	0	9	0	0	1	1
Chestnuts, Chinese, Dried 1 oz (28.35g)	102	1	0	0	22	0	0	2	1
Chestnuts, Chinese, Roasted 1 oz (28.35g)	67	0	0	0	15	0	0	1	1
Chestnuts, European, Boiled and Steamed 1 oz (28.35g)	37	0	0	0	8	0	0	1	8
Chestnuts, European, Dried, Peeled 1 oz (28.35g)	103	1	0	0	22	0	0	1	10
Chestnuts, European, Dried, Unpeeled 1 oz (28.35g)	105	1	0	0	22	3.3	0	2	10
Chestnuts, European, Raw, Unpeeled 1 oz (28.35g)	60	1	0	0	13	2.3	0	1	1
Chestnuts, European, Roasted 1 oz (28.35g)	69	1	0	0	15	1.4	3	1	1
Chestnuts, Japanese, Boiled and Steamed 1 oz (28.35g)	16	0	0	0	4	0	0	0	1

Food Serving size	Cal.	(g) Total Fat	(g) Sat. Fat	(mg) Chol.	(g) Carb.	(g) Fiber	(g) Sug.	(g) Prot.	(mg) Sod.
Chestnuts, Japanese, Dried 1 oz (28.35g)	102	0	0	0	23	0	0	1	10
Chestnuts, Japanese, Roasted 1 oz (28.35g)	56	0	0	0	13	0	0	1	5
Chia Seeds, Dried 1 oz (28.35g)	139	9	1	0	12	10.7	0	4	5
Coconut Meat, Dried (Desiccated), Creamed 1 oz (28.35g)	194	20	17	0	6	0	0	2	10
Coconut Meat, Dried (Desiccated), Not Sweetened 1 oz (28.35g)	185	18	16	0	7	4.6	2	2	10
Coconut Meat, Dried (Desiccated), Sweetened, Flaked, Canned 4 oz (114g)	505	36	32	0	47	5.1	0	4	23
Coconut Meat, Dried (Desiccated), Sweetened, Shredded 1 package (7 oz) (199g)	997	71	63	0	95	9	86	6	521
Coconut Meat, Dried (Desiccated), Toasted 1 oz (28.35g)	168	13	12	0	13	0	0	2	10
Cumin Seed 1 tsp, whole (2.1g)	8	0	0	0	1	0.2	0	0	4
Ginkgo Nuts, Canned 1 oz (14 kernels) (28.35g)	31	0	0	0	6	2.6	0	1	87
Ginkgo Nuts, Dried 1 oz (28.35g)	97	1	0	0	20	0	0	3	4
Hazelnuts or Filberts 1 cup, ground (75g)	471	46	3	0	13	7.3	3	11	0
Hazelnuts or Filberts, Blanched 1 oz (28.35g)	178	17	1	0	5	3.1	1	4	0
Hazelnuts or Filberts, Dry Roasted, Without Salt 1 oz (28.35g)	183	18	1	0	5	2.7	1	4	0
Hickory Nuts, Dried 1 oz (28.35g)	186	18	2	0	5	1.8	0	4	0
Lotus Seeds, Dried 1 oz (42 medium seeds) (28.35g)	94	1	0	0	18	0	0	4	1
Macadamia Nuts, Dry Roasted, with Salt 1 oz (10-12 kernels) (28.35g)	203	22	3	0	4	2.3	1	2	75

Food Serving size	Cal.	(g) Total Fat	(g) Sat. Fat	(mg) Chol.	(g) Carb.	(g) Fiber	(g) Sug.	(g) Prot.	(mg) Sod.
Macadamia Nuts, Dry Roasted, Without Salt									
1 oz (10-12 kernels) (28.35g)	204	22	3	0	4	2.3	1	2	1
Mixed Nuts, Dry Roasted, with Peanuts, with Salt									
1 oz (28.35g)	168	15	2	0	7	2.6	1	5	190
Mixed Nuts, Dry Roasted, with Peanuts, Without Salt									
1 oz (28.35g)	168	15	2	0	7	2.6	0	5	3
Mixed Nuts, Oil Roasted, with Peanuts, Without Salt									
1 tbsp (8.9g)	55	5	1	0	2	0.9	0	1	1
Mixed Nuts, Oil Roasted, Without Peanuts, Without Salt									
1 oz (28.35g)	174	16	3	0	6	1.6	0	4	3
Mixed Nuts, Without Peanuts, Oil Roasted, with Salt									
1 oz (28.35g)	174	16	3	0	6	1.6	1	4	87
Nuts, Coconut Cream, Canned, Sweetened									
1 cup (296g)	1057	48	46	0	158	0.6	152	3	107
Nuts, Mixed Nuts, with Peanuts, Oil Roasted, with Salt Added									
1 oz (28.35g)	175	16	2	0	6	2.6	1	5	119
Nuts, Pilinuts, Dried									
1 oz (15 kernels) (28.35g)	204	23	9	0	1	0	0	3	1
Nuts, Pine Nuts, Dried									
1 oz (167 kernels) (28.35g)	191	19	1	0	4	1	1	4	1
Peanut Butter with Omega-3, Creamy									
1 tbsp (16g)	97	9	2	0	3	1	0	4	57
Peanut Butter, Chunk Style, with Salt									
1 cup (258g)	1520	129	20	0	56	20.6	22	62	1254
Peanut Butter, Chunk Style, Without Salt									
2 tbsp (32g)	188	16	3	0	7	2.6	3	8	5
Peanut Butter, Chunky, Vitamin and Mineral Fortified									
1 cup (258g)	1530	133	21	0	46	14.7	28	67	944
Peanut Butter, Reduced Sodium									
1 tbsp (16g)	94	8	1	0	3	1.1	0	4	32
Peanut Butter, Smooth Style, with Salt									
1 cup (258g)	1543	133	26	0	58	12.9	27	57	1099
Peanut Butter, Smooth Style, Without Salt									
2 tbsp (32g)	188	16	3	0	6	1.9	3	8	5

Food Serving size	Cal.	(g) Total Fat	(g) Sat. Fat	(mg) Chol.	(g) Carb.	(g) Fiber	(g) Sug.	(g) Prot.	(mg) Sod.
Peanut Butter, Smooth, Vitamin and Mineral Fortified									
2 tbsp (32g)	189	16	3	0	6	1.8	3	8	134
Peanut Flour, Defatted									
1 oz (28.35g)	93	0	0	0	10	4.5	2	15	51
Peanut Flour, Lowfat									
1 oz (28.35g)	121	6	1	0	9	4.5	0	10	0
Peanut Spread, Reduced Sugar									
2 tbsp (31g)	202	17	3	0	4	2.4	1	8	139
Peanuts, All Types, Cooked, Boiled, with Salt									
1 cup, shelled (180g)	572	40	5	0	38	15.8	4	24	1352
Peanuts, All Types, Dry-roasted, with Salt									
1 peanut (1g)	6	0	0	0	0	0.1	0	0	8
Peanuts, All Types, Dry-Roasted, Without Salt									
1 oz (28.35g)	166	14	2	0	6	2.3	1	7	2
Peanuts, All Types, Oil-roasted, with Salt									
1 cup, halves and whole (144g)	863	76	13	0	22	13.5	6	40	461
Peanuts, All Types, Oil-roasted, Without Salt									
1 oz, shelled (28.35g)	170	15	2	0	4	2.7	1	8	2
Peanuts, Spanish, Oil-roasted, with Salt									
1 oz (28.35g)	164	14	2	0	5	2.5	0	8	123
Peanuts, Spanish, Oil-roasted, Without Salt									
1 oz (28.35g)	164	14	2	0	5	2.5	0	8	2
Peanuts, Valencia, Oil-roasted, with Salt									
1 oz (28.35g)	167	15	2	0	5	2.5	0	8	219
Peanuts, Valencia, Oil-roasted, Without Salt									
1 oz (28.35g)	167	15	2	0	5	2.5	0	8	2
Peanuts, Virginia, Oil-roasted, with Salt									
1 oz (28.35g)	164	14	2	0	6	2.5	0	7	123
Peanuts, Virginia, Oil-roasted, Without Salt									
1 oz (28.35g)	164	14	2	0	6	2.5	0	7	2
Pecans									
1 cup, halves (99g)	684	71	6	0	14	9.5	4	9	0
Pecans, Dry Roasted, with Salt									
1 oz (28.35g)	201	21	2	0	4	2.7	1	3	109

Food Serving size	Cal.	(g) Total Fat	(g) Sat. Fat	(mg) Chol.	(g) Carb.	(g) Fiber	(g) Sug.	(g) Prot.	(mg) Sod.
Pecans, Dry Roasted, Without Salt									
1 oz (28.35g)	199	21	2	0	4	2.7	1	3	0
Pecans, Oil Roasted, with Salt									
1 oz (15 halves) (28.35g)	203	21	2	0	4	2.7	1	3	111
Pecans, Oil Roasted, Without Salt									
1 oz (15 halves) (28.35g)	203	21	2	0	4	2.7	1	3	0
Pine Nuts, Pinyon, Dried									
10 nuts (1g)	6	1	0	0	0	0.1	0	0	1
Pistachio Nuts, Dry Roasted, with Salt									
1 oz (49 kernels) (28.35g)	160	13	2	0	8	2.8	2	6	121
Pistachio Nuts, Dry Roasted, Without Salt									
1 oz (49 kernels) (28.35g)	161	13	2	0	8	2.8	2	6	2
Safflower Seed Kernels, Dried									
1 oz (28.35g)	147	11	1	0	10	0	0	5	1
Safflower Seed Meal, Part Defatted									
1 oz (28.35g)	97	1	0	0	14	0	0	10	1
Seeds, Flaxseed									
1 tbsp, whole (10.3g)	55	4	0	0	3	2.8	0	2	3
Sesame Butter, Paste									
1 tbsp (16g)	94	8	1	0	4	0.9	0	3	2
Sesame Butter, Tahini, from Raw and Stone Ground Kernels									
1 oz (28.35g)	162	14	2	0	7	2.6	0	5	21
Sesame Butter, Tahini, from Roasted Kernels (Most Common Type)									
1 oz (28.35g)	169	15	2	0	6	2.6	0	5	33
Sesame Butter, Tahini, from Unroasted Kernels									
1 oz (28.35g)	172	16	2	0	5	2.6	0	5	0
Sesame Butter, Tahini, Kernels Unspecified									
1 tbsp (15g)	89	8	1	0	3	0.7	0	3	5
Sesame Seed Kernels, Dried (Decort)									
1 tbsp (8g)	50	5	1	0	1	0.9	0	2	4
Sesame Seed Kernels, Toasted, with Salt (Decort)									
1 oz (28.35g)	161	14	2	0	7	4.8	0	5	167
Sesame Seed Kernels, Toasted, Without Salt (Decort)									
1 oz (28.35g)	161	14	2	0	7	4.8	0	5	11

Food Serving size	Cal.	(g) Total Fat	(g) Sat. Fat	(mg) Chol.	(g) Carb.	(g) Fiber	(g) Sug.	(g) Prot.	(mg) Sod.
Sesame Seeds, Whole, Dried									
1 tbsp (9g)	52	4	1	0	2	1.1	0	2	1
Sesame Seeds, Whole, Roasted and Toasted									
1 oz (28.35g)	158	13	2	0	7	3.9	0	5	3
Sunflower Seed Butter, with Salt									
1 oz (28.35g)	175	16	1	0	7	1.6	3	5	94
Sunflower Seed Butter, Without Salt									
1 oz (28.35g)	175	16	1	0	7	1.6	3	5	1
Sunflower Seed Flour, Part Defatted									
1 tbsp (4g)	13	0	0	0	1	0.2	0	2	0
Sunflower Seed Kernels, Dried									
1 cup (140g)	818	72	6	0	28	12	4	29	13
Sunflower Seed Kernels, Dry Roasted, with Salt									
1 oz (28.35g)	165	14	1	0	7	2.6	1	5	116
Sunflower Seed Kernels, Dry Roasted, Without Salt									
1 oz (28.35g)	165	14	1	0	7	3.1	1	5	1
Sunflower Seed Kernels, Oil Roasted, with Salt									
1 oz (28.35g)	168	15	2	0	6	3	1	6	116
Sunflower Seed Kernels, Oil Roasted, Without Salt									
1 oz (28.35g)	168	15	2	0	6	3	1	6	1
Sunflower Seed Kernels, Toasted, with Salt									
1 oz (28.35g)	175	16	2	0	6	3.3	0	5	174
Sunflower Seed Kernels, Toasted, Without Salt									
1 oz (28.35g)	175	16	2	0	6	3.3	0	5	1
Walnuts, Black, Dried									
1 tbsp (7.8g)	48	5	0	0	1	0.5	0	2	0
Walnuts, English									
1 cup, ground (80g)	523	52	5	0	11	5.4	2	12	2
Watermelon Seed Kernels, Dried									
1 oz (28.35g)	158	13	3	0	4	0	0	8	28

Seafood

Abalone, Mixed Species, Cooked, Fried									
3 oz (85g)	161	6	1	80	9	0	0	17	502

Food Serving size	Cal.	(g) Total Fat	(g) Sat. Fat	(mg) Chol.	(g) Carb.	(g) Fiber	(g) Sug.	(g) Prot.	(mg) Sod.
Anchovy, European, Canned in Oil, Drained Solid									
1 anchovy (4g)	8	0	0	3	0	0	0	1	147
Bass, Fresh Water, Mixed Species, Cooked, Dry Heat									
3 oz (85g)	124	4	1	74	0	0	0	21	77
Bass, Striped, Cooked, Dry Heat									
3 oz (85g)	105	3	1	88	0	0	0	19	75
Bluefish, Cooked, Dry Heat									
3 oz (85g)	135	5	1	65	0	0	0	22	65
Burbot, Cooked, Dry Heat									
3 oz (85g)	98	1	0	65	0	0	0	21	105
Butterfish, Cooked, Dry Heat									
3 oz (85g)	159	9	0	71	0	0	0	19	97
Carp, Cooked, Dry Heat									
1 fillet (170g)	275	12	2	143	0	0	0	39	107
Catfish, Channel, Cooked, Breaded and Fried									
3 oz (85g)	195	11	3	60	7	0.6	0	15	238
Catfish, Channel, Farmed, Cooked, Dry Heat									
3 oz (85g)	122	6	1	56	0	0	0	16	101
Catfish, Channel, Wild, Cooked, Dry Heat									
3 oz (85g)	89	2	1	61	0	0	0	16	43
Caviar, Black and Red, Granular									
1 oz (28.35g)	75	5	1	167	1	0	0	7	425
Clam, Mixed Species, Canned, Drained Solid									
3 oz (85g)	121	1	0	43	5	0	0	21	95
Clam, Mixed Species, Canned, Liquid									
3 oz (85g)	2	0	0	3	0	0	0	0	183
Clam, Mixed Species, Cooked, Breaded and Fried									
20 small (188g)	380	21	5	115	19	0	0	27	684
Clam, Mixed Species, Cooked, Moist Heat									
20 small (190g)	281	4	0	127	10	0	0	49	213
Cod, Atlantic, Canned, Solids and Liquid									
1 can (312g)	328	3	1	172	0	0	0	71	680
Cod, Atlantic, Cooked, Dry Heat									
1 fillet (180g)	189	2	0	99	0	0	0	41	140

Food Serving size	Cal.	(g) Total Fat	(g) Sat. Fat	(mg) Chol.	(g) Carb.	(g) Fiber	(g) Sug.	(g) Prot.	(mg) Sod.
Cod, Atlantic, Dried and Salted 1 piece (5-1/2" x 1-1/2" x 1/2") (80g)	232	2	0	122	0	0	0	50	5622
Cod, Pacific, Cooked, Dry Heat 3 oz (85g)	72	0	0	48	0	0	0	16	316
Crab, Alaska King, Cooked, Moist Heat 3 oz (85g)	82	1	0	45	0	0	0	16	911
Crab, Alaska King, Imitation, Made from Surimi 3 oz (85g)	81	0	0	17	13	0.4	5	6	715
Crab, Blue, Canned 1 oz (28.35g)	24	0	0	27	0	0	0	5	112
Crab, Blue, Cooked, Moist Heat 1 cup (not packed) (135g)	112	1	0	131	0	0	0	24	533
Crab, Blue, Crab Cakes 1 cake (60g)	93	5	1	90	0	0	0	12	198
Crab, Dungeness, Cooked, Moist Heat 1 crab (127g)	140	2	0	97	1	0	0	28	480
Crab, Queen, Cooked, Moist Heat 3 oz (85g)	98	1	0	60	0	0	0	20	587
Crayfish, Mixed Species, Farmed, Cooked, Moist Heat 3 oz (85g)	74	1	0	116	0	0	0	15	82
Crayfish, Mixed Species, Wild, Cooked, Moist Heat 3 oz (85g)	70	1	0	113	0	0	0	14	80
Croaker, Atlantic, Cooked, Breaded and Fried 3 oz (85g)	188	11	3	71	6	0.3	0	15	296
Cusk, Cooked, Dry Heat 3 oz (85g)	95	1	0	45	0	0	0	21	34
Cuttlefish, Mixed Species, Cooked, Moist Heat 3 oz (85g)	134	1	0	190	1	0	0	28	632
Dolphinfish, Cooked, Dry Heat 3 oz (85g)	93	1	0	80	0	0	0	20	96
Drum, Fresh Water, Cooked, Dry Heat 3 oz (85g)	130	5	1	70	0	0	0	19	82

Food Serving size	Cal.	(g) Total Fat	(g) Sat. Fat	(mg) Chol.	(g) Carb.	(g) Fiber	(g) Sug.	(g) Prot.	(mg) Sod.
Eel, Mixed Species, Cooked, Dry Heat 1 oz, with bone (yield after bone removed) (22g)									
	52	3	1	35	0	0	0	5	14
Fish Broth 1 fl oz (30.5g)	5	0	0	0	0	0	0	1	97
Flatfish (Flounder and Sole Species), Cooked, Dry Heat 3 oz (85g)	73	2	0	48	0	0	0	13	309
Gefilte Fish, Commercial, Sweet Recipe 1 piece (42g)	35	1	0	13	3	0	0	4	220
Grouper, Mixed Species, Cooked, Dry Heat 1 fillet (202g)	238	3	1	95	0	0	0	50	107
Haddock, Cooked, Dry Heat 3 oz (85g)	77	0	0	56	0	0	0	17	222
Haddock, Smoked 1 cubic inch, boneless (17g)	20	0	0	13	0	0	0	4	130
Halibut, Atlantic and Pacific, Cooked, Dry Heat .5 fillet (159g)	176	3	1	95	0	0	0	36	130
Halibut, Greenland, Cooked, Dry Heat 3 oz (85g)	203	15	3	50	0	0	0	16	88
Herring, Atlantic, Cooked, Dry Heat 3 oz (85g)	173	10	2	65	0	0	0	20	98
Herring, Atlantic, Kippered 1 cubic inch, boneless (17g)	37	2	0	14	0	0	0	4	156
Herring, Atlantic, Pickled 1 oz, boneless (28.35g)	74	5	1	4	3	0	2	4	247
Herring, Pacific, Cooked, Dry Heat 3 oz (85g)	213	15	4	84	0	0	0	18	81
Jellyfish, Dried, Salted 1 cup (58g)	21	1	0	3	0	0	0	3	5620
Ling, Cooked, Dry Heat 3 oz (85g)	94	1	0	43	0	0	0	21	147
Lingcod, Cooked, Dry Heat 3 oz (85g)	93	1	0	57	0	0	0	19	65
Lobster, Northern, Cooked, Moist Heat 3 oz (85g)	76	1	0	124	0	0	0	16	413

Food Serving size	Cal.	(g) Total Fat	(g) Sat. Fat	(mg) Chol.	(g) Carb.	(g) Fiber	(g) Sug.	(g) Prot.	(mg) Sod.
Mackerel, Atlantic, Cooked, Dry Heat									
3 oz (85g)	223	15	4	64	0	0	0	20	71
Mackerel, Jack, Canned, Drained Solid									
1 oz, boneless (28.35g)	44	2	1	22	0	0	0	7	107
Mackerel, King, Cooked, Dry Heat									
3 oz (85g)	114	2	0	58	0	0	0	22	173
Mackerel, Pacific and Jack, Mixed Species, Cooked, Dry Heat									
1 cubic inch, boneless (17g)	34	2	0	10	0	0	0	4	19
Mackerel, Salted									
1 cup, cooked (136g)	415	34	10	129	0	0	0	25	6052
Mackerel, Spanish, Cooked, Dry Heat									
3 oz (85g)	134	5	2	62	0	0	0	20	56
Milkfish, Cooked, Dry Heat									
3 oz (85g)	162	7	0	57	0	0	0	22	78
Monkfish, Cooked, Dry Heat									
3 oz (85g)	82	2	0	27	0	0	0	16	20
Mullet, Striped, Cooked, Dry Heat									
3 oz (85g)	128	4	1	54	0	0	0	21	60
Octopus, Common, Cooked, Moist Heat									
3 oz (85g)	139	2	0	82	4	0	0	25	391
Oyster, Eastern, Canned									
1 cup, undrained (248g)	169	6	2	136	10	0	0	18	278
Oyster, Eastern, Cooked, Breaded and Fried									
6 medium (88g)	175	11	3	62	10	0	0	8	367
Oyster, Eastern, Farmed, Cooked, Dry Heat									
6 medium (59g)	47	1	0	22	4	0	0	4	96
Oyster, Eastern, Farmed, Raw									
6 medium (84g)	50	1	0	21	5	0	0	4	150
Oyster, Eastern, Wild, Cooked, Dry Heat									
6 medium (59g)	47	2	0	37	2	0	1	5	78
Oyster, Eastern, Wild, Cooked, Moist Heat									
6 medium (42g)	43	1	0	33	2	0	1	5	70
Oyster, Pacific, Cooked, Moist Heat									
3 oz (85g)	139	4	1	85	8	0	0	16	180

Food Serving size	Cal.	(g) Total Fat	(g) Sat. Fat	(mg) Chol.	(g) Carb.	(g) Fiber	(g) Sug.	(g) Prot.	(mg) Sod.
Oyster, Pacific, Raw 3 oz (85g)	69	2	0	43	4	0	0	8	90
Perch, Mixed Species, Cooked, Dry Heat 3 oz (85g)	99	1	0	98	0	0	0	21	67
Pike, Northern, Cooked, Dry Heat .5 fillet (155g)	175	1	0	78	0	0	0	38	76
Pike, Walleye, Cooked, Dry Heat 3 oz (85g)	101	1	0	94	0	0	0	21	55
Pollock, Atlantic, Cooked, Dry Heat .5 fillet (151g)	178	2	0	137	0	0	0	38	166
Pollock, Walleye, Cooked, Dry Heat 3 oz (85g)	94	1	0	73	0	0	0	20	88
Pompano, Florida, Cooked, Dry Heat 3 oz (85g)	179	10	4	54	0	0	0	20	65
Pout, Ocean, Cooked, Dry Heat 3 oz (85g)	87	1	0	57	0	0	0	18	66
Rockfish, Pacific, Mixed Species, Cooked, Dry Heat 3 oz (85g)	93	1	0	52	0	0	0	19	76
Roe, Mixed Species, Cooked, Dry Heat 3 oz (85g)	173	7	2	407	2	0	0	24	99
Sablefish, Cooked, Dry Heat 3 oz (85g)	213	17	3	54	0	0	0	15	61
Sablefish, Smoked 3 oz (85g)	218	17	4	54	0	0	0	15	626
Salmon, Atlantic, Farmed, Cooked, Dry Heat .5 fillet (178g)	367	22	4	112	0	0	0	39	109
Salmon, Atlantic, Wild, Cooked, Dry Heat .5 fillet (154g)	280	13	2	109	0	0	0	39	86
Salmon, Chinook, Cooked, Dry Heat .5 fillet (154g)	356	21	5	131	0	0	0	40	92
Salmon, Chinook, Smoked (Lox), Regular 3 oz (85g)	99	4	1	20	0	0	0	16	1700
Salmon, Chum, Canned, Without Salt, Drained Solid with Bone 3 oz (85g)	120	5	1	33	0	0	0	18	64

Food Serving size	Cal.	(g) Total Fat	(g) Sat. Fat	(mg) Chol.	(g) Carb.	(g) Fiber	(g) Sug.	(g) Prot.	(mg) Sod.
Salmon, Chum, Cooked, Dry Heat .5 fillet (154g)	237	7	2	146	0	0	0	40	99
Salmon, Coho, Farmed, Cooked, Dry Heat 3 oz (85g)	151	7	2	54	0	0	0	21	44
Salmon, Coho, Wild, Cooked, Dry Heat .5 fillet (178g)	247	8	2	98	0	0	0	42	103
Salmon, Coho, Wild, Cooked, Moist Heat .5 fillet (155g)	285	12	2	88	0	0	0	42	82
Salmon, Pink, Canned, Solids with Bone and Liquid 1 can, drained solids (total) (315g)	435	16	3	261	0	0	0	73	1200
Salmon, Pink, Canned, Without Salt, Solids with Bone and Liquid 1 can (454g)	631	27	7	250	0	0	0	90	341
Salmon, Pink, Cooked, Dry Heat .5 fillet (124g)	190	7	1	68	0	0	0	30	112
Salmon, Sockeye, Canned, Drained Solid with Bone 3 oz (85g)	141	6	1	37	0	0	0	20	306
Salmon, Sockeye, Canned, Without Salt, Drained Solid with Bone 1 can (369g)	565	27	6	162	0	0	0	76	277
Salmon, Sockeye, Cooked, Dry Heat 3 oz (85g)	144	6	1	54	0	0	0	22	114
Sardine, Atlantic, Canned in Oil, Drained Solid with Bone 1 oz (28.35g)	59	3	0	40	0	0	0	7	143
Sardine, Pacific, Canned in Tomato Sauce, Drained Solid with Bone 1 can (370g)	685	39	10	226	2	0.4	2	77	1532
Scallop, Mixed Species, Cooked, Breaded and Fried 2 large (31g)	67	3	1	17	3	0	0	6	144
Scallop, Mixed Species, Imitation, Made from Surimi 3 oz (85g)	84	0	0	19	9	0	0	11	676
Scup, Cooked, Dry Heat 3 oz (85g)	115	3	0	57	0	0	0	21	46
Sea Bass, Mixed Species, Cooked, Dry Heat 3 oz (85g)	105	2	1	45	0	0	0	20	74
Sea Trout, Mixed Species, Cooked, Dry Heat 3 oz (85g)	113	4	1	90	0	0	0	18	63

Food Serving size	Cal.	(g) Total Fat	(g) Sat. Fat	(mg) Chol.	(g) Carb.	(g) Fiber	(g) Sug.	(g) Prot.	(mg) Sod.
Shark, Mixed Species, Cooked, Batter-dipped and Fried									
3 oz (85g)	194	12	3	50	5	0	0	16	104
Shrimp, Mixed Species, Canned									
1 oz (28.35g)	28	0	0	71	0	0	0	6	220
Shrimp, Mixed Species, Cooked, Breaded and Fried									
4 large (30g)	73	4	1	41	3	0.1	0	6	103
Shrimp, Mixed Species, Cooked, Moist Heat									
4 large (22g)	26	0	0	46	0	0	0	5	208
Shrimp, Mixed Species, Imitation, Made from Surimi									
3 oz (85g)	86	1	0	31	8	0	0	11	599
Smelt, Rainbow, Cooked, Dry Heat									
3 oz (85g)	105	3	0	77	0	0	0	19	65
Snapper, Mixed Species, Cooked, Dry Heat									
1 fillet (170g)	218	3	1	80	0	0	0	45	97
Spiny Lobster, Mixed Species, Cooked, Moist Heat									
3 oz (85g)	122	2	0	77	3	0	0	22	193
Squid, Mixed Species, Cooked, Fried									
3 oz (85g)	149	6	2	221	7	0	0	15	260
Sturgeon, Mixed Species, Cooked, Dry Heat									
1 cup, cooked (136g)	184	7	2	105	0	0	0	28	94
Sturgeon, Mixed Species, Smoked									
3 oz (85g)	147	4	1	68	0	0	0	27	628
Sunfish, Pumpkin Seed, Cooked, Dry Heat									
3 oz (85g)	97	1	0	73	0	0	0	21	88
Swordfish, Cooked, Dry Heat									
1 piece (106g)	182	8	2	83	0	0	0	25	103
Tilefish, Cooked, Dry Heat									
3 oz (85g)	125	4	1	54	0	0	0	21	50
Trout, Mixed Species, Cooked, Dry Heat									
3 oz (85g)	162	7	1	63	0	0	0	23	57
Trout, Rainbow, Farmed, Cooked, Dry Heat									
3 oz (85g)	143	6	1	60	0	0	0	20	52
Trout, Rainbow, Wild, Cooked, Dry Heat									
3 oz (85g)	128	5	1	59	0	0	0	19	48

Food Serving size	Cal.	(g) Total Fat	(g) Sat. Fat	(mg) Chol.	(g) Carb.	(g) Fiber	(g) Sug.	(g) Prot.	(mg) Sod.
Tuna Salad 1 cup (205g)	383	19	3	27	19	0	0	33	824
Tuna, Fresh, Bluefin, Cooked, Dry Heat 3 oz (85g)	156	5	1	42	0	0	0	25	43
Tuna, Light, Canned in Oil, Drained Solid 1 oz (28.35g)	56	2	0	5	0	0	0	8	100
Tuna, Light, Canned in Oil, Without Salt, Drained Solid 1 can (171g)	339	14	3	31	0	0	0	50	86
Tuna, Light, Canned in Water, Drained Solid 3 oz (85g)	73	1	0	31	0	0	0	17	210
Tuna, Light, Canned in Water, Without Salt, Drained Solid 1 can (165g)	191	1	0	50	0	0	0	42	83
Tuna, Skipjack, Fresh, Cooked, Dry Heat .5 fillet (154g)	203	2	1	92	0	0	0	43	72
Tuna, White, Canned in Oil, Drained Solid 1 can (178g)	331	14	2	55	0	0	0	47	705
Tuna, White, Canned in Oil, Without Salt, Drained Solid 1 can (178g)	331	14	3	55	0	0	0	47	89
Tuna, White, Canned in Water, Drained Solid 1 can (172g)	220	5	1	72	0	0	0	41	648
Tuna, White, Canned in Water, Without Salt, Drained Solid 1 can (172g)	220	5	1	72	0	0	0	41	86
Tuna, Yellowfin, Fresh, Cooked, Dry Heat 3 oz (85g)	111	1	0	40	0	0	0	25	46
Turbot, European, Cooked, Dry Heat .5 fillet (154g)	194	6	0	99	0	0	0	33	305
Whitefish, Mixed Species, Cooked, Dry Heat 1 fillet (154g)	265	12	2	119	0	0	0	38	100
Whitefish, Mixed Species, Smoked 1 oz, boneless (28.35g)	31	0	0	9	0	0	0	7	289
Whiting, Mixed Species, Cooked, Dry Heat .5 fillet (153g)	147	4	1	70	0	0	0	27	130
Wolffish, Atlantic, Cooked, Dry Heat 3 oz (85g)	105	3	0	50	0	0	0	19	93

Food Serving size	Cal.	(g) Total Fat	(g) Sat. Fat	(mg) Chol.	(g) Carb.	(g) Fiber	(g) Sug.	(g) Prot.	(mg) Sod.
Yellowtail, Mixed Species, Cooked, Dry Heat 3 oz (85g)	159	6	0	60	0	0	0	25	43

Eggs

Food Serving size	Cal.	Total Fat	Sat. Fat	Chol.	Carb.	Fiber	Sug.	Prot.	Sod.
Egg Substitute, Liquid or Frozen, Fat Free 1 cup (240g)	115	0	0	0	5	0	5	24	478
Egg Substitute, Powder .7 oz (20g)	89	3	1	114	4	0	4	11	160
Egg, White, Dried, Flakes, Glucose Reduced .5 lb (227g)	797	0	0	0	9	0	9	175	2624
Egg, White, Dried, Powder, Glucose Reduced 1 tbsp (7g)	26	0	0	0	0	0	0	6	87
Egg, White, Dried, Stabilized, Glucose Reduced 1 tbsp (7g)	25	0	0	1	0	0	0	6	71
Egg, Whole, Cooked, Fried 1 large (46g)	90	7	2	184	0	0	0	6	95
Egg, Whole, Cooked, Hard-boiled 1 tbsp (8.5g)	13	1	0	32	0	0	0	1	11
Egg, Whole, Cooked, Omelet 1 large (61g)	94	7	2	191	0	0	0	6	95
Egg, Whole, Cooked, Scrambled 1 tbsp (13.7g)	20	2	0	38	0	0	0	1	20
Egg, Whole, Dried 1 tbsp (13.7g)	30	2	1	82	0	0	0	2	24
Egg, Whole, Dried, Stabilized, Glucose Reduced 1 tbsp (5g)	31	2	1	101	0	0	0	2	27
Egg, Yolk, Dried 1 tbsp (4g)	27	2	1	92	0	0	0	1	7
Egg, Yolk, Frozen, Salted, Pasteurized .5 lb (227g)	624	52	16	2070	4	0	0	32	7915
Egg, Yolk, Raw, Fresh 1 cup (243g)	782	64	23	2637	9	0	1	39	117
Egg, Yolk, Raw, Frozen .5 lb (227g)	688	58	18	2145	3	0	1	35	152

Food Serving size	Cal.	(g) Total Fat	(g) Sat. Fat	(mg) Chol.	(g) Carb.	(g) Fiber	(g) Sug.	(g) Prot.	(mg) Sod.
Egg, Yolk, Raw, Fozen, Pasteurized									
.5 lb (227g)	13	0	0	0	0	0	0	3	47
Egg, Yolk, Raw, Frozen, Sugared									
.5 lb (227g)	697	52	16	2082	25	0	23	31	159

Soy Products

Food Serving size	Cal.	(g) Total Fat	(g) Sat. Fat	(mg) Chol.	(g) Carb.	(g) Fiber	(g) Sug.	(g) Prot.	(mg) Sod.
Soy Protein Concentrate, Crude Protein Basis (N x 6.25), Acid Wash									
1 oz (28.35g)	93	0	0	0	7	1.6	0	18	255
Soy Protein Concentrate, Produced by Alcohol Extraction									
1 oz (28.35g)	94	0	0	0	9	1.6	6	16	1
Soy Protein Concentrated, Produced by Acid Wash									
1 oz (28.35g)	94	0	0	0	9	1.6	6	16	255
Soy Protein Isolate									
1 oz (28.35g)	96	1	0	0	2	1.6	0	23	285
Soy Protein Isolate, Potassium									
1 oz (28.35g)	92	0	0	0	3	1.6	0	23	14
Soy Protein Isolate, Potassium, Crude Protein Basis									
1 oz (28.35g)	91	0	0	0	1	0.6	0	25	14
Soy Protein Isolate, Protein Technologies International, Proplus									
1 oz (28.35g)	108	1	0	0	0	0	0	24	11
Soy Protein Isolate, Protein Technologies International, Supro									
1 oz (28.35g)	110	1	0	0	0	0	0	25	337
Soybean, Curd, Cheese									
1 cup (225g)	340	18	3	0	16	0	0	28	45
Soybeans, Green, Cooked, Boiled, Drained, with Salt									
1 cup (180g)	254	12	1	0	20	7.6	0	22	450
Soybeans, Green, Cooked, Boiled, Drained, Without Salt									
1 cup (180g)	254	12	1	0	20	7.6	0	22	25
Soybeans, Green, Raw									
1 cup (256g)	376	17	2	0	28	10.8	0	33	38
Soybeans, Mature Seeds, Cooked, Boiled, with Salt									
1 cup (172g)	298	15	2	0	17	10.3	5	29	408
Soybeans, Mature Seeds, Dry Roasted									
1 cup (172g)	776	37	5	0	56	13.9	0	68	3

Food Serving size	Cal.	(g) Total Fat	(g) Sat. Fat	(mg) Chol.	(g) Carb.	(g) Fiber	(g) Sug.	(g) Prot.	(mg) Sod.
Soybeans, Mature Seeds, Roasted, No Salt Added 1 cup (172g)	810	44	6	0	58	30.4	0	61	7
Soybeans, Mature Seeds, Roasted, Salted 1 cup (172g)	810	44	6	0	58	30.4	7	61	280
Soybeans, Mature Seeds, Sprouted, Cooked, Raw 10 sprouts (10g)	12	1	0	0	1	0.1	0	1	1
Soybeans, Mature Seeds, Sprouted, Cooked, Steamed 1 cup (94g)	76	4	1	0	6	0.8	0	8	9
Soybeans, Mature Seeds, Sprouted, Cooked, Steamed, with Salt 1 cup (94g)	76	4	1	0	6	0.8	0	8	231
Soybeans, Mature, Cooked, Boiled, Without Salt 1 tbsp (10.7g)	19	1	0	0	1	0.6	0	2	0
Tempeh 1 cup (166g)	320	18	4	0	16	0	0	31	15

Tofu Products

Food Serving size	Cal.	(g) Total Fat	(g) Sat. Fat	(mg) Chol.	(g) Carb.	(g) Fiber	(g) Sug.	(g) Prot.	(mg) Sod.
Mori-nu, Tofu, Silken, Firm 1 slice (84g)	52	2	0	0	2	0.1	1	6	30
Mori-nu, Tofu, Silken, Lite Extra Firm 1 slice (84g)	32	1	0	0	1	0	0	6	82
Mori-nu, Tofu, Silken, Lite Firm 1 slice (84g)	31	1	0	0	1	0	0	5	71
Mori-nu, Tofu, Silken, Soft 1 slice (84g)	46	2	0	0	2	0.1	1	4	4
Mori-nu, Yofu, Silken, Extra Firm 1 slice (84g)	46	2	0	0	2	0.1	1	6	53
Tofu, Dried-frozen (Koyadofu) 1 piece (17g)	82	5	1	0	2	1.2	0	8	1
Tofu, Dried-frozen (Koyadofu), Prepared with Calcium Sulfate 1 piece (17g)	80	5	1	0	2	0.2	0	8	1
Tofu, Extra Firm, Prepared with Nigari .2 block (91g)	83	5	0	0	2	0.4	0	9	7
Tofu, Firm, Prepared with Calcium Sulfate and Magnesium Chloride (Nigari) .25 block (81g)	57	3	1	0	1	0.7	0	7	10

Food Serving size	Cal.	(g) Total Fat	(g) Sat. Fat	(mg) Chol.	(g) Carb.	(g) Fiber	(g) Sug.	(g) Prot.	(mg) Sod.
Tofu, Fried									
1 piece (13g)	35	3	0	0	1	0.5	0	2	2
Tofu, Fried, Prepared with Calcium Sulfate									
1 piece (13g)	35	3	0	0	1	0.5	0	2	2
Tofu, Hard, Prepared with Nigari									
.25 block (122g)	178	12	2	0	5	0.7	0	15	2
Tofu, Okara									
1 cup (122g)	94	2	0	0	15	0	0	4	11
Tofu, Salted and Fermented (Fuyu)									
1 block (11g)	13	1	0	0	1	0	0	1	316
Tofu, Salted and Fermented (Fuyu), Prepared with Calcium Sulfate									
1 block (11g)	13	1	0	0	1	0	0	1	316
Tofu, Soft, Prepared with Calcium Sulfate and Magnesium Chloride (Nigari)									
1 cubic inch (18g)	11	1	0	0	0	0	0	1	1
VitaSoy USA, Nasoya Lite Firm Tofu									
1 serving (79g)	43	1	0	0	1	0.5	0	7	27
VitaSoy USA, Organic Nasoya Extra Firm Tofu									
1 serving (79g)	77	4	1	0	2	1	0	8	3
VitaSoy USA, Organic Nasoya Firm Tofu									
1 serving (79g)	66	3	0	0	2	0.6	0	7	3
VitaSoy USA, Organic Nasoya Super Firm Cubed Tofu									
.2 package (79g)	96	5	1	0	3	1.7	0	10	5
VitaSoy USA, VitaSoy Light Vanilla Soymilk									
1 serving (243g)	73	2	0	0	10	0.2	7	4	119
VitaSoy USA, VitaSoy Organic Classic Original Soy Milk									
1 serving (243g)	114	4	1	0	11	1	5	8	160
VitaSoy USA, VitaSoy Organic Creamy Original Soy Milk									
1 serving (243g)	107	4	0	0	11	1	5	7	160

Fats and Oils

Why Eat Fats and Oils?

Fats and oils are not a food group, but they do provide essential nutrients. Most of the fats you eat should be polyunsaturated (PUFA) or monounsaturated (MUFA) fats. Some fatty acids are necessary for health; these are called "essential fatty acids." The MUFAs and PUFAs found in fish, nuts, and vegetable oils do not raise LDL ("bad") cholesterol levels in the blood. Omega-3 fatty acids are in this group. Additionally, these oils may reduce the risk of heart disease and some cancers. Saturated fats, on the other hand, may raise LDL cholesterol and increase risk of heart disease. Recent studies found that all saturated fat is not harmful to heart health, the saturated fat found in nuts, nut butters, and coconut included. Aside from essential fatty acids, fats and oils are important because they are a source of fat-soluble vitamins A, D, E, and K.

Daily Goal

6 teaspoons for an adult on a 2,000-calorie diet
One-teaspoon equivalents:
    1 tablespoon oil = 2.5 teaspoons
    1 tablespoon mayonnaise = 2.5 teaspoons
    2 tablespoons Italian dressing = 2 teaspoons
    4 large olives = ½ teaspoon
    1 oz nuts = 3 teaspoons
    2 tablespoons peanut butter = 4 teaspoons
    8 olives = 1 teaspoon

Shopping Tips

- Choose fats and oils high in monounsaturated and polyunsaturated fatty acids, such as fish, nuts, seeds, and vegetable oils.
- Limit solid fats, such as butter, stick margarine, shortening, and animal fats.
- Choose fats high in omega-3, such as olive oil, soy oil, walnuts, and flaxseeds.
- Use products with 3 grams or less saturated fat per serving listed on the nutrition facts label. This will help you adhere to the healthy heart recommendation to keep saturated fats to 10% or less of total daily calories.

Shopping List Essentials

Olive oil	Soybean oil	Nuts	Seeds
Canola oil	Tub margarine	Avocadoes	Olives

Red Flags

While consuming some fats and oils is healthy, they still contain calories. In fact, oils and solid fats both contain about 120 calories per tablespoon. To balance total calorie intake, the amount of fats and oils consumed needs to be limited to about 30% of total calories. Vegetable oils (soy and corn) often do not have a healthy ratio of omega-3 to omega-6 fatty acids and can be replaced with sunflower, safflower, and avocado oil. Also, avoid trans fats, which are clearly identified on the nutrition facts label. Research has shown that trans fats increase the risk of heart disease.

Preparation Pointer

Add nuts and seeds to salads. Add ¼ avocado to salads and sandwiches. Reduce the amount of oil used in cooking by using broth (low-fat, low-sodium) as a substitution whenever possible. Cut the fat in dressings, sauces, and marinades by replacing some of the oil with citrus juice, mustard, or flavored vinegars. Mix water with yogurt for a creamy base. When baking, use unsweetened applesauce, ¾ to 1 cup for every 1 cup oil being replaced. When you stir-fry, use cooking oil spray to reduce the fat added by the cooking oil.

Food Serving size	Cal.	(g) Total Fat	(g) Sat. Fat	(mg) Chol.	(g) Carb.	(g) Fiber	(g) Sug.	(g) Prot.	(mg) Sod.
Olives									
Olives, Pickled, Canned or Bottled, Green 1 olive (2.7g)	3	0	0	0	0	0.1	0	0	31
Olives, Ripe, Canned (Jumbo-Super Colossal) 1 jumbo (8.3g)	7	1	0	0	0	0.2	0	0	61
Olives, Ripe, Canned (Small-Extra Large) 1 large (4.4g)	5	0	0	0	0	0.1	0	0	32
Butter/Margarine									
Butter Oil, Anhydrous 1 cup (205g)	1796	204	127	525	0	0	0	1	4
Butter Replacement, Without Fat, Powder 1 cup (80g)	298	1	0	2	71	0	2	2	960
Butter, Whipped, with Salt 1 tbsp (9.4g)	67	8	5	21	0	0	0	0	62
Butter, with Salt 1 tbsp (14.2g)	102	12	7	31	0	0	0	0	91
Butter, Without Salt 1 tbsp (14.2g)	102	12	7	31	0	0	0	0	2
Fat, Beef Tallow 1 cup (205g)	1849	205	102	223	0	0	0	0	0
Fat, Chicken 1 cup (205g)	1845	205	61	174	0	0	0	0	0
Fat, Duck 1 cup (205g)	1808	205	68	205	0	0	0	0	0
Fat, Goose 1 cup (205g)	1845	205	57	205	0	0	0	0	0
Fat, Turkey 1 tsp (4.3g)	39	4	1	4	0	0	0	0	0
Margarine Spread, Approximately 48% Fat, Tub 1 tbsp (14g)	59	7	1	0	0	0	0	0	90
Margarine, 80% Fat, Stick, Including Regular and Hydrogenated Corn and Soybean Oils 1 tbsp (14g)	100	11	2	0	0	0	0	0	92

Food Serving size	Cal.	(g) Total Fat	(g) Sat. Fat	(mg) Chol.	(g) Carb.	(g) Fiber	(g) Sug.	(g) Prot.	(mg) Sod.
Margarine, 80% Fat, Tub, Canola Harvest Soft Spread									
1 tbsp (1 NLEA serving) (14g)	102	11	2	0	0	0	0	0	100
Margarine, Industrial, Non-diary, Cottonseed, Soy Oil (Part Hydrogenated)									
1 tbsp (14g)	100	11	3	0	0	0	0	0	123
Margarine, Industrial, Soy and Part Hydrogenated Soy Oil, Baking, Sauces, Candy									
1 cup (227g)	1621	182	37	0	2	0	0	0	2011
Margarine, Margarine-like Vegetable Oil Spread, 67-70% Fat, Tub									
1 tbsp (1 NLEA serving) (14g)	85	10	2	0	0	0	0	0	75
Margarine, Regular, 80% Fat, Composite, Stick, with Salt									
1 cup (227g)	1628	183	34	0	2	0	0	0	1705
Margarine, Regular, 80% Fat, Composite, Tub, with Salt									
1 cup (227g)	1619	182	32	0	2	0	0	0	1491
Margarine, Regular, 80% Fat, Composite, Tub, with Salt, with Added Vitamin D									
1 tbsp (14g)	100	11	2	0	0	0	0	0	92
Margarine, Regular, 80% Fat, Composite, Tub, Without Salt									
1 cup (227g)	1619	182	32	0	2	0	0	0	64
Margarine, Regular, Hard, Soybean (Hydrogenated)									
1 stick (113g)	812	91	19	0	1	0	0	1	1066
Margarine, Vegetable Oil Spread, 70% Fat, Soybean and Part Hydrogenated Soybean, Stick									
1 tbsp (1 NLEA serving) (14g)	88	10	2	0	0	0	0	0	98
Margarine-like Shortening, Industrial, Soy (Part Hydrogenated), Cottonseed and Soy									
1 tbsp (14g)	88	10	3	0	0	0	0	0	121
Margarine-like Spread with Yogurt, 70% Fat, Stick, with Salt									
1 tbsp (14g)	88	10	2	0	0	0	0	0	83
Margarine-like Spread with Yogurt, Approximately 40% Fat, Tub, with Salt									
1 tbsp (14g)	46	5	1	0	0	0	0	0	88
Margarine-like Spread, Benecol Light Spread									
1 tbsp (1 NLEA serving) (14g)	50	5	1	0	1	0	0	0	94
Margarine-like Spread, Smart Balance Light Buttery Spread									
1 tbsp (14g)	47	5	1	0	0	0	0	0	81

Food Serving size	Cal.	(g) Total Fat	(g) Sat. Fat	(mg) Chol.	(g) Carb.	(g) Fiber	(g) Sug.	(g) Prot.	(mg) Sod.
Margarine-like Spread, Smart Balance Omega Plus Spread									
1 tbsp (14g)	85	10	3	3	0	0	0	0	102
Margarine-like Spread, Smart Balance Regular Buttery Spread									
1 tbsp (14g)	82	9	2	0	0	0	0	0	90
Margarine-like Spread, Smart Beat, Smart Squeeze									
1 tbsp (14g)	7	0	0	0	1	0	0	0	116
Margarine-like Spread, Smart Beat, Super Light Without Saturated Fat									
1 tbsp (14g)	22	2	0	0	0	0	0	0	106
Margarine-like, Butter-margarine Blend, 80% Fat, Stick, Without Salt									
1 tbsp (14g)	101	11	4	12	0	0	0	0	4
Margarine-like, Margarine-butter Blend, Soybean Oil and Butter									
1 cup (227g)	1650	182	32	27	2	0	0	1	1632
Margarine-like, Vegetable Oil Spread, 20% Fat, Without Salt									
1 cup (205g)	359	40	6	0	1	0	0	0	0
Margarine-like, Vegetable Oil Spread, Stick or Tub, Sweetened									
1 tbsp (14g)	75	7	1	0	2	0	0	0	76
Margarine-like, Vegetable Oil, Spread, 20% Fat, with Salt									
1 cup (240g)	420	47	7	0	1	0	0	0	1759
Margarine-like, Vegetable Oil, Spread, 60% Fat, Stick, with Salt, with Added Vitamin D									
1 cup (229g)	NA	75	8	2	0	0	0	0	110
Margarine-like, Vegetable Oil, Spread, 60% Fat, Stick/tub/bottle, with Salt, with Added Vitamin D									
1 cup (229g)	1225	135	23	2	0	0	0	1	1798
Margarine-like, Vegetable Oil, Spread, 60% Fat, Tub, with Salt, with Added Vitamin D									
1 cup (229g)	1221	137	28	2	2	0	0	0	1798
Margarine-like, Vegetable Oil, Spread, Fat Free, Tub									
1 cup (233g)	103	7	5	0	10	0	0	0	1351
Margarine-like, Vegetable Oil-butter Spread, Reduced Calorie, Tub with Salt									
1 tbsp (14g)	63	7	2	10	0	0	0	0	85
Margarine-like, Vegetable Oil-butter Spread, Tub, with Salt									
1 tbsp (14g)	51	6	1	0	0	0	0	0	110
Meat Drippings (Lard, Beef Tallow, Mutton Tallow)									
1 oz (28.35g)	252	28	13	29	0	0	0	0	155

Food Serving size	Cal.	(g) Total Fat	(g) Sat. Fat	(mg) Chol.	(g) Carb.	(g) Fiber	(g) Sug.	(g) Prot.	(mg) Sod.
Oil, Cocoa Butter									
1 cup (218g)	1927	218	130	0	0	0	0	0	0
Oil, Pam Cooking Spray, Original									
1 spray, about 1/3 second (1 NLEA serving) (0.3g)	0	0	0	0	0	0	0	0	0

Salad Dressings

Food Serving size	Cal.	Total Fat	Sat. Fat	Chol.	Carb.	Fiber	Sug.	Prot.	Sod.
Creamy Dressing, Made with Sour Cream and/or Buttermilk and Oil, Reduced Calorie									
1 cup (245g)	392	34	5	0	17	0	9	4	2744
Creamy Dressing, Made with Sour Cream and/or Buttermilk and Oil, Reduced Calorie, Fat Free									
1 cup (264g)	282	7	1	0	53	0	0	4	2368
Creamy Dressing, with Sour Cream and/or Buttermilk and Oil, Reduced Calorie, Cholesterol Free									
1 cup (234g)	328	19	3	0	37	0	0	2	2181
Mayonnaise, Reduced Fat, with Olive Oil									
1 cup (232g)	838	93	12	77	0	0	0	1	1856
Mayonnaise Dressing, No Cholesterol									
1 cup (239g)	1644	186	26	0	1	0	90	0	1162
Oil, Almond									
1 cup (218g)	1927	218	18	0	0	0	0	0	0
Oil, Apricot Kernel									
1 cup (218g)	1927	218	14	0	0	0	0	0	0
Oil, Avocado									
1 cup (218g)	1927	218	25	0	0	0	0	0	0
Oil, Babassu									
1 cup (218g)	1927	218	177	0	0	0	0	0	0
Oil, Canola									
1 cup (218g)	1927	218	16	0	0	0	0	0	0
Oil, Coconut									
1 cup (218g)	1879	218	189	0	0	0	0	0	0
Oil, Cooking and Salad, Enova, 80% Diglycerides									
1 cup (214g)	1892	214	10	0	0	0	0	0	0
Oil, Corn or Canola									
1 cup (224g)	1980	224	18	0	0	0	14	0	0

Food Serving size	Cal.	(g) Total Fat	(g) Sat. Fat	(mg) Chol.	(g) Carb.	(g) Fiber	(g) Sug.	(g) Prot.	(mg) Sod.
Oil, Corn, Industrial and Retail, All Purpose Salad or Cooking									
1 cup (218g)	1962	218	28	0	0	0	0	0	0
Oil, Corn, Peanut, and Olive									
1 teaspoon (4.5g)	40	5	1	0	0	0	3	0	0
Oil, Cottonseed, Salad or Cooking									
1 cup (218g)	1927	218	56	0	0	0	0	0	0
Oil, Cupu Assu									
1 cup (218g)	1927	218	116	0	0	0	0	0	0
Oil, Fish Oil, Cod Liver									
1 tbsp (13.6g)	123	14	3	78	0	0	0	0	0
Oil, Fish Oil, Salmon									
1 tsp (4.5g)	41	5	1	22	0	0	0	0	0
Oil, Flaxseed									
1 cup (218g)	1927	218	20	0	0	0	0	0	0
Oil, Flaxseed, Contains Added Sliced Flaxseed									
1 cup (219g)	1923	217	20	0	1	0	0	1	13
Oil, Grape Seed									
1 cup (218g)	1927	218	21	0	0	0	0	0	0
Oil, Hazelnut									
1 cup (218g)	1927	218	16	0	0	0	0	0	0
Oil, Industrial, Canola (Part Hydrogenated) Oil for Deep Fat Frying									
1 tablespoon (4.5g)	40	5	0	0	0	0	0	0	0
Oil, Industrial, Canola for Salads, Woks, and Light Frying									
1 teaspoon (4.5g)	40	5	0	0	0	0	0	0	0
Oil, Industrial, Canola with Antifoaming Agent									
1 cup (218g)	1927	218	17	0	0	0	0	0	0
Oil, Industrial, Canola, Hi Oleic									
1 cup (218g)	1962	218	15	0	0	0	0	0	0
Oil, Industrial, Coconut									
1 cup (218g)	1927	218	187	0	0	0	0	0	0
Oil, Industrial, Coconut (Hydrogenated), for Toppings and Whiteners									
1 cup (218g)	1918	217	204	0	0	0	0	0	15
Oil, Industrial, Coconut, Confection Fat, Ice Cream Coatings									
1 cup (218g)	1927	218	189	0	0	0	0	0	11

Food Serving size	Cal.	(g) Total Fat	(g) Sat. Fat	(mg) Chol.	(g) Carb.	(g) Fiber	(g) Sug.	(g) Prot.	(mg) Sod.
Oil, Industrial, Cottonseed, Fully Hydrogentated									
1 cup (218g)	1927	218	204	0	0	0	0	0	0
Oil, Industrial, Mid Oleic, Sunflower									
1 teaspoon (4.5g)	40	5	0	0	0	0	0	0	0
Oil, Industrial, Palm and Palm Kernel, Filling Fat (Non-hydrogenated)									
1 cup (218g)	1918	217	156	0	0	0	0	0	13
Oil, Industrial, Palm Kernel (Hydrogenated), Filling Fat									
1 cup (218g)	1927	218	192	0	0	0	0	0	13
Oil, Industrial, Palm Kernel, Confection Fat									
1 cup (218g)	1927	218	191	0	0	0	0	0	13
Oil, Industrial, Soy (Part Hydrogenated) and Soy, Pourable Frying									
1 cup (218g)	1927	218	33	0	0	0	0	0	0
Oil, Industrial, Soy (Part Hydrogenated) for Non-diary Butter Flavor									
1 cup (218g)	1927	218	39	0	0	0	0	0	0
Oil, Industrial, Soy (Part Hydrogenated), All Purpose									
1 cup (218g)	1927	218	54	0	0	0	0	0	0
Oil, Industrial, Soy (Part Hydrogenated), for Popcorn and Flavoring Vegetables									
1 cup (218g)	1927	218	39	0	0	0	0	0	0
Oil, Industrial, Soy, Refined, for Woks and Light Frying									
1 cup (218g)	1927	218	33	0	0	0	0	0	0
Oil, Industrial, Soy, Ultra Lo Linolenic									
1 cup (218g)	1927	218	32	0	0	0	0	0	0
Oil, Mustard									
1 cup (218g)	1927	218	25	0	0	0	0	0	0
Oil, Nutmeg, Butter									
1 cup (218g)	1927	218	196	0	0	0	0	0	0
Oil, Oat									
1 cup (218g)	1927	218	43	0	0	0	0	0	0
Oil, Olive, Salad or Cooking									
1 cup (216g)	1909	216	30	0	0	0	0	0	4
Oil, Palm									
1 cup (216g)	1909	216	106	0	0	0	0	0	0
Oil, Peanut, Salad or Cooking									
1 cup (216g)	1909	216	37	0	0	0	0	0	0

Food Serving size	Cal.	(g) Total Fat	(g) Sat. Fat	(mg) Chol.	(g) Carb.	(g) Fiber	(g) Sug.	(g) Prot.	(mg) Sod.
Oil, Poppy Seed 1 cup (218g)	1927	218	29	0	0	0	0	0	0
Oil, Rice Bran 1 cup (218g)	1927	218	43	0	0	0	0	0	0
Oil, Safflower, Salad or Cooking, Hi Oleic 1 cup (218g)	1927	218	16	0	0	0	0	0	0
Oil, Safflower, Salad or Cooking, Linoleic (Over 70%) 1 cup (218g)	1927	218	14	0	0	0	0	0	0
Oil, Salad or Cooking 1 cup (216g)	1909	216	30	0	0	0	0	0	4
Oil, Sesame, Salad or Cooking 1 cup (218g)	1927	218	31	0	0	0	0	0	0
Oil, Soybean Lecithin 1 cup (218g)	1663	218	33	0	0	0	0	0	0
Oil, Soybean, Salad or Cooking 1 cup (218g)	1927	218	34	0	0	0	0	0	0
Oil, Sunflower, Hi Oleic (70% and Over) 1 cup (218g)	1927	218	21	0	0	0	0	0	0
Oil, Sunflower, Linoleic (Approximately 65%) 1 cup (218g)	1927	218	22	0	0	0	0	0	0
Oil, Sunflower, Linoleic (Less than 60%) 1 cup (218g)	1927	218	22	0	0	0	0	0	0
Oil, Sunflower, Linoleic (Partially Hydrogenated) 1 cup (218g)	1927	218	28	0	0	0	0	0	0
Oil, Tomato Seed 1 cup (218g)	1927	218	43	0	0	0	0	0	0
Oil, Vegetable, Natreon Canola, Hi Stability, Non Trans, Hi Oleic (70%) 1 tbsp (14g)	124	14	1	0	0	0	0	0	0
Oil, Walnut 1 cup (218g)	1927	218	20	0	0	0	0	0	0
Oil, Wheat Germ 1 tbsp (13.6g)	120	14	3	0	0	0	0	0	0
Vegetable Oil, Palm Kernel 1 cup (218g)	1879	218	178	0	0	0	0	0	0

Food Serving size	Cal.	(g) Total Fat	(g) Sat. Fat	(mg) Chol.	(g) Carb.	(g) Fiber	(g) Sug.	(g) Prot.	(mg) Sod.
Salad Dressing, Bacon and Tomato									
1 cup (240g)	782	84	13	10	5	0.5	4	4	2172
Salad Dressing, Blue or Roquefort Cheese, Low Calorie									
1 cup (245g)	243	18	6	2	7	0	0	12	2301
Salad Dressing, Buttermilk, Lite									
1 serving (2 tbsp) (30g)	61	4	0	5	6	0.3	6	0	336
Salad Dressing, Caesar Dressing, Regular									
1 cup (235g)	1274	136	21	92	8	1.2	1	5	2841
Salad Dressing, Caesar, Low Calorie									
1 cup (240g)	264	11	2	5	45	0.2	0	1	2755
Salad Dressing, Cole Slaw									
1 cup (250g)	975	84	12	65	60	0.3	0	2	1775
Salad Dressing, Cole Slaw Dressing, Reduced Fat									
1 cup (269g)	885	54	8	67	108	1.1	0	0	4304
Salad Dressing, French Dressing, Commercial, Regular									
1 cup (250g)	1143	112	14	0	39	0	40	2	2090
Salad Dressing, French Dressing, Commercial, Regular, Without Salt									
1 tablespoon (15g)	69	7	1	0	2	0	2	0	0
Salad Dressing, French Dressing, Fat Free									
1 cup (256g)	338	1	0	0	82	5.6	42	1	2184
Salad Dressing, French Dressing, Reduced Calorie									
1 cup (260g)	520	34	5	0	70	0	0	1	2179
Salad Dressing, French Dressing, Reduced Fat									
1 cup (260g)	577	30	2	0	81	3.9	44	2	2179
Salad Dressing, French Dressing, Reduced Fat, Without Salt									
1 cup (260g)	606	35	3	0	76	2.9	74	2	78
Salad Dressing, French, Cottonseed, Oil, Home Recipe									
1 cup (220g)	1388	154	40	0	7	0	0	0	1448
Salad Dressing, French, Home Recipe									
1 cup (220g)	1388	154	28	0	7	0	0	0	1448
Salad Dressing, Green Goddess, Regular									
1 cup (245g)	1046	106	15	98	18	0.2	0	5	2124
Salad Dressing, Home Recipe, Cooked									
1 cup (255g)	400	24	7	145	38	0	23	11	1872

Food Serving size	Cal.	(g) Total Fat	(g) Sat. Fat	(mg) Chol.	(g) Carb.	(g) Fiber	(g) Sug.	(g) Prot.	(mg) Sod.
Salad Dressing, Home Recipe, Vinegar and Oil									
1 cup (250g)	1123	125	23	0	6	0	6	0	3
Salad Dressing, Honey Mustard Dressing, Reduced Calorie									
2 tbsp (1 serving) (30g)	62	3	0	0	8	0.2	5	0	210
Salad Dressing, Italian Dressing, Fat Free									
1 cup (231g)	109	2	1	5	20	1.4	20	2	2608
Salad Dressing, Italian Dressing, Reduced Calorie									
1 cup (216g)	432	43	6	0	14	0.4	0	1	2320
Salad Dressing, Italian Dressing, Reduced Fat									
1 cup (240g)	245	16	2	0	24	0	22	1	2138
Salad Dressing, Italian Dressing, Reduced Fat, Without Salt									
1 cup (240g)	182	15	1	14	11	0	11	1	72
Salad Dressing, Kraft, Mayonnaise, Fat Free Mayonnaise									
1 tbsp (16g)	11	0	0	2	2	0.3	1	0	120
Salad Dressing, Kraft, Mayonnaise, Light Mayonnaise									
1 tbsp (15g)	50	5	1	5	1	0	1	0	95
Salad Dressing, Kraft, Miracle Whip Free Non-fat Dressing									
1 tbsp (16g)	13	0	0	1	2	0.3	2	0	126
Salad Dressing, Kraft, Miracle Whip Light Dressing									
1 tbsp (16g)	37	3	0	4	2	0	2	0	131
Salad Dressing, Mayonnaise, Imitation, Soybean Without Cholesterol									
1 cup (225g)	1085	107	17	0	36	0	14	0	794
Salad Dressing, Mayonnaise, Light									
1 tablespoon (15g)	36	3	1	2	1	0	1	0	124
Salad Dressing, Mayonnaise, Light, Smart Balance, Omega Plus Light									
1 tbsp (1 NLEA serving) (14g)	47	5	0	5	1	0	1	0	119
Salad Dressing, Mayonnaise, Soybean and Safflower Oil, with Salt									
1 cup (220g)	1577	175	19	130	6	0	1	2	1250
Salad Dressing, Mayonnaise, Soybean Oil, with Salt									
1 cup (220g)	1580	175	26	84	7	0	2	2	1250
Salad Dressing, Mayonnaise, Soybean Oil, Without Salt									
1 cup (220g)	1577	175	26	130	6	0	0	2	66
Salad Dressing, Mayonnaise-like, Fat Free									
1 cup (256g)	215	7	2	23	40	4.9	0	1	2017

Food Serving size	Cal.	(g) Total Fat	(g) Sat. Fat	(mg) Chol.	(g) Carb.	(g) Fiber	(g) Sug.	(g) Prot.	(mg) Sod.
Salad Dressing, Mayonnaise-type, Regular with Salt									
1 cup (220g)	1496	165	26	92	1	0	1	2	1397
Salad Dressing, Peppercorn Dressing, Commercial, Regular									
1 fl oz (26g)	147	16	3	13	1	0	0	0	287
Salad Dressing, Ranch Dressing, Commercial, Regular									
1 serving (30g)	126	13	2	8	2	0	1	0	270
Salad Dressing, Ranch Dressing, Fat Free									
1 tablespoon (14g)	17	0	0	1	4	0	1	0	126
Salad Dressing, Ranch Dressing, Reduced Fat									
1 serving (2 tbsp) (30g)	59	4	0	5	6	0.3	1	0	336
Salad Dressing, Russian Dressing									
1 cup (245g)	870	64	6	0	78	1.7	43	2	2776
Salad Dressing, Russian Dressing, Low Calorie									
1 cup (260g)	367	10	2	16	72	0.8	57	1	2257
Salad Dressing, Sesame Seed Dressing, Regular									
1 cup (245g)	1085	111	15	0	21	2.5	20	8	2450
Salad Dressing, Spray-style Dressing, Assorted Flavors									
1 serving (approximately 10 sprays) (8g)	13	1	0	0	1	0	1	0	88
Salad Dressing, Sweet and Sour									
1 cup (250g)	38	0	0	0	9	0	0	0	520
Salad Dressing, Thousand Island Dressing, Commercial, Regular									
1 cup (250g)	948	88	13	65	37	2	38	3	2405
Salad Dressing, Thousand Island Dressing, Fat Free									
1 cup (256g)	338	4	1	13	75	8.4	43	1	2017
Salad Dressing, Thousand Island Dressing, Reduced Fat									
1 cup (245g)	478	28	2	27	59	2.9	42	2	2340
Vinegar, Balsamic									
1 tbsp (16g)	14	0	0	0	3	0	2	0	4
Vinegar, Cider									
1 cup (239g)	50	0	0	0	2	0	1	0	12
Vinegar, Distilled									
1 cup (238g)	43	0	0	0	0	0	0	0	5
Vinegar, Red Wine									
1 cup (239g)	45	0	0	0	1	0	0	0	19

Snacks and Sweets

Why Eat Snacks?

Snacks are important to keep you energized throughout the day, especially when the time between meals is longer than 4 hours. This is the amount of time it takes for the food you eat to be digested, metabolized, and assimilated into your body cells, where it is used for energy and other maintenance tasks. After about 4 hours, your body will start sending hunger messages and may start slowing down, so a snack between meals can help you stay alert and control hunger. Avoiding extreme hunger may help you choose more appropriate portion sizes at meals. The important thing is to make nutritious snack choices that don't contain empty calories.

Daily Goal

Plan two healthy snacks each day.
Avoid "empty calories" in added sugar and solid fats.

Shopping Tips

- Keep nuts and seeds handy.
- Prepare cut-up fruits and vegetables and store in the refrigerator.
- Air-popped corn is a whole grain snack.
- Whole grain cereal makes a good snack.
- Low-fat or fat-free yogurt is a good choice, providing protein and calcium.

Shopping List Essentials

Nuts, dry-roasted or raw   Fruits
Seeds, dry-roasted or raw   Vegetables
Popcorn   Yogurt
Dried fruit

Red Flags

Avoid "empty calories" in added sugar and solid fats. "Empty calorie" foods and beverages provide calories but few or no nutrients. Solid fats can be butter or shortening used in baked or fried foods, or they can be other fats added in processing that result in trans fats. Check ingredients lists for the term "partially hydrogenated fats." This indicates the presence of trans fats—even when the Nutrition Facts say "0 grams trans fat." Be wary of snack bars and protein bars that may contain high amounts of fats and calories. Many snack/protein bars are more like candy bars than nutritious snacks.

Preparation Pointer

Even the healthiest snack choices need to be portion controlled. Break down large containers of nuts, pretzels, crackers, and dried fruit into single servings (snack-size, zip-seal plastic bags work well, as do reusable small plastic containers with snap-on lids) before storing. For snacking, raw vegetables go well with low-fat dips like hummus, yogurt-dill sauce, or ranch-style dressing.

Food Serving size	Cal.	(g) Total Fat	(g) Sat. Fat	(mg) Chol.	(g) Carb.	(g) Fiber	(g) Sug.	(g) Prot.	(mg) Sod.
Candies									
Candies, 5th Avenue Candy Bar 1 bar, snack size (16g)	77	4	1	1	10	0.5	8	1	36
Candies, Almond Joy Bites 18 pieces (40g)	225	14	8	4	23	1.7	21	2	16
Candies, Almond Joy, Candy Bar 1 bar, snack size (19g)	91	5	3	1	11	1	9	1	27
Candies, Butterscotch 3 pieces (16g)	63	1	0	1	14	0	13	0	63
Candies, Caramello Candy Bar 1 bar, 1.6 oz (45g)	208	10	6	12	29	0.5	26	3	55
Candies, Caramels 1 piece (10.1g)	39	1	0	1	8	0	7	0	25
Candies, Caramels, Chocolate-flavor Roll 1 piece (6.6g)	26	0	0	0	6	0	4	0	3
Candies, Carob, Unsweetened 1 bar (3 oz) (87g)	470	27	25	1	49	3.3	30	7	93
Candies, Chocolate Covered, Caramel with Nuts 1 piece (14g)	66	3	1	0	8	0.6	0	1	3
Candies, Confectioner's Coating, Butterscotch 1 oz (28.35g)	153	8	7	0	19	0	19	1	25
Candies, Dark Chocolate Coated Coffee Beans 1 serving, 28 pieces (40g)	216	12	6	5	24	3	17	3	10
Candies, Divinity, Prepared from Recipe 1 piece (11g)	40	0	0	0	10	0	9	0	4
Candies, Fudge, Chocolate Marshmallow, Prepared from Recipe 1 recipe, yields (60 pieces) (1229g)	5567	215	131	307	877	20.9	787	28	1045
Candies, Fudge, Chocolate, Prepared from Recipe 1 piece (17g)	70	2	1	2	13	0.3	12	0	8
Candies, Fudge, Peanut Butter, Prepared from Recipe 1 piece (16g)	62	1	0	0	12	0.1	12	1	19
Candies, Hard 1 piece (6g)	24	0	0	0	6	0	4	0	2

Food Serving size	Cal.	(g) Total Fat	(g) Sat. Fat	(mg) Chol.	(g) Carb.	(g) Fiber	(g) Sug.	(g) Prot.	(mg) Sod.
Candies, Hard, Dietetic or Low Calorie (Sorbitol)									
1 piece (3g)	12	0	0	0	3	0	0	0	0
Candies, Heath Bites									
15 pieces (39g)	207	12	6	7	25	0.8	23	2	96
Candies, Hershey, Kit Kat Big Kat Bar									
1 bar, king size 2.8 oz (79g)	411	22	14	7	50	1.5	43	5	51
Candies, Hershey, Reesesticks Crispy Wafers, Peanut Butter, Milk Chocolate									
1 serving, 1.5 oz (42g)	219	13	6	3	23	1.4	17	4	111
Candies, Hershey's Golden Almond Solitaires									
13 pieces (41g)	234	15	6	5	19	1.8	15	5	21
Candies, Hershey's Milk Chocolate with Almond Bites									
17 pieces (39g)	215	14	7	7	20	1.4	17	4	29
Candies, Hershey's Pot of Gold Almond Bar									
1 bar, 2.8 oz (78g)	450	30	13	10	36	3	30	10	50
Candies, Kit Kat Wafer Bar									
1 bar, miniature (.35 oz) (10g)	52	3	2	1	6	0.1	5	1	5
Candies, Krackel Chocolate Bar									
1 bar, 2 oz (56g)	287	15	9	6	36	1.2	29	4	110
Candies, Mars Snack US, Cocoavia Blueberry and Almond Chocolate Bar									
1 serving, 0.78 oz bar (22g)	116	6	3	0	13	2	9	1	2
Candies, Mars Snack US, Pop'ables 3 Musketeers Bite Size									
1 serving, 15 pieces (41g)	182	6	4	3	31	0.5	27	1	71
Candies, Mars Snack US, Starburst Fruit Chews, Fruit and Cream									
1 serving, fun size (8 chews) (40g)	163	3	3	0	33	0	23	0	1
Candies, Mars Snackfood US, 3 Musketeers Bar									
1 serving, 2 fun size bars (28g)	122	4	2	1	22	0.4	19	1	54
Candies, Mars Snackfood US, Cocoavia Chocolate Bar									
1 serving, 0.78 oz bar (22g)	119	6	3	0	14	1.9	9	1	2
Candies, Mars Snackfood US, Cocoavia Chocolate Covered Almonds									
1 serving, 1 oz pack (28g)	160	10	3	0	14	2.9	8	3	3
Candies, Mars Snackfood US, Cocoavia Crispy Chocolate Bar									
1 serving, 0.7 oz bar (20g)	103	5	3	0	12	1.6	7	2	8
Candies, Mars Snackfood US, Dove Dark Chocolate									
1 serving, 7 pieces (42g)	218	14	8	3	25	3.2	19	2	2

Food Serving size	Cal.	(g) Total Fat	(g) Sat. Fat	(mg) Chol.	(g) Carb.	(g) Fiber	(g) Sug.	(g) Prot.	(mg) Sod.
Candies, Mars Snackfood US, Dove Milk Chocolate									
1 serving, 5 pieces (40g)	218	13	8	7	24	1	22	2	25
Candies, Mars Snackfood US, M&M's Crispy Chocolate Candies									
1 serving, 1.6 oz bag (47g)	223	9	5	6	34	0.9	28	2	64
Candies, Mars Snackfood US, M&M's Milk Chocolate Candies									
1 box (1.48 oz) (42g)	207	9	5	6	30	1.2	27	2	26
Candies, Mars Snackfood US, M&M's Minis Milk Chocolate Candies									
1 serving, 0.50 oz box (15g)	75	4	2	2	10	0.4	9	1	10
Candies, Mars Snackfood US, M&M's Peanut Chocolate Candies									
1 package, fun size (18g)	93	5	2	1	11	0.7	9	2	9
Candies, Mars Snackfood US, Mars Almond Bar									
1 bar (1.76 oz) (50g)	234	12	4	9	31	1	26	4	85
Candies, Mars Snackfood US, Milky Way Bar									
1 bar, fun size (17g)	78	3	2	2	12	0.2	10	1	28
Candies, Mars Snackfood US, Milky Way Caramel, Dark Chocolate Covered									
1 serving, 5 pieces (44g)	202	9	6	7	30	1.2	24	2	108
Candies, Mars Snackfood US, Milky Way Caramel, Milk Chocolate Covered									
1 serving, 5 pieces (44g)	204	8	6	9	30	0.3	26	2	120
Candies, Mars Snackfood US, Pop Milky Way Bite Size									
1 serving, 13 pieces (39g)	181	7	3	4	28	0.4	24	1	57
Candies, Mars Snackfood US, Pop Snickers Bite Size Candies									
1 serving, 13 pieces (39g)	187	9	4	5	24	0.9	20	3	87
Candies, Mars Snackfood US, Skittles Original Bite Size Candies									
1 cup (205g)	830	9	8	0	186	0	155	0	31
Candies, Mars Snackfood US, Skittles Sours Original									
1 serving, 1.80 oz bag (51g)	205	2	2	0	46	0	37	0	7
Candies, Mars Snackfood US, Skittles Tropical Bite Size Candies									
1 serving, fun size bag (20g)	81	1	0	0	18	0	15	0	3
Candies, Mars Snackfood US, Skittles Wild Berry Bite Size									
1 serving, fun size bag (20g)	80	1	1	0	18	0	15	0	3
Candies, Mars Snackfood US, Snickers Almond Bar									
1 serving, 1.76 oz bar (50g)	236	11	4	7	32	1.3	27	3	78
Candies, Mars Snackfood US, Snickers Bar									
1 bar, fun size (15g)	74	4	1	2	9	0.3	8	1	36

Food Serving size	Cal.	(g) Total Fat	(g) Sat. Fat	(mg) Chol.	(g) Carb.	(g) Fiber	(g) Sug.	(g) Prot.	(mg) Sod.
Candies, Mars Snackfood US, Snickers Cruncher									
1 bar, fun size (15g)	73	4	2	1	9	0.3	7	1	28
Candies, Mars Snackfood US, Snickers Munch Bar									
1 serving, 1.42 oz bar (40g)	214	14	4	10	17	1.9	12	6	143
Candies, Mars Snackfood US, Starburst Fruit Chews, Original Fruit									
1 serving, 2.07 oz pack (59g)	241	5	5	0	49	0	34	0	1
Candies, Mars Snackfood US, Starburst Fruit Chews, Tropical									
1 serving, 2.07 oz pack (59g)	241	5	5	0	49	0	34	0	1
Candies, Mars Snackfood US, Starburst Sour Fruit Chews									
1 serving, 2.07 oz pack (59g)	236	5	4	0	47	0	33	0	53
Candies, Mars Snackfood US, Twix Caramel Cookie Bars									
1 package (2.06 oz, 2 bars) (58g)	291	14	11	4	38	0.6	28	3	115
Candies, Mars Snackfood US, Twix Peanut Butter Cookie Bars									
1 package (2.06 oz, 2 bars) (58g)	311	19	9	3	31	1.8	21	5	131
Candies, Mars, M&M's Almond Chocolate Candies									
1 serving, about 1/4 cup (42g)	219	12	4	3	25	2.4	0	3	19
Candies, Mars, M&M's Peanut Butter Chocolate Candies									
1 cup (203g)	1074	60	38	14	115	8.1	0	21	432
Candies, Mars, Milky Way Midnight Bar									
1 bar, fun size (19g)	84	3	2	2	14	0.6	0	1	32
Candies, Marshmallows									
10 miniatures (7g)	22	0	0	0	6	0	4	0	6
Candies, Milk Chocolate									
1 bar, miniature (7g)	37	2	1	2	4	0.2	4	1	6
Candies, Milk Chocolate Coated Peanuts									
10 pieces (40g)	208	13	6	4	20	1.9	15	5	16
Candies, Milk Chocolate Coated Raisins									
10 pieces (10g)	39	1	1	0	7	0.3	6	0	4
Candies, Milk Chocolate, with Almonds									
1 bar (1.55 oz) (44g)	231	15	8	8	23	2.7	19	4	33
Candies, Milk Chocolate, with Rice Cereal									
1 bar (1.45 oz) (45g)	230	13	7	10	27	1.5	23	3	39

Food Serving size	Cal.	(g) Total Fat	(g) Sat. Fat	(mg) Chol.	(g) Carb.	(g) Fiber	(g) Sug.	(g) Prot.	(mg) Sod.
Candies, Mounds Candy Bar 1 package, 1.9 oz (53g)	258	14	11	1	31	2	24	2	77
Candies, Mr. Goodbar Chocolate Bar 1 bar (2.6 oz) (73g)	393	24	10	7	40	2.8	34	7	30
Candies, Nestle, 100 Grand Bar 1 bar, miniature (21g)	98	4	2	3	15	0.2	11	1	43
Candies, Nestle, After Eight Mints 1 piece (8.4g)	36	1	1	0	7	0.2	6	0	0
Candies, Nestle, Raisinets Chocolate Covered Raisins 1 serving, fun size (48g)	203	8	5	5	34	1.1	28	2	16
Candies, Nougat, with Almonds 1 piece (14g)	56	0	0	0	13	0.5	0	0	5
Candies, Peanut Bar 1 bar (1.4 oz) (40g)	209	13	2	0	19	1.6	17	6	62
Candies, Praline, Prepared from Recipe 1 recipe, yields (907g)	4399	235	20	0	540	31.7	506	30	435
Candies, Reese's Bites 16 pieces (39g)	203	12	7	3	22	1.2	19	4	70
Candies, Reese's Fast Break, Candy Bar 1 serving, 1 bar (56g)	277	13	5	5	36	2	30	5	180
Candies, Reese's Nutrageous Candy Bar 2 bars (34g)	176	11	3	1	18	1.3	14	4	48
Candies, Reese's Peanut Butter Cups 1 package, 1.6 oz 2 cups (45g)	232	14	5	3	25	1.6	21	5	161
Candies, Reese's Pieces Candy 10 pieces (8g)	40	2	1	0	5	0.2	4	1	16
Candies, Reese's, Fast Break, Milk Chocolate Peanut Butter and Soft Nuggets 2 oz, bar (56g)	265	13	5	2	34	1.6	30	5	185
Candies, Rolo Caramels in Milk Chocolate 7 pieces (42g)	199	9	6	5	29	0.4	27	2	79
Candies, Semisweet Chocolate 1 cup, large chips (182g)	874	55	32	0	116	10.7	99	8	20
Candies, Semisweet Chocolate, Made with Butter 1 cup, large chips (182g)	868	54	32	33	115	10.7	0	8	20

Food Serving size	Cal.	(g) Total Fat	(g) Sat. Fat	(mg) Chol.	(g) Carb.	(g) Fiber	(g) Sug.	(g) Prot.	(mg) Sod.
Candies, Sesame Crunch									
1 piece (1.8g)	9	1	0	0	1	0.1	1	0	3
Candies, Skor Toffee Bar									
1 bar, 1.4 oz (39g)	209	13	7	21	24	0.5	23	1	124
Candies, Special Dark Chocolate Bar									
1 bar, 2.6 oz (73g)	406	24	0	4	44	4.7	35	4	4
Candies, Sugar-coated Almonds									
1 piece (3.5g)	17	1	0	0	2	0.1	2	0	0
Candies, Sweet Chocolate									
1 bar (1.45 oz) (41g)	208	14	8	0	25	2.3	21	2	7
Candies, Sweet Chocolate Coated Fondant									
1 patty, small (11g)	40	1	1	0	9	0.2	8	0	3
Candies, Symphony, Milk Chocolate Bar									
1 bar, 2.4 oz (68g)	361	21	12	16	39	1.2	37	6	69
Candies, Taffy, Prepared from Recipe									
1 piece (15g)	60	0	0	1	14	0	10	0	8
Candies, Toffee, Prepared from Recipe									
1 piece (12g)	67	4	2	12	8	0	8	0	16
Candies, Tootsie Roll, Chocolate Flavor Roll									
1 piece (6.6g)	26	0	0	0	6	0	4	0	3
Candies, Truffles, Prepared from Recipe									
1 recipe, yield, recipe makes 49 1" x 1" pieces (612g)	3121	207	113	324	275	15.3	234	38	416
Candies, Twizzlers Cherry Bites									
18 pieces (40g)	135	1	0	0	32	0	0	1	104
Candies, Twizzlers Nibs Cherry Bits									
27 pieces (40g)	139	1	0	0	32	0.2	21	1	78
Candies, Twizzlers Strawberry Twists Candy									
4 pieces, from 5 oz package (38g)	133	1	0	0	30	0	15	1	109
Candies, Whatchamacallit Candy Bar									
1 bar, 1.7 oz (48g)	237	11	8	6	30	0.9	23	4	144
Candies, White Chocolate									
1 bar (3 oz) (85g)	458	27	17	18	50	0.2	50	5	77

Food Serving size	Cal.	(g) Total Fat	(g) Sat. Fat	(mg) Chol.	(g) Carb.	(g) Fiber	(g) Sug.	(g) Prot.	(mg) Sod.
Candies, York Bites 15 pieces (39g)	154	3	2	0	32	0.8	29	1	18
Candies, York Peppermint Pattie 1 patty, 1.5 oz (43g)	165	3	2	0	35	0.9	27	1	12
Heinz, Weight Watchers, Chocolate Éclair, Frozen 1 eclair, frozen (59g)	142	4	1	28	24	1.2	10	3	177
McKee Baking, Little Debbie Nut Bar, Wafer with Peanut Butter, Chocolate Covered 1 serving (57g)	312	19	4	0	31	0	19	5	127
Snacks, Farley Candy, Farley Fruit Snacks, with Vitamins A, C, and E 1 pouch (26g)	89	0	0	0	21	0	0	1	9
Snacks, General Mills, Betty Crocker Fruit Roll Ups, Berry Flavored with Vitamin C 2 rolls (28g)	104	1	0	0	24	0	11	0	89
Snacks, M&M Mars, Kudos Whole Grain Bar, M&M's Milk Chocolate 1 bar (24g)	100	3	2	1	18	0.6	0	1	82
Snacks, M&M Mars, Kudos Whole Grain Bar, Peanut Butter 1 bar (28g)	130	6	3	1	18	0.7	0	2	75
Snacks, M&M Mars, Kudos Whole Grain Bars, Chocolate Chip 1 bar (28g)	118	4	1	38	20	0.7	11	1	69
Snacks, Sunkist, Sunkist Fruit Roll, Strawberry with Vitamins A, C, and E 1 roll (21g)	72	0	0	0	17	1.6	0	0	23

Jellies, Jams, and Preserves

Food Serving size	Cal.	(g) Total Fat	(g) Sat. Fat	(mg) Chol.	(g) Carb.	(g) Fiber	(g) Sug.	(g) Prot.	(mg) Sod.
Candies, Gumdrops, Dietetic or Low Calorie (Sorbitol) 1 piece (5g)	8	0	0	0	4	0.9	0	0	0
Candies, Gumdrops, Starch Jelly Pieces 10 gumdrops (36g)	143	0	0	0	36	0	21	0	16
Candies, Jelly Beans 10 large (1 oz) (28g)	105	0	0	0	26	0.1	20	0	14
Cranberry-Orange Relish, Canned 1 cup (275g)	490	0	0	0	127	0	0	1	88
Desserts, Flan, Caramel Custard, Prepared from Recipe 1 recipe, yield (1531g)	2220	62	28	1378	349	0	354	69	811
Gelatin Dessert, Dry Mix 1 portion, amount to make 1/2 cup (21g)	80	0	0	0	19	0	18	2	98

Food Serving size	Cal.	(g) Total Fat	(g) Sat. Fat	(mg) Chol.	(g) Carb.	(g) Fiber	(g) Sug.	(g) Prot.	(mg) Sod.
Gelatin Dessert, Dry Mix, Prepared with Water									
.5 cup (135g)	84	0	0	0	19	0	18	2	101
Gelatin Dessert, Dry Mix, Reduced Calorie with Aspartame									
1 serving (6.4g)	13	0	0	0	5	0	0	1	55
Gelatin Dessert, Dry Mix, Reduced Calorie with Aspartame, Added Phosphorus, Potassium, Sodium, and Vitamin C									
1 package (0.35 oz) (10g)	35	0	0	0	3	0	0	6	275
Gelatin Dessert, Dry Mix, Reduced Calorie with Aspartame, No Added Sodium									
1 package (0.35 oz) (10g)	35	0	0	0	3	0	0	6	16
Gelatin Dessert, Dry Mix, Reduced Calorie with Aspartame, Prepared with Water									
1 package, yield (2 cups) (469g)	94	0	0	0	20	0	0	4	225
Gelatin Dessert, Dry Mix, with Added Vitamin C, Sodium-citrate, and Salt									
1 portion, amount to make 1/2 cup (21g)	80	0	0	0	19	0	0	2	103
Gelatins, Dry Powder, Unsweetened									
1 package (1 oz) (28g)	94	0	0	0	0	0	0	24	55
Jams and Preserves									
1 packet (0.5 oz) (14g)	39	0	0	0	10	0.2	7	0	4
Jams and Preserves, Apricot									
1 packet (0.5 oz) (14g)	34	0	0	0	9	0	6	0	6
Jams and Preserves, Dietetic (with Sodium Saccharin), Any Flavor									
1 tbsp (14g)	18	0	0	0	8	0.4	1	0	0
Jellies									
1 packet (0.5 oz) (14g)	37	0	0	0	10	0.1	7	0	4
Jellies, Reduced Sugar, Home Preserved									
1 tbsp (19g)	34	0	0	0	9	0.2	2	0	0
Marmalade, Orange									
1 tbsp (20g)	49	0	0	0	13	0.1	12	0	11
Pectin, Unsweetened, Dry Mix									
1 package (1.75 oz) (50g)	163	0	0	0	45	4.3	0	0	100
Pie Fillings, Apple, Canned									
.125 can (74g)	74	0	0	0	19	0.7	10	0	35
Pie Fillings, Blueberry, Canned									
1 cup (262g)	474	1	0	0	116	6.8	124	1	31

Food Serving size	Cal.	(g) Total Fat	(g) Sat. Fat	(mg) Chol.	(g) Carb.	(g) Fiber	(g) Sug.	(g) Prot.	(mg) Sod.
Pie Fillings, Cherry, Canned .125 can (74g)	85	0	0	0	21	0.4	0	0	13
Pie Fillings, Cherry, Low Calorie 1 cup (264g)	140	0	0	0	32	3.2	0	2	32

Misc. Candies (Gums, etc.)

Chewing Gum 10 Chiclets (16g)	58	0	0	0	15	0.4	11	0	0
Chewing Gum, Sugarless 1 piece (2g)	5	0	0	0	2	0	0	0	0
Snacks, Beef Sticks, Smoked 1 stick (20g)	110	10	4	27	1	0	0	4	306

Chips and Pretzels

Banana Chips 3 oz (85g)	441	29	25	0	50	6.5	30	2	5
Cheese Puffs and Twists, Corn Based, Baked, Low Fat 1 oz (28.35g)	122	3	1	0	21	3	2	2	240
Corn-based, Extruded, Chips, Barbecue Flavor 1 bag (7 oz) (198g)	1036	65	9	0	111	10.3	0	14	1511
Corn-based, Extruded, Chips, Barbecue Flavor, with Enriched Masa Flour 1 oz (28.35g)	148	9	1	0	16	0	0	2	216
Corn-based, Extruded, Chips, Plain 1 bag (7 oz) (198g)	1026	56	7	0	125	10.5	2	12	1079
Corn-based, Extruded, Chips, Unsalted 1 bag, single serving (28g)	156	9	1	0	16	1.2	3	2	4
Corn-based, Extruded, Cones, Nacho Flavor 1 oz (28.35g)	152	9	8	1	16	0.3	0	2	270
Corn-based, Extruded, Onion Flavor 2 oz (57g)	284	13	2	0	37	2.2	3	4	542
Corn-based, Extruded, Puffs or Twists, Cheese Flavor 32 pieces (28g)	158	10	2	2	15	0.5	1	2	255
Corn-based, Extruded, Puffs or Twists, Cheese Flavor, Unenriched 1 bag (8 oz) (227g)	1267	81	13	9	123	5	6	13	2034

Food Serving size	Cal.	(g) Total Fat	(g) Sat. Fat	(mg) Chol.	(g) Carb.	(g) Fiber	(g) Sug.	(g) Prot.	(mg) Sod.
Cornnuts, Barbecue-flavor 2 oz (57g)	249	8	1	0	41	4.8	0	5	342
Cornnuts, Nacho-flavor 2 oz (57g)	250	8	1	1	41	4.6	0	5	361
Cornnuts, Plain 2 oz (57g)	254	9	1	0	41	3.9	0	5	362
Doo Dads Snack Mix, Original Flavor .5 cup (28g)	128	5	1	0	18	1.9	0	3	356
Fritolay, SunChips, Multigrain Snack, Original Flavor 1 oz (28.35g)	139	6	1	0	19	1.9	0	2	93
Fritolay, SunChips, Multigrain, French Onion Flavor 1 oz (28.35g)	141	6	1	1	19	2.2	0	2	132
Fritolay, SunChips, Multigrain, Harvest Cheddar 1 oz (28.35g)	139	6	1	1	18	2.3	0	2	153
M&M Mars, Combo Snacks, Cheddar Cheese Pretzel 10 pieces (30g)	139	5	3	0	20	0	0	3	466
Plaintain Chips, Salted 1 oz (28.35g)	151	8	2	0	18	1	0	1	57
Popcorn, Air-popped 1 oz (28.35g)	110	1	0	0	22	4.1	0	4	2
Popcorn, Air-popped, White Popcorn 1 oz (28.35g)	108	1	0	0	22	4.3	0	3	1
Popcorn, Cakes 2 cakes (20g)	77	1	0	0	16	0.6	0	2	58
Popcorn, Caramel-coated, with Peanuts 2 oz (57g)	228	4	1	0	46	2.2	26	4	168
Popcorn, Caramel-coated, Without Peanuts 1 oz (28.35g)	122	4	1	1	22	1.5	15	1	58
Popcorn, Cheese Flavor 1 oz (28.35g)	149	9	2	3	15	2.8	0	3	252
Popcorn, Micowave, Low Fat and Low Sodium 1 oz (28.35g)	122	3	0	0	21	4	0	4	139
Popcorn, Microwave, 94% Fat Free 1 oz (28.35g)	120	3	0	0	20	4	0	4	251

Food Serving size	Cal.	(g) Total Fat	(g) Sat. Fat	(mg) Chol.	(g) Carb.	(g) Fiber	(g) Sug.	(g) Prot.	(mg) Sod.
Popcorn, Microwave, Low Fat									
1 oz (28.35g)	114	2	0	0	22	3.9	0	3	178
Popcorn, Microwave, Regular (Butter) Flavor, with Partially Hydrogenated Oil									
1 oz (28.35g)	149	8	2	1	16	2.8	0	2	219
Popcorn, Oil-popped, Microwave									
1 oz (28.35g)	165	12	2	0	13	2.3	0	2	300
Popcorn, Oil-popped, White Popcorn									
1 oz (28.35g)	142	8	1	0	16	2.8	0	3	251
Popcorn, Sugar Syrup, Caramel, Fat Free									
1 oz (28.35g)	108	0	0	0	26	0.7	18	1	81
Popcorn, Unpopped Kernels									
1 oz (28.35g)	106	1	0	0	21	3.6	0	3	2
Popovers, Dry Mix, Unenriched									
1 package (6 oz) (170g)	631	7	2	0	121	0	0	18	1540
Potato Chips, Barbecue Flavor									
1 bag (7 oz) (198g)	972	64	16	0	105	8.7	0	15	1485
Potato Chips, Cheese Flavor									
1 bag (6 oz) (170g)	843	46	15	7	98	8.8	0	14	1348
Potato Chips, Fat Free, Made with Olestra									
1 oz (28.35g)	78	0	0	0	18	1.9	0	2	157
Potato Chips, Fat Free, Salted									
1 bag (8 oz) (227g)	860	1	0	0	190	17	8	22	1460
Potato Chips, from Dried Potatoes, Fat Free, with Olestra									
1 oz (28.35g)	72	0	0	0	16	2.1	0	1	122
Potato Chips, Light									
1 bag (6 oz) (170g)	801	35	7	0	114	10	0	12	836
Potato Chips, Made from Dried Potatoes, Cheese Flavor									
1 can (6.25 oz) (191g)	1052	71	18	8	97	6.5	0	13	1442
Potato Chips, Made from Dried Potatoes, Light									
1 can (6 oz) (170g)	853	44	11	0	110	5.4	1	8	699
Potato Chips, Made from Dried Potatoes, Plain									
1 can (7 oz) (198g)	1107	76	19	0	103	6.1	2	9	768
Potato Chips, Made from Dried Potatoes, Sour Cream and Onion Flavor									
1 can (6.75 oz) (198g)	1083	73	19	6	102	2.4	0	13	1426

Food Serving size	Cal.	(g) Total Fat	(g) Sat. Fat	(mg) Chol.	(g) Carb.	(g) Fiber	(g) Sug.	(g) Prot.	(mg) Sod.
Potato Chips, Plain, Made with Partially Hydrogenated Soybean Oil, Salted									
1 bag (8 oz) (227g)	1217	79	12	0	120	10.9	0	16	1348
Potato Chips, Plain, Made with Partially Hydrogenated Soybean Oil, Unsalted									
1 bag (8 oz) (227g)	1217	79	12	0	120	10.9	0	16	18
Potato Chips, Plain, Salted									
1 bag (8 oz) (227g)	1230	83	9	0	115	10	1	15	1192
Potato Chips, Plain, Unsalted									
1 bag (8 oz) (227g)	1217	79	25	0	120	10.9	0	16	18
Potato Chips, Sour Cream and Onion Flavor									
1 bag (7 oz) (198g)	1051	67	18	14	102	10.3	0	16	1238
Potato Chips, White, Restructured, Baked									
10 chips (12g)	56	2	0	0	9	0.6	0	1	76
Potato Chips, Without Salt, Reduced Fat									
1 oz (28.35g)	138	6	1	0	19	1.7	0	2	2
Pretzels, Hard, Confectioner's Coating, Chocolate Flavor									
1 pretzel (11g)	50	2	1	0	8	0	0	1	63
Pretzels, Hard, Plain, Made with Enriched Flour, Unsalted									
10 twists (60g)	229	2	0	0	48	1.7	1	5	173
Pretzels, Hard, Plain, Made with Unenriched Flour, Salted									
10 twists (60g)	229	2	0	0	48	1.7	0	5	1029
Pretzels, Hard, Plain, Made with Unenriched Flour, Unsalted									
10 twists (60g)	229	2	0	0	48	1.7	0	5	173
Pretzels, Hard, Plain, Salted									
10 twists (60g)	228	2	0	0	48	1.8	2	6	814
Pretzels, Hard, Whole Wheat									
2 oz (57g)	206	1	0	0	46	4.4	0	6	116
Pretzels, Soft									
1 medium (115g)	389	4	1	3	80	2	0	9	926
Pretzels, Soft, Unsalted									
1 medium (115g)	389	4	1	3	82	2	0	9	794
Soy Chips or Crisps, Salted									
1 oz (28.35g)	109	2	0	0	15	1	0	8	239
Sweet Potato Chips									
1 oz (28.35g)	141	7	1	0	18	1	0	1	10

Food Serving size	Cal.	(g) Total Fat	(g) Sat. Fat	(mg) Chol.	(g) Carb.	(g) Fiber	(g) Sug.	(g) Prot.	(mg) Sod.
Taro Chips									
10 chips (23g)	115	6	1	0	16	1.7	1	1	79
Tortilla Chips, Light (Baked with Less Oil)									
10 chips (16g)	74	2	0	0	12	0.9	7	1	137
Tortilla Chips, Low Fat, Baked, Without Fat									
1 oz (28.35g)	118	2	0	0	23	1.5	0	3	119
Tortilla Chips, Low Fat, Made with Olestra, Nacho Cheese									
1 oz (28.35g)	90	1	0	1	18	1.8	1	2	171
Tortilla Chips, Low Fat, Unsalted									
1 oz (28.35g)	118	2	0	0	23	1.5	0	3	4
Tortilla Chips, Nacho Cheese									
1 oz (28.35g)	146	7	1	0	18	1.3	1	2	174
Tortilla Chips, Nacho Flavor, Made with Enriched Masa Flour									
1 oz (28.35g)	141	7	1	1	18	1.5	0	2	201
Tortilla Chips, Nacho Flavor, Reduced Fat									
1 bag (6 oz) (170g)	757	26	5	5	122	8.2	0	15	1705
Tortilla Chips, Ranch Flavor									
1 bag (7 oz) (198g)	992	49	7	0	124	7.9	6	14	1028
Tortilla Chips, Taco Flavor									
1 bag (8 oz) (227g)	1090	55	11	11	143	12	0	18	1786
Tortilla Chips, Unsalted, White Corn									
1 bag, single serving (28g)	141	7	1	0	18	1.5	1	2	4
Tortillas, Ready-to-bake or Fry, Corn									
1 enchilada (19g)	41	1	0	0	8	1.2	0	1	9
Tortillas, Ready-to-bake or Fry, Corn, Without Salt									
1 tortilla, medium (approx 6" dia) (26g)	58	1	0	0	12	1.4	0	1	3
Tostada Shells, Corn									
3 pieces (mean serving weight, aggregated over brands) (37g)	175	9	3	0	24	2.1	0	2	243
Tostada with Guacamole									
2 pieces (261g)	360	23	10	39	32	0	0	12	799
Trail Mix, Regular									
1 oz (28.35g)	131	8	2	0	13	0	0	4	65

Food Serving size	Cal.	(g) Total Fat	(g) Sat. Fat	(mg) Chol.	(g) Carb.	(g) Fiber	(g) Sug.	(g) Prot.	(mg) Sod.
Trail Mix, Regular, Unsalted									
1 oz (28.35g)	131	8	2	0	13	0	0	4	3
Trail Mix, Regular, with Chocolate Chips, Salted Nuts, and Seeds									
1 oz (28.35g)	137	9	2	1	13	0	0	4	34
Trail Mix, Regular, with Chocolate Chips, Unsalted Nuts, and Seeds									
1 oz (28.35g)	137	9	2	1	13	0	0	4	8
Trail Mix, Tropical									
1 oz (28.35g)	115	5	2	0	19	0	0	2	3

Sugars, Syrups, and Toppings

Food Serving size	Cal.	(g) Total Fat	(g) Sat. Fat	(mg) Chol.	(g) Carb.	(g) Fiber	(g) Sug.	(g) Prot.	(mg) Sod.
Candies, Confectioner's Coating, Peanut Butter									
1 oz (28.35g)	150	8	4	0	13	1.4	11	5	71
Candies, Confectioner's Coating, Yogurt									
1 cup, chips (170g)	887	46	41	2	109	0	106	10	150
Chocolate Syrup									
1 cup (300g)	837	3	2	0	195	7.8	149	6	216
Chocolate-flavored Hazelnut Spread									
1 serving, 2 tbsp (37g)	200	11	11	0	23	2	20	2	15
Frostings, Chocolate, Creamy, Dry Mix									
1 package (388g)	1509	20	0	0	357	9.3	0	5	295
Frostings, Chocolate, Creamy, Ready-to-eat									
2 tbsp, creamy (41g)	163	7	2	0	26	0.4	24	0	75
Frostings, Coconut-nut, Ready-to-eat									
.083 package (38g)	165	9	3	0	20	1	15	1	74
Frostings, Cream Cheese Flavor, Ready-to-eat									
2 tbsp, whipped (24g)	100	4	1	0	16	0	15	0	46
Frostings, Glaze, Prepared from Recipe									
1 recipe, yield (327g)	1115	2	1	3	274	0	263	1	20
Frostings, White, Fluffy, Dry Mix, Prepared with Water									
.083 package (26g)	63	0	0	0	16	0	0	0	41
Honey									
1 tbsp (21g)	64	0	0	0	17	0	17	0	1
Ice Cream Cones, Cake or Wafer-type									
1 cone (4g)	17	0	0	0	3	0.1	0	0	10

Food Serving size	Cal.	(g) Total Fat	(g) Sat. Fat	(mg) Chol.	(g) Carb.	(g) Fiber	(g) Sug.	(g) Prot.	(mg) Sod.
Ice Cream Cones, Sugar, Rolled-type 1 cone (10g)	40	0	0	0	8	0.2	3	1	25
Molasses 1 serving, 1 tbsp (20g)	58	0	0	0	15	0	11	0	7
Sugar, Brown 1 cup, unpacked (145g)	551	0	0	0	142	0	141	0	41
Sugar, Granulated 1 tsp (4.2g)	16	0	0	0	4	0	4	0	0
Sugar, Maple 1 oz (28.35g)	100	0	0	0	26	0	24	0	3
Sugar, Powdered 1 cup, sifted (100g)	389	0	0	0	100	0	98	0	2
Sweeteners, Tabletop, Aspartame, Equal, Packets 1 serving, 1 packet (1g)	4	0	0	0	1	0	1	0	0
Sweeteners, Tabletop, Fructose, Dry, Powder 1 tsp (4.2g)	15	0	0	0	4	0	2	0	1
Sweeteners, Tabletop, Saccharin 1 serving, 1 packet (0.8g)	3	0	0	0	1	0	0	0	3
Sweeteners, Tabletop, Sucralose, Splenda Packets 1 serving, 1 packet (1g)	3	0	0	0	1	0	1	0	0
Syrup, Chocolate, Fudge-type 2 tbsp (38g)	133	3	2	0	24	1.1	13	2	131
Syrup, Chocolate, Hershey's Genuine Chocolate Flavor Lite Syrup 2 tbsp (35g)	54	0	0	0	12	0	10	0	35
Syrup, Corn, Dark 1 tbsp (20g)	57	0	0	0	16	0	5	0	31
Syrup, Corn, High Fructose 1 tbsp (19g)	53	0	0	0	14	0	5	0	0
Syrup, Corn, Light 1 tbsp (22g)	62	0	0	0	17	0	6	0	14
Syrup, Grenadine 1 tsp (6.7g)	18	0	0	0	4	0	0	0	2
Syrup, Malt 1 tbsp (24g)	76	0	0	0	17	0	17	1	8

Food Serving size	Cal.	(g) Total Fat	(g) Sat. Fat	(mg) Chol.	(g) Carb.	(g) Fiber	(g) Sug.	(g) Prot.	(mg) Sod.
Syrup, Maple 1 tbsp (20g)	52	0	0	0	13	0	12	0	2
Syrup, Sorghum 1 tbsp (21g)	61	0	0	0	16	0	16	0	2
Syrup, Table Blends, Cane and 15% Maple 1 tbsp (20g)	56	0	0	0	14	0	14	0	21
Syrup, Table Blends, Corn, Refiner and Sugar 1 tbsp (20g)	64	0	0	0	17	0	0	0	14
Syrup, Table Blends, Pancake 1 tbsp (20g)	47	0	0	0	12	0	4	0	16
Syrup, Table Blends, Pancake, Reduced Calorie 1 tbsp (15g)	25	0	0	0	7	0	5	0	27
Syrup, Table Blends, Pancake, with 2% Maple 1 tbsp (20g)	53	0	0	0	14	0	8	0	12
Syrup, Table Blends, Pancake, with 2% Maple, with Potassium 1 tbsp (20g)	53	0	0	0	14	0	0	0	12
Syrup, Table Blends, Pancake, with Butter 1 tbsp (20g)	59	0	0	1	15	0	0	0	20
Toppings, Butterscotch or Caramel 2 tbsp (41g)	103	0	0	0	27	0.4	0	1	143
Toppings, Marshmallow Cream 1 jar (198g)	638	1	0	0	156	0.2	93	2	158
Toppings, Nuts in Syrup 2 tbsp (41g)	184	9	1	0	24	0.9	15	2	17
Toppings, Pineapple 2 tbsp (42g)	106	0	0	0	28	0.2	9	0	18
Toppings, Strawberry 2 tbsp (42g)	107	0	0	0	28	0.3	11	0	9
Vanilla Extract 1 tbsp (13g)	37	0	0	0	2	0	2	0	1
Vanilla Extract, Imitation, Alcohol 1 tbsp (13g)	31	0	0	0	0	0	0	0	1
Vanilla Extract, Imitation, No Alcohol 1 tbsp (13g)	7	0	0	0	2	0	2	0	0

Beverages

Why Drink Beverages?

Beverages provide hydration and may provide additional nutrients (calcium in milk and vitamin C in orange juice). Water is the body's principle component and makes up 60% of your body weight. Every system in your body depends on water. Even mild dehydration can drain you of energy and cause a headache. Drinking is most often how water enters the body; however, water also enters the body through some foods, especially vegetables and fruits.

Daily Goal

Recommendations for daily water intake vary by age, gender, activity level, and health status. Young children and older adults may dehydrate more rapidly. An adult male on a 2,000-calorie diet may require up to 15, 8-ounce cups of beverages each day. An adult woman may need approximately 11, 8-ounce cups of fluids per day. Women who are expecting or breast feeding may need as much as 13 cups of fluids per day.

Shopping Tips

- Plain water is best for hydration.
- Choose 100% juices rather than juice drinks.
- Drink fat-free (skim) milk.
- Limit the use of sports drinks to vigorous physical activity lasting longer than one hour.

Shopping List Essentials

Bottled water
Milk, fat-free (skim)
100% fruit juice

Red Flags

Drinks can be high in calories and sugars. Make sure that your juice choices are not made with added sugars. A beverage like soda that only has sugar calories is an example of an "empty calories" choice. Diet sodas should be consumed in moderation, since research has pointed to sugar substitutes as a possible disruptor to the mechanisms in the body that help maintain a healthy weight. Energy drinks and some sports drinks containing caffeine and other stimulants may be an inappropriate beverage choice for most people. These beverages have extra calories and contribute to obesity and tooth decay. You need water for hydration but try not to drink calories with your water.

Preparation Pointer

For a healthy alternative to flavored waters and sugary beverages, prepare caffeine-free fruit and herbal teas, several servings at a time, and store in a pitcher in the fridge for convenience. Seltzers are a healthy alternative to soda and do not contain the sodium found in club soda. Try cutting your juice consumption and upping your water intake by mixing 4 oz of your favorite juice with water of equal or greater amount.

Food Serving size	Cal.	(g) Total Fat	(g) Sat. Fat	(mg) Chol.	(g) Carb.	(g) Fiber	(g) Sug.	(g) Prot.	(mg) Sod.
Alcoholic Beverages/Wines									
Alcoholic Beverage, Crème de Menthe, 72 Proof									
1 jigger, 1.5 fl oz (50g)	186	0	0	0	21	0	21	0	3
Alcoholic Beverage, Distilled, All (Gin, Rum, Vodka, Whiskey) 90 Proof									
1 jigger, 1.5 oz (42g)	110	0	0	0	0	0	0	0	0
Alcoholic Beverage, Distilled, All (Gin, Rum, Vodka, Whiskey) 94 Proof									
1 jigger, 1.5 oz (42g)	116	0	0	0	0	0	0	0	0
Alcoholic Beverage, Distilled, Gin, 90 Proof									
1 jigger, 1.5 fl oz (42g)	110	0	0	0	0	0	0	0	1
Alcoholic Beverage, Distilled, Rum, 80 Proof									
1 jigger, 1.5 fl oz (42g)	97	0	0	0	0	0	0	0	0
Alcoholic Beverage, Distilled, Vodka, 80 Proof									
1 jigger, 1.5 fl oz (42g)	97	0	0	0	0	0	0	0	0
Alcoholic Beverage, Distilled, Whiskey, 86 Proof									
1 jigger, 1.5 fl oz (42g)	105	0	0	0	0	0	0	0	0
Beer, Light 1 can or bottle (12 fl oz) (354g)	103	0	0	0	6	0	0	1	14
Beer, Light, Bud Light									
12 fl oz (354g)	103	0	0	0	5	0	0	1	11
Beer, Light, Budweiser Select									
12 fl oz (355g)	99	0	0	0	3	0	0	1	11
Beer, Light, Michelob Ultra									
12 fl oz (354g)	96	0	0	0	3	0	0	1	11
Beer, Regular, All									
1 can (356g)	153	0	0	0	13	0	0	2	14
Beer, Regular, Budweiser									
12 fl oz (357g)	146	0	0	0	11	0	0	1	11
Daiquiri, Canned									
1 can (6.8 fl oz, 200 ml) (207g)	259	0	0	0	32	0	0	0	83
Daiquiri, Prepared from Recipe									
1 cocktail (2 fl oz) (60g)	112	0	0	0	4	0.1	3	0	3
Liqueur, Coffee, 53 Proof									
1 jigger, 1.5 fl oz (52g)	175	0	0	0	24	0	20	0	4

Food Serving size	Cal.	(g) Total Fat	(g) Sat. Fat	(mg) Chol.	(g) Carb.	(g) Fiber	(g) Sug.	(g) Prot.	(mg) Sod.
Liqueur, Coffee, 63 Proof 1 jigger, 1.5 fl oz (52g)	160	0	0	0	17	0	17	0	4
Liqueur, Coffee, with Cream, 34 Proof 1 jigger, 1.5 fl oz (47g)	154	7	5	27	10	0	9	1	43
Pina Colada, Canned 1 can (6.8 fl oz, 200 ml) (222g)	526	17	15	0	61	0.2	0	1	158
Pina Colada, Prepared from Recipe 1 cocktail (4.5 fl oz) (141g)	245	3	2	0	32	0.4	31	1	8
Rice (Sake) 1 fl oz (29.1g)	39	0	0	0	1	0	0	0	1
Tequila Sunrise, Canned 1 can (6.8 fl oz, 200 ml) (211g)	232	0	0	0	24	0	0	1	120
Whiskey Sour Mix, Bottled 2 fl oz (65g)	57	0	0	0	14	0	14	0	66
Whiskey Sour Mix, Bottled, with Added Potassium and Sodium 1 fl oz (32.3g)	27	0	0	0	7	0	0	0	11
Whiskey Sour Mix, Powder 1 packet (17g)	65	0	0	0	17	0	17	0	47
Whiskey Sour, Canned 1 can (6.8 fl oz, 200 ml) (209g)	249	0	0	0	28	0.2	0	0	92
Whiskey Sour, Prepared from Bottled Mix 1 portion (2 oz mix + 1.5 oz whiskey) (106g)	162	0	0	0	14	0	14	0	65
Whiskey Sour, Prepared from Bottled Mix, with Added Potassium and Sodium 1 portion (2 oz mix + 1.5 oz whiskey) (106g)	158	0	0	0	14	0	0	0	21
Whiskey Sour, Prepared with Water, Whiskey and Powder Mix 1 packet, prepared (103g)	169	0	0	0	16	0	16	0	48
Wine, Cooking 1 fl oz (29g)	15	0	0	0	2	0	0	0	182
Wine, Dessert, Dry 1 glass (3.5 fl oz) (103g)	157	0	0	0	12	0	1	0	9
Wine, Dessert, Sweet 1 glass (3.5 fl oz) (103g)	165	0	0	0	14	0	8	0	9

Food Serving size	Cal.	(g) Total Fat	(g) Sat. Fat	(mg) Chol.	(g) Carb.	(g) Fiber	(g) Sug.	(g) Prot.	(mg) Sod.
Wine, Light 1 serving, 5 fl oz (148g)	73	0	0	0	2	0	3	0	10
Wine, Non-alcoholic 1 fl oz (29g)	2	0	0	0	0	0	0	0	2
Wine, Table, All 1 fl oz (29.5g)	24	0	0	0	1	0	0	0	1
Wine, Table, Red 1 serving, 5 fl oz (147g)	125	0	0	0	4	0	1	0	6
Wine, Table, Red, Burgundy 1 serving, 5 fl oz (148g)	127	0	0	0	5	0	0	0	0
Wine, Table, Red, Cabernet Franc 1 serving, 5 fl oz (147g)	122	0	0	0	4	0	0	0	0
Wine, Table, Red, Cabernet Sauvignon 1 serving, 5 fl oz (147g)	122	0	0	0	4	0	0	0	0
Wine, Table, Red, Carignane 1 serving, 5 fl oz (147g)	109	0	0	0	4	0	0	0	0
Wine, Table, Red, Claret 1 serving, 5 fl oz (147g)	122	0	0	0	4	0	0	0	0
Wine, Table, Red, Merlot 1 serving, 5 fl oz (147g)	122	0	0	0	4	0	1	0	6
Wine, Table, Red, Pinot Noir 1 serving, 5 fl oz (147g)	121	0	0	0	3	0	0	0	0
Wine, Table, Red, Sangiovese 1 serving, 5 fl oz (147g)	126	0	0	0	4	0	0	0	0
Wine, Table, Red, Syrah 1 serving, 5 fl oz (147g)	122	0	0	0	4	0	0	0	0
Wine, Table, Red, Zinfandel 1 serving, 5 fl oz (147g)	129	0	0	0	4	0	0	0	0
Wine, Table, White, Chardonnay 1 serving, 5 fl oz (147g)	123	0	0	0	3	0	1	0	7
Wine, Table, White, Chenin Blanc 1 serving, 5 fl oz (148g)	118	0	0	0	5	0	0	0	0
Wine, Table, White, Fume Blanc 1 serving, 5 fl oz (147g)	121	0	0	0	3	0	0	0	0

Food Serving size	Cal.	(g) Total Fat	(g) Sat. Fat	(mg) Chol.	(g) Carb.	(g) Fiber	(g) Sug.	(g) Prot.	(mg) Sod.
Wine, Table, White, Muscat									
1 serving, 5 fl oz (150g)	123	0	0	0	8	0	0	0	0
Wine, Table, White, Pinot Blanc									
1 serving, 5 fl oz (147g)	119	0	0	0	3	0	0	0	0
Wine, Table, White, Pinot Gris (Grigio)									
1 serving, 5 fl oz (147g)	122	0	0	0	3	0	0	0	0
Wine, Table, White, Riesling									
1 serving, 5 fl oz (148g)	118	0	0	0	6	0	0	0	0
Wine, Table, White, Sauvignon Blanc									
1 serving, 5 fl oz (147g)	119	0	0	0	3	0	0	0	0
Wine, Table, White, Late Harvest									
1 serving, 5 fl oz (154 g)	172	0	0	0	21	0	0	0	0

Non-alcoholic

Food Serving size	Cal.	(g) Total Fat	(g) Sat. Fat	(mg) Chol.	(g) Carb.	(g) Fiber	(g) Sug.	(g) Prot.	(mg) Sod.
Bean Beverage									
1 fl oz (28.8g)	10	0	0	0	2	0	0	1	1
Beverage, Fruit Juice Drink, Reduced Sugar, with Vitamin E Added									
1 ml (1.1g)	0	0	0	0	0	0	0	0	0
Beverage, Instant Breakfast Powder, Chocolate Sugar-free, Not Reconstituted									
1 envelope (20g)	72	1	0	9	8	0.4	0	7	143
Beverage, Instant Breakfast Powder, Chocolate, Not Reconstituted									
1 envelope (37g)	132	1	0	4	24	0.1	0	7	142
Beverage, Milkshake Mix, Dry, Not Chocolate									
1 envelope (21g)	69	1	0	3	11	0.3	0	5	164
Beverage, Vegetables and Fruit Juice Blend, with Added Vitamins A, C, and E									
1 serving, 8 oz (246g)	113	0	0	0	27	0	26	1	71
Chocolate Syrup, Prepared with Whole Milk									
1 cup (8 fl oz) (282g)	254	8	5	25	36	0.8	32	9	133
Chocolate-flavor Beverage Mix for Milk, Powder, with Added Nutrients									
1 serving (22g)	88	0	1	0	20	1	18	1	30
Chocolate-flavor Beverage Mix for Milk, Powder, Without Added Nutrients									
1 portion (2-3 heaping tsp) (22g)	89	1	0	0	20	1.1	18	1	46
Chocolate-flavor Beverage Mix with Added Nutrients, Prepared with Whole Milk									
1 serving (266g)	237	8	5	27	32	1.1	31	9	133

Food Serving size	Cal.	(g) Total Fat	(g) Sat. Fat	(mg) Chol.	(g) Carb.	(g) Fiber	(g) Sug.	(g) Prot.	(mg) Sod.
Chocolate-flavor Beverage Mix, Powder, Prepared with Whole Milk									
1 cup (8 fl oz) (266g)	226	9	5	24	32	1.1	0	9	154
Chocolate-flavor Drink, Whey and Milk-based									
1 fl oz (30.5g)	15	0	0	0	3	0.2	1	0	28
Clam and Tomato Juice, Canned									
1 can (5.5 oz) (166g)	80	0	0	0	18	0.7	5	1	601
Cocktail Mix, Non-alcoholic, Concentrated, Frozen									
1 fl oz (36g)	103	0	0	0	26	0	3	0	0
Coconut milk, Canned (Liquid Expressed from Grated Meat and Water)									
1 tbsp (15g)	30	3	3	0	0	0	0	0	2
Coconut Milk, Frozen (Liquid Expressed from Grated Meat and Water)									
1 tbsp (15g)	30	3	3	0	1	0	0	0	2
Coconut Milk, Raw (Liquid Expressed from Grated Meat and Water)									
1 tbsp (15g)	35	4	3	0	1	0.3	1	0	2
Coconut Water (Liquid from Coconuts)									
1 tbsp (15g)	3	0	0	0	1	0.2	0	0	16
Corn Beverage									
1 fl oz (30.2g)	12	0	0	0	3	0.1	0	0	42
Eggnog									
1 fl oz (31.8g)	28	1	1	19	3	0	3	1	17
Eggnog-flavor Mix, Powder, Prepared with Whole Milk									
1 cup (8 fl oz) (272g)	258	8	5	30	39	0	34	8	150
Fruit Punch Drink, Frozen Concentrate, Prepared with Water									
1 fl oz (30.9g)	14	0	0	0	4	0	0	0	2
Fruit Punch Drink, with Added Nutrients, Canned									
1 fl oz (31g)	15	0	0	0	4	0.1	3	0	12
Fruit Punch Juice Drink, Frozen Concentrate									
1 can (12 fl oz) (423g)	740	3	0	0	182	0.8	0	1	42
Fruit Punch Juice Drink, Frozen Concentrate, Prepared with Water									
1 serving, 8 fl oz (234g)	98	0	0	0	27	0	27	0	12
Fruit Punch-flavor Drink, Powder, Without Added Sodium, Prepared with Water									
1 fl oz (32.8g)	12	0	0	0	3	0	3	0	2
Fruit-flavored Drink Mix, Powder, Unsweetened									
2 tsp, rounded (25g)	57	0	0	0	23	0	0	0	682

Food Serving size	Cal.	(g) Total Fat	(g) Sat. Fat	(mg) Chol.	(g) Carb.	(g) Fiber	(g) Sug.	(g) Prot.	(mg) Sod.
Fruit-flavored Drink, Dry Powder Mix, Low Calorie, with Aspartame									
1 tsp (8g)	17	0	0	0	7	0	0	0	32
Fruit-flavored Drink, Powder, with High Vitamin C with Other Added Vitamins, Low Calorie									
1 tsp (2g)	5	0	0	0	2	0	0	0	0
Grape Drink, Canned									
1 cup (8 fl oz) (250g)	153	0	0	0	39	0	33	0	40
Horchata, Dry Mix, Unprepared, Variety of Brands, All with Morro Seeds									
1 cup (118g)	487	9	2	0	93	4.7	46	9	4
Malt Beverage									
1 fl oz (29.6g)	11	0	0	0	2	0	2	0	4
Malted Drink Mix, Chocolate, Powder									
1 serving (3 heaping tsp or 1 envelope) (21g)	86	1	1	0	18	1	14	1	40
Malted Drink Mix, Chocolate, Powder, Prepared with Whole Milk									
1 cup (8 fl oz) (265g)	228	9	5	29	28	0	22	10	191
Malted Drink Mix, Chocolate, with Added Nutrients, Powder									
1 serving (4 tbsp or 1 envelope) (21g)	82	1	0	0	18	1	15	1	125
Malted Drink Mix, Chocolate, with Added Nutrients, Powder, Prepared with Whole Milk									
1 cup (8 fl oz) (265g)	231	9	5	27	30	1.1	28	9	231
Malted Drink Mix, Natural, Powder									
1 serving (3 heaping tsp or 1 envelope) (21g)	90	2	1	5	15	0	10	3	85
Malted Drink Mix, Natural, Powder, Prepared with Whole Milk									
1 cup (8 fl oz) (265g)	233	10	5	32	27	0.3	25	10	209
Malted Drink Mix, Natural, with Added Nutrients, Powder									
1 serving (4 tbsp or 1 envelope) (21g)	78	0	0	0	18	0.4	13	2	54
Malted Drink Mix, Natural, with Added Nutrients, Powder, Prepared with Whole Milk									
1 cup (8 fl oz) (265g)	228	9	5	29	28	0	22	10	191
Meal Supplement Drink, Nestle, Supligen, Canned, Peanut Flavor									
1 cup (158g)	160	5	1	0	23	0	0	6	85

Food Serving size	Cal.	(g) Total Fat	(g) Sat. Fat	(mg) Chol.	(g) Carb.	(g) Fiber	(g) Sug.	(g) Prot.	(mg) Sod.
Water, Tap, Drinking 1 cup, 8 fl oz (237g)	0	0	0	0	0	0	0	0	9
Water, Tap, Municipal 1 cup, 8 fl oz (237g)	0	0	0	0	0	0	0	0	7
Water, Tap, Well 1 cup, 8 fl oz (237g)	0	0	0	0	0	0	0	0	12

Bottled Waters

Food Serving size	Cal.	(g) Total Fat	(g) Sat. Fat	(mg) Chol.	(g) Carb.	(g) Fiber	(g) Sug.	(g) Prot.	(mg) Sod.
Water, Bottled, Non-carbonated, Crystal Geyser 1 bottle, 8 fl oz in packages of 8 (237g)	0	0	0	0	0	0	0	0	2
Water, Bottled, Non-carbonated, Dannon 1 bottle, 11.2 fl oz in package of 12 (331g)	0	0	0	0	0	0	0	0	0
Water, Bottled, Non-carbonated, Dasani 1 bottle, 16.9 fl oz in packages of 6 and 24 (500g)	0	0	0	0	0	0	0	0	0
Water, Bottled, Non-carbonated, Evian 1 bottle, 11.2 fl oz in package of 6 (331g)	0	0	0	0	0	0	0	0	0
Water, Bottled, Non-carbonated, Naya 1 fl oz (29.6g)	0	0	0	0	0	0	0	0	0
Water, Bottled, Perrier 1 bottle, 6.5 fl oz (192g)	0	0	0	0	0	0	0	0	2
Water, Bottled, Poland Spring 1 bottle, 16.9 fl oz in packages of 6 and 24 (500g)	0	0	0	0	0	0	0	0	5
Water, Non-carbonated, Fruit Flavors, Sweetened, with Low Calorie Sweetener 1 fl oz (29.6g)	0	0	0	0	0	0	0	0	1
Water, with Added Vitamins and Minerals, Sweetened, Fruit Flavors 1 serving (237g)	52	0	0	0	13	0	13	0	0
Water, with Corn Syrup and/or Sugar and Low Calorie Sweetener, Fruit Flavor 1 pouch (200g)	36	0	0	0	9	0	9	0	16

Food Serving size	Cal.	(g) Total Fat	(g) Sat. Fat	(mg) Chol.	(g) Carb.	(g) Fiber	(g) Sug.	(g) Prot.	(mg) Sod.

Coffees, Teas, and Cocoas

Cocoa Mix, Nestle, Hot Cocoa Mix, Rich Chocolate with Marshmallows

1 serving, 1 envelope (20g)	80	3	3	0	15	0.7	13	1	160

Cocoa Mix, Nestle, Rich Chocolate Hot Cocoa Mix

1 serving, 1 envelope (20g)	80	3	2	0	15	0.8	12	1	170

Cocoa Mix, Powder

1 serving (3 heaping tsp or 1 envelope) (28g)

	111	1	1	0	23	1	18	2	141

Cocoa Mix, Powder, Prepared with Water

1 fl oz (34.3g)	19	0	0	0	4	0.2	3	0	25

Cocoa Mix, Swiss Miss, No Sugar Added, Powder

1 envelope Swiss Miss (.53 oz) (15g)

	57	0	0	0	11	1.1	6	2	131

Cocoa Mix, with Aspartame, Low Calorie, Powder, with Added Calcium, No Added Sodium or Vitamin A

1 packet (0.675 oz) (19g)	68	1	0	2	11	0.2	11	5	124

Cocoa Mix, with Aspartame, Powder, Prepared with Water

1 fl oz (32.1g)	9	0	0	0	2	0.2	1	0	23

Cocoa, Dry Powder, Hi-fat or Breakfast, Plain

1 tbsp (5.4g)	26	1	1	0	3	1.6	0	1	1

Cocoa, Dry Powder, Unsweetened

1 tbsp (5.4g)	12	1	0	0	3	1.8	0	1	1

Cocoa, Dry Powder, Unsweetened, Hershey's European Style Cocoa

1 tbsp (5g)	20	1	0	0	3	1	0	1	0

Cocoa, Dry Powder, Unsweetened, Processed with Alkali

1 tbsp (5.4g)	12	1	0	0	3	1.6	0	1	1

Coffee and Cocoa (Mocha) Powder, with Whitener and Low Calorie Sweetener

1 tsp, dry (6.4g)	16	1	1	0	5	0.3	0	1	32

Coffee and Cocoa (Mocha) Powder, with Whitener and Low Calorie Sweetener, Decaffeinated

1 tsp, dry (6.4g)	16	1	1	0	5	0.3	2	1	32

Coffee Substitute, Cereal Grain Beverage, Powder

1 tsp (1 serving) (3g)	11	0	0	0	2	0.7	0	0	2

Coffee Substitute, Cereal Grain Beverage, Powder, Prepared with Whole Milk

6 fl oz (185g)	120	6	4	24	10	0.2	0	6	91

Food Serving size	Cal.	(g) Total Fat	(g) Sat. Fat	(mg) Chol.	(g) Carb.	(g) Fiber	(g) Sug.	(g) Prot.	(mg) Sod.
Coffee Substitute, Cereal Grain Beverage, Prepared with Water									
1 serving, 6 fl oz (180g)	11	0	0	0	2	0.7	0	0	9
Coffee Substitute, Roasted Grain Beverage, Natural Touch Kaffree Roma, Powder									
1 tsp, rounded (1 serving) (2g)	7	0	0	0	2	0	0	0	3
Coffee, Brewed from Grounds, Prepared with Tap Water									
6 fl oz (178g)	2	0	0	0	0	0	0	0	4
Coffee, Brewed from Grounds, Prepared with Tap Water, Decaffeinated									
6 fl oz (178g)	0	0	0	0	0	0	0	0	4
Coffee, Dry, Powder, with Whitener, Reduced Calorie									
1 tsp, dry (1.7g)	9	0	0	0	1	0	0	0	14
Coffee, Instant, Decaffeinated, Powder									
1 tsp, rounded (1.8g)	4	0	0	0	1	0	0	0	0
Coffee, Instant, Decaffeinated, Powder, Prepared with Water									
1 fl oz (29.9g)	1	0	0	0	0	0	0	0	1
Coffee, Instant, Regular, Powder									
1 packet (2g)	7	0	0	0	2	0	0	0	1
Coffee, Instant, Regular, Powder, Half the Caffeine									
1 packet (2g)	7	0	0	0	1	0	0	0	1
Coffee, Instant, Regular, Prepared with Water									
1 serving, 6 fl oz (179g)	4	0	0	0	1	0	0	0	7
Coffee, Instant, with Chicory, Prepared with Water									
1 serving, 6 fl oz (179g)	5	0	0	0	1	0	0	0	13
Coffee, Instant, with Sugar, Cappuccino-flavor Powder									
4 teaspoon (1 serving) (13g)	53	1	0	0	11	0.2	9	0	23
Coffee, Instant, with Sugar, French-flavor, Powder									
4 teaspoon (1 serving) (13g)	63	3	1	0	9	0	5	1	72
Coffee, Instant, with Sugar, Mocha-flavor, Powder									
1 serving, 2 tbsp (13g)	60	2	1	0	10	0.2	8	1	41
Tea, Black, Brewed, Prepared with Tap Water									
6 fl oz (178g)	2	0	0	0	1	0	0	0	5
Tea, Brewed, Prepared with Distilled Water									
6 fl oz (178g)	2	0	0	0	1	0	0	0	0
Tea, Brewed, Prepared with Tap Water									
1 fl oz (29.6g)	0	0	0	0	0	0	0	0	1

Food Serving size	Cal.	(g) Total Fat	(g) Sat. Fat	(mg) Chol.	(g) Carb.	(g) Fiber	(g) Sug.	(g) Prot.	(mg) Sod.
Tea, Brewed, Prepared with Tap Water, Decaffeinated 6 fl oz (178g)	2	0	0	0	1	0	0	0	5
Tea, Herb, Chamomile, Brewed 6 fl oz (178g)	2	0	0	0	0	0	0	0	2
Tea, Herb, Other than Chamomile, Brewed 6 fl oz (178g)	2	0	0	0	0	0	0	0	2
Tea, Instant, Sweetened with Sodium Saccharin, Lemon-flavored, Powder 4 tbsp (1/4 cup) (14.4g)	49	0	0	0	12	0	0	0	59
Tea, Instant, Sweetened with Sodium Saccharin, Lemon-flavored, Powder, Decaffeinated 2 tsp (1.6g)	5	0	0	0	1	0	0	0	7
Tea, Instant, Sweetened with Sodium Saccharin, Lemon-flavored, Prepared 1 fl oz (29.8g)	1	0	0	0	0	0	0	0	2
Tea, Instant, Sweetened with Sugar, Lemon-flavored, with Vitamin C, Powder 1 serving (3 heaping tsp) (23g)	89	0	0	0	22	0	0	0	1
Tea, Instant, Sweetened with Sugar, Lemon-flavored, Without Vitamin C, Powder 1 serving (3 heaping tsp) (23g)	92	0	0	0	23	0.2	22	0	1
Tea, Instant, Sweetened with Sugar, Lemon-flavored, Without Vitamin C, Powder, Decaffeinated 1 serving (3 heaping tsp) (23g)	89	0	0	0	23	0	22	0	1
Tea, Instant, Sweetened with Sugar, Lemon-flavored, Without Vitamin C, Powder, Prepared 1 cup (8 fl oz) (259g)	91	0	0	0	22	0.3	22	0	5
Tea, Instant, Unsweetened, Lemon-flavored, Powder 2 tbsp, rounded (11.3g)	39	0	0	0	9	0.6	1	1	6
Tea, Instant, Unsweetened, Powder, Prepared 1 fl oz (29.7g)	0	0	0	0	0	0	0	0	1
Tea, Ready-to-drink, Arizona Iced Tea, with Lemon Flavor 1 serving, 8 fl oz (227g)	89	0	0	0	22	0	22	0	9
Tea, Ready-to-drink, Lipton Brisk Iced Tea, with Lemon Flavor 1 serving, 8 fl oz (245g)	86	0	0	0	22	0	21	0	51
Tea, Ready-to-drink, Nestle, Cool Nestea Iced tea, with Lemon Flavor 1 serving, 8 fl oz (245g)	88	0	0	0	22	0	22	0	51

Food Serving size	Cal.	(g) Total Fat	(g) Sat. Fat	(mg) Chol.	(g) Carb.	(g) Fiber	(g) Sug.	(g) Prot.	(mg) Sod.

Energy and Sports Drinks

Food Serving size	Cal.	Total Fat	Sat. Fat	Chol.	Carb.	Fiber	Sug.	Prot.	Sod.
Drink Mix, Quaker Oats, Gatorade, Orange Flavor, Powder 1 scoop, powder (23g)	89	0	0	0	22	0	19	0	14
Energy Drink, Amp 1 serving (240g)	110	0	0	0	29	0	29	1	65
Energy Drink, Amp, Sugar-free 1 serving, 8 fl oz (240g)	5	0	0	0	2	0	0	0	74
Energy Drink, Full Throttle 1 serving, 8 fl oz (240g)	110	0	0	0	29	0	29	1	84
Energy Drink, Monster 1 serving (240g)	101	0	0	0	27	0	27	0	180
Energy Drink, Red Bull, Sugar Free, with Added Caffeine, Niacin, Panto, Vitamins B6 and B12 1 serving, 8.3 fl oz can (250g)	13	0	0	0	2	0	0	1	98
Energy Drink, Red Bull, with Added Caffeine, Niacin, Panto, Vitamins B6 and B12 1 can, 12 fl oz (369g)	166	0	0	0	40	0	37	1	140
Energy Drink, Vault, Citrus Flavor 1 oz (31g)	15	0	0	0	4	0	4	0	4
Ensure Plus, Liquid Nutrition 1 fl oz (31.5g)	44	1	0	1	6	0	0	2	30
Fluid Replacement, Electrolyte Solin (Including Pedialyte) 1 fl oz (31.2g)	3	0	0	0	1	0	0	0	32
Protein Supplement, Milk-based, Muscle Milk, Powder 1 tbsp (11g)	45	2	0	2	2	0.8	1	5	36
Quaker Oats, Propel Fitness Water, Fruit-flavored, Non-carbonated 1 bottle, 16.9 fl oz in packages of 6 (501g)	25	0	0	0	6	0	6	0	65
Rice Drink, Unsweetened, with Added Calcium, Vitamins A and D 8 fl oz (approximate weight, 1 serving) (240g)	113	2	0	0	22	0.7	13	1	94
Sports Drink, Coca-Cola, Powerade, Lemon-lime Flavor, Ready-to-drink 8 fl oz (244g)	78	0	0	0	19	0	15	0	54
Sports Drink, Fruit-flavored, Low Calorie, Ready-to-drink 1 fl oz (30g)	3	0	0	0	1	0	0	0	11

Food Serving size	Cal.	(g) Total Fat	(g) Sat. Fat	(mg) Chol.	(g) Carb.	(g) Fiber	(g) Sug.	(g) Prot.	(mg) Sod.
Sports Drink, Pepsico, Gatorade, Fruit-flavored, Ready-to-drink									
8 fl oz (244g)	63	0	0	0	16	0	13	0	95

Soft Drinks and Sodas and Drink Mixes

Food Serving size	Cal.	Total Fat	Sat. Fat	Chol.	Carb.	Fiber	Sug.	Prot.	Sod.
Carbonated Beverage, Chocolate-flavored Soda									
1 can or bottle (16 fl oz) (492g)	207	0	0	0	53	0	53	0	433
Carbonated Beverage, Club Soda									
1 can or bottle (16 fl oz) (474g)	0	0	0	0	0	0	0	0	100
Carbonated Beverage, Cola, Contains Caffeine									
1 can, 12 fl oz (368g)	136	0	0	0	35	0	33	0	15
Carbonated Beverage, Cola, with Higher Caffeine									
1 can, 12 fl oz (368g)	151	0	0	0	39	0	39	0	15
Carbonated Beverage, Cola, Without Caffeine									
1 can, 12 fl oz (368g)	151	0	0	0	39	0	39	0	15
Carbonated Beverage, Cream Soda									
1 can or bottle (16 fl oz) (494g)	252	0	0	0	66	0	66	0	59
Carbonated Beverage, Dr. Pepper-type, Contains Caffeine									
1 can or bottle (16 fl oz) (491g)	201	0	0	0	51	0	0	0	49
Carbonated Beverage, Ginger Ale									
1 can or bottle (16 fl oz) (488g)	166	0	0	0	43	0	42	0	34
Carbonated Beverage, Grape Soda									
1 can or bottle (12 fl oz) (372g)	160	0	0	0	42	0	0	0	56
Carbonated Beverage, Lemon-lime Soda, Contains Caffeine									
1 can, 12 fl oz (369g)	151	0	0	0	38	0	38	0	37
Carbonated Beverage, Local, Other than Cola or Dr Pepper, with Saccharin, Without Caffeine									
1 can (12 fl oz) (355g)	0	0	0	0	0	0	0	0	57
Carbonated Beverage, Low calorie, Not Cola or Dr Pepper-type, with Aspartame, Contains Caffeine									
1 can (12 fl oz) (355g)	0	0	0	0	0	0	0	0	21
Carbonated Beverage, Low Calorie, Other than Cola or Dr Pepper, Without Caffeine									
1 can (12 fl oz) (355g)	0	0	0	0	0	0	0	0	21

Food Serving size	Cal.	(g) Total Fat	(g) Sat. Fat	(mg) Chol.	(g) Carb.	(g) Fiber	(g) Sug.	(g) Prot.	(mg) Sod.
Carbonated Beverage, Orange 1 can or bottle (16 fl oz) (496g)									
	238	0	0	0	61	0	0	0	60
Carbonated Beverage, Reduced Sugar, Cola, Contains Caffeine and Sweeteners 1 can (8 fl oz) (355g)	71	0	0	0	18	0	18	0	14
Carbonated Beverage, Root Beer 1 can or bottle (16 fl oz) (493g)									
	202	0	0	0	52	0	52	0	64
Carbonated Beverage, Sprite, Lemon-lime, Without Caffeine 1 can, 12 fl oz (369g)	148	0	0	0	37	0	33	0	33
Carbonated Beverage, Tonic Water 1 bottle (11 fl oz) (336g)	114	0	0	0	30	0	30	0	40
Carob-flavor Beverage Mix, Powder 1 tbsp (12g)	45	0	0	0	11	1	0	0	12
Carob-flavor Beverage Mix, Powder, Prepared with Whole Milk 1 cup (8 fl oz) (256g)	192	8	5	26	22	1	0	8	118
Lemonade, Powder 1 cup (218g)	820	2	0	0	213	0.9	206	0	111
Lemonade, Powder, Prepared with Water 1 serving, 1 cup 8 fl oz (264g)	37	0	0	0	9	0	9	0	16
Lemonade-flavor Drink, Powder .5 scoop, (2 tbsp) (29g)	110	0	0	0	28	0	28	0	38
Lemonade-flavor Drink, Powder, Prepared with Water 1 serving, 1 cup 8 fl oz (255g)	69	0	0	0	18	0	18	0	33
Shake, Fast Food, Chocolate 1 small, 12 fl oz (282g)	358	10	7	37	58	5.4	52	10	274
Shake, Fast Food, Strawberry 1 small, 12 fl oz (282g)	319	8	5	31	53	1.1	0	10	234
Shake, Fast Food, Vanilla 1 cup, (8 fl oz) (166g)	246	11	7	38	33	1.5	23	6	134
Strawberry-flavored Beverage Mix, Powder 1 serving (2-3 heaping tsp) (22g)									
	86	0	0	0	22	0	21	0	8
Strawberry-flavored Beverage Mix, Powder, Prepared with Whole Milk 1 cup (8 fl oz) (266g)	234	8	5	32	33	0	0	8	128

Mixed Dishes

Why Eat Mixed Dishes?

Mixed dishes are convenient and enjoyable to eat but they don't fit neatly into one food group. For example, a cheese pizza provides nutrients from several food groups: the crust from the grains group, the tomato sauce from the vegetable group, and the cheese from the dairy group. Frozen and shelf-stable, partially prepared foods are convenient and can be healthy.

Daily Goal

Compare each mixed food selection to ChooseMyPlate. A prepared entrée should have:

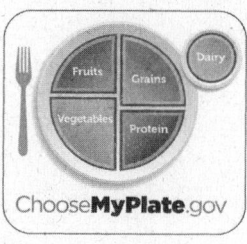

ChooseMyPlate.gov

    300 to 500 calories
    10 g or more protein
    30% or less fat calories (10 to 28 grams total fat)
    10% or less saturated fat (1 to 2 grams)
    480 mg or less sodium

Shopping Tips

- Most prepared entrées don't include a serving of dairy. If the calcium level is below 10% Daily Value, plan to have an 8 oz glass of milk along with it.
- Fresh fruits and vegetables are usually lacking in prepared meals. Plan a side salad or vegetable.
- Purchase fruit for a sweet ending to the meal.
- Choose mixed dishes with sauces in separate packets so that you can decide how much to use.
- Look for low-sodium soups.

Shopping List Essentials

Healthy frozen dinners and prepackaged entrées
Low-sodium soups
Whole grain-based entrées: brown rice, quinoa, whole grain pasta
Vegetables
Fruits

Red Flags

Some mixed foods can contain a lot of fat or sugar, which adds empty calories. Mixed dishes are also usually high in sodium. Look for those that claim "Healthy." These have limits on fat, saturated fat, and sodium and must contain a good source of at least one positive nutrient. See the guidelines for "Healthy" on page vi.

Preparation Pointer

Home-cooked mixed dishes allow you to use the most nutrient dense ingredients without the extra sodium, fat, and sugar found in packaged foods. Mixed dishes often can be prepared in bulk for multiple meals or frozen for later use. Consider soups, stews, and casseroles loaded with vegetables, using lean animal (chicken or fish) or vegetable protein (beans or lentils) sources.

Food Serving size	Cal.	(g) Total Fat	(g) Sat. Fat	(mg) Chol.	(g) Carb.	(g) Fiber	(g) Sug.	(g) Prot.	(mg) Sod.
Soups									
Beef Stew, Canned Entrée									
1 cup (1 serving) (196g)	194	11	4	25	15	1.8	5	9	760
Campbell's Bowls, 98% Fat Free New England Clam Chowder									
1 cup (245g)	110	2	1	10	17	1	1	6	480
Campbell's Brown Sugar and Bacon Flavor Baked Beans									
1 serving (130g)	160	2	1	5	30	8.1	13	5	471
Campbell's Chunky Microwavable Bowls, Beef with Country Vegetables, Ready-to-serve									
1 serving, 1 cup (245g)	149	3	1	20	21	4.9	3	10	899
Campbell's Chunky Microwavable Bowls, Chicken Dumplings Soup									
1 serving, 1 cup (245g)	191	9	2	25	18	2.9	2	8	889
Campbell's Chunky Microwavable Bowls, Old Fashioned Vegetable Beef, Ready-to-serve									
1 serving, 1 cup (245g)	100	1	0	10	14	2.9	4	7	880
Campbell's Chunky Microwavable Bowls, Sirloin Burger with Country Vegetables, Ready-to-serve									
1 serving, 1 cup (245g)	140	4	1	15	18	2.9	4	8	801
Campbell's Chunky Soups, Baked Potato Cheddar Bacon Bits Soup									
1 cup (245g)	191	9	3	10	23	2	3	5	789
Campbell's Chunky Soups, Baked Potato with Steak and Cheese Soup									
1 cup (245g)	201	10	2	15	21	2.9	3	8	840
Campbell's Chunky Soups, Barbecue Seasoned Burger Soup									
1 serving (245g)	206	6	2	15	28	4.9	10	10	899
Campbell's Chunky Soups, BBQ Seasoned Pork Soup									
1 serving (245g)	167	4	1	15	22	4.9	5	12	921
Campbell's Chunky Soups, Chicken Broccoli Cheese and Potato Soup									
1 cup (245g)	211	11	4	20	20	2.9	6	7	880
Campbell's Chunky Soups, Chicken Corn Chowder									
1 cup (245g)	201	10	3	15	20	2	3	7	860
Campbell's Chunky Soups, Chicken Mushroom Chowder									
1 serving (245g)	191	9	1	25	19	2.9	4	8	850
Campbell's Chunky Soups, Classic Chicken Noodle Soup									
1 can (526g)	247	7	2	42	28	5.3	2	18	1710

Food Serving size	Cal.	(g) Total Fat	(g) Sat. Fat	(mg) Chol.	(g) Carb.	(g) Fiber	(g) Sug.	(g) Prot.	(mg) Sod.
Campbell's Chunky Soups, Fajita Chicken with Rice and Beans Soup									
1 cup (245g)	130	1	0	15	23	2	7	7	850
Campbell's Chunky Soups, Firehouse — Hot Spicy Beef Bean Chili									
1 cup (245g)	233	8	4	25	25	5.9	7	15	870
Campbell's Chunky Soups, Grilled Chicken Sausage Gumbo Soup									
1 cup (245g)	140	3	1	20	21	2	4	7	850
Campbell's Chunky Soups, Grilled Chicken Vegetable and Pasta Soup									
1 cup (245g)	100	2	0	15	14	2	2	6	880
Campbell's Chunky Soups, Grilled Sirloin Steak and Hearty Vegetables Soup									
1 cup (245g)	125	2	1	10	19	3.9	4	8	889
Campbell's Chunky Soups, Healthy Request									
1 cup (245g)	130	3	1	10	20	2	0	5	409
Campbell's Chunky Soups, Healthy Request Chicken Noodle Soup									
1 cup (245g)	100	2	0	20	14	2	3	7	394
Campbell's Chunky Soups, Healthy Request, Beef Barley Soup									
1 serving (245g)	140	2	1	15	21	4.9	0	9	480
Campbell's Chunky Soups, Healthy Request, Microwavable Bowls, Chicken Noodle Soup									
1 serving (245g)	120	2	1	15	17	1	0	7	409
Campbell's Chunky Soups, Healthy Request, Microwavable Bowls, Grilled Chicken Sausage Gumbo Soup									
1 cup (245g)	130	3	1	10	18	2	0	7	409
Campbell's Chunky Soups, Healthy Request, Vegetable Soup									
1 cup (245g)	120	1	0	0	24	3.9	8	4	409
Campbell's Chunky Soups, Hearty Bean 'n' Ham Soup									
1 cup (245g)	181	2	0	10	30	8.1	5	11	779
Campbell's Chunky Soups, Hearty Beef Barley Soup									
1 cup (245g)	159	2	0	10	26	3.9	5	9	789
Campbell's Chunky Soups, Hearty Chicken with Vegetables Soup									
1 serving (245g)	110	2	0	15	17	2.9	3	6	711
Campbell's Chunky Soups, Hearty Vegetable with Pasta Soup									
1 cup (245g)	125	2	0	5	23	2.9	9	4	931
Campbell's Chunky Soups, Herb Roasted Chicken with Potatoes and Garlic Soup									
1 serving (245g)	113	1	1	15	17	2.9	4	8	870

Food Serving size	Cal.	(g) Total Fat	(g) Sat. Fat	(mg) Chol.	(g) Carb.	(g) Fiber	(g) Sug.	(g) Prot.	(mg) Sod.
Campbell's Chunky Soups, Honey Roasted Ham with Potatoes Soup									
1 serving (245g)	135	2	1	15	20	2.9	7	8	811
Campbell's Chunky Soups, Italian Sausage and Peppers Soup									
1 serving (245g)	152	5	1	20	20	2.9	8	7	801
Campbell's Chunky Soups, Manhattan Clam Chowder									
1 cup (245g)	127	4	1	5	19	2.9	4	5	831
Campbell's Chunky Soups, New England Clam Chowder									
1 can (519g)	420	20	0	21	47	6.2	0	13	1832
Campbell's Chunky Soups, Old Fashioned Potato Ham Chowder									
1 cup (245g)	191	11	4	20	17	2.9	1	6	801
Campbell's Chunky Soups, Old Fashioned Vegetable Beef Soup									
1 can (529g)	259	7	2	32	33	6.9	6	17	1830
Campbell's Chunky Soups, Pepper Steak Soup									
1 serving (245g)	118	1	0	15	18	2.9	4	8	801
Campbell's Chunky Soups, Pork Roast with Carrots and Potatoes Soup									
1 serving (245g)	123	3	1	15	16	2.9	3	8	889
Campbell's Chunky Soups, Rigatoni and Meat									
1 cup (245g)	211	7	3	20	25	2.9	0	11	801
Campbell's Chunky Soups, Roadhouse — Beef Bean Chili									
1 cup (245g)	233	8	4	25	25	5.9	7	15	880
Campbell's Chunky Soups, Salisbury Steak, Mushroom and Onion Soup									
1 serving (245g)	140	5	2	15	19	2	6	7	801
Campbell's Chunky Soups, Savory Chicken White Wild Rice Soup									
1 cup (245g)	110	2	0	10	18	2	1	7	811
Campbell's Chunky Soups, Savory Pot Roast Soup									
1 cup (245g)	120	1	0	10	20	2	4	7	789
Campbell's Chunky Soups, Savory Vegetable Soup									
1 cup (245g)	108	1	0	0	22	3.9	6	3	769
Campbell's Chunky Soups, Sizzlin' Steak — Grilled Steak with Chili Beans									
1 cup (245g)	198	3	1	15	27	7.1	9	16	870
Campbell's Chunky Soups, Slow Roasted Beef with Mushrooms Soup									
1 cup (245g)	118	1	1	15	18	2.9	5	8	831
Campbell's Chunky Soups, Smoked Chicken with Roasted Corn Chowder									
1 serving (245g)	206	10	2	15	19	4.9	3	10	889

Food Serving size	Cal.	(g) Total Fat	(g) Sat. Fat	(mg) Chol.	(g) Carb.	(g) Fiber	(g) Sug.	(g) Prot.	(mg) Sod.
Campbell's Chunky Soups, Split Pea 'n' Ham Soup									
1 cup (245g)	191	2	1	10	30	4.9	5	12	779
Campbell's Chunky Soups, Steak 'n' Potato Soup									
1 cup (245g)	120	2	0	15	18	2.9	1	8	921
Campbell's Chunky Soups, Tantalizin' Turkey–Turkey Chili Beans Soup									
1 serving (245g)	191	2	1	15	27	8.1	9	15	880
Campbell's Chunky Soups, Turkey Pot Pie									
1 cup (245g)	201	8	1	34	21	3.9	0	11	801
Campbell's Healthy Request, Chicken Noodle Soup, Condensed									
1 serving, 1/2 cup (126g)	59	2	1	13	8	1.3	1	3	421
Campbell's Healthy Request, Chicken with Rice Soup, Condensed									
1 serving, 1/2 cup (126g)	58	1	1	5	9	1	1	2	410
Campbell's Healthy Request, Cream of Celery Soup, Condensed									
1 serving, 1/2 cup (124g)	69	2	0	5	12	1	2	1	410
Campbell's Healthy Request, Cream of Chicken Soup, Condensed									
1 serving, 1/2 cup (124g)	62	2	0	5	9	0.5	1	4	430
Campbell's Healthy Request, Cream of Mushroom Soup, Condensed									
1 serving, 1/2 cup (124g)	68	2	0	0	11	1.2	2	2	405
Campbell's Healthy Request, Homestyle Chicken Noodle Soup, Condensed									
1 serving, 1/2 cup (126g)	64	1	0	9	10	0.8	1	3	399
Campbell's Healthy Request, Minestrone Soup, Condensed									
1 serving, 1/2 cup (120g)	76	0	0	0	14	2.9	4	3	390
Campbell's Healthy Request, Tomato Juice									
1 serving (243g)	51	0	0	0	11	1.9	0	2	481
Campbell's Healthy Request, Vegetable Soup, Condensed									
1 serving, 1/2 cup (126g)	100	1	0	0	20	3	5	4	410
Campbell's Homestyle Butternut Squash Bisque									
1 serving (245g)	110	3	2	10	19	1	12	1	649
Campbell's Homestyle New England Clam Chowder									
1 can (519g)	363	22	4	21	29	4.2	0	12	1884
Campbell's Low Sodium Soups, Chicken Broth									
1 serving, 1 container (298g)	30	1	1	6	1	0	1	3	140
Campbell's Low Sodium Soups, Chicken with Noodle Soup									
1 serving, 1 container (305g)	159	5	2	31	17	2.1	4	12	140

Food Serving size	Cal.	(g) Total Fat	(g) Sat. Fat	(mg) Chol.	(g) Carb.	(g) Fiber	(g) Sug.	(g) Prot.	(mg) Sod.
Campbell's Low Sodium Soups, Cream of Mushroom Soup									
1 serving, 1 container (298g)	161	8	3	15	19	0	6	3	60
Campbell's Organic Tomato Juice									
1 serving (243g)	51	0	0	0	10	1.9	0	2	680
Campbell's Pace, Diced Green Chilies, Green Chilies									
1 serving (30g)	8	0	0	0	2	1	0	0	100
Campbell's Pace, Dry Taco Seasoning Mix									
2 tbsp (1 serving) (5.3g)	9	0	0	0	3	0.9	1	0	403
Campbell's Pace, Jalapenos Nacho Sliced Peppers									
1 serving (30g)	4	0	0	0	1	1	0	0	300
Campbell's Pace, Pico de Gallo									
2 tbsp (32g)	10	0	0	0	3	0	0	0	150
Campbell's Pace, Salsa Refried Beans									
1 serving (120g)	72	0	0	0	14	4	4	4	590
Campbell's Pace, Salsa Verde									
2 tbsp (32g)	15	0	0	0	2	0	0	0	230
Campbell's Pace, Spicy Jalapeno Refried Beans									
1 serving (120g)	76	0	0	0	14	5	4	5	590
Campbell's Pace, Tequila Lime Salsa									
2 tbsp (32g)	15	0	0	0	3	0	0	0	190
Campbell's Pace, Traditional Refried Beans									
1 serving (120g)	80	0	0	0	13	5	3	5	690
Campbell's Pace, Triple Pepper Salsa									
2 tbsp (32g)	15	0	0	0	3	1	0	1	190
Campbell's Pork and Beans									
1 serving (130g)	140	1	1	5	25	7	8	6	439
Campbell's Prego Pasta, Heart Smart, Traditional Sauce									
.5 cup (130g)	70	1	0	0	13	3	0	2	360
Campbell's Red and White, Microwavable Bowls, Chicken Rice Soup									
1 serving (245g)	74	1	0	5	14	1	1	2	801
Campbell's Red and White, Microwavable Bowls, Creamy Tomato Soup									
1 serving (245g)	157	5	1	5	25	2.9	16	3	750
Campbell's Red and White, Microwavable Bowls, Tomato Soup									
1 serving (245g)	108	0	0	0	24	2.9	18	3	789

Food Serving size	Cal.	(g) Total Fat	(g) Sat. Fat	(mg) Chol.	(g) Carb.	(g) Fiber	(g) Sug.	(g) Prot.	(mg) Sod.
Campbell's Red and White, Microwavable Bowls, Vegetable Beef Soup									
1 serving (245g)	83	0	0	10	15	2.9	2	5	880
Campbell's Red and White, 25% Less Sodium, Chicken Noodle Soup, Condensed									
1 serving, 1/2 cup (126g)	62	2	1	15	8	1	1	4	562
Campbell's Red and White, 25% Less Sodium, Cream of Mushroom Soup, Condensed									
1 serving, 1/2 cup (124g)	110	8	1	5	8	2	1	2	650
Campbell's Red and White, 25% Less Sodium, Tomato Soup, Condensed									
1 serving, 1/2 cup (124g)	91	0	0	0	20	1	12	2	480
Campbell's Red and White, 98% Fat Free Cream of Broccoli Soup, Condensed									
1 serving, 1/2 cup (124g)	69	2	0	5	10	2	1	2	701
Campbell's Red and White, 98% Fat Free Cream of Mushroom Soup, Condensed									
1 serving, 1/2 cup (124g)	60	3	0	5	9	1	0	1	480
Campbell's Red and White, 98% Fat Free, Broccoli Cheese Soup, Condensed									
1 serving, 1/2 cup (124g)	69	2	1	5	12	1	3	2	480
Campbell's Red and White, 98% Fat Free, Cream of Celery Soup, Condensed									
1 serving, 1/2 cup (124g)	69	3	1	5	9	2	1	1	480
Campbell's Red and White, 98% Fat Free, Cream of Chicken Soup, Condensed									
1 serving, 1/2 cup (124g)	68	3	1	5	9	0.5	1	2	713
Campbell's Red and White, Batman Fun Shapes Soup, Condensed									
1 serving, 1/2 cup (126g)	71	2	1	5	10	1	1	3	580
Campbell's Red and White, Bean with Bacon Soup, Condensed									
1 serving, 1/2 cup (128g)	160	3	2	5	25	8.1	4	8	860
Campbell's Red and White, Beef Broth, Condensed									
1 serving, 1/2 cup (124g)	15	0	0	0	1	0	1	3	861
Campbell's Red and White, Beef Consommé, Condensed									
1 serving, 1/2 cup (124g)	20	0	0	0	1	0	1	4	810
Campbell's Red and White, Beef Noodle Soup, Condensed									
1 serving, 1/2 cup (126g)	71	2	1	10	8	1	1	4	820
Campbell's Red and White, Beef with Vegetable and Barley Soup, Condensed									
1 serving, 1/2 cup (126g)	89	1	1	10	15	3	2	5	890
Campbell's Red and White, Beefy Mushroom Soup, Condensed									
1 serving, 1/2 cup (126g)	50	2	1	5	6	0	1	3	890
Campbell's Red and White, Broccoli Cheese Soup, Condensed									
1 serving, 1/2 cup (124g)	100	5	2	5	12	0	3	2	820

Food Serving size	Cal.	(g) Total Fat	(g) Sat. Fat	(mg) Chol.	(g) Carb.	(g) Fiber	(g) Sug.	(g) Prot.	(mg) Sod.
Campbell's Red and White, Chicken Alphabet Soup, Condensed									
1 serving, 1/2 cup (126g)	71	1	1	5	12	1	1	3	480
Campbell's Red and White, Chicken and Dumplings Soup, Condensed									
1 serving, 1/2 cup (126g)	71	2	1	10	10	1	1	3	760
Campbell's Red and White, Chicken and Stars Soup, Condensed									
1 serving, 1/2 cup (126g)	71	2	1	5	11	1	1	3	480
Campbell's Red and White, Chicken Barley with Mushroom Soup, Condensed									
1 serving (126g)	89	1	1	5	16	3	0	4	719
Campbell's Red and White, Chicken Broth, Condensed									
1 serving, 1/2 cup (124g)	20	1	0	5	1	0	1	1	770
Campbell's Red and White, Chicken Gumbo Soup, Condensed									
1 serving, 1/2 cup (126g)	60	1	1	5	10	1	2	2	869
Campbell's Red and White, Chicken Noodle Soup, Condensed									
1 serving, 1/2 cup (126g)	58	2	0	10	7	0	0	3	840
Campbell's Red and White, Chicken NOODLEO'S Soup, Condensed									
1 serving, 1/2 cup (126g)	89	2	1	20	15	1	2	3	480
Campbell's Red and White, Chicken Vegetable Soup, Condensed									
1 serving, 1/2 cup (126g)	79	1	1	5	15	2	3	3	890
Campbell's Red and White, Chicken with Rice Soup, Condensed									
1 serving, 1/2 cup (126g)	71	1	1	5	13	1	1	2	610
Campbell's Red and White, Chicken Won Ton Soup, Condensed									
1 serving, 1/2 cup (126g)	50	1	1	5	8	0	1	3	869
Campbell's Red and White, Cream of Mushroom with Roasted Garlic Soup, Condensed									
1 serving, 1/2 cup (124g)	69	3	1	5	10	2	1	2	480
Campbell's Red and White, Cream of Onion Soup, Condensed									
1 serving, 1/2 cup (124g)	100	6	2	5	10	3	4	1	800
Campbell's Red and White, Cream of Potato Soup, Condensed									
1 serving, 1/2 cup (124g)	88	2	0	1	16	1.6	2	2	749
Campbell's Red and White, Cream of Shrimp Soup, Condensed									
1 serving, 1/2 cup (124g)	100	6	2	20	8	0	0	3	861
Campbell's Red and White, Creamy Chicken Noodle Soup, Condensed									
1 serving, 1/2 cup (124g)	120	7	2	15	11	4	1	4	870
Campbell's Red and White, Creamy Chicken Verde Soup, Condensed									
1 serving, 1/2 cup (124g)	110	7	2	10	10	3	1	2	780

Food Serving size	Cal.	(g) Total Fat	(g) Sat. Fat	(mg) Chol.	(g) Carb.	(g) Fiber	(g) Sug.	(g) Prot.	(mg) Sod.
Campbell's Red and White, Curly Noodle Soup, Condensed									
1 serving, 1/2 cup (126g)	79	2	1	15	11	1	1	4	480
Campbell's Red and White, Danny Phantom Shaped Pasta									
1 serving, 1/2 cup (126g)	71	2	1	5	10	1	1	4	559
Campbell's Red and White, Dora the Explorer Soup, Condensed									
1 serving, 1/2 cup (126g)	79	2	1	5	13	1	3	3	480
Campbell's Red and White, Double Noodle in Chicken Broth Soup, Condensed									
1 serving, 1/ 2 cup (126g)	110	2	1	10	20	1	1	3	480
Campbell's Red and White, Fiesta Nacho Cheese Soup, Condensed									
1 serving, 1/2 cup (124g)	120	8	3	10	10	1	2	3	790
Campbell's Red and White, French Onion Soup, Condensed									
1 serving, 1/2 cup (126g)	45	1	1	5	6	1	4	2	650
Campbell's Red and White, Golden Mushroom Soup, Condensed									
1 serving, 1/2 cup (124g)	81	*3	1	0	10	1	1	2	650
Campbell's Red and White, Goldfish Pasta with Chicken Soup									
1 serving, 1/2 cup (126g)	79	2	1	5	12	1	1	3	480
Campbell's Red and White, Mega Noodle in Chicken Broth, Condensed									
1 serving, 1/2 cup (126g)	89	2	1	15	15	1	1	3	480
Campbell's Red and White, Microwavable Bowls, Chicken Noodle Soup									
1 serving (245g)	74	2	0	15	10	1	0	4	870
Campbell's Red and White, Minestrone Soup, Condensed									
1 serving, 1/2 cup (126g)	89	1	1	5	17	3	3	4	650
Campbell's Red and White, New England Clam Chowder, Condensed									
1 serving, 1/2 cup (126g)	89	2	1	5	13	1	1	4	650
Campbell's Red and White, Old Fashioned Tomato Rice Soup, Condensed									
1 serving, 1/2 cup (126g)	110	2	1	0	23	1	10	1	770
Campbell's Red and White, Oyster Stew, Condensed									
1 serving, 1/2 cup (126g)	79	6	3	20	3	0	0	3	910
Campbell's Red and White, Pepper Pot Soup, Condensed									
1 serving, 1/2 cup (126g)	89	4	1	25	9	1	1	5	980
Campbell's Red and White, Scotch Broth, Condensed									
1 serving, 1/2 cup (124g)	60	1	0	5	10	2	1	3	861
Campbell's Red and White, Shrek Shaped Pasta with Chicken in Chicken Broth									
1 serving (126g)	79	2	1	5	12	1	0	3	480

Food Serving size	Cal.	(g) Total Fat	(g) Sat. Fat	(mg) Chol.	(g) Carb.	(g) Fiber	(g) Sug.	(g) Prot.	(mg) Sod.
Campbell's Red and White, Souper Shapes									
1 serving (126g)	79	2	1	5	11	1	0	4	480
Campbell's Red and White, Southwest Style Pepper Jack Special, Condensed									
1 serving, 1/2 cup (124g)	110	6	2	5	13	4	3	2	880
Campbell's Red and White, Southwestern-Style Chicken Vegetable Soup, Condensed									
1 serving, 1/2 cup (126g)	110	1	1	5	21	4	3	5	830
Campbell's Red and White, Split Pea with Ham and Bacon Soup, Condensed									
1 serving, 1/2 cup (128g)	180	2	1	5	30	4	4	10	850
Campbell's Red and White, Tomato Bisque, Condensed									
1 serving, 1/2 cup (126g)	130	4	1	5	23	1	15	2	879
Campbell's Red and White, Tomato Soup, Condensed									
1 serving, 1/2 cup (124g)	91	0	0	0	20	1	12	2	480
Campbell's Red and White, Vegetable Beef Soup, Condensed									
1 serving, 1/2 cup (126g)	82	0	1	5	15	3	2	5	890
Campbell's Red and White, Vegetable Soup, Condensed									
1 serving, 1/2 cup (126g)	100	1	1	5	21	3	7	4	650
Campbell's Red and White, Vegetarian Vegetable Soup, Condensed									
1 serving, 1/2 cup (126g)	89	1	0	0	18	2	6	3	650
Campbell's Select Gold Label Soups, Blended Red Pepper Black Bean Soup									
1 serving (245g)	120	1	1	5	23	3.9	10	3	821
Campbell's Select Gold Label Soups, Creamy Portobello Mushroom Soup									
1 serving (245g)	103	4	3	10	14	2	2	3	789
Campbell's Select Gold Label Soups, Golden Butternut Squash Soup									
1 serving (245g)	91	1	1	5	18	2.9	8	2	811
Campbell's Select Gold Label Soups, Italian Tomato and Basil Soup									
1 serving (245g)	91	0	0	0	19	2.9	0	3	769
Campbell's Select Gold Label Soups, Southwestern Corn Chowder									
1 serving (245g)	149	3	0	0	26	2	0	3	620
Campbell's Select Microwavable Bowls, Chicken with Egg Noodles Soup									
1 cup (245g)	120	4	1	25	12	1	2	8	480
Campbell's Select Microwavable Bowls, Healthy Request, Mexican Style Tortilla									
1 cup (245g)	130	2	0	10	20	2	0	8	409

Food Serving size	Cal.	(g) Total Fat	(g) Sat. Fat	(mg) Chol.	(g) Carb.	(g) Fiber	(g) Sug.	(g) Prot.	(mg) Sod.
Campbell's Select Microwavable Bowls, Italian Sausage Pasta and Pepperoni Soup									
1 serving (245g)	130	6	2	15	15	2	5	7	870
Campbell's Select Microwavable Bowls, Italian Style Wedding Soup									
1 cup (245g)	130	4	2	15	16	2	3	7	480
Campbell's Select Microwavable Bowls, Mexican Style Chicken Tortilla Soup									
1 cup (245g)	127	2	1	20	19	2	3	8	480
Campbell's Select Microwavable Bowls, Minestrone Soup									
1 cup (245g)	96	1	0	5	19	2.9	5	4	480
Campbell's Select Microwavable Bowls, Savory Chicken and Long Grain Rice Soup									
1 cup (245g)	110	1	0	15	15	1	3	6	480
Campbell's Select Soup, 98% Fat Free, New England Clam Chowder									
1 cup (245g)	110	2	1	10	17	1	1	6	480
Campbell's Select Soup, Beef with Roasted Barley Soup									
1 cup (245g)	132	1	0	10	21	2	4	9	480
Campbell's Select Soup, Chicken and Pasta with Roasted Garlic Soup									
1 serving (245g)	113	1	0	15	18	2	2	8	821
Campbell's Select Soup, Chicken Vegetable Medley Soup									
1 cup (245g)	120	1	0	20	19	1	4	7	480
Campbell's Select Soup, Creamy Chicken Alfredo Soup									
1 cup (245g)	221	13	4	20	15	1	1	10	480
Campbell's Select Soup, Harvest Tomato with Basil Soup									
1 cup (245g)	100	0	0	0	22	2	0	3	480
Campbell's Select Soup, Healthy Request									
1 serving (245g)	100	2	1	15	13	2	0	7	480
Campbell's Select Soup, Healthy Request, Mexican Style Chicken Tortilla									
1 cup (245g)	140	2	1	15	22	2	2	8	409
Campbell's Select Soup, Italian Sausage with Pasta Pepperoni Soup									
1 cup (245g)	159	7	2	15	18	2	3	7	480
Campbell's Select Soup, Italian Style Wedding Soup									
1 cup (245g)	130	5	3	15	13	1	3	7	480
Campbell's Select Soup, Mediterranean Meatball Bowtie Pasta Soup									
1 cup (245g)	120	4	1	20	15	2	3	7	480

Food Serving size	Cal.	(g) Total Fat	(g) Sat. Fat	(mg) Chol.	(g) Carb.	(g) Fiber	(g) Sug.	(g) Prot.	(mg) Sod.
Campbell's Select Soup, Mexican Style Chicken Tortilla Soup									
1 cup (245g)	110	2	1	10	15	2	3	7	480
Campbell's Select Soup, Minestrone Soup									
1 cup (245g)	100	0	0	0	20	2.9	5	5	480
Campbell's Select Soup, New England Clam Chowder									
1 cup (245g)	179	10	2	10	17	1	1	6	480
Campbell's Select Soup, Potato Broccoli Cheese Soup									
1 cup (245g)	149	9	1	5	15	2.9	3	3	480
Campbell's Select Soup, Roasted Chicken with Long Grain Wild Rice Soup									
1 cup (245g)	110	0	0	15	20	1	2	6	480
Campbell's Select Soup, Savory White Bean with Roasted Ham Soup									
1 cup (245g)	169	1	0	5	30	7.1	4	9	480
Campbell's Select Soup, Slow Roasted Beef and Vegetable Soup									
1 cup (245g)	100	0	0	10	16	2	4	7	480
Campbell's Select Soup, Split Pea with Roasted Ham Soup									
1 cup (245g)	149	1	0	5	29	4.9	5	9	480
Campbell's Select Soup, Tomato Garden Soup									
1 cup (245g)	100	0	0	5	21	2	10	3	480
Campbell's Select Soup, Vegetable Medley Soup									
1 cup (245g)	81	0	0	0	16	2.9	6	3	480
Campbell's Soup On The Go, 25% Less Sodium, Chicken with Mini Noodles Soup									
1 container (305g)	79	2	1	9	11	2.1	0	4	729
Campbell's Soup On The Go, 25% Less Sodium, Classic Tomato									
1 container (305g)	119	0	0	0	27	2.1	0	3	659
Campbell's Soup On The Go, Blended Vegetable Medley Soup									
1 container (305g)	101	1	1	6	19	4	9	3	891
Campbell's Soup On The Go, Cheesy Potato with Bacon Flavor Soup									
1 container (305g)	131	6	2	9	16	0.9	4	2	891
Campbell's Soup On The Go, Chicken and Stars Soup									
1 container (305g)	70	1	1	6	10	2.1	1	3	891
Campbell's Soup On The Go, Chicken with Mini Noodles Soup									
1 container (305g)	79	2	1	9	11	2.1	2	4	979
Campbell's Soup On The Go, Classic Tomato Soup									
1 container (305g)	140	0	0	0	31	2.1	20	3	641

Food Serving size	Cal.	(g) Total Fat	(g) Sat. Fat	(mg) Chol.	(g) Carb.	(g) Fiber	(g) Sug.	(g) Prot.	(mg) Sod.
Campbell's Soup On The Go, Creamy Broccoli Soup 1 container (305g)	159	11	3	6	13	3.1	4	2	881
Campbell's Soup On The Go, Creamy Chicken Soup 1 container (305g)	131	9	2	6	10	2.1	1	3	881
Campbell's Soup On The Go, Creamy Tomato Soup 1 container (305g)	180	5	2	6	30	2.1	22	3	650
Campbell's Soup On The Go, Italian Style Wedding Soup 1 container (305g)	73	3	1	9	10	0.9	3	3	860
Campbell's Soup On The Go, New England Clam Chowder 1 container (305g)	159	11	3	6	13	3.1	2	2	891
Campbell's Soup On The Go, Vegetable Beef Soup 1 container (305g)	61	1	1	6	10	0.9	5	3	930
Campbell's Soup On The Go, Velvety Potato Soup 1 container (305g)	156	7	1	6	21	4	5	2	869
Campbell's SpaghettiOs A to Z 1 cup (1 serving) (252g)	169	1	0	5	35	3	55	6	600
Campbell's SpaghettiOs in Meat Sauce 1 cup (1 serving) (252g)	174	2	1	10	31	3	0	8	890
Campbell's SpaghettiOs Original 1 cup (1 serving) (252g)	169	1	0	5	35	3	187	6	600
Campbell's SpaghettiOs Original, Easy Open 1 can (1 serving) (213g)	149	1	1	4	31	3	2	5	479
Campbell's SpaghettiOs with Meatballs 1 cup (1 serving) (252g)	239	7	2	20	32	4	7	11	600
Campbell's SpaghettiOs with Meatballs, Easy Open 1 can (1 serving) (206g)	179	5	2	21	24	3.1	19	9	490
Campbell's Supper Bakes Meal Kits, Lemon Chicken with Herb Rice 1 serving (NLEA serving) (94g)	197	1	1	5	43	2	16	4	780
Campbell's Swanson Broth, Certified Organic Vegetable Broth 1 serving (235g)	12	0	0	0	3	0	2	0	550
Campbell's Swanson Broth, Vegetable Broth 1 serving (235g)	12	0	0	0	3	0	2	0	940
Campbell's Swanson, Chicken a la King 1 can (1 serving) (298g)	212	12	3	21	12	2.1	33	14	1371

Food Serving size	Cal.	(g) Total Fat	(g) Sat. Fat	(mg) Chol.	(g) Carb.	(g) Fiber	(g) Sug.	(g) Prot.	(mg) Sod.
Campbell's Swanson, Chicken and Dumplings									
1 cup (1 serving) (247g)	230	10	5	35	24	2	20	11	990
Campbell's Tomato Juice									
1 serving (243g)	51	0	0	0	10	1.9	0	2	680
Campbell's Tomato Juice, Low Sodium									
1 serving (243g)	51	0	0	0	10	1.9	0	2	141
Campbell's V8 60% Vegetable Juice, V8 V-lite									
1 serving (243g)	34	0	0	0	7	1	0	1	360
Campbell's V8 Splash Juice Drinks, Berry Blend									
1 serving, 8 oz (243g)	70	0	0	0	18	0	18	0	51
Campbell's V8 Splash Juice Drinks, Diet Berry Blend									
1 serving, 8 oz (243g)	10	0	0	0	3	0	1	0	34
Campbell's V8 Splash Juice Drinks, Diet Fruit Medley									
1 serving, 8 oz (238g)	10	0	0	0	3	0	2	0	31
Campbell's V8 Splash Juice Drinks, Diet Strawberry Kiwi									
1 serving (238g)	10	0	0	0	3	0	2	0	31
Campbell's V8 Splash Juice Drinks, Diet Tropical Blend									
1 serving, 8 oz (238g)	10	0	0	0	3	0	1	0	36
Campbell's V8 Splash Juice Drinks, Fruit Medley									
1 serving, 8 oz (243g)	80	0	0	0	19	0	19	0	51
Campbell's V8 Splash Juice Drinks, Strawberry Kiwi									
1 serving, 8 oz (243g)	70	0	0	0	18	0	18	0	51
Campbell's V8 Splash Juice Drinks, Tropical Blend									
1 serving, 8 oz (243g)	70	0	0	0	18	0	18	0	51
Campbell's V8 Splash Smoothies, Peach Mango									
1 serving, 8 oz (245g)	91	0	0	0	19	0	18	3	71
Campbell's V8 Splash Smoothies, Strawberry Banana									
1 serving, 8 oz (245g)	91	0	0	0	20	0	18	3	71
Campbell's V8 Splash Smoothies, Tropical Colada									
1 serving, 8 oz (246g)	101	0	0	0	21	1	18	3	49
Campbell's V8 Vegetable Juice, Calcium Enriched V8									
1 serving (243g)	51	0	0	0	11	1.9	0	2	481
Campbell's V8 Vegetable Juice, Essential Antioxidants V8									
1 serving (243g)	51	0	0	0	11	1.9	0	2	481

Food Serving size	Cal.	(g) Total Fat	(g) Sat. Fat	(mg) Chol.	(g) Carb.	(g) Fiber	(g) Sug.	(g) Prot.	(mg) Sod.
Campbell's V8 Vegetable Juice, Hi Fiber V8									
1 serving (243g)	61	0	0	0	13	5.1	0	2	481
Campbell's V8 Vegetable Juice, Low Sodium Spicy Hot									
1 serving (243g)	51	0	0	0	11	1.9	0	2	141
Campbell's V8 Vegetable Juice, Low Sodium V8									
1 serving (243g)	51	0	0	0	10	1.9	0	2	141
Campbell's V8 Vegetable Juice, Organic V8									
1 serving (243g)	49	0	0	0	11	1.9	0	1	481
Campbell's V8 Vegetable Juice, Spicy Hot V8									
1 serving (243g)	51	0	0	0	10	1.9	0	2	481
Campbell's V8 V-Fusion Juices, Acai Berry									
1 serving, 8 oz (246g)	111	0	0	0	27	0	26	0	69
Campbell's V8 V-Fusion Juices, Peach Mango									
1 serving, 8 oz (246g)	121	0	0	0	28	0	26	1	69
Campbell's V8 V-Fusion Juices, Strawberry Banana									
1 serving, 8 oz (246g)	121	0	0	0	29	0	25	1	69
Campbell's V8 V-Fusion Juices, Tropical									
1 serving, 8 oz (246g)	121	0	0	0	28	0	25	1	81
Chili Con Carne with Beans, Canned Entrée									
1 cup (246g)	298	13	4	32	28	9.6	6	17	1043
Chili with Beans, Canned									
1 tbsp (16g)	18	1	0	3	2	0.7	0	1	84
Oriental Mix, Rice-based									
2 oz (57g)	288	15	2	0	29	7.5	2	10	235
Soup, Bean with Bacon, Dry, Mix, Prepared with Water									
1 cup (8 fl oz) (265g)	106	2	1	3	16	9	1	5	928
Soup, Beans with Frankfurters, Canned, Condensed									
1 can (11.25 oz) (319g)	453	17	5	29	53	14.7	0	24	2651
Soup, Beans with Frankfurters, Canned, Prepared with Equal Volume of Water									
1 can (11.25 oz), prepared (607g)	455	17	5	30	53	0	0	24	2653
Soup, Beef Broth or Bouillon, Canned, Ready-to-serve									
1 can, 14.5 oz (435g)	30	1	0	0	0	0	0	5	1618
Soup, Beef Broth or Bouillon, Powder, Dry									
1 packet (6g)	13	1	0	1	1	0	1	1	1560

Food Serving size	Cal.	(g) Total Fat	(g) Sat. Fat	(mg) Chol.	(g) Carb.	(g) Fiber	(g) Sug.	(g) Prot.	(mg) Sod.
Soup, Beef Broth or Bouillon, Powder, Prepared with Water									
1 fl oz (30g)	1	0	0	0	0	0	0	0	115
Soup, Beef Broth, Bouillon, Consommé, Prepared with Equal Volume of Water									
1 can (10.5 oz), prepared (586g)	70	0	0	0	4	0	0	13	1547
Soup, Beef Broth, Cubed, Dry									
1 cube (3.6g)	5	0	0	0	0	0	0	1	720
Soup, Beef Broth, Cubed, Prepared with Water									
1 fl oz (30g)	1	0	0	0	0	0	0	0	78
Soup, Beef Mushroom, Canned, Condensed									
1 can (10.75 oz) (305g)	186	7	4	15	16	0.6	0	14	2162
Soup, Beef Mushroom, Canned, Prepared with Equal Volume of Water									
1 can (10.75 oz), prepared (593g)	178	7	4	18	15	0.6	0	14	2289
Soup, Beef Noodle, Canned, Condensed									
1 can (10.75 oz) (305g)	204	8	3	12	22	1.8	6	12	1992
Soup, Beef Noodle, Canned, Prepared with Equal Volume of Water									
1 can (10.75 oz), prepared (593g)	202	7	3	12	21	1.8	6	11	1927
Soup, Beef Noodle, Dry, Mix									
1 packet (9.2g)	30	1	0	1	4	0.2	0	2	774
Soup, Beef Stroganoff, Canned, Chunky Style, Ready-to-serve									
1 cup (240g)	235	11	6	50	22	1.4	4	12	1044
Soup, Beef with Vegetables and Barley, Canned, Condensed, Single Brand									
1 package, yields (312g)	190	4	1	19	26	0	0	12	2206
Soup, Black Bean, Canned, Condensed									
1 can (11 oz), undiluted (312g)	284	4	1	0	48	21.2	8	15	3026
Soup, Black Bean, Canned, Prepared with Equal Volume of Water									
1 can (11 oz), prepared (600g)	276	4	1	0	46	20.4	7	15	2922
Soup, Bouillon Cubes and Granules, Low Sodium, Dry									
1 cube (3.6g)	16	1	0	0	2	0	1	1	38
Soup, Broccoli Cheese, Canned, Condensed, Commercial									
1 can, 10.7 oz (10.75 oz) (303g)	264	16	5	12	23	5.5	6	6	2003
Soup, Cheese, Canned, Prepared with Equal Volume of Milk									
1 can (11 oz), prepared (609g)	560	35	22	116	39	2.4	0	23	2473

Food Serving size	Cal.	(g) Total Fat	(g) Sat. Fat	(mg) Chol.	(g) Carb.	(g) Fiber	(g) Sug.	(g) Prot.	(mg) Sod.
Soup, Cheese, Canned, Prepared with Equal Volume of Water									
1 can (11 oz), prepared (600g)	378	25	16	72	26	2.4	0	13	2328
Soup, Chicken Broth Cubes, Dry									
1 cube (4.8g)	8	0	0	1	1	0	0	1	960
Soup, Chicken Broth Cubes, Dry, Prepared with Water									
1 cube (6 fl oz prepared) (182g)	9	0	0	0	1	0	0	1	593
Soup, Chicken Broth or Bouillon, Dry									
1 teaspoon (2g)	5	0	0	0	0	0	0	0	478
Soup, Chicken Broth or Bouillon, Dry, Prepared with Water									
1 fl oz (30.1g)	1	0	0	0	0	0	0	0	121
Soup, Chicken Broth, Canned, Condensed									
1 can (10.75 oz) (305g)	95	3	1	3	2	0	1	13	1894
Soup, Chicken Broth, Canned, Less/Reduced Sodium									
1 cup (240g)	17	0	0	0	1	0	1	3	554
Soup, Chicken Broth, Canned, Prepared with Equal Volume of Water									
1 can (10.75 oz), prepared (593g)	95	3	1	0	2	0	2	12	1815
Soup, Chicken Broth, Low Sodium, Canned									
1 cup (240g)	38	1	0	0	3	0	0	5	72
Soup, Chicken Corn Chowder, Chunky, Ready-to-serve, Single Brand									
1 package, yields (539g)	534	34	9	59	40	4.9	0	17	1612
Soup, Chicken Gumbo, Canned, Condensed									
1 can (10.75 oz) (305g)	137	3	1	9	20	4.9	6	6	2114
Soup, Chicken Gumbo, Canned, Prepared with Equal Volume of Water									
1 can (10.75 oz), prepared (593g)	136	3	1	12	20	4.7	6	6	2319
Soup, Chicken Mushroom Chowder, Chunky, Ready-to-serve, Single Brand									
1 package, yields (539g)	431	24	6	32	38	7.5	0	16	1827
Soup, Chicken Mushroom, Canned, Prepared with Equal Volume of Water									
1 can (10.75 oz), prepared (593g)	320	22	6	24	23	0.6	0	11	1939
Soup, Chicken Noodle, Canned, Prepared with Equal Volume of Water									
1 serving, 1 cup (248g)	62	2	1	12	7	0.5	1	3	866
Soup, Chicken Noodle, Dry, Mix									
1 packet (6 fl oz) (11.1g)	42	1	0	8	7	0.4	0	2	404

Food Serving size	Cal.	(g) Total Fat	(g) Sat. Fat	(mg) Chol.	(g) Carb.	(g) Fiber	(g) Sug.	(g) Prot.	(mg) Sod.
Soup, Chicken Noodle, Dry, Mix, Prepared with Water									
1 cup (245g)	56	1	0	10	9	0.2	1	2	561
Soup, Chicken Noodle, Low Sodium, Canned, Prepared with Equal Volume of Water									
1 fl oz (31g)	8	0	0	2	1	0.1	0	0	54
Soup, Chicken Rice, Canned, Chunky, Ready-to-serve									
1 can, 19 oz (539g)	286	7	2	27	29	2.2	3	28	1994
Soup, Chicken Rice, Dry, Mix, Prepared with Water									
1 fl oz (30g)	7	0	0	0	1	0.1	0	0	116
Soup, Chicken Vegetable, Canned, Condensed									
1 can (10.7 oz) (303g)	185	7	2	21	21	2.1	4	9	2139
Soup, Chicken Vegetable, Canned, Prepared with Equal Volume of Water									
1 cup (8 fl oz) (248g)	77	3	1	10	9	1	1	4	972
Soup, Chicken Vegetable, Chunky, Canned, Ready-to-serve									
1 can (19 oz) (539g)	372	11	3	38	42	0	0	28	1870
Soup, Chicken Vegetable, Chunky, Reduced Fat, Ready-to-serve, Single Brand									
1 package, yields (454g)	182	2	1	18	29	0	0	12	872
Soup, Chicken with Dumplings, Canned, Condensed									
1 can (10.5 oz) (298g)	235	13	3	80	15	1.2	1	14	1842
Soup, Chicken with Dumplings, Canned, Prepared with Equal Volume of Water									
1 can (10.5 oz), prepared (586g)	234	13	3	82	15	1.2	2	14	1787
Soup, Chicken with Rice, Canned, Prepared with Equal Volume of Water									
1 serving, 1 cup (243g)	58	2	0	7	7	0.7	0	4	578
Soup, Chicken with Star-shaped Pasta, Canned, Condensed, Single Brand									
1 package, yields (298g)	149	4	1	12	21	0	0	7	2181
Soup, Chicken, Canned, Chunky, Ready-to-serve									
1 cup (245g)	174	6	2	29	17	1.5	2	12	867
Soup, Chicken Rice, Canned, Chunky, Ready-to-serve									
1 can, 19 oz (539g)	286	7	2	27	29	2.2	3	28	1994
Soup, Chili Beef, Canned, Condensed									
1 can (11.25 oz) (319g)	373	8	4	32	60	8	16	16	2514
Soup, Chili Beef, Canned, Prepared with Equal Volume of Water									
1 fl oz (32.6g)	19	0	0	2	3	0.4	1	1	126

Food Serving size	Cal.	(g) Total Fat	(g) Sat. Fat	(mg) Chol.	(g) Carb.	(g) Fiber	(g) Sug.	(g) Prot.	(mg) Sod.
Soup, Chunky Beef with Country Vegetables, Ready-to-serve									
1 serving (243g)	151	3	1	24	21	0	0	10	892
Soup, Chunky Beef, Canned, Ready-to-serve									
1 can (19 oz) (539g)	356	6	3	32	54	3.2	4	21	1822
Soup, Chunky Chicken Noodle, Canned, Ready-to-serve									
1 cup (243g)	100	3	2	12	11	1.9	1	8	744
Soup, Clam Chowder, Manhattan Style, Canned, Chunky, Ready-to-serve									
1 can (19 oz) (539g)	302	8	5	32	42	6.5	9	16	2248
Soup, Clam Chowder, Manhattan, Canned, Condensed									
1 can (10.75 oz) (305g)	186	5	1	6	30	3.7	8	5	2129
Soup, Clam Chowder, Manhattan, Canned, Prepared with Equal Volume of Water									
1 fl oz (31.1g)	9	0	0	0	1	0.2	0	0	70
Soup, Clam Chowder, New England, Canned, Condensed									
1 can (10.7 oz) (303g)	218	6	3	18	31	2.1	1	10	1563
Soup, Clam Chowder, New England, Canned, Prepared with Equal Volume of Low Fat (2%) Milk									
1 fl oz (31.5g)	19	1	0	2	2	0.1	1	1	86
Soup, Clam Chowder, New England, Canned, Prepared with Equal Volume of Water									
1 fl oz (31g)	11	0	0	1	2	0.1	0	0	79
Soup, Consommé with Gelatin, Dry, Mix, Prepared with Water									
1 fl oz (31.1g)	2	0	0	0	0	0	0	0	96
Soup, Crab, Canned, Ready-to-serve									
1 can (13 oz) (369g)	114	2	1	15	16	1.1	0	8	1867
Soup, Cream of Asparagus, Canned, Condensed									
1 can (10.75 oz) (305g)	210	10	3	12	26	1.2	2	6	2040
Soup, Cream of Asparagus, Canned, Prepared with Equal Volume of Milk									
1 can (10.75 oz), prepared (602g)	391	20	8	54	40	1.8	0	15	2528
Soup, Cream of Asparagus, Canned, Prepared with Equal Volume of Water									
1 can (10.75 oz), prepared (593g)	208	10	3	12	26	1.2	0	6	2384
Soup, Cream of Celery, Canned, Condensed									
1 can (10.75 oz) (305g)	220	14	3	34	21	1.8	4	4	1574
Soup, Cream of Celery, Canned, Prepared with Equal Volume of Milk									
1 can (10.75 oz), prepared (602g)	397	24	10	78	35	1.8	0	14	1637

Food Serving size	Cal.	(g) Total Fat	(g) Sat. Fat	(mg) Chol.	(g) Carb.	(g) Fiber	(g) Sug.	(g) Prot.	(mg) Sod.
Soup, Cream of Celery, Canned, Prepared with Equal Volume of Water									
1 can (10.75 oz), prepared (593g)	219	14	3	36	21	1.8	0	4	1506
Soup, Cream of Chicken, Canned, Condensed									
1 can (10.75 oz) (305g)	275	18	5	24	22	0	2	7	2141
Soup, Cream of Chicken, Canned, Condensed, Single Brand									
1 package, yields (305g)	302	20	5	21	23	0	0	7	2403
Soup, Cream of Chicken, Canned, Prepared with Equal Volume of Milk									
1 fl oz (31g)	24	1	1	3	2	0	0	1	112
Soup, Cream of Chicken, Canned, Prepared with Equal Volume of Water									
1 fl oz (30.5g)	15	1	0	1	1	0	0	0	106
Soup, Cream of Chicken, Dry, Mix, Prepared with Water									
1 fl oz (32.6g)	13	1	0	0	2	0	1	0	148
Soup, Cream of Mushroom, Canned, Condensed, Reduced Sodium									
1 cup (251g)	131	4	1	8	20	1.5	5	3	961
Soup, Cream of Mushroom, Canned, Prepared with Equal Volume of Low Fat (2%) Milk									
1 fl oz (31.5g)	21	1	0	1	2	0.1	1	1	112
Soup, Cream of Mushroom, Canned, Prepared with Equal Volume of Water									
1 fl oz (31g)	12	1	0	0	1	0.1	0	0	105
Soup, Cream of Mushroom, Low Sodium, Ready-to-serve, Canned									
1 can (10.75 oz) (305g)	162	11	3	3	14	0.6	5	3	61
Soup, Cream of Onion, Canned, Condensed									
1 can (10.75 oz) (305g)	268	13	4	37	32	1.2	11	7	1943
Soup, Cream of Onion, Canned, Prepared with Equal Volume of Milk									
1 can (10.75 oz), prepared (602g)	452	23	10	78	45	1.8	0	16	2438
Soup, Cream of Onion, Canned, Prepared with Equal Volume of Water									
1 can (10.75 oz), prepared (593g)	261	13	4	36	31	2.4	0	7	2253
Soup, Cream of Potato, Canned, Prepared with Equal Volume of Milk									
1 can (10.75 oz), prepared (602g)	361	16	9	54	42	1.2	0	14	1385
Soup, Cream of Potato, Canned, Prepared with Equal Volume of Water									
1 can (10.75 oz), prepared (593g)	178	6	3	12	28	1.2	0	4	1411

Food Serving size	Cal.	(g) Total Fat	(g) Sat. Fat	(mg) Chol.	(g) Carb.	(g) Fiber	(g) Sug.	(g) Prot.	(mg) Sod.
Soup, Cream of Shrimp, Canned, Condensed 1 can (10.75 oz) (305g)	220	13	8	40	20	0.6	0	7	2089
Soup, Cream of Shrimp, Canned, Prepared with Equal Volume of Low Fat (2%) Milk 1 fl oz (31.6g)	19	1	1	3	2	0	1	1	112
Soup, Cream of Shrimp, Canned, Prepared with Equal Volume of Water 1 can (10.75 oz), prepared (593g)	213	12	8	42	19	0.6	1	7	2319
Soup, Cream of Vegetable, Dry, Powder 1 packet (18g)	80	4	1	0	9	0.5	3	1	892
Soup, Egg Drop, Chinese Restaurant 1 cup (241g)	65	1	0	55	10	1	0	3	892
Soup, Escarole, Canned, Ready-to-serve 1 can (19.5 oz) (553g)	61	4	1	6	4	0	0	3	2278
Soup, Gazpacho, Canned, Ready-to-serve 1 can (13 oz) (369g)	70	0	0	0	7	0.7	2	11	1118
Soup, Healthy Choice Chicken Noodle Soup, Condensed 1 serving, 1 cup (243g)	100	2	1	12	13	1.9	1	9	474
Soup, Healthy Choice, Chicken and Rice Soup, Condensed 1 serving, 1 cup (240g)	89	1	0	17	14	1.9	1	6	434
Soup, Healthy Choice, Garden Vegetable Soup, Condensed 1 serving, 1 cup (246g)	125	1	0	2	25	4.7	5	5	480
Soup, Hot and Sour, Chinese Restaurant 1 cup (233g)	91	3	1	49	10	1.2	0	6	876
Soup, Lentil with Ham, Canned, Ready-to-serve 1 can (20 oz) (567g)	318	6	3	17	46	0	0	21	3016
Soup, Minestrone, Canned, Chunk, Ready-to-serve 1 can (19 oz) (539g)	286	6	3	11	47	12.9	12	11	1552
Soup, Minestrone, Canned, Condensed 1 can (10.5 oz) (298g)	203	6	1	3	27	2.4	4	10	1538
Soup, Minestrone, Canned, Prepared with Equal Volume of Water 1 can (10.5 oz), prepared (586g)	199	6	1	6	27	2.3	0	10	1488
Soup, Mushroom Barley, Canned, Condensed 1 can (10.75 oz) (305g)	186	5	1	0	29	0	0	5	1748

Food Serving size	Cal.	(g) Total Fat	(g) Sat. Fat	(mg) Chol.	(g) Carb.	(g) Fiber	(g) Sug.	(g) Prot.	(mg) Sod.
Soup, Mushroom Barley, Canned, Prepared with Equal Volume of Water									
1 can (10.75 oz), prepared (593g)	178	6	1	0	28	1.8	0	5	2164
Soup, Mushroom with Beef Stock, Canned, Condensed									
1 can (10.75 oz) (305g)	207	10	4	18	23	0.3	7	8	2358
Soup, Mushroom with Beef Stock, Canned, Prepared with Equal Volume of Water									
1 can (10.75 oz), prepared (593g)	208	10	4	18	23	1.8	0	8	2354
Soup, Mushroom, Dry, Mix, Prepared with Water									
1 packet (6 fl oz prepared) (194g)	64	4	1	0	9	0.4	0	1	782
Soup, Onion Dry, Mix									
1 packet (39g)	114	0	0	0	25	2.6	2	3	3132
Soup, Onion, Canned, Prepared with Equal Volume of Water									
1 fl oz (30.4g)	7	0	0	0	1	0.1	0	0	129
Soup, Onion, Dry, Mix, Prepared with Water									
1 fl oz (28.7g)	3	0	0	0	1	0.1	0	0	99
Soup, Oxtail, Dry, Mix, Prepared with Water									
1 cup (244g)	68	2	1	0	9	0.2	2	3	1159
Soup, Oyster Stew, Canned, Prepared with Equal Volume of Milk									
1 can (10.5 oz), prepared (595g)	327	19	12	77	24	0	0	15	2529
Soup, Oyster Stew, Canned, Prepared with Equal Volume of Water									
1 can (10.5 oz), prepared (586g)	141	9	6	35	10	0	0	5	2385
Soup, Pea, Green, Canned, Prepared with Equal Volume of Milk									
1 can (11.25 oz), prepared (616g)	579	17	10	43	78	6.8	0	31	2168
Soup, Pea, Green, Canned, Prepared with Equal Volume of Water									
1 fl oz (32.4g)	20	0	0	0	3	0.6	1	1	109
Soup, Pea, Low Sodium, Prepared with Equal Volume of Water									
1 fl oz (32.4g)	20	0	0	0	3	0.6	1	1	3
Soup, Pepper Pot, Canned, Prepared with Equal Volume of Water									
1 fl oz (30.4g)	12	1	0	1	1	0.1	0	1	117
Soup, Potato Ham Chowder, Chunky, Ready-to-serve, Single Brand									
1 package, yields (539g)	431	28	9	49	30	3.2	0	15	1962

Food Serving size	Cal.	(g) Total Fat	(g) Sat. Fat	(mg) Chol.	(g) Carb.	(g) Fiber	(g) Sug.	(g) Prot.	(mg) Sod.
Soup, Ramen Noodle, Any Flavor, Dry									
1 package (5.8g)	26	1	0	0	3	0.2	0	1	108
Soup, Sirloin Burger with Vegetables, Ready-to-serve, Single Brand									
1 package, yields (539g)	415	20	7	59	37	12.4	0	23	1946
Soup, Split Pea with Ham, Chunky, Reduced Fat, Reduced Sodium, Ready-to-serve, Single Brand									
1 package, yields (539g)	410	6	2	32	61	0	0	28	1849
Soup, Split Pea, Canned, Reduced Sodium, Prepared with Water or Ready-to-serve									
1 cup (253g)	167	2	1	7	28	4.7	4	10	480
Soup, Split Pea, with Ham and Bacon, Canned, Condensed, Single Brand									
1 package, yields (326g)	456	7	2	10	69	9.8	0	28	2377
Soup, Split Pea, with Ham, Canned, Chunky, Ready-to-serve									
1 can (19 oz) (539g)	415	9	4	16	60	9.2	10	25	1622
Soup, Split Pea, with Ham, Canned, Condensed									
1 can (11.5 oz) (326g)	460	11	4	20	68	5.5	0	25	2054
Soup, Split Pea, with Ham, Canned, Prepared with Equal Volume of Water									
1 can (11.5 oz), prepared (614g)	461	11	4	18	68	5.5	0	25	2444
Soup, Stock, Beef, Home-prepared									
1 cup (240g)	31	0	0	0	3	0	1	5	475
Soup, Stock, Chicken, Home-prepared									
1 cup (240g)	86	3	1	7	8	0	4	6	343
Soup, Stock, Fish, Home-prepared									
1 cup (233g)	37	2	0	2	0	0	0	5	363
Soup, Stockpot, Canned, Condensed									
1 can (11 oz), undiluted (312g)	243	9	2	9	28	0	0	12	2546
Soup, Stockpot, Canned, Prepared with Equal Volume of Water									
1 can (11 oz), prepared (600g)	240	9	2	12	28	0	0	12	2544
Soup, Swanson Chicken Broth, 99% Fat Free									
1 serving, 1 cup 8 oz (227g)	9	0	0	0	0	0	0	1	928
Soup, Tomato Beef with Noodle, Canned, Condensed									
1 can (10.75 oz) (305g)	342	10	4	9	51	3.7	0	11	2230

Food Serving size	Cal.	(g) Total Fat	(g) Sat. Fat	(mg) Chol.	(g) Carb.	(g) Fiber	(g) Sug.	(g) Prot.	(mg) Sod.
Soup, Tomato Beef with Noodle, Canned, Prepared with Equal Volume of Water									
1 can (10.75 oz), prepared (593g)	332	10	4	12	50	3.6	4	11	2176
Soup, Tomato Bisque, Canned, Condensed									
1 can (11 oz), undiluted (312g)	300	6	1	12	58	2.5	0	5	2137
Soup, Tomato Bisque, Canned, Prepared with Equal Volume of Milk									
1 can (11 oz), prepared (609g)	481	16	8	55	71	1.2	0	15	2692
Soup, Tomato Bisque, Canned, Prepared with Equal Volume of Water									
1 can (11 oz), prepared (600g)	300	6	1	12	58	1.2	0	6	2544
Soup, Tomato Rice, Canned, Condensed									
1 can (11 oz), undiluted (312g)	290	7	1	3	53	4.1	18	5	1981
Soup, Tomato Rice, Canned, Prepared with Equal Volume of Water									
1 can (11 oz), prepared (600g)	282	6	1	6	51	4.2	18	5	1914
Soup, Tomato Vegetable, Dry, Mix									
1 packet (39g)	127	2	1	1	23	1.2	1	5	2622
Soup, Tomato Vegetable, Dry, Mix, Prepared with Water									
1 cup, 8 fl oz (245g)	54	1	0	0	10	0.7	2	2	323
Soup, Tomato, Canned, Condensed									
1 can (294g)	194	1	0	0	45	3.2	24	4	1108
Soup, Tomato, Canned, Condensed, Reduced Sodium									
1 can, 10.7 oz (303g)	197	2	0	0	41	3.6	25	5	67
Soup, Tomato, Canned, Prepared with Equal Volume of Low Fat (2%) Milk									
1 fl oz (31.5g)	17	0	0	1	3	0.2	2	1	66
Soup, Tomato, Canned, Prepared with Equal Volume of Water, Commercial									
1 fl oz (31g)	9	0	0	0	2	0.2	1	0	59
Soup, Tomato, Dry, Mix, Prepared with Water									
1 cup, 8 fl oz (265g)	101	2	1	5	19	1.1	10	2	943
Soup, Tomato, Low Sodium, with Water									
1 fl oz (31g)	9	0	0	0	2	0.2	1	0	10
Soup, Turkey Noodle, Canned, Condensed									
1 can (10.75 oz) (305g)	168	5	1	12	21	1.8	1	9	1983
Soup, Turkey Noodle, Canned, Prepared with Equal Volume of Water									
1 fl oz (30.5g)	9	0	0	1	1	0.1	0	0	102
Soup, Turkey Vegetable, Canned, Condensed									
1 can (10.5 oz) (298g)	179	7	2	3	21	1.5	3	8	2202

Food Serving size	Cal.	(g) Total Fat	(g) Sat. Fat	(mg) Chol.	(g) Carb.	(g) Fiber	(g) Sug.	(g) Prot.	(mg) Sod.
Soup, Turkey Vegetable, Canned, Prepared with Equal Volume of Water									
1 fl oz (30.1g)	9	0	0	0	1	0.1	0	0	113
Soup, Turkey, Chunky, Canned, Ready-to-serve									
1 can (18.75 oz) (532g)	303	10	3	21	32	0	0	23	2080
Soup, Vegetable Beef, Canned, Condensed									
1 can (10.75 oz) (305g)	192	5	2	12	25	4.9	3	14	2153
Soup, Vegetable Beef, Canned, Condensed, Single Brand									
1 package, yields (298g)	158	2	1	15	23	0	0	11	1654
Soup, Vegetable Beef, Canned, Prepared with Equal Volume of Water									
1 can (10.75 oz), prepared (593g)	184	5	2	12	24	4.7	3	13	2070
Soup, Vegetable Beef, Dry, Mix, Prepared with Water									
1 cup, 8 fl oz (253g)	53	1	1	0	8	0.8	1	3	789
Soup, Vegetable Beef, Microwavable, Ready-to-serve, Single Brand									
1 serving (292g)	128	2	1	9	10	4.4	0	18	1098
Soup, Vegetable Chicken, Canned, Prepared with Water, Low sodium									
1 cup (241g)	166	5	1	17	21	1	3	12	84
Soup, Vegetable Soup, Low Sodium, Condensed, Prepared with Equal Volume of Water									
1 cup (253g)	83	1	0	0	15	2.8	5	3	491
Soup, Vegetable with Beef Broth, Canned, Condensed									
1 can (10.5 oz) (298g)	197	5	1	3	32	3.9	5	7	1535
Soup, Vegetables with Beef Broth, Canned, Prepared with Equal Volume of Water									
1 can (10.5 oz), prepared (586g)	193	5	1	6	31	4.1	5	7	1483
Soup, Vegetarian Vegetable, Canned, Condensed									
1 can (10.5 oz) (298g)	176	5	1	0	29	1.5	9	5	1538
Soup, Vegetarian Vegetable, Canned, Prepared with Equal Volume of Water									
1 can (10.5 oz), prepared (586g)	164	5	1	0	29	1.8	9	5	1981

Sauces and Gravies

Campbell's Au Jus Gravy									
.25 cup (59g)	5	0	0	0	0	0	0	1	230
Campbell's Beef Gravy									
.25 cup (59g)	25	1	0	5	3	0	1	1	270

Food Serving size	Cal.	(g) Total Fat	(g) Sat. Fat	(mg) Chol.	(g) Carb.	(g) Fiber	(g) Sug.	(g) Prot.	(mg) Sod.
Campbell's Brown Gravy, with Onions									
.25 cup (59g)	25	1	0	0	4	0	2	0	330
Campbell's Chunky Soups, Beef Stew - Fully Loaded									
1 cup (245g)	169	5	2	20	20	2.9	0	10	811
Campbell's Prego Pasta, Chunky Garden Combo Italian Sauce, Ready-to-serve									
1 serving, 1/2 cup (130g)	70	1	0	0	13	3	10	2	471
Campbell's, Chicken Gravy									
.25 cup (59g)	40	3	1	5	3	0	1	0	260
Campbell's, Country Style Cream Gravy									
.25 cup (59g)	45	3	1	5	3	0	1	1	190
Campbell's, Country Style Sausage Gravy									
.25 cup (59g)	70	6	1	10	3	0	1	2	270
Campbell's, Fat Free Beef Gravy									
.25 cup (59g)	15	0	0	0	3	0	0	1	300
Campbell's, Fat Free Chicken Gravy									
.25 cup (59g)	15	0	0	5	3	0	0	1	310
Campbell's, Fat Free Turkey Gravy									
.25 cup (60g)	20	0	0	5	4	0	0	1	290
Campbell's, Franco-American, Fat Free Slow Roasted Beef Gravy									
.25 cup (59g)	20	0	0	5	3	0	0	1	300
Campbell's, Franco-American, Fat Free Slow Roasted Chicken Gravy									
.25 cup (59g)	20	0	0	5	4	0	0	1	250
Campbell's, Franco-American, Slow Roasted Beef Gravy									
.25 cup (59g)	25	1	0	5	3	0	0	1	310
Campbell's, Franco-American, Slow Roasted Chicken Gravy									
.25 cup (59g)	20	1	0	5	3	0	0	1	240
Campbell's, Franco-American, Slow Roasted Turkey Gravy									
.25 cup (59g)	25	1	0	5	4	0	0	1	320
Campbell's, Golden Pork Gravy									
.25 cup (59g)	45	3	1	5	3	0	1	1	310
Campbell's, Microwavable Beef Gravy									
.25 cup (59g)	25	1	0	0	3	0	1	1	280
Campbell's, Microwavable Chicken Gravy									
.25 cup (60g)	40	3	1	5	3	0	1	0	260

Food Serving size	Cal.	(g) Total Fat	(g) Sat. Fat	(mg) Chol.	(g) Carb.	(g) Fiber	(g) Sug.	(g) Prot.	(mg) Sod.
Campbell's, Microwavable Turkey Gravy .25 cup (60g)	25	1	0	0	3	0	1	1	270
Campbell's, Mushroom Gravy .25 cup (59g)	20	1	0	5	3	0	1	0	280
Campbell's, Pace, Chipotle Chunky Salsa 2 tbsp (32g)	8	0	0	0	2	1	2	0	230
Campbell's, Pace, Cilantro Chunky Salsa 2 tbsp (32g)	8	0	0	0	2	1	2	0	270
Campbell's, Pace, Enchilada Sauce 1 serving (60g)	24	0	0	0	5	1	4	1	520
Campbell's, Pace, Green Taco Sauce 2 tbsp (16g)	4	0	0	0	1	0	1	0	100
Campbell's, Pace, Lime and Garlic Chunky Salsa 2 tbsp (32g)	12	0	0	0	3	1	2	0	210
Campbell's, Pace, Organic Picante Sauce 2 tbsp (32g)	8	0	0	0	2	1	2	0	220
Campbell's, Pace, Picante Sauce 2 tbsp (32g)	8	0	0	0	2	1	2	0	250
Campbell's, Pace, Red Taco Sauce 1 serving (16g)	8	0	0	0	2	0	1	0	130
Campbell's, Pace, Thick and Chunky Salsa 2 tbsp (32g)	8	0	0	0	2	1	2	0	230
Campbell's, Prego Pasta, Chunky Garden Tomato, Onion and Garlic Italian Sauce, Ready-to-serve 1 serving, 1/2 cup (130g)	94	3	0	0	14	3.1	10	2	489
Campbell's, Prego Sauce, Chunky Garden Mushroom and Green Pepper with Italian Sausage, Ready-to-serve 1 serving, 1/2 cup (130g)	90	3	0	0	13	3	10	2	471
Campbell's, Prego Sauce, Diced Onion and Garlic with Italian Sausage, Ready-to-serve 1 serving, 1/2 cup (130g)	120	4	2	0	18	3	12	2	480
Campbell's, Prego Sauce, Flavored with Italian Sausage, Ready-to-serve 1 serving, 1/2 cup (130g)	81	2	1	5	13	3	10	2	480
Campbell's, Prego Sauce, Fresh Mushroom with Italian Sausage, Ready-to-serve 1 serving, 1/2 cup (130g)	70	1	1	0	13	3	11	2	480

Food Serving size	Cal.	(g) Total Fat	(g) Sat. Fat	(mg) Chol.	(g) Carb.	(g) Fiber	(g) Sug.	(g) Prot.	(mg) Sod.
Campbell's, Prego Sauce, Garlic and Italian Sausage, Ready-to-serve									
1 serving, 1/2 cup (125g)	90	3	1	5	13	3	10	3	480
Campbell's, Prego Sauce, Garlic Supreme with Italian Sausage, Ready-to-serve									
1 serving, 1/2 cup (130g)	111	4	2	0	17	3	13	2	530
Campbell's, Prego Sauce, Heart Smart, Ricotta, Parmesan with Italian Sausage, Ready-to-serve									
1 serving, 1/2 cup (125g)	90	3	1	5	13	3	10	3	360
Campbell's, Prego Sauce, Heart Smart, Roasted Red Peppers and Garlic with Italian Sausage, Ready-to-serve									
1 serving, 1/2 cup (125g)	70	2	0	0	13	3	9	2	360
Campbell's, Prego Sauce, Mini Meatballs and Italian Sausage, Ready-to-serve									
1 serving, 1/2 cup (130g)	100	3	1	5	13	3	10	4	480
Campbell's, Prego Sauce, Mushroom and Garlic with Italian Sausage, Ready-to-serve									
1 serving, 1/2 cup (130g)	81	2	0	0	13	3	10	2	471
Campbell's, Prego Sauce, Mushroom and Parmesan Italian Sausage, Ready-to-serve									
1 serving, 1/2 cup (125g)	130	4	2	5	22	3	13	3	480
Campbell's, Prego Sauce, Organic Mushroom with Italian Sausage, Ready-to-serve									
1 serving, 1/2 cup (125g)	90	3	1	0	13	4	9	2	470
Campbell's, Prego Sauce, Organic Tomato and Basil with Italian Sausage, Ready-to-serve									
1 serving, 1/2 cup (125g)	90	3	0	0	13	4	9	2	470
Campbell's, Prego Sauce, Roasted Garlic and Herb Italian Sausage, Ready-to-serve									
1 serving, 1/2 cup (130g)	90	3	0	0	13	3	9	2	460
Campbell's, Prego Sauce, Roasted Garlic with Parmesan Italian Sausage, Ready-to-serve									
1 serving, 1/2 cup (130g)	100	1	1	5	13	3	10	3	480
Campbell's, Prego Sauce, Tomato, Basil and Garlic with Italian Sausage, Ready-to-serve									
1 serving, 1/2 cup (125g)	80	3	0	0	12	3	9	2	420
Campbell's, Prego Sauce, Traditional Italian, Ready-to-serve									
1 serving, 1/2 cup (130g)	70	1	0	0	13	3	10	2	480
Campbell's, Prego Sauce, Zesty Mushroom with Italian Sausage, Ready-to-serve									
1 serving, 1/2 cup (130g)	111	3	1	0	18	3	12	2	530

Food Serving size	Cal.	(g) Total Fat	(g) Sat. Fat	(mg) Chol.	(g) Carb.	(g) Fiber	(g) Sug.	(g) Prot.	(mg) Sod.
Campbell's, Turkey Gravy .25 cup (59g)	25	1	0	0	3	0	1	.1	270
Cheese Sauce, Prepared from Recipe 1 cup (243g)	479	36	20	92	13	0.2	0	25	1198
Gravy, Au Jus, Canned 1 can (298g)	48	1	0	0	7	0	0	4	1424
Gravy, Au Jus, Dry 1 tsp (3g)	9	0	0	0	1	0	0	0	348
Gravy, Beef, Canned, Ready-to-serve 1 can (291g)	154	7	3	9	14	1.2	1	11	1630
Gravy, Brown Instant, Dry 1 package (454g)	1725	54	27	54	271	14.5	42	39	22941
Gravy, Brown, Dry 1 tbsp (6g)	22	1	0	0	4	0.1	0	1	291
Gravy, Chicken, Canned, Ready-to-serve 1 can (298g)	235	17	4	6	16	1.2	2	6	1264
Gravy, Chicken, Dry 1 serving (8g)	30	1	0	2	5	0	0	1	332
Gravy, Heinz Home Style Savory Beef Gravy 1 serving, 1/4 cup 2 oz (57g)	22	1	0	1	4	0.4	0	1	335
Gravy, Mushroom, Dry, Powder 1 cup (8 fl oz) (21g)	69	1	0	1	14	1	1	2	1382
Gravy, Onion, Dry, Mix 1 cup (8 fl oz) (24g)	77	1	0	0	16	1.4	0	2	1005
Gravy, Pork, Dry, Powder 1 serving (6.7g)	22	1	0	1	4	0.1	1	1	321
Gravy, Turkey, Canned, Ready-to-serve 1 tbsp (14.9g)	8	0	0	0	1	0.1	0	0	86
Gravy, Turkey, Dry 1 serving (7g)	26	1	0	1	5	0	0	.1	307
Guava Sauce, Cooked 1 cup (238g)	86	0	0	0	23	8.6	14	1	10
Kraft, Stove Top Stuffing Mix, Chicken Flavor 1 NLEA serving (makes 1/2 cup prepared) (28g)	107	1	0	1	20	0.7	3	4	429

Food Serving size	Cal.	(g) Total Fat	(g) Sat. Fat	(mg) Chol.	(g) Carb.	(g) Fiber	(g) Sug.	(g) Prot.	(mg) Sod.
Roast Beef Spread 1 serving, .25 cup (57g)	127	9	4	40	2	0.1	0	9	413
Sandwich Spread, Meatless 1 tbsp (15g)	22	1	0	0	1	0.5	0	1	95
Sandwich Spread, Pork, Beef 1 oz (28.35g)	67	5	2	11	3	0.1	0	2	287
Sandwich Spread, with Chopped Pickle, Regular, Unspecified Oils 1 cup (245g)	953	83	12	186	55	1	37	2	2450
Sauce, Barbecue .5 cup (143g)	246	1	0	0	58	1.3	48	1	1469
Sauce, Barbecue, Kraft, Original .5 cup (146g)	251	1	0	0	60	0.6	47	1	1813
Sauce, Barbecue, Low Sodium 1 cup (250g)	375	1	0	0	91	1.5	65	0	333
Sauce, Cheese, Dry, Powder 1 packet (35g)	157	9	4	18	12	0.4	9	8	1299
Sauce, Cheese, Ready-to-serve .25 cup (63g)	110	8	4	18	4	0.3	0	4	522
Sauce, Chili, Peppers, Hot, Immature Greens, Canned 1 cup (245g)	49	0	0	0	12	4.7	6	2	61
Sauce, Fish, Ready-to-serve 1 tbsp (18g)	6	0	0	0	1	0	1	1	1413
Sauce, Hoisin, Ready-to-serve 1 tbsp (16g)	35	1	0	0	7	0.4	4	1	258
Sauce, Homemade, White, Medium .5 cup (125g)	184	13	4	9	11	0.3	5	5	443
Sauce, Homemade, White, Thick .5 cup (125g)	233	17	4	8	15	0.4	5	5	466
Sauce, Homemade, White, Thin .5 cup (125g)	131	8	3	10	9	0.1	6	5	410
Sauce, Mole Poblano, Dry Mix, Single Brand 1 cup, sauce (265g)	1513	110	0	0	111	26.8	0	20	3085
Sauce, Oyster, Ready-to-serve 1 tbsp (18g)	9	0	0	0	2	0.1	0	0	492

Food Serving size	Cal.	(g) Total Fat	(g) Sat. Fat	(mg) Chol.	(g) Carb.	(g) Fiber	(g) Sug.	(g) Prot.	(mg) Sod.
Sauce, Pasta, Spaghetti, Marinara, Ready-to-serve									
1 cup (257g)	65	2	0	3	10	2.4	7	2	553
Sauce, Pasta, Spaghetti, Marinara, Ready-to-serve, Low Sodium									
1 cup (257g)	131	4	0	5	21	4.6	14	4	77
Sauce, Peppers, Hot, Chili, Mature Red, Canned									
1 cup (245g)	51	1	0	0	10	1.7	6	2	61
Sauce, Pizza, Canned, Ready-to-serve									
.25 cup (63g)	34	1	0	0	5	1.3	2	1	219
Sauce, Plum, Ready-to-serve									
1 cup (305g)	561	3	0	0	131	2.1	0	3	1641
Sauce, Ready-to-serve, Pepper, Tabasco									
.25 tsp (1.2g)	0	0	0	0	0	0	0	0	8
Sauce, Salsa, Ready-to-serve									
.5 cup (130g)	38	0	0	0	9	2.3	5	2	917
Sauce, Sofrito, Prepared from Recipe									
.5 cup (103g)	244	19	0	0	6	1.8	0	13	1179
Sauce, Teriyaki, Ready-to-serve									
1 fl oz (36g)	32	0	0	0	6	0	5	2	640
Sauce, Tomato Chili Sauce, Bottled, No Salt, Low Sodium									
1 tbsp (17g)	18	0	0	0	5	0.1	2	0	3
Sauce, Tomato Chili Sauce, Bottled, with Salt									
1 cup (273g)	284	1	0	0	54	16.1	29	7	3653
Sauce, Worcestershire									
1 cup (275g)	215	0	0	0	54	0	28	0	2695
Soy Sauce, Made from Hydrolyzed Vegetable Protein									
1 tsp (6g)	2	0	0	0	0	0	0	0	341
Soy Sauce, Made from Soy (Tamari)									
1 tsp (6g)	4	0	0	0	0	0	0	1	335
Soy Sauce, Made from Soy and Wheat (Shoyu)									
1 tbsp (16g)	8	0	0	0	1	0.1	0	1	902
Soy Sauce, Made from Soy and Wheat (Shoyu), Low Sodium									
1 tbsp (16g)	8	0	0	0	1	0.1	0	1	533
Tomato Products, Canned, Paste, with Salt									
1 can (6 oz) (170g)	139	1	0	0	32	7	21	7	1343

Food Serving size	Cal.	(g) Total Fat	(g) Sat. Fat	(mg) Chol.	(g) Carb.	(g) Fiber	(g) Sug.	(g) Prot.	(mg) Sod.
Tomato Products, Canned, Paste, Without Salt Added									
1 tbsp (16g)	13	0	0	0	3	0.7	2	1	16
Tomato Products, Canned, Puree, with Salt									
1 can (29 oz) (401 x 411) (822g)	312	2	0	0	74	15.6	40	14	3280
Tomato Products, Canned, Puree, Without Salt									
1 can (29 oz) (401 x 411) (822g)	312	2	0	0	74	15.6	40	14	230
Tomato Products, Canned, Sauce									
1 cup (245g)	59	0	0	0	13	3.7	10	3	1284
Tomato Products, Canned, Sauce, Spanish Style									
1 can, 15 oz (303 x 406) (425g)	140	1	0	0	31	6	0	6	2006
Tomato Products, Canned, Sauce, with Herbs and Cheese									
1 can, 15 oz (303 x 406) (425g)	251	8	3	13	44	9.4	0	9	2308
Tomato Products, Canned, Sauce, with Mushrooms									
1 cup (245g)	86	0	0	0	21	3.7	14	4	1107
Tomato Products, Canned, Sauce, with Onions									
1 cup (245g)	103	0	0	0	24	4.4	0	4	1350
Tomato Products, Canned, Sauce, with Onions, Green Peppers, and Celery									
1 can, 15 oz (303 x 406) (411g)	169	3	1	0	36	5.8	30	4	2244
Tomato Products, Canned, Sauce, with Tomato Tidbits									
1 can, 15 oz (303 x 406) (425g)	136	2	0	0	30	6	0	6	64
Tomato Sauce, No Salt									
1 cup (245g)	103	0	0	0	21	3.7	1	3	27
Worthington Saucettes, Canned, Unprepared									
1 link (38g)	83	6	0	1	2	1.1	0	6	202

Frozen Dinners/Meals

Food Serving size	Cal.	(g) Total Fat	(g) Sat. Fat	(mg) Chol.	(g) Carb.	(g) Fiber	(g) Sug.	(g) Prot.	(mg) Sod.
Beef Pot Pie, Frozen Entrée, Prepared									
1 pie, cooked (average weight) (268g)	590	31	11	56	59	2.1	10	19	978
Chicken Pot Pie, Frozen Entrée, Prepared									
1 pie (average weight of prepared pie) (234g)	501	25	8	56	54	2.8	7	14	889

Food Serving size	Cal.	(g) Total Fat	(g) Sat. Fat	(mg) Chol.	(g) Carb.	(g) Fiber	(g) Sug.	(g) Prot.	(mg) Sod.
DiGiorno Pizza, Cheese Topping, Cheese Stuffed Crust, Frozen, Baked									
1 pie, 12″ diameter (688g)	1920	80	39	193	205	13.1	0	93	5545
DiGiorno Pizza, Pepperoni Topping, Thin Crispy Crust, Frozen, Baked									
1 pie, 22.1 oz (548g)	1551	70	27	153	157	15.3	18	72	3633
DiGiorno Pizza, Supreme Topping, Rising Crust, Frozen, Baked									
1 pie, 12″ diameter (876g)	2234	94	35	166	245	20.1	32	103	6237
DiGiorno Pizza, Supreme Topping, Thin Crispy Crust, Frozen, Baked									
1 pie, 24.8 oz (595g)	1517	64	26	119	167	16.7	21	68	3302
Egg Rolls, Chicken, Refrigerated, Heated									
1 oz (28.35g)	56	1	0	4	8	0.7	7	3	159
Egg Rolls, Pork, Refrigerated, Heated									
1 oz (28.35g)	63	2	0	4	8	0.6	6	3	149
Egg Rolls, Vegetable, Refrigerated, Heated									
1 oz (28.35g)	56	1	0	0	9	0.8	7	2	159
Entrees, Crab Cake									
1 cake (60g)	160	10	2	82	5	0.2	0	11	491
Entrees, Fish Fillet, Battered or Breaded and Fried									
1 fillet (91g)	211	11	3	31	15	0.5	0	13	484
French Toast, Frozen, Ready-to-heat									
1 piece (59g)	126	4	1	48	19	0.6	0	4	292
Kellogg, Kellogg's Eggo, Banana Bread Waffles									
1 serving (78g)	212	7	1	0	32	2	5	5	280
Kellogg, Kellogg's Eggo, Buttermilk Pancake									
3 pancakes (NLEA serving) (116g)	270	8	2	13	44	1.3	10	7	589
Kellogg's Eggo Golden Oat Waffles									
1 serving (70g)	139	2	0	1	26	2.5	2	5	270
Kellogg's Eggo Low Fat Blueberry Nutri-Grain Waffles									
1 serving (70g)	146	2	0	0	30	2.5	6	4	414
Kellogg's Eggo Low Fat Homestyle Waffles									
1 serving (70g)	165	2	1	18	31	0.7	2	5	309
Lasagna with Meat and Sauce, Frozen Entrée									
1 serving (297g)	377	14	7	45	38	3.6	11	25	832
Lasagna with Meat and Sauce, Low-Fat, Frozen Entrée									
1 oz (28.35g)	29	1	0	2	4	0.4	1	2	51

Food Serving size	Cal.	(g) Total Fat	(g) Sat. Fat	(mg) Chol.	(g) Carb.	(g) Fiber	(g) Sug.	(g) Prot.	(mg) Sod.
Lasagna, Cheese, Frozen, Prepared									
1 oz (28.35g)	37	2	1	4	4	0.5	1	2	81
Lasagna, Vegetable, Frozen, Baked									
1 cup (226g)	314	14	5	32	32	4.3	44	16	796
Lean Pockets, Ham N Cheddar									
1 each (analytical measurement) (129g)	297	8	3	26	42	2.2	27	13	637
Morningstar Farms Asian Veggie Patties, Frozen, Unprepared									
1 patty (67g)	107	4	1	0	10	2	3	7	486
Morningstar Farms BBQ Riblets, Frozen, Unprepared									
1 piece, with sauce (142g)	223	4	0	0	35	6.8	24	19	815
Morningstar Farms Breakfast Pattie, Made with Organic Soy, Frozen, Unprepared									
1 patty (38g)	78	3	0	1	4	1.6	1	8	240
Morningstar Farms California Turkey Burger, Frozen, Unprepared									
1 patty (64g)	91	5	1	0	7	5	1	9	390
Morningstar Farms Chik Patties, Frozen, Unprepared									
1 patty (71g)	140	5	1	0	16	2.1	1	8	593
Morningstar Farms Chik'n Grill Veggie Patties, Frozen, Unprepared									
1 patty (67g)	79	3	0	0	7	3.8	0	9	348
Morningstar Farms Chik'n Nuggets, Frozen, Unprepared									
4 pieces (86g)	190	9	1	0	19	4.2	2	12	604
Morningstar Farms Garden Veggie Patties, Frozen, Unprepared									
1 patty (67g)	118	4	1	1	9	3	2	12	352
Morningstar Farms Grillers Original, Frozen, Unprepared									
1 patty (64g)	136	6	1	2	5	2.8	1	15	270
Morningstar Farms Grillers Prime, Frozen, Unprepared									
1 patty (71g)	169	9	1	1	4	1.8	0	17	356
Morningstar Farms Grillers Quarter Pound Veggie Burger, Frozen, Unprepared									
1 patty (114g)	252	12	2	1	10	2.9	1	26	489
Morningstar Farms Hot and Spicy Veggie Sausage Patties, Frozen, Unprepared									
1 patty (38g)	71	3	0	0	3	0.9	0	8	209
Morningstar Farms Italian Herb Chik Patties, Frozen, Unprepared									
1 patty (71g)	168	5	1	0	22	2.4	1	10	484
Morningstar Farms Lasagna with Veggie Sausage, Frozen, Unprepared									
1 serving (284g)	304	7	3	11	41	6.5	5	20	591

Food Serving size	Cal.	(g) Total Fat	(g) Sat. Fat	(mg) Chol.	(g) Carb.	(g) Fiber	(g) Sug.	(g) Prot.	(mg) Sod.
Morningstar Farms Maple Flavor Veggie Sausage Patties, Frozen, Unprepared									
1 patty (38g)	84	3	0	0	5	0.8	2	10	249
Morningstar Farms Sausage Style Recipe Crumbles, Frozen, Unprepared									
1 cup (55g)	89	3	0	0	5	2.5	1	11	417
Morningstar Farms Tomato and Basil Pizza Burger, Frozen, Unprepared									
1 patty (67g)	121	6	1	7	7	2.5	2	10	261
Morningstar Farms Veggie Breakfast Bacon Strips, Frozen, Unprepared									
2 strips (16g)	55	4	1	0	2	0.8	0	2	234
Morningstar Farms Veggie Breakfast Sausage Links, Frozen, Unprepared									
2 links (45g)	72	3	0	1	3	1.8	0	9	302
Morningstar Farms Veggie Italian Style Sausage, Frozen, Unprepared									
1 link (64g)	120	6	1	0	7	1.3	1	11	351
Morningstar Farms Veggie Sweet and Sour Chick'n, Frozen, Unprepared									
1 serving (284g)	346	7	1	0	58	3.7	12	14	545
Morningstar Farms, Grillers Burger Style Recipe Crumbles, Frozen, Unprepared									
.667 cup (1 serving) (55g)	77	2	0	0	5	2.6	2	10	235
Morningstar Farms, Grillers Vegan, Frozen, Unprepared									
1 patty (71g)	94	2	0	0	6	3.7	2	12	280
Morningstar Farms, Spicy Black Bean Burger, Frozen, Unprepared									
1 patty (67g)	115	4	1	1	13	4.6	2	11	348
Morningstar Farms, Veggie Breakfast Sausage Patties, Frozen, Unprepared									
1 patty (38g)	80	3	0	1	3	1.6	1	10	255
Onion Rings, Breaded, Partially Fried, Frozen, Unprepared									
1 package (16 oz) (454g)	1171	64	21	0	139	8.2	0	14	1117
Pizza Pepperoni Topping, Regular Crust, Frozen, Cooked									
1 pizza (428g)	1267	65	21	64	122	9.4	14	48	2645
Pizza, Cheese Topping, Regular Crust, Frozen, Cooked									
1 package, 15.1 oz pizza (452g)	1211	56	19	63	131	9.9	17	47	2020
Pizza, Cheese Topping, Rising Crust, Frozen, Cooked									
1 package, 19.7 oz pizza (595g)	1547	52	23	95	196	14.9	21	74	3308
Pizza, Meat and Vegetable Topping, Regular Crust, Frozen, Cooked									
1 package, 22.85 oz pizza (644g)	1777	93	33	103	162	14.2	33	73	3574

Food Serving size	Cal.	(g) Total Fat	(g) Sat. Fat	(mg) Chol.	(g) Carb.	(g) Fiber	(g) Sug.	(g) Prot.	(mg) Sod.
Pizza, Meat and Vegetable Topping, Rising Crust, Frozen, Cooked									
1 package, 30.7 oz pizza (891g)	2415	105	41	169	256	20.5	43	113	5702
Supper Bakes Meal Kit, Creamy Stroganoff Sauce with Pasta									
1 serving (125g)	184	4	2	10	31	1	11	6	650
Supper Bakes Meal Kit, Garlic Chicken with Pasta									
.167 box (NLEA serving) (103g)	227	1	1	5	44	2.1	25	10	763
Supper Bakes Meal Kit, Southwestern-style Chicken with Rice									
1 serving (81g)	153	1	0	5	32	2	20	4	600
Supper Bakes Meal, Cheesy Chicken with Pasta (Chicken Not Included)									
.167 box (NLEA serving size) (85g)	168	4	1	5	27	1	0	6	840
Supper Bakes Meal, Chicken with Stuffing (Chicken Not Included)									
1 box (505g)	960	18	6	30	174	12.1	48	30	4439
Turkey Pot Pie, Frozen Entrée									
1 serving (397g)	699	35	11	64	70	4.4	15	26	1390
Turkey Roast, Boneless, Frozen, Seasoned, Light and Dark Meat, Roasted									
1 box (net weight, 1.72 lb) (782g)	1212	45	15	414	24	0	0	167	5318
Turkey, Stuffing, Mashed Potatoes with Gravy, Assorted Vegetables, Frozen, Microwave									
1 package (422g)	540	16	4	59	69	5.5	107	29	1772
Waffles, Buttermilk, Frozen, Ready-to-heat									
1 waffle, round (38g)	104	4	1	6	16	0.8	2	3	236
Waffles, Buttermilk, Frozen, Ready-to-heat, Microwaved									
1 waffle (35g)	101	3	1	6	15	0.8	2	2	232
Waffles, Buttermilk, Frozen, Ready-to-heat, Toasted									
1 waffle, round (4" dia) (33g)	102	3	1	4	16	0.9	1	2	234
Waffles, Chocolate Chip, Frozen, Ready-to-heat									
2 waffles, round (70g)	195	7	2	15	29	1	9	4	380
Waffles, Plain, Frozen, Ready-to-heat									
1 waffle, square (4" square) (include frozen) (35g)	100	3	1	5	15	0.8	2	2	223
Waffles, Plain, Frozen, Ready-to-heat, Microwave									
1 waffle, round (4" dia) (32g)	95	3	1	5	15	0.8	2	2	218

Food Serving size	Cal.	(g) Total Fat	(g) Sat. Fat	(mg) Chol.	(g) Carb.	(g) Fiber	(g) Sug.	(g) Prot.	(mg) Sod.
Waffles, Plain, Frozen, Ready-to-heat, Toasted									
1 waffle, round (4" dia) (33g)	103	3	1	5	16	0.8	2	2	241
Waffles, Plain, Prepared from Recipe									
1 waffle, round (7" dia) (75g)	218	11	2	52	25	0	0	6	383
Worthington Chic-ketts, Frozen, Unprepared									
2 slices (3/8" thick) (55g)	110	5	1	0	3	0.7	0	13	353
Worthington Chili, Canned, Unprepared									
1 cup (230g)	290	10	2	0	25	7.8	3	24	1042
Worthington Dinner Roasted, Frozen, Unprepared									
1 slice, 3/4" (85g)	181	11	2	1	6	2.6	1	14	570
Worthington Fri Chik Original, Canned, Unprepared									
2 pieces (90g)	144	9	1	1	3	1.4	0	12	361
Worthington Fripats, Frozen, Unprepared									
1 patty (64g)	134	6	1	1	5	1.8	1	15	331
Worthington Leanies, Frozen, Unprepared									
1 link (40g)	100	7	1	1	2	1.5	0	8	431
Worthington Prime Stakes, Canned, Unprepared									
1 piece (92g)	124	7	1	1	7	1.3	0	9	442
Worthington Prosage Links, Frozen, Unprepared									
2 links (45g)	64	2	0	1	2	1.3	0	9	369
Worthington Prosage Roll, Frozen, Unprepared									
1 slice, 5/8" (55g)	144	10	2	1	3	1.9	0	11	367
Worthington Smoked Turkey Roll, Frozen, Unprepared									
1 slice, 3/8" (55g)	138	9	1	0	4	0.6	1	10	472
Worthington Stakelets, Frozen, Unprepared									
1 piece (71g)	150	7	1	1	7	2	1	14	462
Worthington Stripples, Frozen, Unprepared									
2 strips (16g)	55	4	1	0	2	0.8	0	2	234
Worthington Super Links, Canned, Unprepared									
1 link (48g)	105	7	1	0	3	0.9	0	7	340
Worthington Vegetable Steaks, Canned, Unprepared									
2 slices (72g)	81	1	0	0	4	1.6	0	15	300
Worthington Vegetarian Burger, Canned, Unprepared									
.25 cup (55g)	68	2	0	0	3	1.5	0	10	248

Food Serving size	Cal.	(g) Total Fat	(g) Sat. Fat	(mg) Chol.	(g) Carb.	(g) Fiber	(g) Sug.	(g) Prot.	(mg) Sod.
Worthington Wham (Roll), Frozen, Unprepared									
1 slice, 3/8" (55g)	108	6	1	0	3	0	2	10	394

Meal Replacement Bars

Food Serving size	Cal.	(g) Total Fat	(g) Sat. Fat	(mg) Chol.	(g) Carb.	(g) Fiber	(g) Sug.	(g) Prot.	(mg) Sod.
Formulated Bar, Luna Bar, Nutz Over Chocolate									
1 bar (48g)	193	6	3	0	25	2.1	0	10	185
Formulated Bar, Mars Snackfood US, Cocoavia, Chocolate Almond									
1 bar (22g)	76	3	1	0	11	1.1	0	2	57
Formulated Bar, Mars Snackfood US, Cocoavia, Chocolate Blueberry									
1 bar (22g)	72	2	1	0	13	1	0	1	57
Formulated Bar, Mars Snackfood US, Snickers Marathon Chewy Chocolate Peanut Bar									
1 bar (55g)	218	7	3	2	26	1.4	0	13	254
Formulated Bar, Mars Snackfood US, Snickers Marathon Double Chocolate Nut Bar									
1 bar (55g)	189	5	3	2	29	5.8	0	12	183
Formulated Bar, Power Bar, Chocolate									
1 bar (68g)	247	2	1	0	47	3.9	0	10	99
Formulated Bar, Slim-Fast Optima Meal Bar, Milk Chocolate Peanut									
1 bar (55g)	212	5	3	4	33	2.8	0	9	139
Formulated, Wheat-based, All Flavors Except Macadamia, Without Salt									
1 oz (28.35g)	183	18	3	0	6	1.5	0	4	26
Formulated, Wheat-based, Flavor, Macadamia Flavor, Without Salt									
1 oz (28.35g)	175	16	2	0	8	1.5	0	3	13
Formulated, Wheat-based, Unflavored, with Salt									
1 oz (28.35g)	176	16	2	0	7	1.5	0	4	143

Baby Foods/Beverages

Feeding Infants, Toddlers, and Children

Good nutrition is a must to support the rapid growth and development your baby will undergo in the first two years of life. Providing the right foods during this critical time will support good health and encourage enjoyment of new tastes and textures as they grow, as well as build the beginning of healthy eating habits. Use this information to help raise healthy and happy children.

What Is a Healthy Diet for Your Baby, Toddler, and Child?

Breast milk or formula is the only food a newborn needs. Breast-feeding is ideal because it allows you to make the perfect food for your baby. Breast milk is easier to digest, it doesn't need preparation, and it contains growth factors for your baby's development. Breast-feeding also provides your baby protection against many infections and diseases. By 4–6 months of age, a baby is usually ready for solid food as well. Check with your pediatrician. Signs to look for are: birth weight has doubled, your baby holds his or her head steady in an upright position, your baby puts hands and toys in the mouth, and your baby shows interest in your food. Once you have the okay from the pediatrician, begin with baby cereal. The baby will consume less breast milk or formula when eating solid food. Once the baby is comfortable with the cereal you may gradually introduce pureed fruits, vegetables, and proteins. It may be a good idea to introduce some vegetables before fruits since the sweet taste of fruits may make vegetables less appealing. Add one new food at a time so that if you become aware of any adverse reactions (diarrhea, rash, vomiting) you will know which food is causing it. At 8–10 months, babies are usually ready for finely chopped finger foods including soft fruits and vegetables, pasta, cheese, scrambled eggs, dry cereal, and well-cooked meats. Be sure to watch for choking. Do not give your baby cow's milk or honey before one year of age. Cow's milk does not provide the required nutrients and honey in infants can cause botulism. As your baby grows into toddlerhood, keep introducing new foods. To prevent choking, don't give your child hot dogs, grapes, marshmallows, chunks of meat or cheese, or large pieces of fruits and vegetables. Make meals an adventure. Providing new tastes and textures will encourage your child to develop an enjoyment of a wide variety of foods and develop healthy eating habits.

The chart on the next page gives the daily estimated calories and recommended servings of each of the major food groups for infants and children from birth to age 8 (see page 363). Calorie estimates are based on a moderately active child. Food portions are assumed to be nutrient-dense, meaning the foods provide the greatest amount of nutrients.

Why Are Nutrition Facts for Children Different?

Because young children have unique nutritional needs for their growing bodies, yet require fewer calories than the 2,000 that the regular Nutrition Facts labels are based on, the Nutrition Facts for children's foods and beverages are different. First, foods specifically for children less than 4 years do not provide % Daily Values for the macronutrients, carbohydrates and fat, as well as sodium, fiber, cholesterol, saturated fat, and trans fat. Since protein is an important nutrient for growing children, a % Daily Value is provided, along with % Daily Values for vitamins A and C, calcium, and iron. Unfortunately, the % Daily Values are based on a 2,000-calorie diet and are not specific to the needs of children. Also, food labels for children less than 2 years of age do not present information on calories from fat, nor do they include amounts for saturated fat, polyunsaturated fat, monounsaturated fat, and cholesterol. Because fat is essential to growth, it should not be restricted during these early years. In addition, serving sizes for infant foods are based on average amounts that infants under two years usually eat. (See page 358.)

	0 to 4 months	4 to 8 months	8 months to 1 year	1 to 3 years	4 to 8 years
Milk	16 to 45 ounces	28 to 45 ounces	24 to 32 ounces	At least 3 servings per day	2.5 to 3 cups Switch to low-fat milk
Meat	None	3 to 4 tbsp well-cooked finely ground or pureed meats and cheese	1 to 2 ounces	2 (1-ounce) servings per day	2 to 4 adult servings
Fruit	None	2 to 3 tbsp per serving 2 servings per day	2 to 3 tbsp per serving 2 servings per day	2 to 3 servings per day 1 serving = $1/4$ to $1/2$ fruit, $1/4$ to $1/3$ juice (limit juice to no more than four ounces)	1 to 1.5 adult servings
Vegetables	None	2 to 3 tbsp per serving 2 servings per day	2 to 3 tbsp per serving 2 servings per day	2 to 3 servings per day 1 serving = $1/4$ to $1/2$ cup cooked, canned, or chopped raw	1 to 1.5 adult servings
Grains	None	1 to 2 tbsp (dry amount) iron fortified baby cereal (mixed with breast milk or formula) Gradually increase to 3 to 4 tbsp	2 to 6 tbsp	At least 6 servings per day 1 serving = $1/4$ to $1/2$ slice of bread, 2 to 3 crackers, $1/4$ to $1/3$ cup cooked pasta, rice, or cereal	3 to 4 adult servings
Fats/Oils	N/A	N/A	3 to 4 tsp	3 to 4 tsp	3 to 4 adult servings

Adapted from 2015 National Institutes of Health Recommendations for Toddler Nutrition.

Fruit desserts for children less than 2 years old	Fruit desserts for children ages 2 years to 4 years

Nutrition Facts
Serving Size 1 jar (140g)

Amount Per Serving

Calories 110

Total Fat	0g
Trans Fat	0g
Sodium	10mg
Total Carbohydrate	27mg
Dietary Fiber	4g
Sugars	0g
Protein	0g

% Daily Value

Protein 0%	•	Vitamin A 6%
Vitamin C 45%	•	Calcium 2%
Iron 2%		

Nutrition Facts
Serving Size 1 jar (140g)

Amount Per Serving

Calories 110	Calories from Fat 0
Total Fat	0g
Saturated Fat	0g
Trans Fat	0g
Cholesterol	0mg
Sodium	10mg
Total Carbohydrate	27g
Dietary Fiber	4g
Sugars	0g
Protein	0g

% Daily Value

Protein 0%	•	Vitamin A 6%
Vitamin C 45%	•	Calcium 2%
Iron 2%		

How Do the Food Label Reference Values (Daily Values) Compare to the Nutritional Recommendations for Children (DRIs)?

Nutrient Recommendations by Age (DRIs)

Nutrient	Daily Value	2 to 3 years	4 to 8 years
Protein (grams)	50	13	19
Iron (mg)	18	7	10
Calcium (mg)	1,000	700	1,000
Vitamin A (IU)	5,000	1,000	1,333
Vitamin C (mg)	60	15	25

Sources: 2010 Dietary Guidelines and IOM Dietary Reference Intakes 2006 and 2010.

Tips for Raising Healthy Children

1. **Offer a variety of healthy foods.** When children eat a variety of foods, they get the nutrients they need from every food group. They will be more likely to try new foods and to like more foods. This will make it easier to plan family meals.

2. **Start with small portions.** Offer children small, easy-to-eat amounts to make eating easy and more enjoyable. Use smaller bowls, plates, and utensils for your child to eat with. Don't insist that children finish all the food on their plate. Let your child know it is okay to only eat as much as he or she wants. We are born with an internal mechanism that signals we are full—don't mess with it.

3. **Follow a meal and snack schedule.** Regularly scheduled meal and snack times help your child learn how to eat to fuel the body and control hunger. Your child is more likely to eat healthy meals and try new foods if snacks are not offered too close to mealtime.

4. **Make mealtime an enjoyable family time.** Family meals allow your child to focus on the task of eating and give you a chance to model good food behaviors. Studies show children who participate in family meals have healthier eating habits and lower rates of obesity. Sharing in trips to the market, food preparation, serving, and cleaning up adds to family time. Busy schedules may make meals difficult to schedule but it's worth it. You may not be able to eat together all the time, but try to plan a family meal at least once a day. The family should remove all distractions such as televisions, tablets, gaming devices, and phones. Not only will you be available for meaningful conversation, you will be able to focus on the taste and texture of the food, how much you are eating, and when you get full. To involve your child in conversation, ask questions like:

   - What made you feel really happy today?
   - What did you eat at lunch today?
   - What's your favorite veggie? Why?
   - Tell me one thing you learned today?
   - What made you laugh today?

5. **Make food fun for picky eaters.** Picky eating most likely is temporary, so don't get discouraged. Get your child involved in planning, shopping for, and preparing the food. Let them create snacks, salads, or desserts. Have the children search the produce department for the new vegetable or fruit to try that week. Be creative with the food. Try fun and interesting food shapes and names like orange smiles and broccoli trees.

6. **Set a good example.** Your child picks up all of your attitudes and behaviors—including your eating habits. Children love to copy what their parents do. They are likely to mimic your table manners, your likes and dislikes, your willingness to try new foods, and your physical activities.

Food Serving size	Cal.	(g) Total Fat	(g) Sat. Fat	(mg) Chol.	(g) Carb.	(g) Fiber	(g) Sug.	(g) Prot.	(mg) Sod.
Baby Foods/Formulas									
Baby Face, Juice, Fruit Punch, with Calcium									
1 fl oz (31.2g)	16	0	0	0	4	0.1	3	0	1
Baby Food, Apple Yogurt Dessert, Strained									
1 jar, NFS (113g)	108	2	1	7	22	0.6	0	1	23
Baby Food, Apple-Banana Juice									
1 bottle, Earth's Best (4.2 fl oz) (131g)	67	0	0	0	16	0.3	14	0	5
Baby Food, Apple-Cranberry Juice									
1 fl oz (31.2g)	14	0	0	0	4	0	2	0	2
Baby Food, Apples, Diced, Toddler									
1 oz (28.35g)	14	0	0	0	3	0.3	3	0	2
Baby Food, Apples, with Ham, Strained									
1 jar, NFS (113g)	70	1	0	9	12	2	9	3	10
Baby Food, Baked Product, Finger Snacks Cereal									
1 cookie (1.7g)	7	0	0	0	1	0	0	0	6
Baby Food, Banana Apple Dessert, Strained									
1 jar, NFS (113g)	77	0	0	0	18	1.1	10	0	8
Baby Food, Banana Juice, with Low Fat Yogurt									
1 bottle, NFS (126g)	112	1	1	4	22	0.5	0	3	47
Baby Food, Banana, No Tapioca, Strained									
1 jar, NFS (113g)	103	0	0	0	24	1.8	0	1	2
Baby Food, Cereal, High Protein, Prepared with Whole Milk									
1 oz (28.35g)	31	1	0	0	3	0	0	2	14
Baby Food, Cereal, High Protein, with Apples and Oranges, Prepared with Whole Milk									
1 oz (28.35g)	31	1	0	0	4	0	0	2	16
Baby Food, Cereal, High Protein, with Apples and Oranges, Dry									
.5 oz (14.2g)	53	1	0	0	8	1	0	4	15
Baby Food, Cereal, Mixed, Dry									
.5 oz (15g)	57	1	0	0	11	1.1	0	2	0
Baby Food, Cereal, Mixed, Prepared with Whole Milk									
1 oz (28.35g)	27	1	0	3	3	0.2	1	1	12
Baby Food, Cereal, Mixed, with Applesauce and Bananas, Junior									
1 jar (170g)	141	1	0	0	31	2	13	2	5

Food Serving size	Cal.	(g) Total Fat	(g) Sat. Fat	(mg) Chol.	(g) Carb.	(g) Fiber	(g) Sug.	(g) Prot.	(mg) Sod.
Baby Food, Cereal, Mixed, with Applesauce and Bananas, Strained									
1 jar (113g)	93	1	0	0	20	1.4	9	1	3
Baby Food, Cereal, Mixed, with Bananas, Dry									
.5 oz (15g)	59	1	0	0	12	1.2	1	2	0
Baby Food, Cereal, Mixed, with Bananas, Prepared with Whole Milk									
1 oz (28.35g)	24	1	1	3	3	0.1	2	1	13
Baby Food, Cereal, Mixed, with Honey, Prepared with Whole Milk									
1 oz (28.35g)	32	1	0	0	5	0	0	1	13
Baby Food, Cereal, Oatmeal, Dry									
.5 oz (15g)	60	1	0	0	11	1.4	1	2	1
Baby Food, Cereal, Oatmeal, Prepared with Whole Milk									
1 oz (28.35g)	32	1	1	3	4	0.3	0	1	13
Baby Food, Cereal, Oatmeal, with Applesauce and Bananas, Junior									
1 jar (170g)	128	1	0	0	27	1.4	16	2	5
Baby Food, Cereal, Oatmeal, with Applesauce and Bananas, Strained									
1 jar (113g)	84	1	0	0	17	0.9	12	1	3
Baby Food, Cereal, Oatmeal, with Bananas, Dry									
.5 oz (15g)	59	1	0	0	11	0.8	2	2	1
Baby Food, Cereal, Oatmeal, with Bananas, Prepared with Whole Milk									
1 oz (28.35g)	24	1	1	3	3	0.1	2	1	13
Baby Food, Cereal, Oatmeal, with Honey, Dry									
.5 oz (14.2g)	56	1	0	0	10	0	0	2	7
Baby Food, Cereal, Oatmeal, with Honey, Prepared with Whole Milk									
1 oz (28.35g)	32	1	0	0	4	0	0	1	14
Baby Food, Cereal, Rice, Dry									
.5 oz (15g)	59	1	0	0	12	0.1	0	1	1
Baby Food, Cereal, Rice, Prepared with Whole Milk									
1 oz (28.35g)	24	1	1	3	3	0	1	1	12
Baby Food, Cereal, Rice, with Applesauce and Bananas, Strained									
1 oz (28.35g)	23	0	0	0	5	0.3	1	0	1
Baby Food, Cereal, Rice, with Bananas, Dry									
.5 oz (15g)	61	1	0	0	12	0.2	3	1	0
Baby Food, Cereal, Rice, with Bananas, Prepared with Whole Milk									
1 oz (28.35g)	24	1	1	3	3	0	2	1	13

Food Serving size	Cal.	(g) Total Fat	(g) Sat. Fat	(mg) Chol.	(g) Carb.	(g) Fiber	(g) Sug.	(g) Prot.	(mg) Sod.
Baby Food, Cereal, Rice, with Honey, Prepared with Whole Milk									
1 oz (28.35g)	33	1	0	0	5	0	0	1	14
Baby Food, Cereal, Rice, with Mixed Fruit, Junior									
1 oz (28.35g)	23	0	0	0	5	0.2	3	0	3
Baby Food, Cereal, Whole Wheat, with Apples, Dry									
.5 oz (15g)	60	1	0	0	12	1.8	3	2	4
Baby Food, Cereal, with Egg Yolks, Junior									
1 jar (170g)	88	3	1	107	12	1.5	0	3	56
Baby Food, Cereal, with Egg Yolks, Strained									
1 jar (113g)	58	2	1	71	8	1	0	2	37
Baby Food, Cereal, with Eggs, Strained									
1 jar (113g)	66	2	1	58	9	0	0	2	43
Baby Food, Cherry Cobbler, Junior									
1 oz (28.35g)	22	0	0	0	5	0.1	3	0	0
Baby Food, Cookie, Fruit									
1 cookie (8g)	35	1	0	0	6	0.3	2	1	1
Baby Food, Cookies									
1 cookie (6.5g)	28	1	0	1	4	0	2	1	20
Baby Food, Cookies, Arrowroot									
1 cookie (5g)	21	1	0	0	4	0	0	0	16
Baby Food, Corn and Sweet Potatoes, Strained									
1 oz (28.35g)	19	0	0	0	4	0.5	1	0	4
Baby Food, Dessert, Banana Pudding, Strained									
1 jar, NFS (113g)	77	1	0	33	16	0.9	0	1	61
Baby Food, Dessert, Banana Yogurt, Strained									
1 jar, NFS (113g)	89	1	0	1	20	0.6	3	1	16
Baby Food, Dessert, Blueberry Yogurt, Strained									
1 jar, NFS (113g)	87	1	1	5	19	0.5	13	1	16
Baby Food, Dessert, Cherry Vanilla Pudding, Junior									
1 jar (170g)	117	0	0	17	31	0.5	29	0	0
Baby Food, Dessert, Cherry Vanilla Pudding, Strained									
1 jar (113g)	77	0	0	11	20	0.3	10	0	0
Baby Food, Dessert, Custard Pudding, Vanilla, Junior									
1 tbsp (14g)	12	0	0	5	2	0	2	0	4

Food Serving size	Cal.	(g) Total Fat	(g) Sat. Fat	(mg) Chol.	(g) Carb.	(g) Fiber	(g) Sug.	(g) Prot.	(mg) Sod.
Baby Food, Dessert, Custard Pudding, Vanilla, Strained									
1 tbsp (14g)	12	0	0	1	2	0	2	0	0
Baby Food, Dessert, Dutch Apple, Junior									
1 jar (170g)	134	0	0	0	33	2.4	30	0	5
Baby Food, Dessert, Dutch Apple, Strained									
1 jar (113g)	85	0	0	0	22	1.6	20	0	0
Baby Food, Dessert, Fruit Dessert, without Vitamin C, Junior									
1 oz (28.35g)	18	0	0	0	5	0.2	3	0	0
Baby Food, Dessert, Fruit Dessert, without Vitamin C, Strained									
1 oz (28.35g)	17	0	0	0	5	0.2	4	0	0
Baby Food, Dessert, Fruit Pudding, Orange, Strained									
1 jar (113g)	90	1	1	3	20	0.7	0	1	23
Baby Food, Dessert, Fruit Pudding, Pineapple, Strained									
1 oz (28.35g)	23	0	0	0	6	0.2	3	0	0
Baby Food, Dessert, Peach Cobbler, Junior									
1 oz (28.35g)	19	0	0	0	5	0.2	3	0	0
Baby Food, Dessert, Peach Cobbler, Strained									
1 oz (28.35g)	18	0	0	0	5	0.2	3	0	2
Baby Food, Dessert, Peach Melba, Junior									
1 jar (220g)	132	0	0	0	36	0	0	1	20
Baby Food, Dessert, Peach Melba, Strained									
1 jar (113g)	68	0	0	0	19	0	0	0	10
Baby Food, Dessert, Peach Yogurt									
1 jar, NFS (113g)	86	0	0	5	20	0.5	10	1	16
Baby Food, Dessert, Tropical Fruit, Junior									
1 jar (113g)	68	0	0	0	19	0	0	0	8
Baby Food, Dinner, Apples and Chicken, Strained									
1 jar (113g)	73	2	0	6	12	2	9	2	14
Baby Food, Dinner, Beef and Rice, Toddler									
1 jar (170g)	139	5	0	0	15	0	0	9	54
Baby Food, Dinner, Beef Lasagna, Toddler									
1 jar (170g)	131	4	0	0	17	0	0	7	70
Baby Food, Dinner, Beef Noodle, Junior									
1 oz (28.35g)	16	1	0	2	2	0.3	0	1	7

Food Serving size	Cal.	(g) Total Fat	(g) Sat. Fat	(mg) Chol.	(g) Carb.	(g) Fiber	(g) Sug.	(g) Prot.	(mg) Sod.
Baby Food, Dinner, Beef Noodle, Strained									
1 oz (28.35g)	18	1	0	2	2	0.4	0	1	4
Baby Food, Dinner, Beef Stew, Toddler									
1 jar (170g)	87	2	1	22	9	1.9	2	9	180
Baby Food, Dinner, Beef with Vegetables									
1 jar, Beech-Nut Stage 2 (4 oz) (113g)	108	8	3	14	7	2	2	2	43
Baby Food, Dinner, Broccoli and Chicken, Junior									
1 container (162g)	100	4	1	21	10	2.3	2	6	28
Baby Food, Dinner, Chicken and Noodle, with Vegetables, Toddler									
1 jar, NFS (170g)	112	3	1	48	15	1	0	6	400
Baby Food, Dinner, Chicken and Rice									
1 jar, Gerber (4 oz) (113g)	58	1	0	11	10	1.2	1	2	28
Baby Food, Dinner, Chicken Noodle, Junior									
1 oz (28.35g)	16	0	0	3	2	0.3	0	1	10
Baby Food, Dinner, Chicken Noodle, Strained									
1 oz (28.35g)	19	1	0	5	3	0.6	1	1	11
Baby Food, Dinner, Chicken Soup, Strained									
1 tbsp (16g)	8	0	0	1	1	0.2	0	0	3
Baby Food, Dinner, Chicken Stew, Toddler									
1 oz (28.35g)	22	1	0	8	2	0.2	0	1	7
Baby Food, Dinner, Macaroni and Cheese, Junior									
1 jar (170g)	104	3	2	10	14	0.5	2	4	452
Baby Food, Dinner, Macaroni and Cheese, Strained									
1 jar (113g)	76	2	1	8	10	0.8	1	4	134
Baby Food, Dinner, Macaroni and Tomato and Beef, Junior									
1 oz (28.35g)	17	0	0	1	3	0.3	1	1	10
Baby Food, Dinner, Macaroni and Tomato and Beef, Strained									
1 oz (28.35g)	17	0	0	2	3	0.3	1	1	11
Baby Food, Dinner, Macaroni, Beef and Tomato, Sauce, Toddler									
1 tbsp (16g)	13	0	0	1	2	0.2	0	1	6
Baby Food, Dinner, Mixed Vegetables, Junior									
1 jar (170g)	56	0	0	0	14	0	0	2	65
Baby Food, Dinner, Mixed Vegetables, Strained									
1 jar (113g)	46	0	0	0	11	0	0	1	43

Food Serving size	Cal.	(g) Total Fat	(g) Sat. Fat	(mg) Chol.	(g) Carb.	(g) Fiber	(g) Sug.	(g) Prot.	(mg) Sod.
Baby Food, Dinner, Pasta, with Vegetables									
1 jar, Gerber (4 oz) (113g)	68	2	1	6	9	1.7	1	2	12
Baby Food, Dinner, Potatoes, with Cheese and Ham, Toddler									
1 oz (28.35g)	22	1	0	2	3	0.3	0	1	57
Baby Food, Dinner, Spaghetti and Tomato and Meat, Junior									
1 oz (28.35g)	19	0	0	1	3	0.3	1	1	9
Baby Food, Dinner, Spaghetti and Tomato and Meat, Toddler									
1 jar (170g)	128	2	0	0	18	0	0	9	406
Baby Food, Dinner, Sweet Potatoes and Chicken, Strained									
1 jar, Beech-Nut Stage 2 (4 oz) (113g)	84	2	1	12	12	1.5	3	3	25
Baby Food, Dinner, Turkey and Rice, Junior									
1 oz (28.35g)	16	0	0	1	3	0.3	0	1	7
Baby Food, Dinner, Turkey and Rice, Strained									
1 oz (28.35g)	15	0	0	1	2	0.3	0	1	5
Baby Food, Dinner, Turkey, Rice, and Vegetables, Toddler									
1 jar, Beech nut (170g)	102	3	1	12	13	1.4	1	6	39
Baby Food, Dinner, Vegetables and Bacon, Strained									
1 tbsp (16g)	11	0	0	1	1	0.3	0	0	8
Baby Food, Dinner, Vegetables and Beef, Junior									
1 tbsp (16g)	12	1	0	1	1	0.2	0	0	5
Baby Food, Dinner, Vegetables and Beef, Strained									
1 tbsp (16g)	12	1	0	1	1	0.2	0	0	5
Baby Food, Dinner, Vegetables and Chicken, Junior									
1 tbsp (16g)	8	0	0	1	1	0.2	0	0	5
Baby Food, Dinner, Vegetables and Chicken, Strained									
1 tbsp (16g)	9	0	0	2	1	0.3	0	0	4
Baby Food, Dinner, Vegetables and Dumplings and Beef, Junior									
1 jar (170g)	82	1	0	0	14	0	0	4	88
Baby Food, Dinner, Vegetables and Dumplings and Beef, Strained									
1 jar (113g)	54	1	0	0	9	0	0	2	55
Baby Food, Dinner, Vegetables and Ham, Junior									
1 tbsp (16g)	10	0	0	0	1	0.2	0	0	7
Baby Food, Dinner, Vegetables and Ham, Strained									
1 tbsp (16g)	9	0	0	1	1	0.3	0	0	3

Food Serving size	Cal.	(g) Total Fat	(g) Sat. Fat	(mg) Chol.	(g) Carb.	(g) Fiber	(g) Sug.	(g) Prot.	(mg) Sod.
Baby Food, Dinner, Vegetables and Lamb, Junior									
1 jar (170g)	87	3	1	9	12	1.9	2	4	22
Baby Food, Dinner, Vegetables and Lamb, Strained									
1 tbsp (16g)	8	0	0	1	1	0.2	0	0	3
Baby Food, Dinner, Vegetables and Noodles and Turkey, Junior									
1 jar (170g)	88	3	0	0	13	1.9	0	3	29
Baby Food, Dinner, Vegetables and Noodles and Turkey, Strained									
1 jar (113g)	50	1	0	0	8	1.2	0	1	24
Baby Food, Dinner, Vegetables and Turkey, Junior									
1 tbsp (16g)	8	0	0	1	1	0.1	0	0	7
Baby Food, Dinner, Vegetables and Turkey, Strained									
1 tbsp (16g)	8	0	0	1	1	0.2	0	0	3
Baby Food, Dinner, Vegetables and Turkey, Toddler									
1 jar (170g)	136	6	0	0	14	0	0	8	70
Baby Food, Dinner, Vegetables, Noodles and Chicken, Junior									
1 jar (170g)	109	4	0	0	15	1.9	0	3	44
Baby Food, Dinner, Vegetables, Noodles and Chicken, Strained									
1 jar (113g)	71	3.	0	0	9	1.2	0	2	23
Baby Food, Fruit and Vegetable, Apple and Sweet Potato									
1 jar, Gerber (4 oz) (113g)	72	0	0	0	17	1.6	13	0	3
Baby Food, Fruit, Applesauce and Apricots, Strained									
1 oz (28.35g)	12	0	0	0	3	0.5	3	0	0
Baby Food, Fruit, Applesauce and Cherries, Junior									
1 jar (170g)	87	0	0	0	24	1.9	18	0	2
Baby Food, Fruit, Applesauce and Cherries, Strained									
1 jar (113g)	58	0	0	0	16	1.2	12	0	1
Baby Food, Fruit, Applesauce and Pineapple, Junior									
1 jar (170g)	66	0	0	0	18	2.6	0	0	3
Baby Food, Fruit, Applesauce and Pineapple, Strained									
1 jar (113g)	42	0	0	0	11	1.7	0	0	2
Baby Food, Fruit, Applesauce and Raspberry, Junior									
1 jar (170g)	99	0	0	0	26	3.6	22	0	0
Baby Food, Fruit, Applesauce and Raspberry, Strained									
1 jar (113g)	66	0	0	0	18	2.4	15	0	0

Food Serving size	Cal.	(g) Total Fat	(g) Sat. Fat	(mg) Chol.	(g) Carb.	(g) Fiber	(g) Sug.	(g) Prot.	(mg) Sod.
Baby Food, Fruit, Applesauce, Junior 1 oz (28.35g)	10	0	0	0	3	0.5	2	0	0
Baby Food, Fruit, Applesauce, Strained 1 oz (28.35g)	12	0	0	0	3	0.5	3	0	0
Baby Food, Fruit, Applesauce, with Banana, Junior 1 jar, NFS (170g)	112	0	0	0	27	2.7	7	1	5
Baby Food, Fruit, Apricot, with Tapioca, Junior 1 oz (28.35g)	18	0	0	0	5	0.4	0	0	0
Baby Food, Fruit, Apricot, with Tapioca, Strained 1 oz (28.35g)	17	0	0	0	4	0.5	0	0	0
Baby Food, Fruit, Bananas and Pineapple with Tapioca, Junior 1 oz (28.35g)	19	0	0	0	5	0.5	2	0	0
Baby Food, Fruit, Bananas and Pineapple with Tapioca, Strained 1 oz (28.35g)	18	0	0	0	5	0.5	3	0	0
Baby Food, Fruit, Bananas, with Apples and Pears, Strained 1 jar, NFS (113g)	94	0	0	0	22	1.6	14	1	2
Baby Food, Fruit, Bananas, with Tapioca, Junior 1 oz (28.35g)	19	0	0	0	5	0.5	2	0	0
Baby Food, Fruit, Bananas, with Tapioca, Strained 1 oz (28.35g)	16	0	0	0	4	0.5	0	0	0
Baby Food, Fruit, Guava and Papaya, with Tapioca, Strained 1 jar (113g)	71	0	0	0	19	0	0	0	5
Baby Food, Fruit, Papaya and Applesauce, with Tapioca, Strained 1 jar (113g)	79	0	0	0	21	1.6	0	0	6
Baby Food, Fruit, Peaches, Junior 1 oz (28.35g)	18	0	0	0	4	0.4	3	0	1
Baby Food, Fruit, Peaches, Strained 1 oz (28.35g)	18	0	0	0	4	0.4	3	0	1
Baby Food, Fruit, Pears and Pineapple, Junior 1 oz (28.35g)	12	0	0	0	3	0.7	2	0	0
Baby Food, Fruit, Pears and Pineapple, Strained 1 oz (28.35g)	12	0	0	0	3	0.7	2	0	0
Baby Food, Fruit, Pears, Junior 1 oz (28.35g)	12	0	0	0	3	1	2	0	0

Food Serving size	Cal.	(g) Total Fat	(g) Sat. Fat	(mg) Chol.	(g) Carb.	(g) Fiber	(g) Sug.	(g) Prot.	(mg) Sod.
Baby Food, Fruit, Pears, Strained									
1 oz (28.35g)	12	0	0	0	3	1	2	0	0
Baby Food, Fruit, Plums, with Tapioca, without Vitamin C, Junior									
1 oz (28.35g)	21	0	0	0	6	0.3	4	0	0
Baby Food, Fruit, Plums, with Tapioca, without Vitamin C, Strained									
1 oz (28.35g)	20	0	0	0	6	0.3	4	0	0
Baby Food, Fruit, Prunes, with Tapioca, without Vitamin C, Junior									
1 jar (170g)	119	0	0	0	32	4.6	19	1	3
Baby Food, Fruit, Prunes, with Tapioca, without Vitamin C, Strained									
1 oz (28.35g)	20	0	0	0	5	0.8	3	0	1
Baby Food, Fruit, Tutti Frutti, Junior									
1 jar, NFS (170g)	117	1	0	26	27	0.7	1	1	29
Baby Food, Fruit, Tutti Frutti, Strained									
1 jar, NFS (113g)	75	0	0	17	17	0.7	0	0	28
Baby Food, Green Beans, Diced, Toddler									
1 jar (128g)	37	0	0	0	7	1.7	1	2	47
Baby Food, Juice Treats, Fruit Medley, Toddler									
1 packet (28g)	97	0	0	0	24	0	16	0	25
Baby Food, Juice, Apple									
1 jar (127g)	60	0	0	0	15	0.1	14	0	10
Baby Food, Juice, Apple and Cherry									
1 jar (127g)	52	0	0	0	13	0.1	11	0	0
Baby Food, Juice, Apple and Grape									
1 jar (127g)	58	0	0	0	14	0.1	14	0	0
Baby Food, Juice, Apple and Peach									
1 jar (127g)	55	0	0	0	13	0.1	12	0	0
Baby Food, Juice, Apple and Plum									
1 jar (127g)	62	0	0	0	16	0.1	15	0	0
Baby Food, Juice, Apple and Prune									
1 jar (127g)	91	0	0	0	23	0.1	13	0	10
Baby Food, Juice, Apple, with Calcium									
1 serving (189g)	87	0	0	0	21	0.8	17	0	6
Baby Food, Juice, Apple-Cherry									
1 bottle, Heinz Strained (4 fl oz) (125g)	59	0	0	0	14	0.4	0	0	5

Food Serving size	Cal.	(g) Total Fat	(g) Sat. Fat	(mg) Chol.	(g) Carb.	(g) Fiber	(g) Sug.	(g) Prot.	(mg) Sod.
Baby Food, Juice, Apple-Sweet Potato 1 fl oz (30.8g)	15	0	0	0	4	0.2	0	0	2
Baby Food, Juice, Mixed Fruit 1 jar (127g)	60	0	0	0	15	0.1	11	0	10
Baby Food, Juice, Orange 1 jar (127g)	57	0	0	0	13	0.1	10	1	0
Baby Food, Juice, Orange and Apple 1 jar (127g)	55	0	0	0	13	0	0	1	4
Baby Food, Juice, Orange and Apricot 1 jar (127g)	58	0	0	0	14	0.1	0	1	8
Baby Food, Juice, Orange and Banana 1 jar (127g)	64	0	0	0	15	0	0	1	4
Baby Food, Juice, Orange and Pineapple 1 jar (127g)	61	0	0	0	15	0.1	0	1	3
Baby Food, Juice, Orange, Apple, and Banana 1 jar (127g)	60	0	0	0	15	0.1	13	1	0
Baby Food, Juice, Orange-Carrot 1 fl oz (30.8g)	13	0	0	0	3	0.1	0	0	3
Baby Food, Juice, Pear 1 bottle, Earth's Best (4.2 fl oz) (131g)	62	0	0	0	16	0.1	10	0	10
Baby Food, Juice, Prune and Orange 1 jar (127g)	89	0	0	0	21	0	0	1	3
Baby Food, Mashed Cheddar Potatoes and Broccoli, Toddler 1 container (170g)	82	2	1	5	13	1.5	2	2	299
Baby Food, Meat, Beef, Strained 1 tbsp (14.7g)	12	0	0	7	0	0	0	2	6
Baby Food, Meat, Beef, Strained 1 oz (28.35g)	23	1	0	14	1	0	0	3	12
Baby Food, Meat, Beef, with Vegetables, Toddler 1 jar, NFS (179g)	122	4	2	21	16	0.9	2	6	47
Baby Food, Meat, Chicken Sticks, Junior 1 jar (71g)	133	10	3	55	1	0.1	1	10	290
Baby Food, Meat, Chicken, Junior 1 oz (28.35g)	41	3	1	17	0	0	0	4	14

Food Serving size	Cal.	(g) Total Fat	(g) Sat. Fat	(mg) Chol.	(g) Carb.	(g) Fiber	(g) Sug.	(g) Prot.	(mg) Sod.
Baby Food, Meat, Chicken, Strained 1 oz (28.35g)	37	2	1	17	0	0	0	4	14
Baby Food, Meat, Ham, Junior 1 jar (71g)	69	3	1	21	3	0	0	8	31
Baby Food, Meat, Ham, Strained 1 oz (28.35g)	27	1	0	7	1	0	0	3	12
Baby Food, Meat, Lamb, Junior 1 jar (71g)	80	4	2	27	0	0	0	11	30
Baby Food, Mixed Fruit Yogurt, Strained 1 jar, NFS (113g)	85	1	1	0	18	0.5	0	1	18
Baby Food, Oatmeal Cereal, with Fruit, Dry, Instant, Toddler 1 packet (.75 oz) (21g)	84	1	0	0	16	1.6	2	2	0
Baby Food, Peaches, Diced, Toddler 1 jar, Gerber (128g)	65	0	0	0	15	1	12	1	12
Baby Food, Pears, Diced, Toddler 1 jar, Gerber (128g)	73	0	0	0	17	1.5	11	0	8
Baby Food, Ravioli, Cheese-filled, with Tomato Sauce 1 piece (8g)	8	0	0	1	1	0	0	0	23
Baby Food, Rice and Apples, Dry 1 tbsp (2.5g)	10	0	0	0	2	0.1	0	0	0
Baby Food, Teething Biscuits 1 biscuit (11g)	43	0	0	1	8	0.2	1	1	31
Baby Food, Vegetable and Brown Rice, Strained 1 tbsp (14.4g)	10	0	0	0	2	0.2	0	0	2
Baby Food, Vegetable, Beets, Strained 1 tbsp (14g)	5	0	0	0	1	0.3	1	0	12
Baby Food, Vegetable, Butternut Squash and Corn 1 jar, Gerber (4 oz) (113g)	57	1	0	0	10	2.3	3	2	6
Baby Food, Vegetable, Carrots, Junior 1 tbsp (14g)	4	0	0	0	1	0.2	0	0	7
Baby Food, Vegetable, Carrots, Strained 1 tbsp (14g)	4	0	0	0	1	0.2	1	0	10
Baby Food, Vegetable, Corn, Creamed, Junior 1 tbsp (15g)	10	0	0	0	2	0.3	0	0	8

Food Serving size	Cal.	(g) Total Fat	(g) Sat. Fat	(mg) Chol.	(g) Carb.	(g) Fiber	(g) Sug.	(g) Prot.	(mg) Sod.
Baby Food, Vegetable, Corn, Creamed, Strained 1 tbsp (15g)	9	0	0	0	2	0.3	0	0	6
Baby Food, Vegetable, Garden Vegetables, Strained 1 jar (113g)	36	0	0	0	8	1.7	3	3	35
Baby Food, Vegetable, Green Beans and Potatoes 1 jar, Gerber (4 oz) (113g)	70	2	1	6	10	1.6	3	2	20
Baby Food, Vegetable, Green Beans, Junior 1 tbsp (15g)	4	0	0	0	1	0.3	0	0	1
Baby Food, Vegetable, Green Beans, Strained 1 tbsp (15g)	4	0	0	0	1	0.3	0	0	1
Baby Food, Vegetable, Mixed Vegetables, Junior 1 tbsp (15g)	5	0	0	0	1	0.2	0	0	5
Baby Food, Vegetable, Mixed Vegetables, Strained 1 jar (113g)	41	1	0	0	9	1.7	2	1	0
Baby Food, Vegetable, Peas, Strained 1 oz (28.35g)	14	0	0	0	2	0.6	1	1	1
Baby Food, Vegetable, Spinach, Creamed, Strained 1 tbsp (15g)	6	0	0	1	1	0.3	0	0	7
Baby Food, Vegetable, Squash, Junior 1 oz (28.35g)	7	0	0	0	2	0.3	1	0	1
Baby Food, Vegetable, Squash, Strained 1 oz (28.35g)	8	0	0	0	2	0.3	1	0	1
Baby Food, Vegetable, Sweet Potatoes, Junior 1 tbsp (14g)	8	0	0	0	2	0.2	1	0	3
Baby Food, Vegetable, Sweet Potatoes, Strained 1 tbsp (14g)	8	0	0	0	2	0.2	1	0	3
Baby Food, Yogurt, Whole Milk, with Fruit, Multigrain Cereal and Added DHA 1 container (113g)	111	4	2	16	15	0.3	13	4	46
Child Formula, Abbott Nutrition, Pediasure, Ready-to-feed 1 fl oz (31g)	31	1	0	1	3	0	3	1	11
Child Formula, Abbott Nutrition, Pediasure, Ready-to-feed, with Iron 1 fl oz (31g)	31	1	0	1	3	0.2	2	1	11
Child Formula, Mead Johnson, Portagen, with Iron, Powder, Not Reconstituted 1 scoop (9.4g)	43	2	2	0	5	0	5	1	23

Food Serving size	Cal.	(g) Total Fat	(g) Sat. Fat	(mg) Chol.	(g) Carb.	(g) Fiber	(g) Sug.	(g) Prot.	(mg) Sod.
Child Formula, Mead Johnson, Portagen, with Iron, Prepared from Powder									
1 fl oz (31g)	27	1	1	0	3	0	2	1	16
Infant Formula, Abbott Nutrition, Similac, Advance with Iron, Liquid, Concentrate									
1 fl oz (31.4g)	40	2	1	1	4	0	4	1	10
Infant Formula, Abbott Nutrition, Similac, Advance with Iron, Powder									
1 scoop (8.5g)	44	2	1	1	5	0	5	1	11
Infant Formula, Abbott Nutrition, Similac, Advance with Iron, Ready-to-feed									
1 fl oz (30.4g)	20	1	0	1	2	0	2	0	5
Infant Formula, Abbott Nutrition, Similac, Neosure, Ready-to-feed, with ARA and DHA									
1 fl oz (30.5g)	21	1	1	1	2	0	2	1	7
Infant Formula, Abbott Nutrition, Similac, PM 60/40, Powder, Not Reconstituted									
1 scoop (8.7g)	42	2	1	1	4	0	4	1	10
Infant Formula, Abbott Nutrition, Similac, Sensitive (Lactose Free), Liquid Concentrate, with ARA and DHA									
1 fl oz (30.5g)	39	2	1	1	4	0	4	1	12
Infant Formula, Abbott Nutrition, Similac, Sensitive (Lactose Free), Powder, with ARA and DHA									
1 fl oz (30.5g)	159	9	6	5	17	0	17	3	48
Infant Formula, Abbott Nutrition, Similac, Sensitive (Lactose Free), Ready-to-feed, with ARA and DHA									
1 fl oz (30.5g)	21	1	1	1	2	0	2	0	6
Infant Formula, Abbott Nutrition, Similac, Special Care, Advance 24, with Iron, Ready-to-feed, with ARA and DHA									
1 fl oz (30.8g)	21	1	1	1	2	0	2	1	10
Infant Formula, Abbott Nutrition, Similac, with Iron, Liquid Concentrate									
1 fl oz (31.4g)	40	2	1	1	4	0	4	1	10
Infant Formula, Abbott Nutrition, Similac, with Iron, Powder									
1 scoop (8.5g)	44	2	1	1	5	0	5	1	11
Infant Formula, Abbott Nutrition, Similac, with Iron, Ready-to-feed									
1 fl oz (30.4g)	20	1	0	1	2	0	2	0	5
Infant Formula, Abbott, Alimentum Advance, Iron, Powder, Not Reconstituted, with DHA and ARA									
1 scoop (8.7g)	45	2	1	1	5	0	3	1	19
Infant Formula, Mead Johnson, Enfamil, AR Lipil, Powder, with ARA and DHA									
1 serving, 100 ml (106g)	540	28	12	18	59	0	59	13	216

Food Serving size	Cal.	(g) Total Fat	(g) Sat. Fat	(mg) Chol.	(g) Carb.	(g) Fiber	(g) Sug.	(g) Prot.	(mg) Sod.
Infant Formula, Mead Johnson, Enfamil, Low Iron, Powder, Not Reconstituted									
1 scoop (8.3g)	41	2	1	1	4	0	4	1	11
Infant Formula, Mead Johnson, Enfamil, Low Iron, Ready-to-feed									
5 fl oz (152g)	96	5	2	2	11	0	11	2	27
Infant Formula, Mead Johnson, Enfamil, Nutramigen Lipil, with Iron, Powder, Not Reconstituted, with ARA and DHA									
1 scoop (9g)	44	2	1	0	5	0	5	1	21
Infant Formula, Mead Johnson, Enfamil, Nutramigen Lipil, with Iron, Ready-to-feed, with ARA and DHA									
1 fl oz (30.5g)	20	1	0	0	2	0	2	1	9
Infant Formula, Mead Johnson, Enfamil, Nutramigen, with Iron, Liquid Concentrate, Not Reconstituted									
1 fl oz (31.5g)	39	2	1	0	4	0	4	1	19
Infant Formula, Mead Johnson, Enfamil, Nutramigen, with Iron, Powder, Not Reconstituted									
1 scoop (9.6g)	48	2	1	0	5	0	5	1	22
Infant Formula, Mead Johnson, Enfamil, Nutramigen, with Iron, Ready-to-feed									
1 fl oz (30.8g)	20	1	0	0	2	0	2	1	10
Infant Formula, Mead Johnson, Enfamil, Prosobee, Iron, Powder, Not Reconstituted									
1 scoop (8.8g)	41	2	1	0	4	0	4	1	14
Infant Formula, Mead Johnson, Enfamil, Prosobee, Lipil, Liquid Concentrate, Not Reconstituted, with ARA and DHA									
1 fl oz (31.3g)	41	2	1	0	4	0	4	1	14
Infant Formula, Mead Johnson, Enfamil, Prosobee, Lipil, with Iron, Powder, Not Reconstituted, with ARA and DHA									
1 scoop (8.8g)	45	2	1	0	5	0	5	1	15
Infant Formula, Mead Johnson, Enfamil, with Iron, Liquid Concentrate, Not Reconstituted									
1 fl oz (31.4g)	40	2	1	0	4	0	4	1	11
Infant Formula, Mead Johnson, Enfamil, with Iron, Powder									
1 scoop (8.3g)	42	2	1	1	5	0	5	1	12
Infant Formula, Mead Johnson, Enfamil, with Iron, Ready-to-feed									
1 fl oz (30.5g)	19	1	0	0	2	0	2	0	5
Infant Formula, Mead Johnson, Next Step Prosobee, Powder									
1 scoop (9.3g)	45	2	1	0	5	0	5	1	16

Food Serving size	Cal.	(g) Total Fat	(g) Sat. Fat	(mg) Chol.	(g) Carb.	(g) Fiber	(g) Sug.	(g) Prot.	(mg) Sod.
Infant Formula, Mead Johnson, Next Step Prosobee, Prepared from Powder									
1 fl oz (30.5g)	20	1	0	0	2	0	2	1	7
Infant Formula, Mead Johnson, Next Step, Prosobee, Lipil, Powder, with ARA and DHA									
3 scoop (28g)	134	6	2	0	16	0	16	4	48
Infant Formula, Mead Johnson, Next Step, Prosobee, Lipil, Ready-to-feed, with ARA and DHA									
1 fl oz (30.5g)	20	1	0	0	2	0	2	1	7
Infant Formula, Mead Johnson, Nutramigen, Lipil, with Iron, Liquid Concentrate, Not Reconstituted, with ARA and DHA									
1 fl oz (31.6g)	39	2	1	0	4	0	3	1	19
Infant Formula, Mead Johnson, Pregestimil, with Iron, Powder, Not Reconstituted									
1 scoop (8.8g)	42	2	1	0	4	0	4	1	19
Infant Formula, Mead Johnson, Pregestimil, with Iron, Prepared from Powder									
1 fl oz (30.8g)	21	1	1	0	2	0	2	1	10
Infant Formula, Mead Johnson, Prosobee, Lipil, with Iron, Ready-to-feed, with ARA and DHA									
1 fl oz (30.5g)	20	1	0	0	2	0	2	1	7
Infant Formula, Mead Johnson, Prosobee, with Iron, Liquid, Concentrate, Not Reconstituted									
1 fl oz (30.8g)	39	2	1	0	4	0	4	1	14
Infant Formula, Mead Johnson, Prosobee, with Iron, Ready-to-feed									
1 fl oz (30.5g)	19	1	0	0	2	0	2	1	7
Infant Formula, Nestle, Good Start 2 Essentials, with Iron, Liquid Concentrate									
1 fl oz (31.9g)	40	2	1	1	5	0	4	1	16
Infant Formula, Nestle, Good Start 2 Essentials, with Iron, Powder									
1 scoop (9.4g)	44	2	1	1	6	0	4	1	17
Infant Formula, Nestle, Good Start 2 Essentials, with Iron, Ready-to-feed									
1 fl oz (30.5g)	20	1	0	1	2	0	2	0	5
Infant Formula, Nestle, Good Start Essentials Soy, with Iron, Powder									
1 scoop (4.3g)	22	1	0	0	2	0	2	1	8
Infant Formula, Nestle, Good Start Essentials Soy, with Iron, Ready-to-feed									
1 fl oz (30.5g)	20	1	0	0	2	0	2	0	7
Infant Formula, Nestle, Good Start Essentials, Soy, with Iron, Liquid Concentrate									
1 fl oz (31.4g)	40	2	1	0	4	0	4	1	14

Food Serving size	Cal.	(g) Total Fat	(g) Sat. Fat	(mg) Chol.	(g) Carb.	(g) Fiber	(g) Sug.	(g) Prot.	(mg) Sod.
Infant Formula, Nestle, Good Start Supreme, Iron, DHA and ARA, Prepared from Liquid Concentrate									
1 fl oz (31.4g)	21	1	0	1	2	0	2	0	6
Infant Formula, Nestle, Good Start Supreme, with Iron, Liquid, Concentrate, Not Reconstituted									
1 fl oz (31.4g)	39	2	1	1	4	0	3	1	11
Infant Formula, Nestle, Good Start Supreme, with Iron, Powder									
1 scoop (8.7g)	41	2	1	3	5	0	3	1	11
Infant Formula, Nestle, Good Start Supreme, with Iron, Ready-to-feed									
1 fl oz (30.5g)	20	1	0	1	2	0	2	0	5
Infant Formula, Nestle, Good Start Supreme, with Iron, with DHA and ARA, Ready-to-feed									
1 fl oz (30.5g)	20	1	0	1	2	0	2	0	5
Infant Formula, PBM Products, Store Brand, Liquid Concentrate, Not Reconstituted									
1 fl oz (31.4g)	41	2	1	3	4	0	4	1	9
Infant Formula, PBM Products, Store Brand, Powder									
1 scoop (8.4g)	44	2	1	3	5	0	5	1	10
Infant Formula, PBM Products, Store Brand, Ready-to-feed									
1 fl oz (30.4g)	19	1	0	1	2	0	2	0	4
Infant Formula, PBM Products, Store Brand, Soy, Liquid Concentrate									
1 fl oz (31.4g)	40	2	1	0	4	0	4	1	11
Infant Formula, PBM Products, Store Brand, Soy, Powder									
1 scoop (8.7g)	44	2	1	0	5	0	5	1	13
Infant Formula, PBM Products, Store Brand, Soy, Ready-to-feed									
1 fl oz (30.4g)	19	1	0	0	2	0	2	1	5
Infant Formula, PBM Products, Ultra Bright Beginnings, Liquid Concentrate, Not Reconstituted									
1 fl oz (31.4g)	41	2	1	3	4	0	4	1	9
Infant Formula, PBM Products, Ultra Bright Beginnings, Powder									
1 scoop (8.4g)	44	2	1	3	5	0	5	1	10
Infant Formula, PBM Products, Ultra Bright Beginnings, Ready-to-feed									
1 fl oz (30.4g)	19	1	0	1	2	0	2	0	4
Infant Formula, PBM Products, Ultra Bright Beginnings, Soy, Liquid Concentrate									
1 fl oz (31.4g)	40	2	1	0	4	0	4	1	11

Food Serving size	Cal.	(g) Total Fat	(g) Sat. Fat	(mg) Chol.	(g) Carb.	(g) Fiber	(g) Sug.	(g) Prot.	(mg) Sod.
Infant Formula, PBM Products, Ultra Bright Beginnings, Soy, Ready-to-feed									
1 fl oz (30.4g)	19	1	0	0	2	0	2	1	5
Infant Formula, PBM, Ultra Bright Beginnings, Soy, Powder									
1 scoop (8.7g)	44	2	1	0	5	0	5	1	13
Zwieback									
1 piece (7g)	30	1	0	1	5	0.2	1	1	16

Restaurant Chains

Healthy Eating Out

Americans consume approximately one-third of their calories from fast food, restaurant food, or take-out foods. Eating out can be a dietary danger zone, but the nutrition information in this book will help you plan ahead and make sensible choices. The goal is to enjoy your meal with control. The problem with eating out is that you lose control of portion sizes and preparation. Here are some tips for healthy eating in restaurants.

Plan Ahead

Set some reasonable guidelines for your meal.

- Set a calorie guideline and compare the nutrient information for different restaurants in this book.
- Chain restaurants and other retail food providers are required by the U.S. Food and Drug Administration to provide customers with nutrition information. Look for calorie information on menus and menu boards for standard menu items. Other nutrient information (sodium, total carbohydrates, fiber, sugar, total fat, saturated fat, trans fat, cholesterol, and protein) may be available on the restaurant website or by asking your waiter/waitress for a copy. Use the calorie and nutrient information to make healthier choices.
- Decide on portion sizes of chicken, bread, etc. Be sure to have a visual reference, such as the palm of your hand for a 3 to 4 oz portion of meat, a die for 1 oz of cheese, and what 4 oz of wine looks like in a wine glass.
- Decide on which items you are going to include in your meal: salad to start with; only half the bun; wine, but no dessert; only 10 french fries or chips; skip the bread or have bread without butter.

Know your restaurant and be familiar with the menu.

- Check out the restaurants included in this book. If your favorite restaurant is not included, there may be a similar one. A hamburger and french fries don't vary much from one restaurant to another.

- Highlight the healthiest options for each restaurant.
- Decide on dishes at home before you are tempted by the sight of the food or what others are ordering.

Never arrive at a restaurant hungry. Hungry people make bad ordering decisions. Don't skip meals or snacks thinking it will save calories for you to eat more at the restaurant. Eat an apple and drink a glass of water before you go out. This will help you control your hunger and the amount of food you consume.

Ask Questions

If you feel awkward doing this at the table, call the restaurant ahead of time and ask to speak to the chef or a waiter.

How are items prepared? Can they alter the preparation?

- Baked rather than fried?
- Saute in broth rather than oil?
- Sauces and dressings on the side rather than on top?
- Plain bread rather than buttered?

Control Portion Sizes

- Order a main dish from the appetizer menu.
- Plan to take half the entrée home for a future meal. Ask your waiter to put half in a to-go box and just to serve you the other half.
- Stay away from buffets, especially an "all you can eat" buffet.

Savor your food. Try to never finish everything on your plate. Always leave a bite or two to prove to yourself that you are in control of your food rather than the food controlling how much you eat. You don't have to clean your plate! Placing the handles of the utensils or your used napkin in the plate when you have had enough will deter you from continuing to eat.

Course-by-Course Suggestions

Beverages

- Drink plenty of water.
- Alcoholic beverages can stimulate your appetite. Plus, the calories (100 calories for 1 oz liquor or 3 to 4 oz wine, 150 calories for 12 oz) in alcohol can add up fast. Best choice of alcoholic beverage is a glass of wine sipped slowly.
- Stick to water, low-fat milk, tea, and coffee.

Starters

- Soup can fill you up. A clear, broth-based soup with vegetables is good as an appetizer because a soup in general tends to decrease your appetite.

Soup takes a long time to eat, is filling and low in calories, and is good for you. Avoid soups made with cream, which would add unhealthy fat and calories.

- Salads are a great way to start a meal because they can take the edge off your appetite. Order a tossed green or spinach salad with the dressing served on the side. You decide how much salad dressing you will eat. Dipping your fork into the dressing and then spearing some veggies can cut down on the amount of dressing you eat. Avoid bacon bits, cheese, croutons, meats, and prepared salads like potato salad.

  - 1 tablespoon of grated cheese adds 28 calories and 2 grams of fat.

  - 1 tablespoon of bacon bits adds 30 calories and 1 gram of fat.

  - 1 tablespoon of salad dressing adds 60 to 90 calories and 6 to 9 grams of fat.

Entrées

- Choose a baked, broiled, grilled, poached, roasted, or steamed entrée. Ask that dishes be prepared without extra salt, butter, or oil. Meats and vegetables sautéed or stir-fried in a small amount of oil, broth, or water are usually lower in fat.
- Avoid entrées that are high in fat (check out the Red Flag Menu Terms below).
- Choose fish often. Some fish are higher in fat than others, but the type of fat is good for you. Ask that the fish be steamed, grilled, broiled, or poached.
- Choose white meat chicken over dark meat. Ask for the skin to be removed or remove it yourself. Order poultry steamed, poached, roasted, broiled, boiled, grilled, or baked.
- Allow yourself a red meat a few times a week. Be sure to choose lean cuts of meat like loin, flank, or tenderloin.
- Request sauces on the side so that you can determine if they contain fat and then decide how much you will eat. "Dry" is a good term to use when ordering.

Side Dishes

- Choose vegetables and ask for them to be steamed.
- Baked potatoes, boiled new potatoes, and rice also may be good options if they are prepared without added fats.
- Top your baked potato with salsa or plain yogurt instead of butter or sour cream.
- Skip the french fries, potato chips, and onion rings, as well as vegetables slathered in cheese or cream sauces. Some restaurants will let you substitute steamed veggies or fruit for your sides.

Dessert

- Leave a little time for your food to digest before ordering dessert. It takes about 20 minutes for your stomach to feel full and send this message to your brain.

- If you still want dessert, consider splitting the dessert with a friend. Half the dessert is half the calories.
- Healthy dessert choices include berries, melon, sorbet, or frozen yogurt.

Green Flag Menu Terms

Baked, broiled, boiled, poached, grilled, roasted, steamed, lean, dry, fat-free, low-fat, fresh, light, marinated, reduced, vinaigrette, high fiber, whole grain, multi-grain, and vegetarian.

Red Flag Menu Terms

Avoid foods described as fried, creamed or creamy, buttered or buttery, oil, breaded, Alfredo, battered or batter-dipped, gravy, smothered, fried, fricasseed, creamed, sautéed, stir-fried, stuffed, breaded, basted, au gratin, parmigiana, béarnaise or hollandaise, crispy, crunchy, giant, loaded, and super-sized.

Food Serving size	Cal.	(g) Total Fat	(g) Sat. Fat	(mg) Chol.	(g) Carb.	(g) Fiber	(g) Sug.	(g) Prot.	(mg) Sod.

Applebee's

Appetizers

Food Serving size	Cal.	Total Fat	Sat. Fat	Chol.	Carb.	Fiber	Sug.	Prot.	Sod.
Boneless Wings (w/o sauce or dressing)									
	680	35	7	95	52	5	1	39	1760
Add Choice of Sauce: Classic Buffalo									
	200	21	8	0	2	1	1	0	2600
Add Choice of Sauce: Honey BBQ									
	230	0	0	0	55	2	49	1	1010
Add Choice of Sauce: Hot Buffalo									
	210	22	8	0	4	1	1	1	2720
Add Choice of Sauce: Sweet Asian Chile									
	240	2	0	0	54	1	44	3	1860
Add Choice of Dressing: Bleu Cheese Dressing									
	240	25	4.5	25	1	0	1	1	250
Add Choice of Dressing: Ranch Dressing									
	210	22	3.5	15	1	0	1	1	330
Brew Pub Pretzels & Beer Cheese Dip									
	1060	45	15	55	131	8	18	33	3120
Chicken Quesadilla									
	980	59	27	165	61	6	4	51	2800
Double Crunch Bone-In Wings (w/o sauce or dressing)									
	660	44	11	255	10	4	1	55	1220
Add Choice of Sauce: Classic Buffalo									
	200	21	8	0	2	1	1	0	2600
Add Choice of Sauce: Honey BBQ									
	230	0	0	0	55	2	49	1	1010
Add Choice of Sauce: Hot Buffalo									
	210	22	8	0	4	1	1	1	2720
Add Choice of Sauce: Southern BBQ									
	660	35	9	NA	25	2	NA	61	1060
Add Choice of Sauce: Sweet Asian Chile Sauce									
	240	2	0	0	54	1	44	3	1860
Add Choice of Sauce: Thai									
	1060	75	16	255	38	5	22	60	2220

Food Serving size	Cal.	(g) Total Fat	(g) Sat. Fat	(mg) Chol.	(g) Carb.	(g) Fiber	(g) Sug.	(g) Prot.	(mg) Sod.
Add Choice of Dressing: Bleu Cheese Dressing									
	240	25	4.5	25	1	0	1	1	250
Add Choice of Dressing: Ranch Dressing									
	210	22	3.5	15	1	0	1	1	330
Double Crunch Bone-In Wings, Thai									
	1060	75	16	255	38	5	22	60	2220
Grilled Chicken Wonton Tacos									
	490	15	3	125	48	3	25	41	1720
Kobe-Style Meatballs									
	680	43	17	125	43	4	6	32	1900
Mozzarella Sticks									
	910	50	20	80	79	5	10	39	2140
Salsa Verde Pulled Pork Nachos									
	1110	62	23	140	96	8	7	45	4890
Salsa Verde Shredded Brisket Nachos									
	1080	57	21	125	97	8	8	45	4820
Spinach and Artichoke Dip									
	930	53	13	25	94	7	13	21	3880
Sriracha Shrimp									
	670	43	8	120	54	3	8	17	1910
Sweet Potato Fries & Dips									
	1070	64	13	45	118	7	51	7	2450

Appetizers: Bar Snacks

	Cal.	Total Fat	Sat. Fat	Chol.	Carb.	Fiber	Sug.	Prot.	Sod.
Chips and Salsa									
	480	19	3	0	71	6	5	8	2900
Churro S'mores									
	580	10	2.5	0	120	5	70	7	650
Double Crunch Bone-In Wings (w/o sauce or dressing)									
	300	20	5	115	5	2	1	25	560
Add Choice of Sauce: Classic Buffalo Sauce									
	100	11	4	0	1	0	1	0	1300
Add Choice of Sauce: Hot Buffalo Sauce									
	110	11	4	0	2	0	1	0	1370

Food Serving size	Cal.	(g) Total Fat	(g) Sat. Fat	(mg) Chol.	(g) Carb.	(g) Fiber	(g) Sug.	(g) Prot.	(mg) Sod.
Add Choice of Sauce: Honey BBQ Sauce									
	110	0	0	0	28	1	25	1	510
Add Choice of Sauce: Sweet Asian Chile Sauce									
	120	1	0	0	27	1	22	2	930
Add Choice of Dressing: Bleu Cheese Dressing									
	240	25	4.5	25	1	0	1	1	250
Add Choice of Dressing: Ranch Dressing									
	210	22	3.5	15	1	0	1	1	330
Green Bean Crispers									
	530	43	7	20	32	4	4	4	680
Housemade Sweet & Spicy Pickles									
	110	0	0	0	26	1	21	2	1590
Chicken Tortilla Soup									
	240	11	3	25	24	3	3	11	1130
French Onion Soup									
	360	22	13	60	24	2	6	17	1390
Tomato Basil Soup									
	260	16	7	30	24	4	12	6	1170
Today's Soup: Potato Soup									
	470	33	15	75	30	2	2	13	1510
Today's Soup: Broccoli & Cheese Soup									
	390	29	18	100	21	3	7	14	1850
Today's Soup: Chicken Noodle Soup									
	140	4	1.5	30	17	1	3	10	1100
Today's Soup: Portsmouth Clam Chowder									
	380	26	16	100	24	2	1	14	1080
Today's Soup: New England Clam Chowder									
	380	26	16	100	24	2	1	14	1080
Small Caesar Salad									
	300	26	5	20	12	3	3	5	480
House Salad (w/o dressing)									
	230	15	7	35	13	3	4	13	400
Add Choice of Dressing: Bacon Vinaigrette									
	180	10	1.5	0	23	0	22	1	500

Food Serving size	Cal.	(g) Total Fat	(g) Sat. Fat	(mg) Chol.	(g) Carb.	(g) Fiber	(g) Sug.	(g) Prot.	(mg) Sod.
Add Choice of Dressing: Bleu Cheese Dressing									
	240	25	4.5	25	1	0	1	1	250
Add Choice of Dressing: Buttermilk Ranch Dressing									
	210	22	3.5	15	1	0	1	1	330
Add Choice of Dressing: Chili Lime Vinaigrette									
	120	7	1	0	13	0	10	0	500
Add Choice of Dressing: Honey French Dressing									
	210	17	2.5	0	15	0	14	0	330
Add Choice of Dressing: Italian Dressing, Fat Free									
	20	0	0	0	5	0	3	0	370
Add Choice of Dressing: Lemon Olive Oil Vinaigrette									
	150	16	2	0	1	0	1	0	370
Add Choice of Dressing: Mexi Ranch Dressing									
	170	18	3	15	3	0	2	1	550
Add Choice of Dressing: Oriental Dressing									
	250	22	3	0	13	0	13	0	85
Boneless Wings (w/o sauce or dressing)									
	340	17	3.5	45	27	3	1	20	900
Add Choice of Sauce: Classic Buffalo Sauce									
	100	11	4	0	1	0	1	0	1300
Add Choice of Sauce: Hot Buffalo Sauce									
	110	11	4	0	2	0	1	0	1370
Add Choice of Sauce: Honey BBQ Sauce									
	110	0	0	0	28	1	25	1	510
Add Choice of Sauce: Sweet Asian Chile Sauce									
	120	1	0	0	27	1	22	2	930
Add Choice of Dressing: Bleu Cheese Dressing									
	240	25	4.5	25	1	0	1	1	250
Add Choice of Dressing: Ranch Dressing									
	210	22	3.5	15	1	0	1	1	330
Brew Pub Pretzels & Beer Cheese Dip									
	520	20	10	40	62	4	4	22	1750
Chicken Quesadilla									
	610	38	16	85	41	4	4	27	1860

Food Serving size	Cal.	(g) Total Fat	(g) Sat. Fat	(mg) Chol.	(g) Carb.	(g) Fiber	(g) Sug.	(g) Prot.	(mg) Sod.
Chips and Salsa									
	480	19	3	0	71	6	5	8	2900
Churro S'mores									
	580	10	2.5	0	120	5	70	7	650
Double Crunch Bone-In Wings (w/o sauce or dressing)									
	300	20	5	115	5	2	1	25	560
Add Choice of Sauce: Classic Buffalo Sauce									
	100	11	4	0	1	0	1	0	1300
Add Choice of Sauce: Hot Buffalo Sauce									
	110	11	4	0	2	0	1	0	1370
Add Choice of Sauce: Honey BBQ Sauce									
	110	0	0	0	28	1	25	1	510
Add Choice of Sauce: Sweet Asian Chile Sauce									
	120	1	0	0	27	1	22	2	930
Add Choice of Dressing: Bleu Cheese Dressing									
	240	25	4.5	25	1	0	1	1	250
Add Choice of Dressing: Ranch Dressing									
	210	22	3.5	15	1	0	1	1	330
Double Crunch Bone-In Wings, Thai									
	500	35	7	115	19	3	11	27	1050
Green Bean Crispers									
	530	43	7	20	32	4	4	4	680
Grilled Chicken Wonton Tacos									
	370	11	2.5	90	38	2	20	30	1380
Kobe-Style Meatballs									
	680	43	17	125	43	4	6	32	1900
Mozzarella Sticks									
	460	25	10	40	39	3	5	19	1070
Salsa Verde Pulled Pork Nachos									
	550	31	11	70	48	4	3	22	2410
Salsa Verde Shredded Brisket Nachos									
	540	28	11	60	48	4	4	22	2370
Spinach and Artichoke Dip									
	930	53	13	25	94	7	13	21	3880

Food Serving size	Cal.	(g) Total Fat	(g) Sat. Fat	(mg) Chol.	(g) Carb.	(g) Fiber	(g) Sug.	(g) Prot.	(mg) Sod.
Sriracha Shrimp	430	29	5	65	35	2	5	9	1100
Housemade Sweet & Spicy Pickles	110	0	0	0	26	1	21	2	1590
Sweet Potato Fries & Dips	1070	64	13	45	118	7	51	7	2450

Ribs - Without Sides

Food Serving size	Cal.	(g) Total Fat	(g) Sat. Fat	(mg) Chol.	(g) Carb.	(g) Fiber	(g) Sug.	(g) Prot.	(mg) Sod.
Applebee's® Riblets Platter (w/o sauce or fries)	720	46	17	230	12	1	9	66	710
Add Choice of Sauce: Honey BBQ Sauce	380	0	0	0	92	3	82	2	1690
Add Choice of Sauce: Smoky Chipotle Sauce	320	6	4	15	62	1	60	2	1010
Add Choice of Sauce: Sweet Asian Chile Sauce	320	2.5	0	0	72	2	59	5	2480
Applebee's® Riblets Basket (w/o sauce or fries)	410	26	10	145	3	0	2	41	390
Add Choice of Sauce: Honey BBQ Sauce	230	0	0	0	55	2	49	1	1010
Add Choice of Sauce: Smoky Chipotle Sauce	190	4	2.5	10	37	1	36	1	610
Add Choice of Sauce: Sweet Asian Chile Sauce	160	1.5	0	0	36	1	30	2	1240
Double-Glazed Baby Back Ribs - Full Rack (w/o sauce or fries)	920	61	24	275	28	2	23	65	1410
Add Choice of Sauce: Honey BBQ Sauce	150	0	0	0	37	1	33	1	670
Add Choice of Sauce: Smoky Chipotle Sauce	130	2.5	1.5	5	25	1	24	1	410
Add Choice of Sauce: Sweet Asian Chile Sauce	80	0.5	0	0	18	0	15	1	620
Double-Glazed Baby Back Ribs - Half Rack (w/o sauce or fries)	490	32	12	140	17	2	15	33	750

Food Serving size	Cal.	(g) Total Fat	(g) Sat. Fat	(mg) Chol.	(g) Carb.	(g) Fiber	(g) Sug.	(g) Prot.	(mg) Sod.
Add Choice of Sauce: Honey BBQ Sauce									
	80	0	0	0	18	1	16	0	340
Add Choice of Sauce: Smoky Chipotle Sauce									
	60	1.5	1	5	12	0	12	0	200
Add Choice of Sauce: Sweet Asian Chile Sauce									
	80	0.5	0	0	18	0	15	1	620
Choice of Fries: Classic Fries									
	440	20	4	0	59	6	0	5	770
Choice of Fries: BBQ-Spiced Fries									
	440	20	4	0	60	6	1	5	890
Choice of Fries: Sweet Potato Fries									
	340	12	2	0	57	4	19	3	990

Steak - Without Sides

Food Serving size	Cal.	(g) Total Fat	(g) Sat. Fat	(mg) Chol.	(g) Carb.	(g) Fiber	(g) Sug.	(g) Prot.	(mg) Sod.
12 oz New York Strip									
	480	25	10	160	1	0	1	65	1120
12 oz Ribeye									
	500	28	13	170	1	0	1	63	970
7 oz House Sirloin									
	270	15	6	85	1	1	1	34	770
9 oz House Sirloin									
	330	17	7	95	1	1	1	45	1020
Bourbon Street Steak, 7 oz (w/sides)									
	670	40	13	95	39	4	7	39	1470
Bourbon Street Steak, 9 oz (w/sides)									
	730	42	14	110	39	5	8	50	1730
Grilled Onion Sirloin with Stout Gravy									
	600	30	9	85	43	5	7	39	1390
Pepper-Crusted Sirloin & Whole Grains (w/sides)									
	370	10	4	55	43	6	5	28	1540
Shrimp 'N Parmesan Sirloin									
	560	33	16	215	5	2	2	61	2220
Sizzling Double Barrel Whisky Sirloins (w/sides)									
	650	31	11	115	43	6	10	50	2530

Food Serving size	Cal.	(g) Total Fat	(g) Sat. Fat	(mg) Chol.	(g) Carb.	(g) Fiber	(g) Sug.	(g) Prot.	(mg) Sod.
Choice of Sides: Vegetable #1 (yellow squash or zucchini, sugar snap peas & carrotinis)									
	45	0	0	0	9	2	4	2	340
Choice of Sides: Vegetable #2 (zucchini, yellow squash, red peppers, carrotinis & red onion)									
	35	0	0	0	8	2	4	1	320
Choice of Sides: Vegetable #3 (zucchini, yellow squash, broccoli & carrotinis)									
	30	0	0	0	7	2	2	2	340
Choice of Sides: Vegetable #4 (yellow squash or zucchini, broccoli & carrotinis)									
	35	0	0	0	8	3	3	2	350
Choice of Sides: Vegetable #5 (broccoli crown)									
	40	0	0	0	8	3	2	3	210
Choice of Sides: Garlic Broccoli (garlic & broccoli)									
	35	0	0	0	6	3	0	3	300
Choice of Sides: Garlic Mashed Potatoes									
	250	14	2.5	0	29	3	4	5	600
Choice of Sides: Baked Potato									
	340	18	11	55	41	3	2	6	170
Top Your Steak: Crispy Onion Topper									
	190	14	2.5	0	14	1	2	2	125
Top Your Steak: Grilled Onions									
	45	2.5	0.5	0	5	1	2	1	280
Top Your Steak: Sauteed Garlic Mushrooms									
	150	15	7	20	4	1	1	2	140
Top Your Steak: Shrimp 'N Parmesan									
	220	16	9	120	4	1	1	16	1190
Bourbon Street Chicken & Shrimp									
	630	29	8	210	42	4	7	52	2160

Chicken

Cedar Grilled Lemon Chicken									
	590	25	4	115	49	4	15	43	2480
Chicken Tenders Basket									
	1120	63	11	90	99	8	13	40	2640
Chicken Tenders Platter									
	1380	78	14	120	117	10	19	54	3260

Food Serving size	Cal.	(g) Total Fat	(g) Sat. Fat	(mg) Chol.	(g) Carb.	(g) Fiber	(g) Sug.	(g) Prot.	(mg) Sod.
Crispy Brewhouse Chicken									
	1080	62	15	115	80	7	8	50	2710
Fiesta Lime Chicken®									
	1210	69	16	170	92	5	7	56	3440
Hot Shot Whisky Chicken									
	640	28	9	145	44	6	10	53	2090
Riblet and Chicken Tenders Basket (w/o sauce)									
	1180	69	15	145	90	7	14	51	2340
Add Choice of Sauce: Honey BBQ Sauce									
	150	0	0	0	37	1	33	1	670
Add Choice of Sauce: Smoky Chipotle Sauce									
	130	2.5	1.5	5	25	1	24	1	410
Add Choice of Sauce: Sweet Asian Chile Sauce									
	80	0.5	0	0	18	0	15	1	620

Pub Diet

Food Serving size	Cal.	(g) Total Fat	(g) Sat. Fat	(mg) Chol.	(g) Carb.	(g) Fiber	(g) Sug.	(g) Prot.	(mg) Sod.
Cedar Grilled Lemon Chicken									
	590	25	4	115	49	4	15	43	2480
Grilled Onion Sirloin with Stout Gravy									
	600	30	9	85	43	5	7	39	1390
Hot Shot Whisky Chicken									
	640	28	9	145	44	6	10	53	2090
Pepper-Crusted Sirloin & Whole Grains (w/sides)									
	370	10	4	55	43	6	5	28	1540
Savory Cedar Salmon									
	540	32	8	105	25	6	5	42	1790
Shrimp Wonton Stir Fry									
	610	14	2.5	125	97	5	22	25	2270
Thai Shrimp Salad									
	390	19	3	125	33	7	15	23	1490

Pastas

Food Serving size	Cal.	(g) Total Fat	(g) Sat. Fat	(mg) Chol.	(g) Carb.	(g) Fiber	(g) Sug.	(g) Prot.	(mg) Sod.
4-Cheese Mac & Cheese with Honey Pepper Chicken Tenders									
	1700	88	41	275	156	10	55	73	4090
Shrimp Scampi Linguini									
	860	46	19	215	78	7	9	35	3390

Food Serving size	Cal.	(g) Total Fat	(g) Sat. Fat	(mg) Chol.	(g) Carb.	(g) Fiber	(g) Sug.	(g) Prot.	(mg) Sod.
Three-Cheese Chicken Penne									
	880	40	22	160	80	3	5	51	2250

Seafood

Hand-Battered Fish & Chips									
	1490	100	17	120	104	10	9	45	1920
Baked Haddock									
	930	37	16	150	105	6	8	45	1580
Blackened Tilapia									
	460	18	6	75	44	6	9	31	1660
Double Crunch Shrimp									
	1350	64	13	215	156	11	22	38	3530
Hand-Breaded Fish & Chips									
	1540	96	18	240	118	11	10	52	3100
New England Fish & Chips/Hand Battered Fish Fry									
	1970	136	24	160	134	12	10	54	4180
Savory Cedar Salmon									
	540	32	8	105	25	6	5	42	1790
Shrimp Wonton Stir Fry									
	610	14	2.5	125	97	5	22	25	2270
Walleye Fish & Chips, Battered									
	1480	105	19	160	93	11	10	42	2510

More

Loaded Brisket Enchiladas									
	1020	46	18	115	108	8	11	43	3570

Handhelds - Without Sides

American BLT									
	1010	64	20	90	75	4	21	36	2610
Battered Fish Sandwich									
	820	57	10	85	57	3	8	21	1150
Brew Pub Philly									
	1130	69	23	140	73	5	10	51	2680

Food Serving size	Cal.	(g) Total Fat	(g) Sat. Fat	(mg) Chol.	(g) Carb.	(g) Fiber	(g) Sug.	(g) Prot.	(mg) Sod.
Chicken Fajita Rollup									
	1090	63	27	235	66	7	10	67	3600
Clubhouse Grille									
	1120	63	18	135	87	4	31	52	2520
Kickin' Turkey Stacker									
	970	52	14	120	73	4	21	50	1660
Maple Bacon Chicken Piadini									
	1040	49	15	175	87	4	26	65	3640
Triple Hog Dare Ya™									
	1010	60	19	125	72	4	13	46	2650
Choice of Side: BBQ-Spiced Fries									
	440	20	4	0	60	6	1	5	890
Choice of Side: Classic Fries									
	440	20	4	0	59	6	0	5	770
Choice of Side: House Chips									
	420	29	5	0	36	3	0	4	960
Choice of Side: Sweet Potato Fries									
	340	12	2	0	57	4	19	3	990
Choice of Side: Crunchy Onion Rings									
	530	29	5	0	60	3	8	7	1180
Add on: Chili & Cheese (for fries)									
	190	13	7	45	7	2	3	12	580

Burgers - Without Sides

Classic									
	780	50	18	140	44	2	7	39	1180
Add Cheese: American Cheese									
	150	12	7	25	2	0	1	8	480
Add Cheese: Cheddar Cheese									
	90	7	4	20	0	0	0	5	135
Add Cheese: Swiss Cheese									
	160	12	7	40	0	0	0	11	80
Add Cheese: Monterey Jack									
	80	6	4	20	0	0	0	5	115
Cowboy									
	1210	80	28	185	68	4	16	53	2260

Food Serving size	Cal.	(g) Total Fat	(g) Sat. Fat	(mg) Chol.	(g) Carb.	(g) Fiber	(g) Sug.	(g) Prot.	(mg) Sod.
Mushroom Swiss									
	1060	72	28	190	48	3	10	53	1270
Quesadilla									
	1410	106	43	240	46	6	6	69	3240
The All-Day Brunch									
	1190	81	29	335	61	3	12	57	2370
The American Standard									
	1030	71	27	180	48	2	10	50	2010
The Blazin' Texan									
	1050	65	25	195	60	3	20	55	1870
Triple Bacon									
	1190	85	32	220	47	2	10	61	2050
Choice of Side: BBQ-Spiced Fries									
	440	20	4	0	60	6	1	5	890
Choice of Side: Classic Fries									
	440	20	4	0	59	6	0	5	770
Choice of Side: House Chips									
	420	29	5	0	36	3	0	4	960
Choice of Side: Sweet Potato Fries									
	340	12	2	0	57	4	19	3	990
Choice of Side: Crunchy Onion Rings									
	530	29	5	0	60	3	8	7	1180
Add on: Chili & Cheese (for fries)									
	190	13	7	45	7	2	3	12	580

Salads - With Dressing

Food Serving size	Cal.	(g) Total Fat	(g) Sat. Fat	(mg) Chol.	(g) Carb.	(g) Fiber	(g) Sug.	(g) Prot.	(mg) Sod.
Fiesta Chicken Chopped Salad									
	890	45	11	90	84	11	20	38	1650
Grilled Chicken Caesar Salad									
	800	56	11	160	27	6	6	49	1760
Grilled Shrimp 'N Spinach Salad									
	1000	66	10	195	67	12	50	44	2990
Oriental Chicken Salad									
	1390	97	15	60	93	11	42	39	1600

Food Serving size	Cal.	(g) Total Fat	(g) Sat. Fat	(mg) Chol.	(g) Carb.	(g) Fiber	(g) Sug.	(g) Prot.	(mg) Sod.
Oriental Grilled Chicken Salad									
	1280	80	12	115	91	9	56	52	2270
Pecan-Crusted Chicken Salad									
	1340	80	16	95	115	14	64	46	2390
Thai Shrimp Salad									
	390	19	3	125	33	7	15	23	1490

Lunch Combos: Soups

Food Serving size	Cal.	(g) Total Fat	(g) Sat. Fat	(mg) Chol.	(g) Carb.	(g) Fiber	(g) Sug.	(g) Prot.	(mg) Sod.
Chicken Tortilla Soup, Lunch									
	240	11	3	25	24	3	3	11	1130
French Onion Soup, Lunch									
	360	22	13	60	24	2	6	17	1390
Tomato Basil Soup, Lunch									
	240	15	7	30	20	3	12	6	1090
Broccoli & Cheese Soup, Lunch									
	370	29	18	100	16	3	7	14	1770
Chicken Noodle Soup, Lunch									
	120	3.5	1	30	13	1	2	9	1020
New England Clam Chowder, Lunch									
	360	26	15	100	19	1	1	13	1000
Portsmouth Clam Chowder, Lunch									
	380	26	16	100	24	2	1	14	1080
Potato Soup, Lunch									
	450	32	15	75	26	2	2	13	1430

Lunch Combos: Salads

Food Serving size	Cal.	(g) Total Fat	(g) Sat. Fat	(mg) Chol.	(g) Carb.	(g) Fiber	(g) Sug.	(g) Prot.	(mg) Sod.
Caesar Salad, Lunch									
	210	18	4	15	8	2	2	4	340
Fiesta Chicken Chopped Salad, Lunch									
	350	17	4	65	25	3	7	25	870
Grilled Chicken Caesar Salad, Lunch									
	310	20	4.5	75	9	2	2	23	750
Grilled Shrimp 'N Spinach Salad, Lunch									
	270	15	2.5	75	24	4	18	13	1300

Food Serving size	Cal.	(g) Total Fat	(g) Sat. Fat	(mg) Chol.	(g) Carb.	(g) Fiber	(g) Sug.	(g) Prot.	(mg) Sod.
House Salad (w/o dressing)	120	7	2.5	15	9	2	3	6	210
Choice of Dressing: Bacon Vinaigrette	120	7	1	0	16	0	15	1	330
Choice of Dressing: Bleu Cheese Dressing	160	17	3	15	1	0	0	1	170
Choice of Dressing: Buttermilk Ranch Dressing	140	15	2.5	10	1	0	0	0	220
Choice of Dressing: Chili Lime Vinaigrette	80	5	1	0	9	0	7	0	330
Choice of Dressing: Dijon Honey Mustard Dressing	140	12	2	10	9	0	8	0	360
Choice of Dressing: Garlic Caesar Dressing	140	15	2.5	10	1	0	0	1	230
Choice of Dressing: Lemon Olive Oil Vinaigrette	100	11	1.5	0	1	0	0	0	240
Choice of Dressing: Mexi Ranch Dressing	120	12	2	10	2	0	1	1	370
Choice of Dressing: Oriental Dressing	160	14	2	0	9	0	8	0	60
Oriental Chicken Salad, Lunch	440	29	4.5	30	29	3	11	17	670
Spinach Salad, Lunch	240	14	2.5	5	23	4	18	6	720
Thai Shrimp Salad, Lunch	190	10	1.5	50	16	4	8	10	730

Lunch Combos: Handhelds

Food Serving size	Cal.	(g) Total Fat	(g) Sat. Fat	(mg) Chol.	(g) Carb.	(g) Fiber	(g) Sug.	(g) Prot.	(mg) Sod.
American BLT, Lunch	520	32	10	45	40	2	12	18	1440
Chicken Fajita Rollup, Lunch	730	42	16	125	50	5	8	36	2460
Clubhouse Grille, Lunch	570	32	9	70	46	2	17	26	1400

Food Serving size	Cal.	Total Fat (g)	Sat. Fat (g)	Chol. (mg)	Carb. (g)	Fiber (g)	Sug. (g)	Prot. (g)	Sod. (mg)
Kickin' Turkey Stacker, Lunch									
	490	26	7	60	39	2	12	25	970
4-Cheese Mac & Cheese with Honey Pepper Chicken Tenders, Lunch									
	680	31	14	95	72	4	26	28	1510
Honey Pepper Chicken Tenders, Lunch									
	930	36	7	45	127	7	47	26	1710
Three Cheese Chicken Penne, Lunch									
	520	23	12	110	43	2	4	36	1490
Shrimp Scampi Linguini, Lunch									
	440	24	10	95	39	4	4	17	1680

Kid's: Really Hungry

Food Serving size	Cal.	Total Fat (g)	Sat. Fat (g)	Chol. (mg)	Carb. (g)	Fiber (g)	Sug. (g)	Prot. (g)	Sod. (mg)
Chicken Tenders									
	280	15	3	45	16	1	0	21	800
Chicken Griller									
	200	3.5	1	115	3	0	0	39	810
Kraft® Macaroni & Cheese									
	310	9	2.5	15	45	2	8	11	550
Grilled Cheese Sandwich									
	640	35	14	40	60	2	8	21	1340

Kid's: Really Really Hungry

Food Serving size	Cal.	Total Fat (g)	Sat. Fat (g)	Chol. (mg)	Carb. (g)	Fiber (g)	Sug. (g)	Prot. (g)	Sod. (mg)
Cheesy Bread Pizza, Full									
	610	31	17	60	59	3	8	24	1610
Fried Shrimp									
	290	15	3	80	28	1	1	11	720
4 oz Sirloin									
	120	3.5	2.5	50	2	0	1	21	580

Kid's: Sides

Food Serving size	Cal.	Total Fat (g)	Sat. Fat (g)	Chol. (mg)	Carb. (g)	Fiber (g)	Sug. (g)	Prot. (g)	Sod. (mg)
Apple Dippers with Yogurt									
	90	0.5	0	0	22	2	19	2	25
Baby Carrots with Ranch									
	250	22	3.5	15	11	3	6	1	410
Caesar Salad - Kid's									
	210	18	4	15	8	2	2	4	340

Food Serving size	Cal.	(g) Total Fat	(g) Sat. Fat	(mg) Chol.	(g) Carb.	(g) Fiber	(g) Sug.	(g) Prot.	(mg) Sod.
Fries									
	440	20	4	0	59	6	0	5	770
Garlic Mashed Potatoes									
	130	7	1	0	14	1	2	2	300
GoGo squeeZ™ Applesauce									
	60	0	0	0	15	1	12	0	0
House Salad - Kid's (w/o dressing)									
	110	7	2.5	15	7	1	2	6	200
Choice of Dressing: Bacon Vinaigrette									
	180	10	1.5	0	23	0	22	1	500
Choice of Dressing: Bleu Cheese Dressing									
	240	25	4.5	25	1	0	1	1	250
Choice of Dressing: Buttermilk Ranch Dressing									
	210	22	3.5	15	1	0	1	1	330
Choice of Dressing: Chili Lime Vinaigrette									
	120	7	1	0	13	0	10	0	500
Choice of Dressing: Dijon Honey Mustard Dressing									
	210	18	2.5	10	13	1	12	1	540
Choice of Dressing: Garlic Caesar Dressing									
	210	23	3.5	15	2	0	1	1	350
Choice of Dressing: Green Goddess Dressing									
	190	20	3.5	20	2	0	1	1	470
Choice of Dressing: Honey Balsamic Dressing									
	170	13	2	0	13	0	11	0	230
Choice of Dressing: Honey French Dressing									
	210	17	2.5	0	15	0	14	0	330
Choice of Dressing: Italian Dressing, Fat Free									
	20	0	0	0	5	0	3	0	370
Choice of Dressing: Lemon Olive Oil Vinaigrette									
	150	16	2	0	1	0	1	0	370
Choice of Dressing: Mexi Ranch Dressing									
	170	18	3	15	3	0	2	1	550
Choice of Dressing: Oriental Dressing									
	250	22	3	0	13	0	13	0	85

Food Serving size	Cal.	(g) Total Fat	(g) Sat. Fat	(mg) Chol.	(g) Carb.	(g) Fiber	(g) Sug.	(g) Prot.	(mg) Sod.
Mozzarella Sticks	350	19	7	30	31	2	5	15	860
Steamed Broccoli	25	0	0	0	4	3	0	3	25
Vanilla Yogurt with Strawberries	100	1.5	1	5	17	1	16	4	55

Kid's: Drinks

Food Serving size	Cal.	Total Fat	Sat. Fat	Chol.	Carb.	Fiber	Sug.	Prot.	Sod.
Milk, 1%	110	2.5	1.5	10	13	0	12	8	130
Milk, 1%, Chocolate	150	2.5	1.5	10	25	0	23	8	200
Apple Juice	90	0	0	0	23	0	21	0	15
Orange Tangerine Juice	100	0	0	0	25	0	23	0	15
Grape Juice	80	0	0	0	23	0	21	0	15

Kid's: Shakes and Sundaes

Food Serving size	Cal.	Total Fat	Sat. Fat	Chol.	Carb.	Fiber	Sug.	Prot.	Sod.
Chocolate Shake	820	35	20	135	110	2	88	19	350
Strawberry Shake	740	34	20	135	90	0	73	19	340
Oreo® Cookie Shake	840	41	22	135	100	1	74	20	470
Vanilla Shake	680	34	20	135	75	0	60	19	330
Oreo® Cookie Sundae	430	22	13	60	53	1	38	8	210
Sundae w/Chocolate Syrup	420	18	10	65	58	1	47	8	150
Sundae w/Strawberry Sauce	340	17	10	65	39	0	32	7	135

Food Serving size	Cal.	(g) Total Fat	(g) Sat. Fat	(mg) Chol.	(g) Carb.	(g) Fiber	(g) Sug.	(g) Prot.	(mg) Sod.
Desserts									
Apple Chimi Cheesecake									
	890	36	18	120	129	3	84	15	830
Blue Ribbon Brownie									
	1670	78	40	240	220	6	154	28	950
Brownie Bite									
	380	18	9	45	52	2	36	5	220
Churro S'mores									
	580	10	2.5	0	120	5	70	7	650
Cracker Jack® Banana Cheesecake									
	930	54	29	225	98	2	75	12	600
Dessert Shooter - Hot Fudge Sundae									
	460	22	15	65	57	0	44	8	190
Triple Chocolate Meltdown®									
	980	52	34	135	125	5	64	15	540
Add a Soup									
Chili									
	410	24	12	100	18	5	7	29	1030
Chicken Tortilla Soup									
	240	11	3	25	24	3	3	11	1130
French Onion Soup									
	360	22	13	60	24	2	6	17	1390
Tomato Basil Soup									
	260	16	7	30	24	4	12	6	1170
Potato Soup									
	470	33	15	75	30	2	2	13	1510
Broccoli & Cheese Soup									
	390	29	18	100	21	3	7	14	1850
Chicken Noodle Soup									
	140	4	1.5	30	17	1	3	10	1100
Portsmouth Clam Chowder									
	380	26	16	100	24	2	1	14	1080
New England Clam Chowder									
	380	26	16	100	24	2	1	14	1080

Food Serving size	Cal.	(g) Total Fat	(g) Sat. Fat	(mg) Chol.	(g) Carb.	(g) Fiber	(g) Sug.	(g) Prot.	(mg) Sod.
Add a Salad									
Green Goddess Wedge Salad	550	52	11	55	12	3	7	9	1210
Small Caesar Salad	300	26	5	20	12	3	3	5	480
House Salad (w/o dressing)	230	15	7	35	13	3	4	13	400
Choice of Dressing: Bacon Vinaigrette	180	10	1.5	0	23	0	22	1	500
Choice of Dressing: Bleu Cheese Dressing	240	25	4.5	25	1	0	1	1	250
Choice of Dressing: Buttermilk Ranch Dressing	210	22	3.5	15	1	0	1	1	330
Choice of Dressing: Chili Lime Vinaigrette	120	7	1	0	13	0	10	0	500
Choice of Dressing: Dijon Honey Mustard Dressing	210	18	2.5	10	13	1	12	1	540
Choice of Dressing: Italian Dressing, Fat Free	20	0	0	0	5	0	3	0	370
Choice of Dressing: Lemon Olive Oil Vinaigrette	150	16	2	0	1	0	1	0	370
Choice of Dressing: Mexi Ranch Dressing	170	18	3	15	3	0	2	1	550
Choice of Dressing: Oriental Dressing	250	22	3	0	13	0	13	0	85
Add a Side									
Baked Potato - Loaded	410	24	14	65	41	3	3	10	340
Baked Potato - Regular	340	18	11	55	41	3	2	6	170
BBQ Spiced Fries, Side	440	20	4	0	60	6	1	5	890
Chili Cheese Fries, Side	630	33	11	45	65	8	3	17	1350

Food Serving size	Cal.	(g) Total Fat	(g) Sat. Fat	(mg) Chol.	(g) Carb.	(g) Fiber	(g) Sug.	(g) Prot.	(mg) Sod.
Classic Fries, Side									
	440	20	4	0	59	6	0	5	770
Crunchy Onion Rings, Side									
	530	29	5	0	60	3	8	7	1180
Fried Shrimp									
	430	20	4	105	48	3	10	16	1430
Garlic Mashed Potatoes - Loaded									
	470	32	13	60	32	4	6	15	980
Garlic Mashed Potatoes - Regular									
	250	14	2.5	0	29	3	4	5	600
Grilled Shrimp									
	160	9	4	180	4	1	1	16	1280
House Chips, Side									
	420	29	5	0	36	3	0	4	960
Seasonal Vegetables: Vegetable #1 (yellow squash or zucchini, sugar snap peas & carrotinis)									
	45	0	0	0	9	2	4	2	340
Seasonal Vegetables: Vegetable #2 (zucchini, yellow squash, red peppers, carrotinis & red onion)									
	35	0	0	0	8	2	4	1	320
Seasonal Vegetables: Vegetable #3 (zucchini, yellow squash, broccoli & carrotinis)									
	30	0	0	0	7	2	2	2	340
Seasonal Vegetables: Vegetable #4 (yellow squash or zucchini, broccoli & carrotinis)									
	35	0	0	0	8	3	3	2	350
Seasonal Vegetables: Vegetable #5 (broccoli crown)									
	40	0	0	0	8	3	2	3	210
Seasonal Vegetables: Garlic Broccoli (garlic & broccoli)									
	35	0	0	0	6	3	0	3	300
Sweet Potato Fries, Side									
	340	12	2	0	57	4	19	3	990

Beverages

Blackberry Quencher Lemonade									
	160	0	0	0	43	1	39	0	0

Food Serving size	Cal.	(g) Total Fat	(g) Sat. Fat	(mg) Chol.	(g) Carb.	(g) Fiber	(g) Sug.	(g) Prot.	(mg) Sod.
Strawberry Quencher Lemonade									
	170	0	0	0	43	1	39	0	0
Blackberry Honey Quencher Iced Tea									
	100	0	0	0	24	1	23	0	35
Kiwi Iced Tea									
	40	0	0	0	10	0	9	0	30
Mango Iced Tea									
	25	0	0	0	6	0	5	0	30
Pomegranate Iced Tea									
	35	0	0	0	9	0	8	0	30
Raspberry Iced Tea									
	40	0	0	0	10	0	9	0	30
Kiwi Lemonade									
	170	0	0	0	46	0	42	0	0
Mango Lemonade									
	160	0	0	0	42	0	38	0	0
Raspberry Lemonade									
	170	0	0	0	46	0	42	0	0
Mango Frozen Lemonade									
	250	0	0	0	62	5	50	1	10
Strawberry Frozen Lemonade									
	240	0	0	0	60	5	48	1	10
Wildberry Frozen Lemonade									
	250	0	0	0	63	5	50	1	10
Strawberry Shake									
	950	44	25	175	114	0	92	25	450
Cherry Limeade									
	200	0	0	0	52	0	48	0	15
Strawberry Limeade									
	160	0	0	0	41	0	37	0	15
Brewed Iced Tea									
	5	0	0	0	1	0	1	0	5
Hot Tea									
	5	0	0	0	1	0	0	0	5

Food Serving size	Cal.	(g) Total Fat	(g) Sat. Fat	(mg) Chol.	(g) Carb.	(g) Fiber	(g) Sug.	(g) Prot.	(mg) Sod.
Fresh Brewed Decaf Coffee									
	0	0	0	0	0	0	0	0	0
Fresh Brewed Coffee									
	0	0	0	0	0	0	0	0	0
Orange Twister									
	110	0	0	0	31	0	30	0	25
Pepsi									
	100	0	0	0	28	0	28	0	20
Mug Root Beer									
	100	0	0	0	26	0	26	0	15
Sierra Mist									
	100	0	0	0	27	0	27	0	20
Sobe Life Water, Yumberry Pomegranate									
	0	0	0	0	0	0	0	0	70
Wild Cherry Pepsi									
	100	0	0	0	28	0	28	0	20
Caffeine Free Coca Cola									
	100	0	0	0	27	0	27	0	0
Caffeine Free Diet Coke									
	0	0	0	0	0	0	0	0	10
Cherry Coke									
	100	0	0	0	27	0	27	0	0
Coca Cola									
	100	0	0	0	27	0	27	0	0
Coke Zero									
	0	0	0	0	0	0	0	0	0
Diet Coke									
	0	0	0	0	0	0	0	0	10
Fruit Punch, Hi-C									
	100	0	0	0	27	0	27	0	10
FUZE® Raspberry Ice Tea									
	60	0	0	0	15	0	15	0	5
Mellow Yellow									
	110	0	0	0	27	0	27	0	5

Food Serving size	Cal.	(g) Total Fat	(g) Sat. Fat	(mg) Chol.	(g) Carb.	(g) Fiber	(g) Sug.	(g) Prot.	(mg) Sod.
Orange Fanta	100	0	0	0	30	0	27	0	0
Pibb Extra	100	0	0	0	27	0	27	0	15
Barq's Root Beer	110	0	0	0	30	0	30	0	20
Sprite	100	0	0	0	25	0	25	0	20
Strawberry Fanta	110	0	0	0	31	0	31	0	10
Dr. Pepper	100	0	0	0	27	0	26	0	30
IBC Diet Root Beer	0	0	0	0	0	0	0	0	80
IBC Root Beer	110	0	0	0	30	0	29	0	40
Hi-C Pink Lemonade	100	0	0	0	27	0	25	0	45
Minute Maid Lemonade	100	0	0	0	27	0	25	0	45
Minute Maid Light Lemonade	5	0	0	0	0	0	0	0	0
Sun Orchard Lemonade	140	0	0	0	37	0	33	0	0
Half & Half Iced Tea & Lemonade	40	0	0	0	11	0	11	0	25
Sugar Free Lemonade	5	0	0	0	0	0	0	0	95
Tropicana Lemonade	100	0	0	0	27	0	27	0	105
Tropicana Pink Lemonade	100	0	0	0	27	0	27	0	105
Bottled Water	0	0	0	0	0	0	0	0	0

Food Serving size	Cal.	(g) Total Fat	(g) Sat. Fat	(mg) Chol.	(g) Carb.	(g) Fiber	(g) Sug.	(g) Prot.	(mg) Sod.
Perrier Sparkling Water									
	0	0	0	0	0	0	0	0	0
Dew Shine									
	170	0	0	0	41	0	41	0	60

Blimpie

Subs and Wraps

Food Serving size	Cal.	(g) Total Fat	(g) Sat. Fat	(mg) Chol.	(g) Carb.	(g) Fiber	(g) Sug.	(g) Prot.	(mg) Sod.
Blimpie Best, Rg									
	450	18	6	50	47	3	10	25	1330
Blimpie Best, Lg Super Stacked									
	1100	45	16	185	104	6	24	71	4180
Blimpie Best, Rg Super Stacked									
	550	22	8	90	52	3	12	36	2090
Blimpie Trio, Rg Super Stacked									
	520	16	5	95	50	3	11	43	1880
BLT, Lg									
	860	44	10	55	83	5	12	31	1980
BLT, Rg									
	430	22	5	25	43	2	6	15	960
BLT, Rg Super Stacked									
	540	30	8	45	43	2	6	22	1420
Blimpie Burger									
	460	24	10	70	42	1	4	21	1280
Club, Lg									
	820	27	8	85	97	6	18	47	2110
Club, Rg									
	410	13	4	45	49	3	9	23	1050
Club, Rg Wheat									
	410	14	4.5	45	47	6	8	26	1040
Club, Rg no cheese/sauce									
	310	4	1	25	49	3	9	18	1020
Cuban, Lg									
	810	21	9	130	83	3	12	59	3260

Food Serving size	Cal.	(g) Total Fat	(g) Sat. Fat	(mg) Chol.	(g) Carb.	(g) Fiber	(g) Sug.	(g) Prot.	(mg) Sod.
Cuban, Rg	410	11	4.5	65	42	1	6	30	1630
Deli Trio, Rg	330	4.5	1	35	49	3	9	22	1080
Deli Trio, Rg Wheat	320	5	1.5	40	43	6	8	24	1080
French Dip, Lg	780	22	10	130	83	3	7	61	2560
French Dip, Rg	410	11	5	65	46	1	3	30	1650
French Dip, Ciabatta	430	11	4.5	65	49	2	2	31	1820
Grilled Chicken Caesar, Ciabatta	580	20	5	65	62	3	4	34	1480
Ham & Swiss, Lg	820	28	10	95	94	6	20	47	2040
Ham & Swiss, Rg	410	14	5	45	47	3	10	23	1020
Ham & Swiss, Rg Wheat	410	15	5	45	44	6	9	25	970
Ham Rg, no cheese/sauce	310	4.5	1	30	49	3	10	19	980
Ham and Pepper Relish, Rg Wheat	300	6	1.5	30	43	5	10	20	1290
Ham, Salami & Provolone, Lg	930	40	14	110	94	6	19	49	2560
Ham, Salami & Provolone, Rg	460	20	7	55	47	3	9	24	1270
Meatball, Lg	1120	58	26	145	94	7	12	57	3640
Meatball, Rg	560	29	13	75	47	3	6	29	1820
Mediterranean, Ciabatta	450	8	2.5	35	65	3	6	26	1720

Food Serving size	Cal.	(g) Total Fat	Sat. Fat	(mg) Chol.	(g) Carb.	(g) Fiber	(g) Sug.	(g) Prot.	(mg) Sod.
Hot Pastrami, Lg									
	860	33	15	130	81	3	11	61	2790
Turkey and Avocado, Lg									
	720	15	2	60	102	8	17	41	2690
Turkey and Avocado, Rg									
	360	7	1	30	51	4	8	21	1340
Turkey and Cranberry, Lg									
	700	7	1.5	60	116	6	29	40	2440
Turkey and Cranberry, Rg									
	350	4	0.5	30	58	3	14	20	1220
Turkey and Bacon, Lg Super Stacked									
	1240	54	22	135	99	6	20	84	5420
Turkey and Bacon, Rg Super Stacked									
	620	27	11	65	50	3	10	42	2680
Turkey & Provolone, Lg									
	820	26	8	85	94	6	17	50	2740
Turkey & Provolone, Rg									
	410	14	5	45	47	3	9	25	1370
Turkey & Provolone, Rg Wheat									
	410	14	5	45	44	6	7	27	1320
Turkey Rg, no cheese/sauce									
	320	3.5	0.5	30	49	3	8	21	1220
Turkey and Sweet/Spicy Mustard, Rg Wheat									
	320	4.5	1	30	46	6	10	23	1470
Tuscan, Ciabatta									
	490	19	6	50	49	2	5	25	1810
Ultimate Club, Ciabatta									
	580	27	8	70	51	3	7	30	1760
Veggie Supreme, Lg									
	1090	56	28	75	97	7	18	53	3000
Veggie Supreme, Rg									
	550	28	14	35	49	3	9	27	1500
VegiMax, Rg									
	520	21	5	10	55	5	9	28	1290

Food Serving size	Cal.	(g) Total Fat	(g) Sat. Fat	(mg) Chol.	(g) Carb.	(g) Fiber	(g) Sug.	(g) Prot.	(mg) Sod.
VegiMax, Rg Wheat									
	530	22	6	10	52	9	8	29	1240
VegiMax Rg, no cheese/sauce									
	390	8	1	0	55	5	7	23	950
Veggie & Cheese, Lg									
	920	42	18	80	100	7	18	37	3290
Veggie & Cheese, Rg									
	460	21	9	40	50	3	9	19	1420
Veggie & Provolone Rg, no sauce									
	330	9	4	15	49	3	8	14	940
Veggie Salad, Rg Wheat									
	260	5	1	0	44	7	7	11	820
Wrap, Buffalo Chicken Pepperjack									
	680	34	10	75	60	5	5	33	2150
Wrap, Chicken Caesar									
	590	26	8	70	56	4	5	34	1610
Wrap, Chicken Cordon Blimpie									
	620	31	9	85	53	3	3	33	1430
Wrap, Southwestern									
	490	18	4	45	57	4	6	23	1530

Kid's Subs

Food	Cal.	Total Fat	Sat. Fat	Chol.	Carb.	Fiber	Sug.	Prot.	Sod.
3" Ham and Cheese									
	240	9	4.5	15	28	1	4	14	900
3" Tuna									
	260	11	1.5	25	25	1	3	13	450
3" Turkey and Cheese									
	210	5	2	25	27	1	4	14	830

Salads - Dressing not included

Food	Cal.	Total Fat	Sat. Fat	Chol.	Carb.	Fiber	Sug.	Prot.	Sod.
Antipasto									
	250	15	6	55	14	4	7	19	1670
Buffalo Chicken									
	200	8	4.5	60	11	4	4	23	1200
Buffalo Chicken Salad, no cheese									
	150	3.5	1.5	45	11	4	4	19	1110

Food Serving size	Cal.	(g) Total Fat	(g) Sat. Fat	(mg) Chol.	(g) Carb.	(g) Fiber	(g) Sug.	(g) Prot.	(mg) Sod.
Grilled Chicken Caesar									
	190	7	3.5	70	6	3	3	27	610
Garden									
	30	0	0	0	6	3	3	2	15
Tuna									
	270	19	2.5	55	6	3	3	18	370
Ultimate Club									
	270	14	7	65	11	4	7	24	1070
Cole Slaw Salad, side									
	160	9	1.5	5	20	2	17	1	240
Macaroni Salad, side									
	330	22	5	15	28	2	8	5	790
Northwest Potato Salad, side									
	260	17	4	25	22	3	3	3	390
Potato Salad, side									
	230	12	2.5	10	28	3	8	3	490

Soups

Food Serving size	Cal.	(g) Total Fat	(g) Sat. Fat	(mg) Chol.	(g) Carb.	(g) Fiber	(g) Sug.	(g) Prot.	(mg) Sod.
Bean with Ham									
	140	1	0	0	23	11	2	8	1070
Beef Steak & Noodle									
	120	4	1.5	30	14	0	4	8	780
Beef Stew									
	170	4	3.5	45	18	2	2	17	890
Captain's Corn Chowder									
	210	7	2.5	5	29	4	7	6	890
Chicken & Dumpling									
	170	7	3	50	19	3	4	11	970
Chicken Gumbo									
	90	2	0	10	13	2	4	6	1280
Chicken Noodle									
	130	4	1	30	18	2	5	7	1040
Chicken with White & Wild Rice									
	250	10	2.5	30	15	4	4	14	1030

Food Serving size	Cal.	(g) Total Fat	(g) Sat. Fat	(mg) Chol.	(g) Carb.	(g) Fiber	(g) Sug.	(g) Prot.	(mg) Sod.
Chili with Bean & Beef	250	9	5	40	16	18	7	18	1230
Cream of Broccoli with Cheese	250	19	11	55	13	<1	2	7	1040
Cream of Potato	190	9	2.5	< 5	24	3	3	5	860
French Onion	80	4	0.5	0	11	1	6	2	1020
Garden Vegetable	80	1	0	0	14	3	5	5	620
Harvest Vegetable	100	1	0	0	19	3	4	4	920
Italian Style Wedding	130	4	1.5	10	17	0	0	7	900
Minestrone	90	3	0	0	14	4	4	4	1150
New England Clam Chowder	170	3	2	25	28	2	5	7	1060
Pasta Fagioli with Sausage	150	5	1.5	20	22	4	2	7	910
Split Pea with Ham	130	2	0	5	21	6	1	8	1090
Tomato Basil with Raviolini	110	1	0	10	22	0	5	4	720
Vegetable Beef	80	2	0.5	5	13	2	3	4	1010
Yankee Pot Roast	80	2	0.5	10	12	2	2	5	750

Breakfast Items

Food Serving size	Cal.	(g) Total Fat	(g) Sat. Fat	(mg) Chol.	(g) Carb.	(g) Fiber	(g) Sug.	(g) Prot.	(mg) Sod.
Biscuit, Bacon Egg & Cheese	440	25	16	160	37	1	3	18	1610
Biscuit, Egg & Cheese	380	20	15	165	37	1	4	13	1380

Food Serving size	Cal.	(g) Total Fat	(g) Sat. Fat	(mg) Chol.	(g) Carb.	(g) Fiber	(g) Sug.	(g) Prot.	(mg) Sod.
Biscuit, Ham Egg & Cheese									
	420	21	15	185	39	1	5	19	1660
Biscuit, Sausage Egg & Cheese									
	530	34	20	195	37	1	4	19	1690
Bluffin, Plain									
	130	1	0	0	25	2	2	5	240
Bluffin, Bacon Egg & Cheese									
	320	16	7	160	27	2	2	17	1090
Bluffin, Egg & Cheese									
	240	10	5	165	27	2	2	12	770
Bluffin, Ham Egg & Cheese									
	280	10	5	180	29	2	4	17	1050
Bluffin, Sausage Egg & Cheese									
	390	24	10	195	27	2	2	18	1080
Burrito, Bacon Egg & Cheese									
	660	35	14	320	54	3	1	31	2570
Burrito, Egg & Cheese									
	510	24	10	300	54	3	1	21	1930
Burrito, Ham Egg & Cheese									
	580	25	10	330	57	3	4	31	2490
Burrito, Sausage Egg & Cheese									
	800	52	20	355	54	3	1	33	2550
Burrito, Turkey Egg & Cheese									
	560	24	10	320	56	3	2	29	2460
Grilled Breakfast Sandwich, Bacon									
	480	23	10	335	44	1	4	25	1620
Grilled Breakfast Sandwich, Ham									
	480	19	9	355	47	1	7	30	1860
Grilled Breakfast Sandwich, Sausage									
	710	45	18	385	44	1	4	32	1920
Grilled Breakfast Sandwich, Turkey									
	460	18	8	345	46	1	5	28	1830
Egg & Cheese on a Roll									
	220	10	5	150	21	1	2	11	740

Food Serving size	Cal.	(g) Total Fat	(g) Sat. Fat	(mg) Chol.	(g) Carb.	(g) Fiber	(g) Sug.	(g) Prot.	(mg) Sod.
Cinnamon Roll	450	20	9	30	60	2	17	9	730
Bagel	290	1	0	0	58	3	12	11	700
Bagel, Cream Cheese	390	11	6	30	59	3	12	13	780
Biscuit with Sausage Gravy	460	27	14	25	43	2	4	12	1320

Chips

Food Serving size	Cal.	(g) Total Fat	(g) Sat. Fat	(mg) Chol.	(g) Carb.	(g) Fiber	(g) Sug.	(g) Prot.	(mg) Sod.
Cheddar Sour Cream	240	15	4.5	0	21	2	3	3	280
Cheetos Crunchy	160	10	2.5	0	15	1	1	2	290
Doritos Cooler Ranch	240	12	2.5	0	31	2	2	3	300
Doritos Nacho Cheese	240	12	2.5	0	30	2	3	3	330
Fritos	320	20	2	0	30	2	0	4	210
KC Master BBQ	240	15	4.5	0	22	1	3	3	300
Baked BBQ	130	3.5	0	0	25	2	2	2	240
SunChips Multigrain Harvest Cheddar	210	9	1.5	0	28	3	3	3	280
SunChips Multigrain Original	210	9	1	0	29	4	3	3	140
Potato Baked	120	1.5	0	0	26	2	2	2	170
Potato Regular	220	15	4.5	0	22	1	0	3	270
Pretzels Classic Thin Style	220	2	0	0	47	2	2	4	—

Food Serving size	Cal.	(g) Total Fat	(g) Sat. Fat	(mg) Chol.	(g) Carb.	(g) Fiber	(g) Sug.	(g) Prot.	(mg) Sod.
Desserts and Snacks									
Brownie									
	230	10	4	22	28	1	21	3	115
Chocolate Chunk Cookie									
	180	10	5	10	24	1	14	2	125
Oatmeal Raisin Cookie									
	160	8	3.5	15	23	1	12	2	110
Peanut Butter Cookie									
	200	8	4.5	15	20	1	12	4	150
Sugar Cookie									
	320	15	6	30	42	1	23	3	210
White Chocolate Macadamia Nut Cookie									
	190	10	5	10	23	0	15	2	120
Cotton Candy									
	220	0	0	0	56	0	56	3	0
Nachos									
	540	28	4	10	66	6	0	9	890
Pickle									
	25	0	0	0	5	0	0	0	1520
Popcorn, regular									
	590	32	6	0	66	11	1	10	0
Soft Pretzel, plain									
	450	3	0	0	93	3	3	12	480
Soft Pretzel, salted									
	480	4	0	0	93	3	3	12	2010
Soft Pretzel, cinnamon sugar									
	510	4	0	0	102	3	12	12	480
Side, Cheese Sauce									
	80	4.5	1.5	5	8	0	0	2	470
Side, Chili									
	70	2.5	1.5	10	9	5	2	5	350

Sub Component - Meats/Protein

Bacon									
	110	8	2.8	15	0	0	0	7	450

Food Serving size	Cal.	(g) Total Fat	(g) Sat. Fat	(mg) Chol.	(g) Carb.	(g) Fiber	(g) Sug.	(g) Prot.	(mg) Sod.
Buffalo Chicken									
	35	1	0.5	15	1	0	0	6	210
Cappacola									
	20	0.5	0.2	10	0	—	0	3	160
Chicken (Grilled) Strips									
	110	3.5	0.8	50	0	0	0	19	300
Corned Beef									
	35	1	0	15	1	0	1	6	250
Ham									
	35	1	0.3	15	2	—	2	5	280
Meatballs with Sauce									
	220	16	6	45	8	2	2	11	1010
Roast Beef									
	30	1	0.4	15	0	0	0	6	150
Salami									
	35	3	1	10	0	0	0	2	135
Seafood Salad									
	90	4	0.5	20	10	1	2	4	410
Tuna									
	240	18	2.5	55	0	0	0	16	350
Turkey									
	30	0.3	0	12	1	—	1	5	316

Sub Component - Cheeses

Food Serving size	Cal.	(g) Total Fat	(g) Sat. Fat	(mg) Chol.	(g) Carb.	(g) Fiber	(g) Sug.	(g) Prot.	(mg) Sod.
American									
	100	9	5	25	1	—	1	5	510
Smoked Cheddar									
	80	6	4	20	1	—	0	4	380
Parmesan, Shredded									
	50	4	2.2	10	1	0	0	4	150
Pepper Jack									
	80	7	3.9	25	0	0	0	6	135
Provolone									
	80	6	3.8	15	0	—	—	5	190
Swiss									
	80	6	3.5	20	0	0	0	6	45

Food Serving size	Cal.	(g) Total Fat	(g) Sat. Fat	(mg) Chol.	(g) Carb.	(g) Fiber	(g) Sug.	(g) Prot.	(mg) Sod.
Sub Component - Toppings									
Guacamole									
	45	4	0.5	0	2	1	0	0	135
Lettuce, serving									
	5	0	0	0	1	0	1	0	0
Olives, serving									
	15	1.5	0.2	0	1	0	0	0	125
Onion, slices									
	10	0	0	0	3	0	1	0	0
Peppers, Hot Banana Ring									
	0	0	0	0	1	0	0	0	450
Peppers, Jalapeno									
	10	0	0	0	1	0	0	0	490
Peppers, Red Roasted									
	10	0	0	0	2	0	1	0	100
Peppers, Sweet Strips									
	20	0	0	0	5	0	5	0	115
Tomato, slices									
	5	0	0	0	2	0	1	0	0
Sub Component - Breads/Wraps									
Cheddar Jalapeno, Lg									
	540	11	4	15	91	3	8	20	1180
Cheddar Jalapeno, Rg									
	210	4.5	1.5	5	36	1	3	8	470
Ciabatta, serving									
	230	2.5	0	0	43	2	2	8	590
Honey Oat, Lg									
	520	15	3	0	82	10	11	20	810
Honey Oat, Rg									
	260	8	1.5	0	41	5	5	10	400
Marble Rye, Lg									
	480	5	1	0	93	5	4	18	1170
Marble Rye, Rg									
	240	2.5	0.5	0	46	2	2	9	590

Food Serving size	Cal.	(g) Total Fat	(g) Sat. Fat	(mg) Chol.	(g) Carb.	(g) Fiber	(g) Sug.	(g) Prot.	(mg) Sod.
Pretzel, serving	300	4.5	2	0	58	2	7	8	75
Wheat, Lg	430	8	2	0	76	10	5	20	810
Wheat, Rg	210	4	1	0	38	5	3	10	400
White, Lg	430	6	1	0	79	3	7	15	840
White, Rg	210	3	0.5	0	40	1	4	7	420
Zesty Parmesan, Lg	470	9	3.5	10	77	3	7	19	980
Zesty Parmesan, Rg	240	4.5	2	5	39	2	4	9	490
Wrap, Flour	310	8	2.5	0	52	5	1	9	670
Wrap, Spinach	310	8	3	0	52	3	3	9	840

Dressings/Sauces

Food Serving size	Cal.	(g) Total Fat	(g) Sat. Fat	(mg) Chol.	(g) Carb.	(g) Fiber	(g) Sug.	(g) Prot.	(mg) Sod.
Blue Cheese	230	24	4.5	25	2	—	2	2	440
Buttermilk Ranch	150	16	2.5	5	1	—	1	1	250
Creamy Caesar	210	21	3.5	10	2	—	1	1	520
Creamy Italian	180	18	2.5	0	4	0	3	0	420
Dijon Honey Mustard	180	17	2.5	15	8	—	7	1	240
Fat-Free Italian	25	0	—	0	5	0	3	0	390
Light Buttermilk Ranch	70	4	0.5	0	8	—	3	1	310
Light Italian	20	1	0	0	2	—	2	0	770

Food Serving size	Cal.	(g) Total Fat	(g) Sat. Fat	(mg) Chol.	(g) Carb.	(g) Fiber	(g) Sug.	(g) Prot.	(mg) Sod.
Thousand Island	210	20	3	15	6	0	6	0	350
Peppercorn	120	12	2	5	1	0	1	0	210
Blimpie Special Sauce	40	4.5	0	0	0	—	—	0	0
Mayonnaise	100	11	1.5	10	0	0	0	0	100
Mustard, Yellow Deli Style	15	0	0	—	0	0	0	0	170
Mustard, Honey	20	0.5	0	0	4	1	3	1	85
Mustard, Spicy Brown	15	0	0	0	0	—	0	0	170
Oil, Blend	60	6	1	—	0	0	0	0	0
Red Wine Vinegar	5	0	0	0	1	0	0	0	0
Sauce, Red Hot Original	10	0	0	0	2	0	0	0	760

CiCi's Pizza

12" Buffet Pizzas (1 Slice)

Food Serving size	Cal.	(g) Total Fat	(g) Sat. Fat	(mg) Chol.	(g) Carb.	(g) Fiber	(g) Sug.	(g) Prot.	(mg) Sod.
Alfredo	120	3.5	1.5	5	19	<1	<1	4	270
Bacon Cheddar	110	4.5	1.5	5	19	<1	<1	5	350
BBQ	140	2.5	1	5	25	1	6	6	380
Beef	150	4	2	10	20	<1	1	6	380
Buffalo Chicken	140	4.5	1.5	10	19	<1	1	6	460

Food Serving size	Cal.	(g) Total Fat	(g) Sat. Fat	(mg) Chol.	(g) Carb.	(g) Fiber	(g) Sug.	(g) Prot.	(mg) Sod.
Cheese	150	3.5	2	10	20	<1	1	6	330
Classic Chicken	130	4	1.5	10	19	<1	<1	5	350
Ham	150	3.5	1.5	10	20	<1	1	6	370
Ham and Pineapple	150	3.5	1.5	10	21	<1	2	6	350
Macaroni and Cheese	170	2.5	1	5	29	1	2	6	250
Medium Pepperoni Deep Dish	180	6	3	15	19	<1	1.5	7	340
Ole'	70	2	1	<5	11	<1	1	4	240
Pepperoni	160	4.5	2	10	20	<1	1	6	370
Tomato Alfredo	120	3	1.5	<5	19	<1	1	4	290
Vegetable Italiano	70	3.5	1	5	9	0	<1	3.5	210
Veggie	130	2	0.5	<5	20	<1	2	4	280
Zesty Ham and Cheddar	120	3	1	5	19	<1	<1	5	340
Zesty Pepperoni	130	4.5	1.5	5	19	<1	<1	5	340
Zesty Veggie	120	3	1	<5	20	<1	1	4	320

15" Buffet Pizzas (1 Slice)

Food	Cal.	Total Fat	Sat. Fat	Chol.	Carb.	Fiber	Sug.	Prot.	Sod.
Alfredo	170	6	3	10	23	<1	1	6	400
Bacon Cheddar	150	8	2.5	15	25	<1	1	8	560
BBQ	240	6	3	20	36	2	12	11	710

Food Serving size	Cal.	(g) Total Fat	(g) Sat. Fat	(mg) Chol.	(g) Carb.	(g) Fiber	(g) Sug.	(g) Prot.	(mg) Sod.
Beef	210	7	3.5	20	24	1	2	9	560
Ole'	150	4.5	2	10	21	1	2	7	480
Pepperoni	210	8	3.5	20	24	<1	2	9	530
Pepperoni and Jalapeno	210	7	3.5	20	24	<1	2	8	590
Sausage	230	10	4.5	20	24	1	2	8	490
Spinach Alfredo	170	6	2.5	10	23	<1	1	6	380
Tomato Alfredo	160	5	2.5	10	24	<1	2	6	400
Veggie 15"	160	2.5	1	<5	25	1	2	5	340
Zesty Ham and Cheddar	180	6	2	15	23	<1	1	8	520
Zesty Pepperoni	190	7	2.5	15	23	<1	1	7	510
Zesty Veggie	160	4.5	1.5	5	24	<1	2	5	390

A La Carte

BBQ Wings (4 pieces)	270	18	5	115	6	<1	0	22	730
Hot Wings (4 pieces)	280	21	5	115	2	0	0	22	1130
Mild Wings (4 pieces)	320	26	6	115	1	0	0	22	980

Additional Menu Items

Chicken Noodle Soup (4 oz)	60	1.5	0	<5	8	0	1	3	520
Garlic Bread Sticks (1 piece)	100	5	1.5	<5	10	0	0	4	120

Food Serving size	Cal.	(g) Total Fat	(g) Sat. Fat	(mg) Chol.	(g) Carb.	(g) Fiber	(g) Sug.	(g) Prot.	(mg) Sod.
Italian Signature Salad (1/2 cup)									
	35	1	0	0	2	<1	1	<1	280
Pasta (with sauce) (4 oz)									
	240	1	0	0	48	3	6	8	300

Dessert Items

Bavarian Dessert (1 roll)									
	170	3	5	0	32	<1	11	3	210
Cinnamon Rolls (1 roll)									
	140	5	1	0	20	0	20	2	100
Fudge Brownies (1 slice)									
	140	6	1	0	23	<1	15	1	125
Iced Apple Crumb Pizza (1 slice)									
	240	6	1	0	43	<1	15	5	290

Coldstone Creamery

Ice Cream

Amaretto Ice Cream (142g)									
	330	20	12	80	33	0	29	5	80
Amaretto Ice Cream (227g)									
	530	31	20	125	53	0	46	8	130
Banana Ice Cream (142g)									
	310	18	12	70	33	0	28	5	70
Banana Ice Cream (227g)									
	500	29	18	115	53	0	46	8	115
Banana Ice Cream (340g)									
	750	44	28	175	80	<1	68	11	170
Blueberry Ice Cream (227g)									
	510	31	21	120	53	0	49	9	90
Blueberry Ice Cream (340g)									
	760	47	31	185	79	0	74	13	130
Butter Pecan Ice Cream (142g)									
	320	19	12	75	32	0	28	5	105

Food Serving size	Cal.	(g) Total Fat	(g) Sat. Fat	(mg) Chol.	(g) Carb.	(g) Fiber	(g) Sug.	(g) Prot.	(mg) Sod.
Butter Pecan Ice Cream (227g)									
	520	31	20	125	53	0	45	8	170
Butter Pecan Ice Cream (340g)									
	780	47	30	185	79	0	68	12	260
Cake Batter Ice Cream (142g)									
	340	19	12	70	41	0	32	5	180
Cake Batter Ice Cream (227g)									
	550	30	19	115	66	0	51	8	280
Cake Batter Ice Cream (340g)									
	830	45	28	170	99	0	76	12	420
Cheesecake Ice Cream (142g)									
	320	19	13	50	36	0	32	4	85
Cheesecake Ice Cream (227g)									
	510	30	20	75	57	0	51	6	140
Cheesecake Ice Cream (340g)									
	760	45	30	115	86	1	76	10	210
Chocolate Cake Batter Ice Cream (142g)									
	340	19	11	70	42	1	33	5	210
Chocolate Cake Batter Ice Cream (227g)									
	550	30	18	110	68	2	53	9	340
Chocolate Cake Batter Ice Cream (340g)									
	820	45	27	160	101	3	79	13	510
Chocolate Dipped Strawberry (142g)									
	310	19	12	30	32	2	29	5	65
Chocolate Dipped Strawberry (227g)									
	490	30	20	45	51	3	46	8	100
Chocolate Ice Cream (142g)									
	320	20	13	75	33	1	30	6	95
Chocolate Ice Cream (227g)									
	520	32	20	125	53	2	48	9	160
Chocolate Ice Cream (340g)									
	780	48	30	185	79	3	71	13	230
Chocolate Peanut Butter Ice Cream (142g)									
	410	28	13	25	36	3	31	10	200

Food Serving size	Cal.	(g) Total Fat	(g) Sat. Fat	(mg) Chol.	(g) Carb.	(g) Fiber	(g) Sug.	(g) Prot.	(mg) Sod.
Chocolate Peanut Butter Ice Cream (227g)									
	660	45	21	35	58	4	49	16	320
Chocolate Peanut Butter Ice Cream (340g)									
	990	67	31	55	86	6	74	24	480
Cinnamon Bun Ice Cream (142g)									
	350	18	12	45	47	1	37	4	190
Cinnamon Bun Ice Cream (227g)									
	560	28	18	70	75	2	59	7	310
Cinnamon Bun Ice Cream (340g)									
	840	42	28	105	112	2	89	10	460
Cinnamon Ice Cream (142g)									
	330	20	12	80	34	<1	29	5	80
Cinnamon Ice Cream (227g)									
	530	32	20	125	55	1	46	8	125
Cinnamon Ice Cream (340g)									
	790	47	30	185	82	2	69	12	190
Coconut Ice Cream (142g)									
	330	20	12	75	33	0	28	5	80
Coconut Ice Cream (227g)									
	520	31	20	125	52	0	45	8	125
Coconut Ice Cream (340g)									
	780	47	30	185	79	0	68	12	190
Coffee Ice Cream (142g)									
	330	20	12	80	34	0	29	5	80
Coffee Ice Cream (227g)									
	530	31	20	125	54	0	46	8	125
Coffee Ice Cream (340g)									
	790	47	30	185	81	0	69	12	190
Cookie Batter Ice Cream (142g)									
	360	20	12	40	43	0	37	4	270
Cookie Batter Ice Cream (227g)									
	580	33	19	65	68	1	59	7	430
Cookie Batter Ice Cream (340g)									
	860	49	28	100	102	1	89	10	650

Food Serving size	Cal.	(g) Total Fat	(g) Sat. Fat	(mg) Chol.	(g) Carb.	(g) Fiber	(g) Sug.	(g) Prot.	(mg) Sod.
Cotton Candy Ice Cream (142g)									
	330	19	12	75	34	0	28	5	75
Cotton Candy Ice Cream (227g)									
	530	31	20	125	55	0	45	8	120
Dark Chocolate Ice Cream (142g)									
	340	20	12	75	32	3	29	7	95
Dark Chocolate Ice Cream (227g)									
	540	32	20	115	51	5	46	11	150
Dark Chocolate Ice Cream (340g)									
	800	47	30	175	77	7	68	16	230
French Toast Ice Cream (142g)									
	330	19	12	75	35	0	30	5	150
French Toast Ice Cream (227g)									
	530	31	19	120	56	0	49	8	250
French Toast Ice Cream (340g)									
	790	46	29	180	84	0	73	12	370
French Vanilla Ice Cream (142g)									
	340	19	14	100	37	0	33	5	80
French Vanilla Ice Cream (227g)									
	540	30	22	60	60	0	52	8	125
Fudge Brownie Batter Ice Cream (142g)									
	350	19	12	30	43	2	37	5	125
Fudge Brownie Batter Ice Cream (227g)									
	550	30	19	45	69	2	59	8	200
Fudge Brownie Batter Ice Cream (340g)									
	830	45	29	65	103	4	89	12	300
Irish Cream Ice Cream (142g)									
	330	20	13	80	33	0	29	5	80
Irish Cream Ice Cream (227g)									
	530	32	20	125	54	0	46	8	125
Irish Cream Ice Cream (340g)									
	790	47	30	190	80	0	70	12	190
Key Lime Ice Cream (142g)									
	340	20	13	70	39	0	36	5	50

Food Serving size	Cal.	(g) Total Fat	(g) Sat. Fat	(mg) Chol.	(g) Carb.	(g) Fiber	(g) Sug.	(g) Prot.	(mg) Sod.
Key Lime Ice Cream (227g)									
	550	32	21	115	63	0	58	8	80
Key Lime Ice Cream (340g)									
	820	47	31	170	94	0	87	12	120
Macadamia Nut Ice Cream (142g)									
	330	20	12	80	34	0	29	5	75
Macadamia Nut Ice Cream (227g)									
	530	31	20	125	54	0	46	8	125
Macadamia Nut Ice Cream (340g)									
	790	47	30	185	81	0	70	12	190
Mango Ice Cream (142g)									
	310	18	12	70	33	0	28	5	70
Mango Ice Cream (227g)									
	490	29	18	115	53	0	45	7	115
Mango Ice Cream (340g)									
	740	44	28	175	80	0	68	11	170
Mint Ice Cream (142g)									
	330	19	12	75	36	0	31	5	75
Mint Ice Cream (227g)									
	530	30	19	120	57	0	50	8	120
Mocha Ice Cream (142g)									
	320	20	12	75	33	1	29	6	95
Peach Ice Cream (227g)									
	500	23	16	90	71	0	63	7	70
Peach Ice Cream (340g)									
	760	35	23	135	106	0	94	10	105
Peanut Butter Ice Cream (340g)									
	890	58	30	175	79	2	66	18	310
Pecan Praline Ice Cream (142g)									
	330	19	12	75	37	0	31	5	90
Pecan Praline Ice Cream (227g)									
	530	30	19	115	58	0	49	8	150
Pecan Praline Ice Cream (340g)									
	800	45	28	175	88	0	73	11	220

Food Serving size	Cal.	(g) Total Fat	(g) Sat. Fat	(mg) Chol.	(g) Carb.	(g) Fiber	(g) Sug.	(g) Prot.	(mg) Sod.
Pistachio Ice Cream (142g)									
	330	20	12	80	34	0	29	5	85
Pistachio Ice Cream (227g)									
	520	31	20	125	54	0	46	8	135
Pistachio Ice Cream (340g)									
	780	47	30	185	80	0	70	12	200
Pistachio Jello Pudding Ice Cream (142g)									
	350	18	12	45	45	0	41	4	260
Pistachio Jello Pudding Ice Cream (227g)									
	560	29	19	70	73	1	66	6	410
Pistachio Jello Pudding Ice Cream (340g)									
	840	43	28	105	109	1	99	9	620
Pumpkin Ice Cream (142g)									
	290	15	10	60	33	1	28	4	105
Pumpkin Ice Cream (227g)									
	460	24	15	95	53	2	45	7	170
Pumpkin Ice Cream (340g)									
	680	37	23	145	80	3	67	10	260
Raspberry Ice Cream (142g)									
	330	19	12	75	36	0	31	5	75
Raspberry Ice Cream (227g)									
	520	30	19	120	57	0	50	8	125
Raspberry Ice Cream (340g)									
	780	44	28	175	85	0	75	12	180
Sinless Sans Fat Sweet Cream (142g)									
	170	0	0	0	35	1	11	8	160
Sinless Sans Fat Sweet Cream (227g)									
	280	0	0	0	56	1	17	12	260
Sinless Sans Fat Sweet Cream (340g)									
	420	0.5	0	10	83	2	26	18	390
Strawberry Cheesecake Ice Cream (142g)									
	320	21	12	65	39	0	32	5	50
Strawberry Cheesecake Ice Cream (227g)									
	520	33	18	105	63	0	51	8	85

Food Serving size	Cal.	Total Fat (g)	Sat. Fat (g)	Chol. (mg)	Carb. (g)	Fiber (g)	Sug. (g)	Prot. (g)	Sod. (mg)
Strawberry Cheesecake Ice Cream (340g)									
	780	50	28	160	94	1	77	12	125
Strawberry Ice Cream (142g)									
	320	18	12	75	35	0	30	5	75
Strawberry Ice Cream (227g)									
	510	30	19	115	55	0	48	8	120
Strawberry Ice Cream (340g)									
	770	44	28	175	83	0	72	11	180
Sweet Cream Ice Cream (142g)									
	330	20	13	80	33	0	29	5	80
Sweet Cream Ice Cream (227g)									
	530	32	20	125	53	0	46	8	125
Sweet Cream Ice Cream (340g)									
	790	48	30	190	80	0	70	12	190
Vanilla Bean Ice Cream (142g)									
	330	19	12	75	32	0	28	5	75
Vanilla Bean Ice Cream (227g)									
	530	31	19	120	52	0	45	8	120
Vanilla Bean Ice Cream (340g)									
	790	46	29	180	77	0	67	12	180
White Chocolate Ice Cream (142g)									
	320	19	12	75	33	0	28	5	75
White Chocolate Ice Cream (227g)									
	520	31	20	125	53	0	45	8	125
White Chocolate Ice Cream (340g)									
	780	47	29	185	79	0	68	12	180

Sorbet and Yogurt

Food	Cal.	Total Fat	Sat. Fat	Chol.	Carb.	Fiber	Sug.	Prot.	Sod.
Countrytime Pink Lemonade Sorbet (340g)									
	570	0	0	0	142	0	142	0	55
Lemon Sorbet (142g)									
	150	0	0	0	40	0	34	0	15
Lemon Sorbet (227g)									
	250	0	0	0	64	0	54	0	25
Lemon Sorbet (340g)									
	370	0	0	0	96	<1	81	0	35

Food Serving size	Cal.	(g) Total Fat	(g) Sat. Fat	(mg) Chol.	(g) Carb.	(g) Fiber	(g) Sug.	(g) Prot.	(mg) Sod.
Raspberry Sorbet (142g)									
	160	0	0	0	42	0	36	0	15
Raspberry Sorbet (227g)									
	260	0	0	0	67	0	58	0	30
Raspberry Sorbet (340g)									
	390	0	0	0	101	<1	87	0	40
Strawberry Mango Banana Sorbet (142g)									
	220	0	0	0	55	0	52	0	15
Strawberry Mango Banana Sorbet (227g)									
	350	0	0	0	87	1	83	0	25
Strawberry Mango Banana Sorbet (340g)									
	520	0.5	0	0	131	1	125	0	35
Tart and Tangy Berry Yogurt (142g)									
	150	0	0	0	36	0	27	3	65
Tart and Tangy Berry Yogurt (227g)									
	240	0	0	0	58	0	44	5	105
Tart and Tangy Berry Yogurt (340g)									
	360	0	0	0	87	0	66	7	160
Tart and Tangy Yogurt (142g)									
	140	0	0	0	33	0	24	3	70
Tart and Tangy Yogurt (227g)									
	230	0	0	0	53	0	38	5	115
Watermelon Sorbet (142g)									
	160	0	0	0	41	0	35	0	15
Watermelon Sorbet (227g)									
	260	0	0	0	66	0	56	0	25
Watermelon Sorbet (340g)									
	380	0	0	90	99	<1	84	0	40

Dunkin' Donuts

AM Snacks

Brown Sugar Flavored Oatmeal with Dried Fruit Topping									
1 Serving	300	4	1	0	61	6	28	7	470

Food Serving size	Cal.	(g) Total Fat	(g) Sat. Fat	(mg) Chol.	(g) Carb.	(g) Fiber	(g) Sug.	(g) Prot.	(mg) Sod.
Hash Browns									
6 Pieces	140	8	1	0	17	2	0	2	480
Jalapeno Kolache									
1 Kolache	180	8	3	20	20	1	5	10	240
Original Kolache									
1 Kolache	180	9	3	20	20	1	6	10	250
Original Oatmeal with Dried Fruit Topping									
1 Serving	270	4	1	0	54	6	22	7	140

Bagels

Food Serving size	Cal.	(g) Total Fat	(g) Sat. Fat	(mg) Chol.	(g) Carb.	(g) Fiber	(g) Sug.	(g) Prot.	(mg) Sod.
Cinnamon Raisin Bagel									
1 Bagel	320	1	0	0	66	4	14	12	500
Cinnamon Raisin Bagel Twist									
1 Bagel Twist	350	1	0	0	72	4	20	12	510
Everything Bagel									
1 Bagel	340	3	0	0	67	5	7	12	630
Garlic Bagel									
1 Bagel	330	1	0	0	69	5	7	12	630
Multigrain Bagel									
1 Bagel	350	7	0.5	0	63	8	8	15	450
Onion Bagel									
1 Bagel	310	1	0	0	63	3	4	11	500
Plain Bagel									
1 Bagel	310	1	0	0	64	4	7	11	620
Poppy Seed Bagel									
1 Bagel	340	3.5	0.5	0	66	5	7	12	630
Salt Bagel									
1 Bagel	310	1	0	0	64	4	7	11	3380
Sesame Seed Bagel									
1 Bagel	350	4.5	1	0	65	5	7	12	630
Sour Cream and Onion Bagel									
1 Bagel	330	1.5	0	0	66	3	6	13	1050
Sour Cream and Onion Bagel Twist									
1 Bagel Twist	330	1.5	0	0	66	3	6	13	1050

Food Serving size	Cal.	(g) Total Fat	(g) Sat. Fat	(mg) Chol.	(g) Carb.	(g) Fiber	(g) Sug.	(g) Prot.	(mg) Sod.
Whole Wheat Bagel									
1 Bagel	320	2	0	0	61	7	10	13	590

Bakery Sandwiches

Bacon Ancho Chicken Sandwich									
1 Sandwich	640	25	7	65	70	3	7	34	1620
Bacon Ranch Chicken Sandwich									
1 Sandwich	660	27	8	65	69	3	6	34	1620
Chicken Bacon Sandwich on a Croissant									
1 Sandwich	690	37	13	55	59	2	12	29	1300
Chicken Salad on a Croissant									
1 Sandwich	580	39	11	45	42	2	7	16	850
Deluxe Grilled Cheese with Bacon									
1 Sandwich	520	30	12	40	41	1	3	20	1070
Deluxe Grilled Cheese with Ham									
1 Sandwich	530	30	13	55	41	1	4	22	1210
Ham and Cheese Flatbread									
1 Sandwich	290	8	3	35	35	3	8	18	950
Snack 'n Go Chicken Wrap - Breaded Chicken									
1 Wrap	280	15	4	35	21	1	2	15	700
Snack 'n Go Steak Wrap									
1 Wrap	210	11	5	35	15	1	3	12	430
Texas Toast Grilled Cheese									
1 Sandwich	510	30	13	40	41	1	3	18	940
Tuna Salad Sandwich on a Plain Bagel									
1 Sandwich	580	25	3.5	40	68	4	7	22	1120
Turkey Cheddar Bacon Flatbread									
1 Sandwich	380	17	6	60	32	3	4	24	1060

Beverage Flavors

Flavor Shot in Medium Beverage									
1 Shot	10	0	0	0	1	0	0	0	0

Breakfast Sandwiches

Angus Steak and Egg Wake Up Wrap									
1 Wrap	230	14	7	65	13	1	1	14	570

Food Serving size	Cal.	(g) Total Fat	(g) Sat. Fat	(mg) Chol.	(g) Carb.	(g) Fiber	(g) Sug.	(g) Prot.	(mg) Sod.
Bacon, Egg & Cheese on Biscuit									
1 Sandwich	470	27	14	75	38	1	4	18	1310
Bacon, Egg & Cheese on Croissant									
1 Sandwich	490	29	13	80	40	2	6	18	870
Bacon, Egg & Cheese on English Muffin									
1 Sandwich	300	12	5	80	32	7	2	16	630
Bacon, Egg & Cheese on a Plain Bagel									
1 Sandwich	470	12	5	80	67	4	7	23	1140
Chicken Biscuit									
1 Sandwich	540	28	11	35	51	2	6	21	1380
Egg & Cheese on Biscuit									
1 Sandwich	420	23	13	70	37	1	4	14	1100
Egg & Cheese on Croissant									
1 Sandwich	440	25	11	70	40	2	6	14	710
Sausage, Egg & Cheese on a Plain Bagel									
1 Sandwich	620	26	11	115	67	4	7	27	1480
Sliced Turkey Breafast Sandwich									
1 Sandwich	310	9	3.5	90	33	3	3	23	980
Sweet Black Pepper Bacon Sandwich									
1 Sandwich	560	34	14	90	43	2	8	22	1030
Turkey Sausage Flatbread Sandwich									
1 Sandwich	410	20	7	155	35	3	2	24	1000

Coffee

Food Serving size	Cal.	(g) Total Fat	(g) Sat. Fat	(mg) Chol.	(g) Carb.	(g) Fiber	(g) Sug.	(g) Prot.	(mg) Sod.
Blueberry Coffee Small									
10 fl oz	15	0	0	0	2	0	0	0	5
Caramel Coffee Small									
10 fl oz	10	0	0	0	2	0	0	0	5
Caramel Coffee with Cream Large									
20 fl oz	340	12	7	45	53	0	49	6	120
Caramel Coffee with Cream Medium									
14 fl oz	250	9	5	30	40	0	37	4	90
Caramel Coffee with Cream Small									
10 fl oz	170	6	3.5	20	27	0	24	3	60
Caramel Mocha Coffee Large									
20 fl oz	230	0	0	0	53	1	48	3	40

Food Serving size	Cal.	(g) Total Fat	(g) Sat. Fat	(mg) Chol.	(g) Carb.	(g) Fiber	(g) Sug.	(g) Prot.	(mg) Sod.
Caramel Mocha Coffee Medium									
14 fl oz	170	0	0	0	39	1	36	2	30
Caramel Mocha Coffee Small									
10 fl oz	110	0	0	0	26	1	24	2	20
Caramel Mocha Coffee with Cream Large									
20 fl oz	340	12	7	40	55	1	48	5	65
Caramel Mocha Coffee with Cream Medium									
14 fl oz	260	9	6	30	41	1	36	3	50
Caramel Mocha Coffee with Cream Small									
10 fl oz	170	6	3.5	20	27	1	24	2	30
Coconut Coffee Small									
10 fl oz	10	0	0	0	1	0	0	0	5
Coffee Extra Large									
24 fl oz	15	0	0	0	2	0	0	1	15
Coffee Large									
20 fl oz	10	0	0	0	2	0	0	1	15
Coffee Medium									
14 fl oz	10	0	0	0	1	0	0	1	10
Coffee Small									
10 fl oz	5	0	0	0	1	0	0	0	5
Coffee with Cream Large									
20 fl oz	120	11	7	40	4	0	0	2	35
Coffee with Cream Medium									
14 fl oz	90	9	5	30	3	0	0	2	25
Coffee with Cream Small									
10 fl oz	60	6	4	20	2	0	0	1	20
Coffee with Cream XLarge									
24 fl oz	160	14	9	50	5	0	0	3	45
Coffee with Cream and Sugar Large									
20 fl oz	260	11	7	40	39	0	35	2	35
Coffee with Cream and Sugar Medium									
14 fl oz	190	9	5	30	29	0	26	2	25
Coffee with Skim Milk and Sugar Medium									
14 fl oz	120	0	0	0	30	0	28	2	30

Food Serving size	Cal.	(g) Total Fat	(g) Sat. Fat	(mg) Chol.	(g) Carb.	(g) Fiber	(g) Sug.	(g) Prot.	(mg) Sod.
Coffee with Skim Milk and Sugar Small									
10 fl oz	70	0	0	0	20	0	19	2	25
Coffee with Skim Milk and Sugar XLarge									
24 fl oz	210	0	0	0	49	0	47	4	50
Coffee with Splenda Large									
20 fl oz	25	0	0	0	5	0	0	1	15
Coffee with Splenda Medium									
14 fl oz	15	0	0	0	3	0	0	1	10
Coffee with Splenda Small									
10 fl oz	15	0	0	0	3	0	0	0	5
Coffee with Sugar Large									
20 fl oz	150	0	0	0	37	0	35	1	15
Coffee with Sugar Medium									
14 fl oz	110	0	0	0	28	0	26	1	10
Coffee with Sugar Small									
10 fl oz	60	0	0	0	18	0	17	0	5
Coffee with Sugar XLarge									
24 fl oz	180	0	0	0	46	0	43	1	15
Coffee with Whole Milk Large									
20 fl oz	45	2	1	5	5	0	3	3	40
Coffee with Whole Milk Medium									
14 fl oz	35	1.5	1	5	3	0	2	2	30
Coffee with Whole Milk Small									
10 fl oz	25	1	1	5	2	0	1	1	20
Coffee with Whole Milk XLarge									
24 fl oz	60	2.5	1.5	10	6	0	4	3	45
Coffee with Whole Milk and Sugar Large									
20 fl oz	200	2	1	5	44	0	42	3	40
Coffee with Whole Milk and Sugar Medium									
14 fl oz	140	1.5	1	5	30	0	28	2	30
Coffee with Whole Milk and Sugar Small									
10 fl oz	80	1	1	5	20	0	19	1	20
Coffee with Whole Milk and Sugar XLarge									
24 fl oz	230	2.5	1.5	10	49	0	47	3	45

Food Serving size	Cal.	(g) Total Fat	(g) Sat. Fat	(mg) Chol.	(g) Carb.	(g) Fiber	(g) Sug.	(g) Prot.	(mg) Sod.
French Vanilla Coffee Small									
10 fl oz	10	0	0	0	1	0	0	0	5
French Vanilla Swirl Hot Coffee Large									
20 fl oz	230	0	0	5	53	0	49	3	75
French Vanilla Swirl Hot Coffee with Cream Large									
20 fl oz	340	12	7	45	54	0	48	5	95
French Vanilla Swirl Hot Coffee with Cream Medium									
14 fl oz	260	9	5	35	41	0	36	4	70
French Vanilla Swirl Hot Coffee with Cream Small									
10 fl oz	170	6	3.5	20	27	0	24	2	45
Hazelnut Coffee Large									
20 fl oz	25	0	0	0	2	0	0	1	15
Hazelnut Coffee Medium									
14 fl oz	15	0	0	0	1	0	0	1	10
Hazelnut Coffee Small									
10 fl oz	10	0	0	0	1	0	0	0	5
Hazelnut Coffee XLarge									
24 fl oz	30	0	0	0	2	0	0	1	15
Hazelnut Swirl Hot Coffee Large									
20 fl oz	230	0	0	5	53	0	48	3	70
Hazelnut Swirl Hot Coffee Medium									
14 fl oz	170	0	0	5	39	0	36	2	50
Hazelnut Swirl Hot Coffee Small									
10 fl oz	110	0	0	0	26	0	24	2	35
Hazelnut Swirl Hot Coffee XLarge									
24 fl oz	280	0	0	5	66	0	60	4	90
Hazelnut Swirl Hot Coffee with Cream Large									
20 fl oz	340	12	7	45	55	0	48	5	95
Hazelnut Swirl Hot Coffee with Cream Medium									
14 fl oz	260	9	5	35	41	0	36	4	70
Hazelnut Swirl Hot Coffee with Cream Small									
10 fl oz	170	6	3.5	20	27	0	24	2	45
Hazelnut Swirl Hot Coffee with Cream XLarge									
24 fl oz	430	15	9	55	68	0	60	6	115

Food Serving size	Cal.	(g) Total Fat	(g) Sat. Fat	(mg) Chol.	(g) Carb.	(g) Fiber	(g) Sug.	(g) Prot.	(mg) Sod.
Hot Coffee with Almond Milk Large									
20 fl oz	45	1	0	0	8	0	6	1	75
Hot Coffee with Almond Milk Medium									
14 fl oz	30	0.5	0	0	6	0	4	1	50
Hot Coffee with Almond Milk Small									
10 fl oz	20	0	0	0	3	0	2	1	25
Hot Coffee with Almond Milk XLarge									
24 fl oz	60	1.5	0	0	11	1	8	1	95
Mocha Coffee Large									
20 fl oz	230	1	0	0	52	2	46	3	40
Mocha Coffee Medium									
14 fl oz	170	0.5	0	0	39	2	34	2	30
Mocha Coffee Small									
10 fl oz	110	0	0	0	26	1	23	1	20
Mocha Swirl Coffee Extra Large									
24 fl oz	280	1	0.5	0	65	3	57	3	50
Peppermint Mocha Hot Coffee Small									
10 fl oz	120	0	0	0	30	1	26	1	35
Peppermint Mocha Hot Coffee XLarge									
24 fl oz	310	1	0.5	0	75	3	65	3	85
Peppermint Mocha Hot Coffee with Cream Large									
20 fl oz	360	12	8	40	62	2	52	4	90
Peppermint Mocha Hot Coffee with Cream Medium									
14 fl oz	270	9	6	30	46	2	39	3	65
Peppermint Mocha Hot Coffee with Cream Small									
10 fl oz	180	6	4	20	31	1	26	2	45
Peppermint Mocha Hot Coffee with Cream XLarge									
24 fl oz	450	16	10	50	77	3	66	5	110
Pumpkin Swirl Hot Coffee Large									
20 fl oz	220	0	0	0	50	0	48	4	125
Pumpkin Swirl Hot Coffee Medium									
14 fl oz	170	0	0	0	38	0	36	3	95
Pumpkin Swirl Hot Coffee Small									
10 fl oz	110	0	0	0	25	0	24	2	65

Food Serving size	Cal.	(g) Total Fat	(g) Sat. Fat	(mg) Chol.	(g) Carb.	(g) Fiber	(g) Sug.	(g) Prot.	(mg) Sod.
Pumpkin Swirl Hot Coffee XLarge									
24 fl oz	280	0	0	0	63	0	60	5	150
Pumpkin Swirl Hot Coffee with Cream Large									
20 fl oz	340	12	7	40	53	0	48	5	150
Pumpkin Swirl Hot Coffee with Cream Medium									
14 fl oz	250	9	6	30	39	0	36	4	110
Pumpkin Swirl Hot Coffee with Cream Small									
10 fl oz	170	6	3.5	20	26	0	24	3	75
Pumpkin Swirl Hot Coffee with Cream XLarge									
24 fl oz	420	15	9	50	65	0	60	7	180
Raspberry Coffee Small									
10 fl oz	15	0	0	0	2	0	0	0	5
Snickerdoodle Hot Coffee Large									
20 fl oz	230	0	0	5	53	0	49	3	75
Snickerdoodle Hot Coffee Medium									
14 fl oz	170	0	0	5	'39	0	37	3	55
Snickerdoodle Hot Coffee Small									
10 fl oz	110	0	0	0	26	0	25	2	35
Snickerdoodle Hot Coffee XLarge									
24 fl oz	280	0	0	5	66	0	62	4	90
Snickerdoodle Hot Coffee with Cream Large									
20 fl oz	340	12	7	45	55	0	50	5	95
Snickerdoodle Hot Coffee with Cream Medium									
14 fl oz	260	9	5	35	41	0	37	4	70
Snickerdoodle Hot Coffee with Cream Small									
10 fl oz	170	6	3.5	20	27	0	25	2	50
Snickerdoodle Hot Coffee with Cream XLarge									
24 fl oz	430	15	9	55	68	0	62	6	120
Sugar Cookie Hot Coffee Large									
20 fl oz	230	0	0	5	53	0	50	3	75
Sugar Cookie Hot Coffee Medium									
14 fl oz	170	0	0	5	40	0	37	3	55
Sugar Cookie Hot Coffee Small									
10 fl oz	110	0	0	0	27	0	25	2	35

Food Serving size	Cal.	(g) Total Fat	(g) Sat. Fat	(mg) Chol.	(g) Carb.	(g) Fiber	(g) Sug.	(g) Prot.	(mg) Sod.
Sugar Cookie Hot Coffee XLarge									
24 fl oz	290	0	0	5	66	0	62	4	90
Sugar Cookie Hot Coffee with Cream Large									
20 fl oz	350	12	7	45	55	0	50	5	95
Sugar Cookie Hot Coffee with Cream Medium									
14 fl oz	260	9	5	35	41	0	37	4	70
Sugar Cookie Hot Coffee with Cream Small									
10 fl oz	170	6	3.5	20	28	0	25	2	50
Sugar Cookie Hot Coffee with Cream XLarge									
24 fl oz	430	15	9	55	68	0	62	6	120
Toasted Almond Coffee Small									
10 fl oz	10	0	0	0	1	0	0	0	5

Cookies

Chocolate Chip Cookie									
1 Cookie	170	6	3	20	29	1	17	3	190
Oatmeal Raisin Cookie									
1 Cookie	160	5	2.5	15	28	1	19	2	95

Coolatta

Frozen Arnold Palmer Coolatta Large									
32 fl oz	360	0	0	0	95	0	90	0	45
Frozen Arnold Palmer Coolatta Small									
16 fl oz	180	0	0	0	47	0	45	0	20
Frozen Coffee Coolatta Lite Large - 75% fewer calories than our Large Frozen Coffee Coolatta made with Cream									
32 fl oz	170	6	3.5	20	30	0	22	6	100
Frozen Coffee Coolatta Lite Medium - 75% fewer calories than our Medium Frozen Coffee Coolatta made with Cream									
24 fl oz	130	4.5	2.5	15	23	0	17	4	75
Frozen Coffee Coolatta Lite Small - 75% fewer calories than our Small Frozen Coffee Coolatta made with Cream									
16 fl oz	80	3	1.5	10	15	0	11	3	50
Mango Passion Fruit Coolatta Large									
32 fl oz	490	0	0	0	126	0	121	0	55

Food Serving size	Cal.	(g) Total Fat	(g) Sat. Fat	(mg) Chol.	(g) Carb.	(g) Fiber	(g) Sug.	(g) Prot.	(mg) Sod.
Mango Passion Fruit Coolatta Lite Large - 60% fewer calories than our Regular Large Mango Passion Fruit Coolatta									
32 fl oz	170	0	0	0	47	0	36	0	45
Mango Passion Fruit Coolatta Small									
16 fl oz	250	0	0	0	63	0	61	0	30
Minute Maid® Orange Coolatta® Large									
32 fl oz	430	0	0	0	109	0	105	1	35
Minute Maid® Orange Coolatta® Medium									
24 fl oz	330	0	0	0	81	0	79	1	25
Minute Maid® Orange Coolatta® Small									
16 fl oz	220	0	0	0	54	0	52	1	20
Pumpkin Pie Coolatta Large									
32 fl oz	560	13	8	45	104	1	88	10	630
Pumpkin Pie Coolatta Medium									
24 fl oz	420	10	6	35	78	1	66	7	470
Pumpkin Pie Coolatta Small									
16 fl oz	280	7	4	20	52	1	44	5	310
Strawberry Coolatta Lite Large - 55% fewer calories than our Regular Large Strawberry Coolatta									
32 fl oz	190	0	0	0	48	0	41	0	60
Strawberry Coolatta Lite Medium - 55% fewer calories than our Regular Medium Strawberry Coolatta									
24 fl oz	140	0	0	0	36	0	31	0	45
Strawberry Coolatta Lite Small - 55% fewer calories than our Regular Small Strawberry Coolatta									
16 fl oz	100	0	0	0	24	0	20	0	30
Strawberry Coolatta® Large									
32 fl oz	470	0	0	0	115	0	114	0	70
Strawberry Coolatta® Medium									
24 fl oz	350	0	0	0	86	0	85	0	55
Strawberry Coolatta® Small									
16 fl oz	230	0	0	0	57	0	57	0	35
Strawberry Fruit Coolatta® Large									
32 fl oz	490	0	0	0	117	0	117	0	60
Strawberry Fruit Coolatta® Medium									
24 fl oz	370	0	0	0	88	0	88	0	45

Food Serving size	Cal.	(g) Total Fat	(g) Sat. Fat	(mg) Chol.	(g) Carb.	(g) Fiber	(g) Sug.	(g) Prot.	(mg) Sod.
Strawberry Fruit Coolatta® Small									
16 fl oz	250	0	0	0	58	0	58	0	30
Vanilla Bean Coolatta Lite Large - 37% fewer calories than our Regular Large Vanilla Bean Coolatta									
32 fl oz	490	0	0	5	119	0	104	10	330
Vanilla Bean Coolatta Lite Medium - 37% fewer calories than our Regular Medium Vanilla Bean Coolatta									
24 fl oz	370	0	0	5	89	0	78	8	250
Vanilla Bean Coolatta Lite Small - 37% fewer calories than our Regular Small Vanilla Bean Coolatta									
16 fl oz	250	0	0	5	59	0	52	5	170
Vanilla Bean Coolatta® Large									
32 fl oz	850	12	7	45	184	0	174	6	300
Vanilla Bean Coolatta® Medium									
24 fl oz	630	9	5	30	138	0	130	4	220
Vanilla Bean Coolatta® Small									
16 fl oz	420	6	3.5	20	92	0	87	3	150

Cream Cheese

Food Serving size	Cal.	Total Fat	Sat. Fat	Chol.	Carb.	Fiber	Sug.	Prot.	Sod.
Plain Cream Cheese Spread									
1 Unit (50g)	150	15	9	40	3	0	3	3	250
Reduced Fat Plain Cream Cheese Spread - 50% Less Fat than Regular Cream Cheese									
1 Unit (50g)	100	8	5	25	5	0	2	4	250
Reduced Fat Strawberry Cream Cheese Spread - 25% Less Fat than Cream Cheese Spread									
1 Unit (50g)	150	10	6	30	15	0	11	2	200
Reduced Fat Veggie Cream Cheese Spread - 25% Less Fat than Cream Cheese Spread									
1 Unit (50g)	120	10	6	30	6	0	2	2	240

Danish

Food Serving size	Cal.	Total Fat	Sat. Fat	Chol.	Carb.	Fiber	Sug.	Prot.	Sod.
Apple Cheese Danish									
1 Danish	400	19	8	5	53	1	29	5	310
Cheese Danish									
1 Danish	420	21	9	10	52	1	27	5	320

Food Serving size	Cal.	(g) Total Fat	(g) Sat. Fat	(mg) Chol.	(g) Carb.	(g) Fiber	(g) Sug.	(g) Prot.	(mg) Sod.
Strawberry Cheese Danish									
1 Danish	400	19	8	0	52	1	26	5	310

Donuts

Apple Croissant Donut									
1 Croissant Donut	350	16	10	25	47	1	22	5	280
Apple Crumb Donut									
1 Donut	320	15	7	0	42	1	21	3	350
Apple Stick									
1 Stick	420	25	12	30	44	1	20	4	390
Apple Streusel Donut									
1 Donut	340	16	7	0	45	1	23	3	350
Apple n Spice Donut									
1 Donut	260	14	6	0	29	1	9	3	340
Bavarian Creme Donut									
1 Donut	270	15	7	0	31	1	9	4	350
Bismark									
1 Bismark	490	25	10	0	62	1	37	5	350
Blueberry Butternut Donut									
1 Donut	420	17	8	30	60	1	35	4	380
Blueberry Crumb Cake Donut									
1 Donut	380	18	8	30	50	1	27	4	390
Blueberry Crumb Donut									
1 Donut	410	16	8	0	64	1	40	4	340
Boston Kreme Croissant Donut									
1 Croissant Donut	330	16	10	25	43	1	18	5	280
Boston Kreme Donut									
1 Donut	300	16	7	0	37	1	17	3	360
Boston Kreme Drizzle Donut									
1 Donut	310	16	7	0	40	1	19	3	360
Boston Kreme Sprinkles Donut									
1 Donut	320	16	7	0	40	1	18	3	360
Boston Scream Donut									
1 Donut	310	16	7	0	40	1	19	3	360
Bowtie Donut									
1 Donut	270	12	4.5	0	38	1	16	4	270

Food Serving size	Cal.	(g) Total Fat	(g) Sat. Fat	(mg) Chol.	(g) Carb.	(g) Fiber	(g) Sug.	(g) Prot.	(mg) Sod.
Butternut Donut									
1 Donut	410	20	9	25	55	1	33	4	330
Buzzer Beater Donut									
1 Donut	310	15	7	0	41	1	19	3	360
Caramel Cheesecake Square Donut									
1 Donut	360	19	10	10	43	1	20	5	360
Cheesecake Square									
1 Donut	350	17	7	10	45	1	22	5	390
Chocolate Butternut Donut									
1 Donut	410	20	10	0	54	2	31	4	430
Chocolate Coconut Donut									
1 Donut	400	23	12	0	45	2	22	4	420
Chocolate Creme Donut									
1 Donut	320	19	8	0	35	1	14	4	360
Chocolate Crumb Cake Donut									
1 Donut	380	22	9	0	43	2	22	4	490
Chocolate Dipped French Cruller									
1 Donut	310	19	9	50	33	0	20	3	160
Chocolate Dulce de Leche Donut									
1 Donut	340	17	7	0	42	1	20	4	370
Chocolate Frosted Cake Donut									
1 Donut	350	19	9	25	40	1	20	4	340
Chocolate Frosted Coffee Roll									
1 Coffee Roll	400	19	8	0	51	2	18	7	430
Chocolate Frosted Donut									
1 Donut	280	15	7	0	31	1	13	3	340
Chocolate Frosted Donut with Sprinkles									
1 Donut	290	16	7	0	34	1	14	3	340
Chocolate Headlight Donut									
1 Donut	330	18	8	0	39	1	18	4	360
Chocolate Iced Bismark									
1 Bismark	390	19	8	0	52	2	21	5	360
Chocolate Long John									
1 Long John	340	17	7	0	42	2	16	5	320

Food Serving size	Cal.	(g) Total Fat	(g) Sat. Fat	(mg) Chol.	(g) Carb.	(g) Fiber	(g) Sug.	(g) Prot.	(mg) Sod.
Chocolate Peanut Butter Flavored Crème Donut									
1 Donut	360	19	8	0	44	1	24	3	360
Cinnamon Donut									
1 Donut	310	19	9	25	32	1	13	4	320
Cinnamon Guava Donut									
1 Donut	250	14	6	0	28	1	8	3	340
Cinnamon Stick									
1 Stick	380	25	12	30	35	1	13	4	370
Coconut Donut									
1 Donut	400	22	12	25	46	2	25	4	330
Coconut Drizzle Dulce de Leche Donut									
1 Donut	300	17	8	0	33	1	11	4	360
Coconut Guava Donut									
1 Donut	310	16	8	0	39	1	17	3	350
Coffee Roll									
1 Coffee Roll	390	18	7	0	51	2	17	7	410
Crumb Cake Donut									
1 Donut	380	20	9	25	46	1	25	4	330
Double Chocolate Donut									
1 Donut	350	20	9	0	39	2	18	4	440
Eclair									
1 Eclair	380	18	7	0	50	2	22	5	350
Fall Harvest Donut									
1 Donut	290	16	7	0	35	1	15	3	340
Football Donut									
1 Donut	310	16	7	0	39	1	19	3	360
French Apple Donut									
1 Donut	300	15	7	0	38	1	18	3	350
French Cruller									
1 Donut	260	18	9	50	21	0	10	2	140
Frosted Chocolate Creme Donut									
1 Donut	360	19	8	0	42	2	21	4	380
Frosted Maple Creme Donut									
1 Donut	360	19	8	0	44	1	25	3	360

Food Serving size	Cal.	(g) Total Fat	(g) Sat. Fat	(mg) Chol.	(g) Carb.	(g) Fiber	(g) Sug.	(g) Prot.	(mg) Sod.
Frosted Strawberry Dream Donut									
1 Donut	360	19	8	0	44	1	25	3	360
Frosted Vanilla Creme Donut									
1 Donut	360	20	9	0	43	1	24	3	370
Glazed Apple Maple Donut									
1 Donut	310	14	6	0	41	1	17	3	350
Glazed Bavarian Creme Donut									
1 Donut	290	15	7	0	37	1	15	3	350
Glazed Blueberry Donut									
1 Donut	340	16	7	30	43	1	21	4	380
Glazed Caramel Donut									
1 Donut	330	16	7	0	41	1	19	4	350
Glazed Chocolate Creme Donut									
1 Donut	360	19	8	0	44	1	22	4	370
Glazed Chocolate Donut									
1 Donut	340	19	9	0	38	1	17	3	420
Glazed Croissant Donut									
1 Croissant Donut	300	15	10	25	34	1	12	5	260
Glazed Donut									
1 Donut	260	14	6	0	31	1	12	3	330
Glazed Dulce de Leche Donut									
1 Donut	330	16	7	0	41	1	19	4	350
Glazed Guava Donut									
1 Donut	280	14	6	0	36	1	15	3	340
Glazed Jelly Donut									
1 Donut	310	14	6	0	43	1	14	3	340
Glazed Jelly Stick									
1 Stick	480	25	11	30	59	1	37	4	380
Glazed Lemon Donut									
1 Donut	300	15	7	0	39	1	17	3	350
Glazed Old Fashioned Donut									
1 Donut	340	19	8	25	39	1	19	4	320
Glazed Stick									
1 Stick	410	25	11	30	43	1	21	4	370

Food Serving size	Cal.	(g) Total Fat	(g) Sat. Fat	(mg) Chol.	(g) Carb.	(g) Fiber	(g) Sug.	(g) Prot.	(mg) Sod.
Glazed Strawberry Donut									
1 Donut	320	14	6	0	45	1	21	3	350
Glazed Vanilla Creme Donut									
1 Donut	370	19	8	0	44	1	25	3	360
Great White Donut									
1 Donut	330	20	8	0	35	1	17	3	350
Guava Burst Donut									
1 Donut	260	15	7	0	29	1	9	3	340
Guayaba Burst Donut									
1 Donut	300	15	7	0	38	1	15	4	330
Halloween Pumpkin Donut									
1 Donut	360	18	7	0	46	1	26	4	320
Jelly Donut									
1 Donut	270	14	6	0	32	1	15	3	330
Jelly Stick									
1 Stick	440	25	11	30	50	1	29	4	380
Lemon Donut									
1 Donut	260	15	7	0	29	1	10	3	350
Lemon Stick									
1 Stick	430	26	12	30	44	1	21	4	400
Maple Apple Croissant Donut									
1 Croissant Donut	350	16	11	25	45	1	19	5	290
Maple Creme Donut									
1 Donut	330	19	8	0	36	1	17	3	350
Maple Creme Drizzle Donut									
1 Donut	370	19	8	0	47	1	28	3	360
Maple Crumb Cake Donut									
1 Donut	380	20	9	25	45	1	25	4	330
Maple Frosted Coffee Roll									
1 Coffee Roll	400	19	8	0	52	2	19	7	430
Maple Frosted Donut									
1 Donut	270	15	7	0	32	1	14	3	340
Maple Frosted Sprinkles Donut									
1 Donut	290	16	7	0	34	1	15	3	340

Food Serving size	Cal.	(g) Total Fat	(g) Sat. Fat	(mg) Chol.	(g) Carb.	(g) Fiber	(g) Sug.	(g) Prot.	(mg) Sod.
Maple Vanilla Creme Donut									
1 Donut	360	20	8	0	43	1	24	3	360
Marble Frosted Donut									
1 Donut	270	15	7	0	32	1	13	3	340
Old Fashioned Cake Donut									
1 Donut	320	22	10	25	33	1	9	3	300
PEEPS Donut									
1 Donut	310	15	7	0	39	1	20	4	350
Peanut Butter Flavored Creme Donut									
1 Donut	320	19	8	0	36	1	18	3	350
Peanut Butter Flavored Creme and Jelly Donut									
1 Donut	360	19	8	0	44	1	26	3	360
Peanut Donut									
1 Donut	450	26	10	25	48	2	25	7	330
Philly Creme Donut									
1 Donut	360	19	8	0	43	1	22	4	370
Pittsburgh Donut									
1 Donut	430	24	10	0	50	1	31	3	390
Plain Stick Donut									
1 Stick	370	25	11	30	31	1	10	4	370
Play Ball Donut									
1 Donut	340	15	7	0	48	1	20	3	360
Powdered Donut									
1 Donut	320	19	9	25	33	1	14	4	320
Powdered Stick									
1 Stick	390	25	12	30	37	1	15	4	370
Pumpkin Cheesecake Square Donut									
1 Donut	340	15	6	0	48	1	25	4	360
Pumpkin Crumb Cake Donut									
1 Donut	450	23	10	15	56	1	35	4	390
Pumpkin Donut									
1 Donut	360	21	10	15	39	1	20	3	380
Reeses Peanut Butter Square Donut									
1 Donut	370	19	7	0	47	1	26	5	400

Food Serving size	Cal.	(g) Total Fat	(g) Sat. Fat	(mg) Chol.	(g) Carb.	(g) Fiber	(g) Sug.	(g) Prot.	(mg) Sod.
Snickerdoodle Croissant Donut									
1 Croissant Donut	410	19	12	25	54	1	29	5	320
Sour Cream Donut									
1 Donut	350	17	7	10	47	1	26	4	330
Spiced Chocolate Dulce de Leche Donut									
1 Donut	340	17	7	0	42	1	20	4	370
Spiced Dulce de Leche Donut									
1 Donut	290	16	7	0	33	1	11	4	350
Strawberry Donut									
1 Donut	280	15	7	0	34	1	14	3	330
Strawberry Dream Donut									
1 Donut	330	19	8	0	36	1	17	3	350
Strawberry Dream Swirl Donut									
1 Donut	370	19	8	0	47	1	28	3	360
Strawberry Frosted Donut									
1 Donut	280	15	7	0	32	1	14	3	340
Strawberry Frosted Sprinkles Donut									
1 Donut	290	16	7	0	35	1	15	3	340
Strawberry Long John									
1 Long John	340	17	7	0	43	1	18	5	310
Strawberry Shortcake Donut									
1 Donut	320	19	8	0	35	1	16	3	350
Sugared Cake Donut									
1 Donut	310	19	8	25	31	1	13	4	320
Sugared Raised Donut									
1 Donut	230	14	6	0	22	1	4	3	330
Sugared Stick									
1 Stick	380	25	11	30	34	1	14	4	370
Taillight Donut									
1 Donut	340	19	8	0	39	1	20	3	360
Toasted Coconut Donut									
1 Donut	420	24	13	25	47	2	27	4	330
Vanilla Berry Shortcake Donut									
1 Donut	350	19	8	0	43	1	24	3	360

Food Serving size	Cal.	(g) Total Fat	(g) Sat. Fat	(mg) Chol.	(g) Carb.	(g) Fiber	(g) Sug.	(g) Prot.	(mg) Sod.
Vanilla Frosted Coffee Roll									
1 Coffee Roll	400	19	8	0	52	2	19	7	430
Vanilla Frosted Donut									
1 Donut	280	15	7	0	32	1	14	3	340
Vanilla Frosted Sprinkles Donut									
1 Donut	290	16	7	0	35	1	15	3	340
Vanilla Headlight Donut									
1 Donut	340	19	8	0	39	1	20	3	360
Vanilla Long John									
1 Long John	340	17	7	0	43	1	18	5	310
Vanilla Peanut Butter Flavored Creme Donut									
1 Donut	360	19	8	0	44	1	26	3	360

Espresso Beverages

Food Serving size	Cal.	(g) Total Fat	(g) Sat. Fat	(mg) Chol.	(g) Carb.	(g) Fiber	(g) Sug.	(g) Prot.	(mg) Sod.
Caramel Latte Lite Large									
20 fl oz	160	0	0	5	25	0	20	12	170
Caramel Mocha Latte with Milk Small									
10 fl oz	220	6	4	25	35	1	33	7	115
Caramel Mocha Latte with Skim Milk Large									
20 fl oz	350	1	0.5	10	70	1	68	15	200
Caramel Mocha Latte with Skim Milk Medium									
16 fl oz	260	0.5	0	5	53	1	51	11	150
Caramel Mocha Latte with Skim Milk Small									
10 fl oz	170	0	0	5	35	1	34	7	100
Espresso									
1.75 fl oz	5	0	0	0	1	0	0	0	5
Espresso with Sugar									
1.75 fl oz	30	0	0	0	7	0	7	0	5
French Vanilla Swirl Hot Latte with Skim Milk Large									
20 fl oz	350	0	0	10	71	0	69	15	230
French Vanilla Swirl Hot Latte with Skim Milk Medium									
16 fl oz	270	0	0	10	54	0	52	11	170
French Vanilla Swirl Hot Latte with Skim Milk Small									
10 fl oz	180	0	0	5	36	0	35	8	115

Food Serving size	Cal.	(g) Total Fat	(g) Sat. Fat	(mg) Chol.	(g) Carb.	(g) Fiber	(g) Sug.	(g) Prot.	(mg) Sod.
French Vanilla Swirl Iced Latte with Skim Milk Medium									
24 fl oz	270	0	0	10	54	0	52	11	180
Hazelnut Swirl Iced Latte with Skim Milk Medium									
24 fl oz	270	0	0	10	54	0	52	11	180
Hazelnut Swirl Iced Latte with Skim Milk Small									
16 fl oz	180	0	0	5	37	0	35	8	120
Hazelnut Swirl Iced Latte with Whole Milk Large									
32 fl oz	450	12	7	40	71	0	68	14	250
Hazelnut Swirl Iced Latte with Whole Milk Medium									
24 fl oz	340	9	5	30	54	0	52	11	180
Hazelnut Swirl Iced Latte with Whole Milk Small									
16 fl oz	230	6	3.5	20	36	0	35	7	125
Hot Latte with Almond Milk Large									
20 fl oz	160	4.5	0	0	28	2	26	2	260
Hot Latte with Almond Milk Medium									
16 fl oz	120	3	0	0	21	1	20	1	190
Hot Latte with Almond Milk Small									
10 floz	80	2	0	0	14	1	13	1	130
Iced Caramel Latte Lite Large									
32 fl oz	160	0	0	5	26	0	20	12	190
Iced Caramel Latte Lite Medium									
24 fl oz	120	0	0	5	19	0	15	9	140
Iced Caramel Latte Lite Small									
16 floz	80	0	0	5	13	0	10	6	95
Iced Caramel Latte with Milk Large									
32 fl oz	460	12	7	40	73	0	72	14	220
Iced Caramel Latte with Milk Medium									
24 fl oz	350	9	5	30	55	0	54	11	160
Iced Caramel Latte with Milk Small									
16 fl oz	230	6	3.5	20	37	0	37	7	110
Iced Caramel Latte with Skim Milk Large									
32 fl oz	360	0	0	10	73	0	72	15	210
Iced Caramel Latte with Skim Milk Medium									
24 fl oz	270	0	0	10	55	0	55	11	160

Food Serving size	Cal.	(g) Total Fat	(g) Sat. Fat	(mg) Chol.	(g) Carb.	(g) Fiber	(g) Sug.	(g) Prot.	(mg) Sod.
Iced Caramel Latte with Skim Milk Small									
16 fl oz	190	0	0	5	38	0	37	8	110
Iced Caramel Mocha Latte with Milk Large									
32 fl oz	450	12	8	55	70	1	67	14	240
Iced Caramel Mocha Latte with Milk Medium									
24 fl oz	330	9	6	40	52	1	50	11	180
Iced Caramel Mocha Latte with Milk Small									
16 fl oz	220	6	4	25	35	1	33	7	120
Iced Latte with Almond Milk Large									
32 fl oz	160	4.5	0	0	28	2	26	2	280
Iced Latte with Almond Milk Medium									
24 fl oz	120	3	0	0	21	1	20	1	210
Iced Latte with Almond Milk Small									
16 fl oz	80	2	0	0	14	1	13	1	140
Iced Latte with Skim Milk Large									
32 fl oz	140	0	0	10	20	0	20	13	190
Iced Latte with Sugar Large									
32 fl oz	370	12	7	35	54	0	54	12	190
Iced Latte with Sugar Medium									
24 fl oz	280	9	5	25	40	0	40	9	140
Latte with Sugar Large									
20 fl oz	370	12	7	35	54	0	54	12	170
Latte with Sugar Medium									
16 fl oz	280	9	5	25	40	0	40	9	130
Latte with Sugar Small									
10 fl oz	170	6	3.5	25	27	0	27	6	100
Mocha Iced Latte with Skim Milk Large									
32 fl oz	360	1.5	1	5	73	2	67	14	210
Mocha Iced Latte with Skim Milk Medium									
24 fl oz	270	1	0.5	5	55	2	51	11	160
Mocha Iced Latte with Skim Milk Small									
16 fl oz	180	0.5	0	5	37	1	35	7	105
Mocha Latte Large with Milk									
20 fl oz	460	13	7	35	72	2	67	13	200

Food Serving size	Cal.	(g) Total Fat	(g) Sat. Fat	(mg) Chol.	(g) Carb.	(g) Fiber	(g) Sug.	(g) Prot.	(mg) Sod.
Mocha Latte Medium with Milk									
16 fl oz	350	10	6	25	54	2	51	10	150
Mocha Latte Medium with Milk									
16 fl oz	350	10	6	25	54	2	51	10	150
Mocha Latte Small									
10 fl oz	220	6	4	25	35	1	32	7	115
Mocha Latte Small with Milk									
10 fl oz	230	6	3.5	20	37	1	34	7	100
Mocha Latte Small with Milk									
10 fl oz	230	6	3.5	20	37	1	34	7	100
Mocha Latte with Skim Milk Large									
20 fl oz	360	1.5	1	5	73	2	67	14	200
Mocha Latte with Skim Milk Large									
20 fl oz	360	1.5	1	5	73	2	67	14	200
Mocha Latte with Skim Milk									
16 fl oz	270	1	0.5	5	55	2	51	11	150
Mocha Latte with Skim Milk									
16 fl oz	270	1	0.5	5	55	2	51	11	150
Mocha Latte with Skim Milk Small									
10 fl oz	180	0.5	0	5	37	1	35	7	100
Mocha Latte with Skim Milk Small									
10 fl oz	180	0.5	0	5	37	1	35	7	100
Peppermint Mocha Hot Latte with Whole Milk Small									
10 fl oz	240	6	3.5	20	41	1	38	7	115
Peppermint Mocha Iced Latte with Skim Milk Large									
32 fl oz	380	1.5	1	5	80	2	74	14	240
Peppermint Mocha Iced Latte with Skim Milk Medium									
24 fl oz	290	1	0.5	5	60	2	56	10	180
Peppermint Mocha Iced Latte with Skim Milk Small									
16 fl oz	190	0.5	0	5	41	1	38	7	120
Peppermint Mocha Iced Latte with Whole Milk Large									
32 fl oz	480	13	7	35	79	2	73	13	240
Peppermint Mocha Iced Latte with Whole Milk Medium									
24 fl oz	360	10	6	25	60	2	55	10	190

Food Serving size	Cal.	(g) Total Fat	(g) Sat. Fat	(mg) Chol.	(g) Carb.	(g) Fiber	(g) Sug.	(g) Prot.	(mg) Sod.
Peppermint Mocha Iced Latte with Whole Milk Small									
16 fl oz	240	6	3.5	20	41	1	38	7	125
Pumpkin Swirl Hot Latte with Skim Milk Large									
20 fl oz	360	0.5	0	10	71	0	70	16	290
Pumpkin Swirl Hot Latte with Skim Milk Medium									
16 fl oz	270	0	0	5	54	0	53	12	220
Pumpkin Swirl Hot Latte with Skim Milk Small									
10 fl oz	180	0	0	5	37	0	36	8	140
Pumpkin Swirl Hot Latte with Whole Milk Large									
20 fl oz	450	12	7	40	70	0	69	15	290
Pumpkin Swirl Hot Latte with Whole Milk Medium									
16 fl oz	340	9	5	30	53	0	52	11	210
Pumpkin Swirl Hot Latte with Whole Milk Small									
10 fl oz	230	6	3.5	20	36	0	36	7	140
Pumpkin Swirl Iced Latte with Skim Milk Large									
32 fl oz	360	0.5	0	10	71	0	70	16	300
Pumpkin Swirl Iced Latte with Skim Milk Medium									
24 fl oz	270	0	0	5	54	0	53	12	230
Pumpkin Swirl Iced Latte with Skim Milk Small									
16 fl oz	180	0	0	5	37	0	36	8	150
Pumpkin Swirl Iced Latte with Whole Milk Medium									
24 fl oz	340	9	5	30	53	0	52	11	230
Pumpkin Swirl Iced Latte with Whole Milk Small									
16 fl oz	230	6	3.5	20	36	0	36	8	150
Snickerdoodle Hot Latte with Skim Milk Large									
20 fl oz	360	0	0	10	73	0	70	15	230
Snickerdoodle Hot Latte with Whole Milk Medium									
16 fl oz	350	9	5	30	54	0	52	11	170
Snickerdoodle Hot Latte with Whole Milk Small									
10 fl oz	230	6	3.5	20	37	0	36	7	115
Snickerdoodle Iced Latte with Skim Milk Large									
32 fl oz	360	0	0	10	73	0	70	15	240
Snickerdoodle Iced Latte with Skim Milk Medium									
24 fl oz	270	0	0	10	55	0	53	11	180

Food Serving size	Cal.	(g) Total Fat	(g) Sat. Fat	(mg) Chol.	(g) Carb.	(g) Fiber	(g) Sug.	(g) Prot.	(mg) Sod.
Snickerdoodle Iced Latte with Skim Milk Small									
16 fl oz	180	0	0	5	37	0	36	8	125
Snickerdoodle Iced Latte with Whole Milk Medium									
24 fl oz	350	9	5	30	54	0	52	11	180
Snickerdoodle Iced Latte with Whole Milk Small									
16 fl oz	230	6	3.5	20	37	0	36	7	125
Sugar Cookie Hot Latte with Skim Milk Large									
20 fl oz	360	0	0	10	73	0	70	15	230
Sugar Cookie Hot Latte with Skim Milk Medium									
16 fl oz	270	0	0	10	55	0	53	11	170
Sugar Cookie Hot Latte with Skim Milk Small									
10 fl oz	190	0	0	5	38	0	36	8	115
Sugar Cookie Iced Latte with Skim Milk Medium									
24 fl oz	270	0	0	10	55	0	53	11	180
Sugar Cookie Iced Latte with Skim Milk Small									
16 fl oz	190	0	0	5	38	0	36	8	125
Sugar Cookie Iced Latte with Whole Milk Large									
32 fl oz	460	12	7	40	73	0	69	14	250
Sugar Cookie Iced Latte with Whole Milk Medium									
24 fl oz	350	9	5	30	55	0	53	11	180
Sugar Cookie Iced Latte with Whole Milk Small									
16 fl oz	230	6	3.5	20	37	0	36	7	125
Vanilla Latte Lite Large									
20 fl oz	160	0	0	10	26	0	20	13	180
Vanilla Latte Lite Medium									
16 fl oz	120	0	0	5	20	0	15	10	130
Vanilla Latte Lite Small									
10 fl oz	80	0	0	5	13	0	10	6	90

Coolatta

Food Serving size	Cal.	(g) Total Fat	(g) Sat. Fat	(mg) Chol.	(g) Carb.	(g) Fiber	(g) Sug.	(g) Prot.	(mg) Sod.
Frozen Caramel Coffee Coolatta with Cream Large									
32 fl oz	990	47	29	165	141	0	130	9	180
Frozen Caramel Coffee Coolatta with Cream Medium									
24 fl oz	740	35	22	125	106	0	97	7	130

Food Serving size	Cal.	(g) Total Fat	(g) Sat. Fat	(mg) Chol.	(g) Carb.	(g) Fiber	(g) Sug.	(g) Prot.	(mg) Sod.
Frozen Caramel Coffee Coolatta with Cream Small									
16 fl oz	490	23	15	80	71	0	65	5	90
Frozen Caramel Coffee Coolatta with Milk Large									
32 fl oz	670	8	4.5	30	144	0	141	10	180
Frozen Caramel Coffee Coolatta with Skim Milk Small									
16 fl oz	300	0	0	5	72	0	71	5	90
Frozen Coffee Coolatta with Skim Milk Small									
16 fl oz	210	0	0	0	50	0	49	4	80
Frozen French Vanilla Swirl Coffee Coolatta with Cream Large									
32 fl oz	990	46	29	165	141	0	128	9	200
Frozen French Vanilla Swirl Coffee Coolatta with Cream Medium									
24 fl oz	740	35	22	120	106	0	96	7	150
Frozen French Vanilla Swirl Coffee Coolatta with Cream Small									
16 fl oz	490	23	14	80	70	0	64	5	100
Frozen Hazelnut Swirl Coffee Coolatta with Skim Milk Medium									
24 fl oz	450	0	0	5	108	0	105	8	160
Frozen Hazelnut Swirl Coffee Coolatta with Skim Milk Small									
16 fl oz	300	0	0	5	72	0	70	5	105
Frozen Hazelnut Swirl Coffee Coolatta with Whole Milk Large									
32 fl oz	670	8	4.5	30	144	0	139	10	210
Frozen Hazelnut Swirl Coffee Coolatta with Whole Milk Medium									
24 fl oz	500	6	3.5	20	108	0	104	8	160
Frozen Hazelnut Swirl Coffee Coolatta with Whole Milk Small									
16 fl oz	330	4	2.5	15	72	0	70	5	105
Frozen Mocha Coffee Coolatta with Cream Large									
32 fl oz	990	47	29	160	141	2	125	8	170
Frozen Pumpkin Swirl Coffee Coolatta with Skim Milk Medium									
24 fl oz	450	0	0	5	107	0	105	9	200
Frozen Pumpkin Swirl Coffee Coolatta with Skim Milk Small									
16 fl oz	300	0	0	5	71	0	70	6	135
Frozen Pumpkin Swirl Coffee Coolatta with Whole Milk Large									
32 fl oz	670	8	4.5	25	142	0	139	11	270
Frozen Pumpkin Swirl Coffee Coolatta with Whole Milk Medium									
24 fl oz	500	6	3.5	20	107	0	104	8	200

Food Serving size	Cal.	(g) Total Fat	(g) Sat. Fat	(mg) Chol.	(g) Carb.	(g) Fiber	(g) Sug.	(g) Prot.	(mg) Sod.
Frozen Pumpkin Swirl Coffee Coolatta with Whole Milk Small									
16 fl oz	330	4	2.5	15	71	0	70	5	135
Frozen Snickerdoodle Coffee Coolatta with Skim Milk Medium									
24 fl oz	450	0	0	5	108	0	106	8	160
Frozen Snickerdoodle Coffee Coolatta with Skim Milk Small									
16 fl oz	300	0	0	5	72	0	71	5	105
Frozen Snickerdoodle Coffee Coolatta with Whole Milk Large									
32 fl oz	670	8	4.5	30	144	0	141	10	210
Frozen Snickerdoodle Coffee Coolatta with Whole Milk Medium									
24 fl oz	500	6	3.5	20	108	0	105	8	160
Frozen Snickerdoodle Coffee Coolatta with Whole Milk Small									
16 fl oz	330	4	2.5	15	72	0	70	5	105
Frozen Sugar Cookie Coffee Coolatta with Cream Large									
32 fl oz	990	47	29	165	142	0	129	9	210
Frozen Sugar Cookie Coffee Coolatta with Cream Medium									
24 fl oz	740	35	22	120	106	0	97	7	150
Frozen Sugar Cookie Coffee Coolatta with Cream Small									
16 fl oz	500	23	14	80	71	0	65	5	105
Frozen Sugar Cookie Coffee Coolatta with Skim Milk Large									
32 fl oz	610	0	0	10	145	0	141	11	210
Frozen Sugar Cookie Coffee Coolatta with Skim Milk Medium									
24 fl oz	450	0	0	5	109	0	106	8	160
Frozen Sugar Cookie Coffee Coolatta with Skim Milk Small									
16 fl oz	300	0	0	5	73	0	71	5	105
Frozen Sugar Cookie Coffee Coolatta with Whole Milk Large									
32 fl oz	670	8	5	30	141	0	141	10	210
Frozen Sugar Cookie Coffee Coolatta with Whole Milk Medium									
24 fl oz	500	6	4	20	108	0	106	8	160
Frozen Sugar Cookie Coffee Coolatta with Whole Milk Small									
16 fl oz	340	4	3	15	72	0	70	5	105

Hot Macciato

Food Serving size	Cal.	(g) Total Fat	(g) Sat. Fat	(mg) Chol.	(g) Carb.	(g) Fiber	(g) Sug.	(g) Prot.	(mg) Sod.
French Vanilla Swirl Hot Macchiato with Skim Milk Large									
20 fl oz	310	0	0	10	66	0	61	11	180
French Vanilla Swirl Hot Macchiato with Skim Milk Medium									
16 fl oz	240	0	0	5	49	0	46	8	135

Food Serving size	Cal.	(g) Total Fat	(g) Sat. Fat	(mg) Chol.	(g) Carb.	(g) Fiber	(g) Sug.	(g) Prot.	(mg) Sod.
French Vanilla Swirl Hot Macchiato with Skim Milk Small									
10 fl oz	160	0	0	5	33	0	30	6	95
French Vanilla Swirl Hot Macchiato with Whole Milk Large									
20 fl oz	380	8	4.5	30	65	0	60	10	180
Hot Macchiato with Whole Milk Large									
20 fl oz	160	8	4.5	25	14	0	14	8	125
Hot Macchiato with Whole Milk Medium									
16 fl oz	120	6	3.5	20	11	0	11	6	95
Hot Macchiato with Whole Milk Small									
10 fl oz	80	4	2.5	10	7	0	7	4	65
Hot Pumpkin Swirl Macchiato with Skim Milk Large									
20 fl oz	320	0.5	0	5	66	0	63	12	240
Hot Pumpkin Swirl Macchiato with Skim Milk Medium									
16 fl oz	240	0	0	5	50	0	47	9	180
Hot Pumpkin Swirl Macchiato with Skim Milk Small									
10 fl oz	160	0	0	5	33	0	31	6	125
Hot Pumpkin Swirl Macchiato with Whole Milk Large									
20 fl oz	390	8	5	25	66	0	62	11	240
Hot Pumpkin Swirl Macchiato with Whole Milk Medium									
16 fl oz	290	6	3.5	20	49	0	47	8	180
Hot Pumpkin Swirl Macchiato with Whole Milk Small									
10 fl oz	200	4	2.5	15	33	0	31	6	125
Mocha Swirl Hot Macchiato with Skim Milk Large									
20 fl oz	310	1	0.5	5	65	2	58	10	150
Mocha Swirl Hot Macchiato with Skim Milk Medium									
16 fl oz	240	1	0.5	5	49	2	43	8	115
Snickerdoodle Hot Macchiato with Skim Milk Large									
20 fl oz	320	0	0	10	66	0	62	11	180
Snickerdoodle Hot Macchiato with Skim Milk Medium									
16 fl oz	240	0	0	5	50	0	47	8	140
Snickerdoodle Hot Macchiato with Skim Milk Small									
10 fl oz	160	0	0	5	33	0	31	6	95
Snickerdoodle Hot Macchiato with Whole Milk Large									
20 fl oz	380	8	4.5	30	65	0	62	11	190

Food Serving size	Cal.	(g) Total Fat	(g) Sat. Fat	(mg) Chol.	(g) Carb.	(g) Fiber	(g) Sug.	(g) Prot.	(mg) Sod.
Snickerdoodle Hot Macchiato with Whole Milk Medium									
16 fl oz	290	6	3.5	20	49	0	46	8	140
Snickerdoodle Hot Macchiato with Whole Milk Small									
10 fl oz	190	4	2.5	15	33	0	31	5	95
Sugar Cookie Hot Macchiato with Skim Milk Large									
20 fl oz	320	0	0	10	66	0	62	11	180
Sugar Cookie Hot Macchiato with Skim Milk Medium									
16 fl oz	240	0	0	5	50	0	47	8	140
Sugar Cookie Hot Macchiato with Skim Milk Small									
10 fl oz	160	0	0	5	34	0	31	6	95
Sugar Cookie Hot Macchiato with Whole Milk Large									
20 fl oz	380	8	4.5	30	66	0	62	10	190
Sugar Cookie Hot Macchiato with Whole Milk Medium									
16 fl oz	290	6	3.5	20	50	0	47	8	140
Sugar Cookie Hot Macchiato with Whole Milk Small									
10 fl oz	190	4	2.5	15	33	0	31	5	95

Hot Specialty Beverages

Food Serving size	Cal.	(g) Total Fat	(g) Sat. Fat	(mg) Chol.	(g) Carb.	(g) Fiber	(g) Sug.	(g) Prot.	(mg) Sod.
Apple Cider Large									
20 fl oz	260	0	0	0	66	0	66	0	130
Apple Cider Medium									
14 fl oz	180	0	0	0	45	0	45	0	90
Apple Cider Small									
10 fl oz	120	0	0	0	31	0	31	0	60
Apple Cider XLarge									
24 fl oz	320	0	0	0	80	0	80	0	160

Hot Tea

Food Serving size	Cal.	(g) Total Fat	(g) Sat. Fat	(mg) Chol.	(g) Carb.	(g) Fiber	(g) Sug.	(g) Prot.	(mg) Sod.
Black Tea Large									
20 fl oz	0	0	0	0	0	0	0	0	20
Black Tea Medium									
14 fl oz	0	0	0	0	0	0	0	0	10
Black Tea Small									
10 fl oz	0	0	0	0	0	0	0	0	10
Black Tea XLarge									
24 fl oz	0	0	0	0	0	0	0	0	20

Food Serving size	Cal.	(g) Total Fat	(g) Sat. Fat	(mg) Chol.	(g) Carb.	(g) Fiber	(g) Sug.	(g) Prot.	(mg) Sod.
Black Tea with Cream Large 20 fl oz	110	11	7	40	2	0	0	2	40
Black Tea with Cream Medium 14 fl oz	90	9	5	30	2	0	0	1	30
Black Tea with Cream Small 10 fl oz	60	6	3.5	20	1	0	0	1	20
Black Tea with Milk Large 20 fl oz	35	2	1	5	3	0	3	2	40
Black Tea with Milk Medium 14 fl oz	30	1.5	1	5	2	0	2	1	30
Black Tea with Milk Small 10 fl oz	20	1	0.5	5	1	0	1	1	20
Black Tea with Milk XLarge 24 fl oz	45	2.5	1.5	10	4	0	4	2	50
Black Tea with Milk and Sugar Large 20 fl oz	170	2	1	5	38	0	38	2	45
Black Tea with Skim Milk and Sugar XLarge 24 fl oz	200	0	0	0	47	0	47	3	55
Black Tea with Sugar Large 20 fl oz	130	0	0	0	35	0	35	0	20
Black Tea with Sugar Medium 14 fl oz	100	0	0	0	26	0	26	0	15
Black Tea with Sugar Small 10 fl oz	60	0	0	0	17	0	17	0	5
Black Tea with Sugar Xlarge 24 fl oz	170	0	0	0	44	0	43	0	20
Decaffeinated Tea with Cream and Sugar XLarge 24 fl oz	310	14	9	50	46	0	44	2	50
Decaffeinated Tea with Milk Large 20 fl oz	35	2	1	5	3	0	3	2	40
Decaffeinated Tea with Milk Medium 14 fl oz	30	1.5	1	5	2	0	2	1	30
Decaffeinated Tea with Milk Small 10 fl oz	20	1	0.5	5	1	0	1	1	20

Food Serving size	Cal.	(g) Total Fat	(g) Sat. Fat	(mg) Chol.	(g) Carb.	(g) Fiber	(g) Sug.	(g) Prot.	(mg) Sod.
Decaffeinated Tea with Milk XLarge									
24 fl oz	45	2.5	1.5	10	4	0	4	2	50
Decaffeinated Tea with Milk and Sugar Large									
20 fl oz	170	2	1	5	38	0	38	2	45
Decaffeinated Tea with Milk and Sugar Medium									
14 fl oz	130	1.5	1	5	28	0	28	1	30
Decaffeinated Tea with Milk and Sugar Small									
10 fl oz	80	1	0.5	5	19	0	19	1	20
Decaffeinated Tea with Milk and Sugar XLarge									
24 fl oz	220	2.5	1.5	10	47	0	47	2	50
Decaffeinated Tea with Skim Milk Large									
20 fl oz	20	0	0	0	3	0	3	2	40
Decaffeinated Tea with Skim Milk Medium									
14 fl oz	15	0	0	0	2	0	2	2	30
Decaffeinated Tea with Skim Milk Small									
10 fl oz	10	0	0	0	2	0	2	1	20
Decaffeinated Tea with Skim Milk XLarge									
24 fl oz	25	0	0	0	4	0	4	3	50
Decaffeinated Tea with Skim Milk and Sugar Large									
20 fl oz	160	0	0	0	38	0	38	2	45
Decaffeinated Tea with Sugar Medium									
14 fl oz	100	0	0	0	26	0	26	0	15
Decaffeinated Tea with Sugar Small									
10 fl oz	70	0	0	0	17	0	17	0	10
Decaffeinated Tea with Sugar XLarge									
24 fl oz	170	0	0	0	44	0	43	0	20
Green Tea Large									
20 fl oz	0	0	0	0	0	0	0	0	20
Green Tea Medium									
14 fl oz	0	0	0	0	0	0	0	0	10
Green Tea Small									
10 fl oz	0	0	0	0	0	0	0	0	5
Green Tea XLarge									
24 fl oz	0	0	0	0	0	0	0	0	20

Food Serving size	Cal.	(g) Total Fat	(g) Sat. Fat	(mg) Chol.	(g) Carb.	(g) Fiber	(g) Sug.	(g) Prot.	(mg) Sod.
Green Tea with Cream Large									
20 fl oz	110	11	7	40	2	0	0	2	40
Green Tea with Cream Medium									
14 fl oz	90	9	5	30	2	0	0	1	30
Green Tea with Cream Small									
10 fl oz	60	6	3.5	20	1	0	0	1	20
Green Tea with Cream XLarge									
24 fl oz	140	14	9	50	3	0	0	2	50
Green Tea with Cream and Sugar Large									
20 fl oz	250	11	7	40	37	0	35	2	40
Green Tea with Cream and Sugar Medium									
14 fl oz	190	9	5	30	28	0	26	1	30
Green Tea with Cream and Sugar Small									
10 fl oz	120	6	3.5	20	18	0	17	1	20
Green Tea with Cream and Sugar XLarge									
24 fl oz	310	14	9	50	46	0	44	2	50
Green Tea with Milk Large									
20 fl oz	35	2	1	5	3	0	3	2	40
Green Tea with Milk Medium									
14 fl oz	30	1.5	1	5	2	0	2	1	30
Green Tea with Milk Small									
10 fl oz	20	1	0.5	5	1	0	1	1	20
Green Tea with Milk XLarge									
24 fl oz	45	2.5	1.5	10	4	0	4	2	50
Green Tea with Milk and Sugar Large									
20 fl oz	170	2	1	5	38	0	38	2	45
Green Tea with Milk and Sugar Medium									
14 fl oz	130	1.5	1	5	28	0	28	1	30
Green Tea with Milk and Sugar Small									
10 fl oz	80	1	0.5	5	19	0	19	1	20
Green Tea with Milk and Sugar XLarge									
24 fl oz	220	2.5	1.5	10	47	0	47	2	50
Green Tea with Skim Milk and Sugar XLarge									
24 fl oz	200	0	0	0	47	0	47	3	55

Food Serving size	Cal.	(g) Total Fat	(g) Sat. Fat	(mg) Chol.	(g) Carb.	(g) Fiber	(g) Sug.	(g) Prot.	(mg) Sod.
Green Tea with Sugar Large									
20 fl oz	130	0	0	0	35	0	35	0	20
Green Tea with Sugar Medium									
14 fl oz	100	0	0	0	26	0	26	0	15
Green Tea with Sugar Small									
10 fl oz	70	0	0	0	17	0	17	0	10
Green Tea with Sugar XLarge									
24 fl oz	170	0	0	0	44	0	43	0	20

Iced Coffee

Food Serving size	Cal.	(g) Total Fat	(g) Sat. Fat	(mg) Chol.	(g) Carb.	(g) Fiber	(g) Sug.	(g) Prot.	(mg) Sod.
Caramel Iced Coffee Large									
32 fl oz	230	0	0	5	52	0	49	5	100
Caramel Iced Coffee Medium									
24 fl oz	170	0	0	0	39	0	37	4	75
Caramel Iced Coffee Small									
16 fl oz	110	0	0	0	26	0	24	2	50
Caramel Iced Coffee with Cream Large									
32 fl oz	340	12	7	45	54	0	49	6	125
Caramel Iced Coffee with Cream Medium									
24 fl oz	260	9	5	30	41	0	37	5	90
Caramel Iced Coffee with Cream Small									
16 fl oz	170	6	3.5	20	27	0	24	3	60
Caramel Mocha Iced Coffee Large									
32 fl oz	230	0	0	0	54	1	48	4	45
Caramel Mocha Iced Coffee Medium									
24 fl oz	180	0	0	0	41	1	36	3	35
Caramel Mocha Iced Coffee Small									
16 fl oz	120	0	0	0	27	1	24	2	25
Caramel Mocha Iced Coffee with Cream Large									
32 fl oz	350	12	7	40	56	1	48	5	70
Caramel Mocha Iced Coffee with Cream Medium									
24 fl oz	260	9	6	30	42	1	36	4	50
Caramel Mocha Iced Coffee with Cream Small									
16 fl oz	180	6	3.5	20	28	1	24	3	35

Food Serving size	Cal.	(g) Total Fat	(g) Sat. Fat	(mg) Chol.	(g) Carb.	(g) Fiber	(g) Sug.	(g) Prot.	(mg) Sod.
French Vanilla Swirl Iced Coffee Large									
32 fl oz	230	0	0	5	54	0	48	4	75
French Vanilla Swirl Iced Coffee Medium									
24 fl oz	170	0	0	5	40	0	36	3	55
French Vanilla Swirl Iced Coffee Small									
16 fl oz	120	0	0	0	27	0	24	2	40
French Vanilla Swirl Iced Coffee with Cream Large									
32 fl oz	350	12	7	45	56	0	48	5	100
French Vanilla Swirl Iced Coffee with Cream Medium									
24 fl oz	260	9	5	35	42	0	36	4	70
French Vanilla Swirl Iced Coffee with Cream Small									
16 fl oz	170	6	3.5	20	28	0	24	3	50
Hazelnut Swirl Iced Coffee Large									
32 fl oz	230	0	0	5	54	0	48	4	75
Hazelnut Swirl Iced Coffee Medium									
24 fl oz	170	0	0	5	41	0	36	3	55
Hazelnut Swirl Iced Coffee Small									
16 fl oz	120	0	0	0	27	0	24	2	40
Hazelnut Swirl Iced Coffee with Cream Large									
32 fl oz	350	12	7	45	56	0	48	5	100
Hazelnut Swirl Iced Coffee with Cream Medium									
24 fl oz	260	9	5	35	42	0	36	4	70
Hazelnut Swirl Iced Coffee with Cream Small									
16 fl oz	180	6	3.5	20	28	0	24	3	50
Iced Coffee Large									
32 fl oz	20	0	0	0	3	0	0	1	15
Iced Coffee Medium									
24 fl oz	15	0	0	0	2	0	0	1	10
Iced Coffee Small									
16 fl oz	10	0	0	0	2	0	0	1	10
Iced Coffee with Almond Milk Medium									
24 fl oz	35	0.5	0	0	7	0	4	1	50
Iced Coffee with Almond Milk Small									
16 fl oz	20	0	0	0	4	0	2	1	30

Food Serving size	Cal.	(g) Total Fat	(g) Sat. Fat	(mg) Chol.	(g) Carb.	(g) Fiber	(g) Sug.	(g) Prot.	(mg) Sod.
Iced Coffee with Cream Large									
32 fl oz	130	11	7	40	5	0	0	3	40
Iced Coffee with Cream Medium									
24 fl oz	100	9	5	30	4	0	0	2	30
Iced Coffee with Cream Small									
16 fl oz	70	6	4	20	3	0	0	1	20
Iced Coffee with Cream and Sugar Large									
32 fl oz	270	11	7	40	40	0	35	3	40
Iced Coffee with Cream and Sugar Medium									
24 fl oz	200	9	5	30	30	0	26	2	30
Iced Coffee with Cream and Sugar Small									
16 fl oz	120	6	4	20	20	0	17	1	20
Iced Coffee with Milk Large									
32 fl oz	50	2	1	5	6	0	3	3	45
Iced Coffee with Milk Medium									
24 fl oz	40	1.5	1	5	5	0	2	2	30
Iced Dunkin' Dark® Roast Coffee with Cream and Sugar Large									
32 fl oz	250	12	7	40	40	0	35	3	40
Iced Dunkin' Dark® Roast Coffee with Cream and Sugar Medium									
24 fl oz	190	9	5	30	30	0	26	2	30
Iced Dunkin' Dark® Roast Coffee with Cream and Sugar Small									
16 fl oz	130	6	3.5	20	20	0	17	1	20
Iced Dunkin' Dark® Roast Coffee with Skim Milk and Splenda Large									
32 fl oz	60	0	0	0	10	0	3	3	50
Iced Dunkin' Dark® Roast Coffee with Skim Milk and Splenda Medium									
24 fl oz	40	0	0	0	8	0	2	3	35
Iced Dunkin' Dark® Roast Coffee with Skim Milk and Splenda Small									
16 fl oz	30	0	0	0	5	0	1	2	25
Mocha Iced Coffee with Cream Large									
32 fl oz	350	12	8	40	56	2	46	5	70
Mocha Iced Coffee with Cream Medium									
24 fl oz	260	9	6	30	42	2	34	3	50
Mocha Iced Coffee with Cream Small									
16 fl oz	180	6	4	20	28	1	23	2	35

Food Serving size	Cal.	(g) Total Fat	(g) Sat. Fat	(mg) Chol.	(g) Carb.	(g) Fiber	(g) Sug.	(g) Prot.	(mg) Sod.
Peppermint Mocha Iced Coffee Large									
32 fl oz	260	1	0	0	61	2	52	3	70
Peppermint Mocha Iced Coffee Medium									
24 fl oz	190	0.5	0	0	46	2	39	2	55
Peppermint Mocha Iced Coffee Small									
16 fl oz	130	0	0	0	31	1	26	1	35
Peppermint Mocha Iced Coffee with Cream Large									
32 fl oz	370	12	8	40	63	2	52	4	95
Peppermint Mocha Iced Coffee with Cream Medium									
24 fl oz	280	9	6	30	47	2	39	3	70
Peppermint Mocha Iced Coffee with Cream Small									
16 fl oz	190	6	4	20	32	1	26	2	50
Pumpkin Swirl Iced Coffee Large									
32 fl oz	240	0	0	0	55	0	51	5	135
Pumpkin Swirl Iced Coffee Medium									
24 fl oz	180	0	0	0	41	0	38	4	100
Pumpkin Swirl Iced Coffee Small									
16 fl oz	120	0	0	0	28	0	25	2	70
Pumpkin Swirl Iced Coffee with Cream Large									
32 fl oz	360	12	7	40	57	0	51	6	160
Pumpkin Swirl Iced Coffee with Cream Medium									
24 fl oz	270	9	6	30	43	0	38	5	120
Pumpkin Swirl Iced Coffee with Cream Small									
16 fl oz	180	6	3.5	20	29	0	25	3	80
Snickerdoodle Iced Coffee Large									
32 fl oz	240	0	0	5	54	0	49	4	75
Snickerdoodle Iced Coffee Medium									
24 fl oz	180	0	0	5	41	0	37	3	55
Snickerdoodle Iced Coffee Small									
16 fl oz	120	0	0	0	27	0	25	2	40
Snickerdoodle Iced Coffee with Cream Large									
32 fl oz	350	12	7	45	56	0	50	5	100
Snickerdoodle Iced Coffee with Cream Medium									
24 fl oz	260	9	5	35	42	0	37	4	75

Food Serving size	Cal.	(g) Total Fat	(g) Sat. Fat	(mg) Chol.	(g) Carb.	(g) Fiber	(g) Sug.	(g) Prot.	(mg) Sod.
Snickerdoodle Iced Coffee with Cream Small									
16 fl oz	180	6	3.5	20	28	0	25	3	50
Sugar Cookie Iced Coffee Medium									
24 fl oz	180	0	0	5	41	0	37	3	55
Sugar Cookie Iced Coffee Small									
16 fl oz	120	0	0	0	27	0	25	2	40
Sugar Cookie Iced Coffee with Cream Large									
32 fl oz	350	12	7	45	56	0	50	5	100
Sugar Cookie Iced Coffee with Cream Medium									
24 fl oz	260	9	5	35	42	0	37	4	75
Sugar Cookie Iced Coffee with Cream Small									
16 fl oz	180	6	3.5	20	28	0	25	3	50

Iced Macchiato

Food Serving size	Cal.	(g) Total Fat	(g) Sat. Fat	(mg) Chol.	(g) Carb.	(g) Fiber	(g) Sug.	(g) Prot.	(mg) Sod.
French Vanilla Swirl Iced Macchiato with Skim Milk Large									
32 fl oz	310	0	0	10	66	0	61	11	190
French Vanilla Swirl Iced Macchiato with Whole Milk Large									
32 fl oz	380	8	4.5	30	65	0	60	10	190
French Vanilla Swirl Iced Macchiato with Whole Milk Medium									
24 fl oz	280	6	3.5	20	49	0	45	8	150
French Vanilla Swirl Iced Macchiato with Whole Milk Small									
16 fl oz	190	4	2.5	15	33	0	30	5	100
Hazelnut Swirl Iced Macchiato with Skim Milk Large									
32 fl oz	310	0	0	10	66	0	61	11	190
Hazelnut Swirl Iced Macchiato with Skim Milk Medium									
24 fl oz	240	0	0	5	50	0	46	8	140
Hazelnut Swirl Iced Macchiato with Skim Milk Small									
16 fl oz	160	0	0	5	33	0	30	6	100
Iced Caramel Swirl Macchiato with Whole Milk Medium									
24 fl oz	290	6	3.5	20	49	0	49	8	125
Iced Caramel Swirl Macchiato with Whole Milk Small									
16 fl oz	190	4	2.5	15	33	0	33	5	85
Mocha Swirl Iced Macchiato with Whole Milk Large									
32 fl oz	380	9	5	25	65	2	58	10	160

Food Serving size	Cal.	(g) Total Fat	(g) Sat. Fat	(mg) Chol.	(g) Carb.	(g) Fiber	(g) Sug.	(g) Prot.	(mg) Sod.
Mocha Swirl Iced Macchiato with Whole Milk Medium									
24 fl oz	280	7	4	20	49	2	43	7	125
Mocha Swirl Iced Macchiato with Whole Milk Small									
16 fl oz	190	4.5	2.5	10	33	1	29	5	85
Peppermint Mocha Iced Macchiato with Skim Milk Small									
16 fl oz	160	0.5	0	0	36	1	31	5	95
Peppermint Mocha Iced Macchiato with Whole Milk Large									
32 fl oz	390	9	5	25	70	2	62	9	190
Peppermint Mocha Iced Macchiato with Whole Milk Medium									
24 fl oz	290	7	4	20	53	2	46	7	140
Peppermint Mocha Iced Macchiato with Whole Milk Small									
16 fl oz	200	4.5	2.5	10	35	1	31	5	100
Snickerdoodle Iced Macchiato with Skim Milk Large									
32 fl oz	320	0	0	10	66	0	62	11	190
Snickerdoodle Iced Macchiato with Skim Milk Medium									
24 fl oz	240	0	0	5	50	0	47	8	150
Snickerdoodle Iced Macchiato with Skim Milk Small									
16 fl oz	160	0	0	5	33	0	31	6	100
Snickerdoodle Iced Macchiato with Whole Milk Large									
32 fl oz	380	8	4.5	30	65	0	62	11	200
Snickerdoodle Iced Macchiato with Whole Milk Medium									
24 fl oz	290	6	3.5	20	49	0	46	8	150
Snickerdoodle Iced Macchiato with Whole Milk Small									
16 fl oz	190	4	2.5	15	33	0	31	5	100
Sugar Cookie Iced Macchiato with Skim Milk Large									
32 fl oz	320	0	0	10	22	0	62	11	190
Sugar Cookie Iced Macchiato with Skim Milk Medium									
24 fl oz	240	0	0	5	17	0	47	8	150
Sugar Cookie Iced Macchiato with Skim Milk Small									
16 fl oz	160	0	0	5	11	0	31	6	100
Sugar Cookie Iced Macchiato with Whole Milk Large									
32 fl oz	380	8	4.5	30	66	0	62	10	200
Sugar Cookie Iced Macchiato with Whole Milk Medium									
24 fl oz	290	6	3.5	20	50	0	47	8	150

Food Serving size	Cal.	(g) Total Fat	(g) Sat. Fat	(mg) Chol.	(g) Carb.	(g) Fiber	(g) Sug.	(g) Prot.	(mg) Sod.
Sugar Cookie Iced Macchiato with Whole Milk Small									
16 fl oz	190	4	2.5	15	33	0	31	5	100

Iced Specialty Beverages

Iced Apple Cider Large									
32 fl oz	260	0	0	0	66	0	66	0	140
Iced Apple Cider Medium									
24 fl oz	180	0	0	0	45	0	45	0	95
Iced Apple Cider Small									
16 fl oz	120	0	0	0	31	0	31	0	65

Iced Tea

Iced Green Tea Sweetened Large									
32 fl oz	150	0	0	0	37	0	34	0	10
Iced Green Tea Sweetened Medium									
24 fl oz	110	0	0	0	27	0	26	0	5
Iced Green Tea Sweetened Small									
16 fl oz	70	0	0	0	18	0	17	0	0
Iced Green Tea Unsweetened Large									
32 fl oz	10	0	0	0	2	0	0	0	10
Iced Green Tea Unsweetened Medium									
24 fl oz	5	0	0	0	2	0	0	0	5
Iced Tea Sweetened Peach Flavored Large									
32 fl oz	160	0	0	0	40	0	34	0	10
Iced Tea Sweetened Peach Flavored Medium									
24 fl oz	120	0	0	0	30	0	25	0	5
Iced Tea Sweetened Peach Flavored Small									
16 fl oz	80	0	0	0	20	0	17	0	0
Iced Tea Sweetened Raspberry Flavored Large									
32 fl oz	160	0	0	0	40	0	34	0	10
Iced Tea Sweetened Raspberry Flavored Medium									
24 fl oz	120	0	0	0	29	0	25	0	5
Iced Tea Sweetened Raspberry Flavored Small									
16 fl oz	80	0	0	0	20	0	17	0	0
Iced Tea Sweetened Small									
16 fl oz	70	0	0	0	18	0	17	0	0

Food Serving size	Cal.	(g) Total Fat	(g) Sat. Fat	(mg) Chol.	(g) Carb.	(g) Fiber	(g) Sug.	(g) Prot.	(mg) Sod.
Iced Tea Unsweetened Blueberry Flavored Large									
32 fl oz	25	0	0	0	3	0	0	0	10
Iced Tea Unsweetened Blueberry Flavored Medium									
24 fl oz	15	0	0	0	2	0	0	0	5
Iced Tea Unsweetened Blueberry Flavored Small									
16 fl oz	10	0	0	0	2	0	0	0	0
Iced Tea Unsweetened Peach Flavored Large									
32 fl oz	25	0	0	0	6	0	0	0	10
Iced Tea Unsweetened Peach Flavored Medium									
24 fl oz	20	0	0	0	5	0	0	0	5
Iced Tea Unsweetened Peach Flavored Small									
16 fl oz	15	0	0	0	3	0	0	0	0
Iced Tea Unsweetened Raspberry Flavored Large									
32 fl oz	25	0	0	0	6	0	0	0	10
Iced Tea Unsweetened Raspberry Flavored Medium									
24 fl oz	20	0	0	0	4	0	0	0	5
Iced Tea Unsweetened Raspberry Flavored Small									
16 fl oz	10	0	0	0	3	0	0	0	0
Iced Tea Unsweetened Large									
32 fl oz	10	0	0	0	2	0	0	0	10
Iced Tea Unsweetened Medium									
24 fl oz	5	0	0	0	2	0	0	0	5
Iced Tea Unsweetened Small									
16 fl oz	5	0	0	0	1	0	0	0	0
Sweet Tea - Medium									
24 fl oz	230	0	0	0	60	0	58	0	5
Sweet Tea - Small									
16 fl oz	160	0	0	0	40	0	39	0	5
Sweet Tea Blueberry Flavored Large									
32 fl oz	340	0	0	0	84	0	81	0	10
Sweet Tea Blueberry Flavored Medium									
24 fl oz	250	0	0	0	63	0	60	0	5
Sweet Tea Blueberry Flavored Small									
16 fl oz	170	0	0	0	42	0	40	0	5

Food Serving size	Cal.	(g) Total Fat	(g) Sat. Fat	(mg) Chol.	(g) Carb.	(g) Fiber	(g) Sug.	(g) Prot.	(mg) Sod.
Sweet Tea Lemonade Large									
32 fl oz	370	0	0	0	94	0	92	0	55
Sweet Tea Lemonade Medium									
24 fl oz	280	0	0	0	71	0	69	0	40
Sweet Tea Lemonade Small									
16 fl oz	190	0	0	0	47	0	46	0	25
Sweet Tea Peach Flavored Large									
32 fl oz	340	0	0	0	87	0	81	0	10
Sweet Tea Peach Flavored Medium									
24 fl oz	260	0	0	0	66	0	60	0	5
Sweet Tea Peach Flavored Small									
16 fl oz	170	0	0	0	44	0	40	0	5
Sweet Tea Raspberry Flavored Large									
32 fl oz	340	0	0	0	87	0	81	0	10
Sweet Tea Raspberry Flavored Medium									
24 fl oz	250	0	0	0	65	0	60	0	5
Sweet Tea Raspberry Flavored Small									
16 fl oz	170	0	0	0	43	0	40	0	5

Muffins

Food Serving size	Cal.	Total Fat	Sat. Fat	Chol.	Carb.	Fiber	Sug.	Prot.	Sod.
Blueberry Muffin									
1 Muffin	460	15	3	60	76	2	44	6	450
Chocolate Chip Muffin									
1 Muffin	550	21	6	65	83	2	50	7	470
Coffee Cake Muffin									
1 Muffin	590	24	8	65	86	1	51	7	480
Corn Muffin									
1 Muffin	460	16	3	70	72	1	31	7	770
Honey Bran Raisin Muffin									
1 Muffin	440	13	2.5	55	74	4	40	7	410
Pumpkin Muffin									
1 Muffin	550	24	5	50	78	3	41	7	480
Reduced Fat Blueberry Muffin - 25% Less Fat than Our Regular Blueberry Muffin									
1 Muffin	410	10	2	55	75	2	40	7	620

Food Serving size	Cal.	(g) Total Fat	(g) Sat. Fat	(mg) Chol.	(g) Carb.	(g) Fiber	(g) Sug.	(g) Prot.	(mg) Sod.
Munchkins									
Boston Kreme Munchkin									
1 Munchkin	70	4.5	2	0	7	0	2	1	85
Butternut Munchkin									
1 Munchkin	90	3.5	2	5	12	0	8	1	50
Chocolate Butternut Munchkin									
1 Munchkin	90	4	2	0	12	0	7	1	95
Cinnamon Munchkin									
1 Munchkin	60	3.5	1.5	5	6	0	3	1	65
Coconut Munchkin									
1 Munchkin	80	4.5	2.5	5	10	0	5	1	50
Fall Munchkin									
1 Munchkin	90	3.5	1.5	5	14	0	9	1	50
Glazed Blueberry Munchkin									
1 Munchkin	70	3.5	1.5	5	9	0	5	1	50
Glazed Chocolate Munchkin									
1 Munchkin	70	3.5	1.5	0	8	0	4	1	95
Glazed Munchkin									
1 Munchkin	70	4	2	0	7	0	3	1	80
Glazed Old Fashioned Munchkin									
1 Munchkin	70	3.5	1.5	5	9	0	4	1	50
Jelly Munchkin									
1 Munchkin	70	4	2	0	8	0	4	1	80
Old Fashioned Munchkin									
1 Munchkin	60	3.5	1.5	5	6	0	2	1	50
Powdered Munchkin									
1 Munchkin	60	3.5	1.5	5	7	0	3	1	50
Pumpkin Munchkin									
1 Munchkin	60	2.5	1	5	9	0	4	1	75
Sugared Raised Munchkin									
1 Munchkin	60	4	2	0	5	0	1	1	80
Toasted Coconut Munchkin									
1 Munchkin	90	5	3	5	10	1	6	1	50

Food Serving size	Cal.	(g) Total Fat	(g) Sat. Fat	(mg) Chol.	(g) Carb.	(g) Fiber	(g) Sug.	(g) Prot.	(mg) Sod.
Other Bakery									
Apple Fritter 1 Fritter	420	19	8	0	58	2	24	6	380
Biscuit 1 Biscuit	320	17	10	0	35	1	3	6	740
Blueberry Coffee Cake 1/8 Cake	190	6	1.5	20	31	1	17	3	170
Brownie 1 Brownie	440	23	5	55	58	1	49	3	250
Chocolate Chip Coffee Cake 1/8 Cake	230	9	2.5	25	34	1	20	3	180
English Muffin 1 Muffin	140	0.5	0	0	30	6	1	4	110
Flatbread 1 Flatbread	160	3	0.5	0	29	3	2	5	270
French Roll 1 Roll	260	1.5	0	0	52	2	2	9	550
Glazed Fritter 1 Fritter	410	17	7	0	60	2	27	6	380
Homestyle Apple Pie 1 Pie	280	14	5	0	36	1	15	3	240
Original Coffee Cake 1/8 Cake	230	9	3	25	33	1	20	3	180
Plain Croissant 1 Croissant	340	18	8	0	37	1	5	6	350
Pretzel Twist 1 Twist	280	2.5	1	0	54	2	2	10	1340
Pumpkin Coffee Cake 1/8 Cake	210	9	2	20	30	1	17	2	170
Other Frozen Beverages									
Frozen Dunkaccino Small 16 fl oz	400	8	6	15	78	1	71	5	160
Frozen Hot Chocolate 16 fl oz	400	7	5	10	80	2	73	5	170

Food Serving size	Cal.	(g) Total Fat	(g) Sat. Fat	(mg) Chol.	(g) Carb.	(g) Fiber	(g) Sug.	(g) Prot.	(mg) Sod.
Frozen Mint Hot Chocolate 16 floz	400	7	5	10	80	2	73	5	160
S'mores Hot Chocolate 16 fl oz	400	7	5	10	80	2	73	5	160
Salted Caramel Hot Chocolate 16 fl oz	400	7	5	10	79	2	73	5	220

Other Hot Beverages

Food Serving size	Cal.	(g) Total Fat	(g) Sat. Fat	(mg) Chol.	(g) Carb.	(g) Fiber	(g) Sug.	(g) Prot.	(mg) Sod.
Dunkaccino® Large 20 fl oz	490	22	16	15	73	1	52	4	470
Dunkaccino® Medium 14 fl oz	350	15	11	10	52	1	37	3	330
Dunkaccino® Small 10 fl oz	240	10	8	5	36	0	25	2	230
Dunkaccino® XLarge 24 fl oz	530	23	17	15	79	1	56	4	510
Mint Hot Chocolate Large 20 fl oz	410	13	12	0	73	3	57	3	410
Mint Hot Chocolate Medium 14 fl oz	300	10	9	0	53	2	42	3	300
Mint Hot Chocolate Small 10 fl oz	210	7	6	0	37	1	29	2	210
Mint Hot Chocolate XLarge 24 fl oz	500	16	14	0	88	3	69	4	500
Original Hot Chocolate Large 20 fl oz	460	14	13	0	82	3	63	3	480
Original Hot Chocolate Medium 14 fl oz	330	10	9	0	58	2	45	2	340
Original Hot Chocolate Small 10 fl oz	220	7	6	0	40	2	30	2	230
Original Hot Chocolate XLarge 24 fl oz	500	15	14	0	89	3	68	4	520
S'mores Hot Chocolate Large 20 fl oz	450	13	13	0	80	3	59	2	460

Food Serving size	Cal.	(g) Total Fat	(g) Sat. Fat	(mg) Chol.	(g) Carb.	(g) Fiber	(g) Sug.	(g) Prot.	(mg) Sod.
S'mores Hot Chocolate Medium 14 fl oz	340	10	9	0	60	2	44	2	340
S'mores Hot Chocolate Small 10 fl oz	220	7	6	0	40	2	30	1	230
S'mores Hot Chocolate Xlarge 24 fl oz	550	16	15	0	98	4	73	3	560
Salted Caramel Hot Chocolate Large 20 fl oz	420	14	13	0	71	2	55	4	640
Salted Caramel Hot Chocolate Medium 14 fl oz	310	10	9	0	52	1	40	3	470
Salted Caramel Hot Chocolate Small 10 fl oz	220	7	6	0	36	1	28	2	330
Salted Caramel Hot Chocolate XLarge 24 fl oz	520	17	15	0	86	2	67	4	780
Turbo Hot Chocolate Large 20 fl oz	450	15	14	0	81	3	62	4	560
Turbo Hot Chocolate Medium 14 fl oz	320	11	10	0	58	2	44	3	400
Turbo Hot Chocolate Small 10 fl oz	220	7	7	0	39	2	30	2	270

Smoothie

Strawberry Banana Smoothie Small 16 fl oz	250	2.5	1.5	10	54	2	45	5	95
Tropical Mango Smoothie Small 16 fl oz	260	2	1	10	57	1	50	5	90

Specialty Beverage

Vanilla Chai 14 fl oz	330	8	6	10	54	0	46	10	150

Wake-Up Wraps

Bacon, Egg & Cheese Wake-Up Wrap 1 Wrap	180	9	4	40	14	1	1	9	520
Egg & Cheese Wake-Up Wrap 1 Wrap	150	8	3.5	40	13	1	1	7	420

Food Serving size	Cal.	(g) Total Fat	(g) Sat. Fat	(mg) Chol.	(g) Carb.	(g) Fiber	(g) Sug.	(g) Prot.	(mg) Sod.
Egg White Veggie Wake-Up Wrap									
1 Wrap	150	7	3	15	14	1	1	9	360
Ham, Egg & Cheese Wake-Up Wrap									
1 Wrap	170	8	3.5	45	14	1	1	10	560
Sausage, Egg & Cheese Wake-Up Wrap									
1 Wrap	260	17	7	60	14	1	1	12	660
Sweet Black Pepper Bacon Wake-Up Wrap									
1 Wrap	210	11	4.5	75	16	1	2	12	590

KFC

Chicken

Food	Cal.	Total Fat	Sat. Fat	Chol.	Carb.	Fiber	Sug.	Prot.	Sod.
Original Recipe® Chicken - Whole Wing									
	140	8	1.5	50	5	0	0	11	450
Original Recipe® Chicken - Breast									
	320	14	3	145	13	2	0	36	1130
Original Recipe® Chicken Breast Without Skin or Breading									
	130	2	0.5	90	0	0	0	29	520
Original Recipe® Chicken - Drumstick									
	120	7	1.5	60	3	0	0	11	380
Original Recipe® Chicken - Thigh									
	290	21	5	100	8	1	0	18	850
Extra Crispy™ Chicken - Whole Wing									
	210	15	2.5	60	8	0	0	12	490
Extra Crispy™ Chicken - Breast									
	490	29	4.5	110	20	1	0	35	1140
Extra Crispy™ Chicken - Drumstick									
	160	10	1.5	55	5	0	0	13	390
Extra Crispy™ Chicken - Thigh									
	370	26	4.5	85	15	1	0	18	760
Spicy Crispy Chicken - Whole Wing									
	160	12	2	40	6	0	0	9	410
Spicy Crispy Chicken - Breast									
	520	34	5	110	23	1	0	29	1220

Food Serving size	Cal.	(g) Total Fat	(g) Sat. Fat	(mg) Chol.	(g) Carb.	(g) Fiber	(g) Sug.	(g) Prot.	(mg) Sod.
Spicy Crispy Chicken - Drumstick									
	150	10	1.5	45	5	0	0	11	410
Spicy Crispy Chicken - Thigh									
	350	27	4.5	75	11	0	0	15	810
Kentucky Grilled Chicken® - Whole Wing									
	80	4.5	1.5	50	1	0	0	10	250
Kentucky Grilled Chicken® - Breast									
	220	7	2	135	0	0	0	40	730
Kentucky Grilled Chicken® - Drumstick									
	90	4	1	60	0	0	0	13	290
Kentucky Grilled Chicken® - Thigh									
	170	10	3	90	0	0	0	19	530

Strips

Extra Crispy™ Tenders (3)									
	380	20	2.5	85	17	3	0	33	940
Extra Crispy™ Tenders (2)									
	250	13	1.5	60	11	2	0	22	630
Extra Crispy™ Tenders (1) - Kids									
	130	7	1	30	6	1	0	11	310

Bites

Original Recipe® Bites (4) - Kids									
	130	6	1	40	5	1	0	15	440
Original Recipe® Bites (6)									
	200	9	1.5	60	7	1	0	22	660
Original Recipe® Bites (10)									
	330	15	2.5	105	12	2	0	37	1100

Wings

Hot Wings™ (1)									
	70	4	1	20	3	0	0	4	160
HBBQ Hot Wings™ (1)									
	80	4	1	20	8	0	2	4	270
Fiery Buffalo Hot Wings™ (1)									
	70	4	1	20	5	0	0	4	290

Food Serving size	Cal.	(g) Total Fat	(g) Sat. Fat	(mg) Chol.	(g) Carb.	(g) Fiber	(g) Sug.	(g) Prot.	(mg) Sod.
Sandwiches									
Chicken Littles®	310	18	2.5	40	23	2	4	14	590
Chicken Littles® Without Sauce	210	8	1	30	23	2	4	14	510
Crispy Twister®	610	32	6	70	52	5	4	29	1260
Crispy Twister® Without Sauce	490	19	3.5	60	51	5	3	28	1130
Honey BBQ Sandwich	320	3.5	1	70	47	3	21	24	770
Colonel's Original Sandwich	450	20	3.5	60	41	3	7	25	1110
Doublicious®	530	27	7	75	42	3	7	30	1390
Pot Pie, Bowls, Value Boxes & Go Cup									
Chicken Pot Pie	790	45	37	75	66	3	7	29	1970
KFC Famous Bowls® - Mashed Potato with Gravy	650	26	6	70	73	6	3	32	2040
Snack-Size Bowl	280	13	3.5	40	27	3	1	16	790
Original Recipe® Bites Snack Box	420	21	3.5	40	39	3	0	19	1240
Extra Crispy™ Tenders Go Cup	540	28	4	60	46	4	0	26	1440
Original Recipe® Bites Go Cup	420	21	3.5	40	40	3	0	19	1250
Chicken Littles® Go Cup	600	33	5	40	58	4	4	18	1400
Grilled Drumstick Value Box	380	19	3.5	60	34	2	0	17	1090
OR Drumstick Value Box	400	22	4	45	37	2	0	15	1110

Food Serving size	Cal.	(g) Total Fat	(g) Sat. Fat	(mg) Chol.	(g) Carb.	(g) Fiber	(g) Sug.	(g) Prot.	(mg) Sod.
EC Drumstick Value Box									
	450	25	4	55	39	3	0	16	1190
Grilled Thigh Value Box									
	460	25	5	90	34	2	0	23	1330
OR Thigh Value Box									
	540	32	7	80	42	2	0	20	1540
EC Thigh Value Box									
	660	41	7	85	49	3	0	22	1560

Salads & More

Food Serving size	Cal.	(g) Total Fat	(g) Sat. Fat	(mg) Chol.	(g) Carb.	(g) Fiber	(g) Sug.	(g) Prot.	(mg) Sod.
Crispy Chicken Caesar Salad Without Dressing & Croutons									
	330	17	4	70	16	4	3	29	810
Caesar Side Salad Without Dressing & Croutons									
	40	2	1	5	2	1	1	3	90
Crispy Chicken BLT Salad Without Dressing									
	350	18	3.5	75	18	5	5	30	990
House Side Salad Without Dressing									
	15	0	0	0	3	1	2	1	10
Heinz Buttermilk Ranch Dressing (1)									
	160	17	2	10	1	0	1	0	220
Hidden Valley® The Original Ranch® Fat Free Dressing (1)									
	35	0	0	0	8	0	2	1	410
Parmesan Garlic Croutons Pouch (1)									
	70	3	0	0	8	0	0	1	160

Sides (Individual)

Food Serving size	Cal.	(g) Total Fat	(g) Sat. Fat	(mg) Chol.	(g) Carb.	(g) Fiber	(g) Sug.	(g) Prot.	(mg) Sod.
Green Beans									
	25	0	0	0	4	2	1	1	260
Mashed Potatoes with Gravy									
	120	4	1	0	19	1	0	2	530
Mashed Potatoes Without Gravy									
	90	3	0.5	0	15	1	0	2	320
Gravy (with Bites)									
	50	2.5	1	5	7	0	0	1	410
Macaroni and Cheese									
	170	6	1.5	5	22	2	2	5	830

Food Serving size	Cal.	(g) Total Fat	(g) Sat. Fat	(mg) Chol.	(g) Carb.	(g) Fiber	(g) Sug.	(g) Prot.	(mg) Sod.
Potato Wedges									
	290	15	2.5	0	35	2	0	4	810
Corn on the Cob (3")									
	70	0.5	0	0	16	2	3	2	0
BBQ Baked Beans									
	210	1.5	0	0	41	8	18	8	780
Cole Slaw									
	170	10	1.5	5	19	3	14	1	170
Biscuit									
	180	8	6	0	23	1	2	4	530
Sweet Kernel Corn									
	100	0.5	0	0	21	2	3	3	0
KFC® Cornbread Muffin									
	210	9	1.5	35	28	0	11	3	240

Other

Food Serving size	Cal.	(g) Total Fat	(g) Sat. Fat	(mg) Chol.	(g) Carb.	(g) Fiber	(g) Sug.	(g) Prot.	(mg) Sod.
GoGo squeeZ™ Applesauce									
	60	0	0	0	15	1	12	0	0
KFC® Gizzards									
	190	11	1.5	135	11	0	0	13	500
KFC® Livers									
	150	8	1.5	185	8	0	0	11	480
Country Fried Steak Without Peppered White Gravy									
	360	24	7	35	22	2	0	13	750
Country Fried Steak with Peppered White Gravy									
	390	26	7	35	26	2	0	13	910
Jalapeno Peppers									
	20	1.5	0	0	1	1	0	0	480
Honey Sauce Packet									
	30	0	0	0	8	0	5	0	0
Colonel's Buttery Spread									
	30	3.5	0.5	0	0	0	0	0	30
Bacon Ranch Dipping Sauce Cup									
	140	15	2.5	10	1	0	1	0	220
Creamy Buffalo Dipping Sauce Cup									
	70	7	1	5	2	0	0	0	510

Food Serving size	Cal.	(g) Total Fat	(g) Sat. Fat	(mg) Chol.	(g) Carb.	(g) Fiber	(g) Sug.	(g) Prot.	(mg) Sod.
Orange Ginger Dipping Sauce Cup									
	50	0	0	0	11	0	10	0	220
Sweet and Sour Dipping Sauce Cup									
	45	0	0	0	12	0	10	0	95
Honey Mustard Dipping Sauce Cup									
	120	10	1.5	5	6	0	5	0	110
Creamy Ranch Dipping Sauce Cup									
	100	10	1.5	10	2	0	1	0	240
HBBQ Dipping Sauce Cup									
	40	0	0	0	9	0	8	0	310

Desserts

Food Serving size	Cal.	(g) Total Fat	(g) Sat. Fat	(mg) Chol.	(g) Carb.	(g) Fiber	(g) Sug.	(g) Prot.	(mg) Sod.
Apple Turnover (1)									
	230	10	2.5	0	32	1	12	2	140
Reese's® Peanut Butter Pie Slice									
	310	19	10	5	31	1	22	5	200
Oreo® Cookies and Crème Pie Slice									
	290	16	10	5	34	1	23	3	210
Sweet Life® Oatmeal Raisin Cookie									
	150	6	2.5	10	22	1	13	2	105
Sweet Life® Chocolate Chip Cookie									
	160	8	3.5	10	22	1	15	2	90
Sweet Life® Sugar Cookie									
	160	7	3	10	21	0	10	2	120
Sweet Life® Double Fudge Cookie									
	160	8	3.5	10	21	1	14	2	105

Beverages

Food Serving size	Cal.	(g) Total Fat	(g) Sat. Fat	(mg) Chol.	(g) Carb.	(g) Fiber	(g) Sug.	(g) Prot.	(mg) Sod.
Capri Sun® Roarin' Waters Tropical Fruit (6 fl oz)									
	30	0	0	0	8	0	8	0	15
Milk 1% (7 fl oz)									
	110	2	1.5	10	14	0	13	9	140
Chocolate Milk 1% (7 fl oz)									
	180	2.5	1.5	10	29	0	26	10	210
Milk 2% (10 fl oz)									
	170	6	4	25	17	0	16	12	180

Food Serving size	Cal.	(g) Total Fat	(g) Sat. Fat	(mg) Chol.	(g) Carb.	(g) Fiber	(g) Sug.	(g) Prot.	(mg) Sod.
Pepsi® (16 fl oz)									
	200	0	0	0	56	0	56	0	40
Diet Pepsi® (16 fl oz)									
	0	0	0	0	0	0	0	0	50
Diet Pepsi® (20 fl oz)									
	0	0	0	0	0	0	0	0	60
Pepsi MAX® (16 fl oz)									
	0	0	0	0	0	0	0	0	50
Pepsi MAX® (20 fl oz)									
	0	0	0	0	0	0	0	0	60
Wild Cherry Pepsi® (16 fl oz)									
	200	0	0	0	56	0	56	0	40
Wild Cherry Pepsi® (20 fl oz)									
	250	0	0	0	69	0	69	0	55
Sierra Mist® (16 fl oz)									
	200	0	0	0	54	0	54	0	40
Sierra Mist® (20 fl oz)									
	250	0	0	0	68	0	68	0	50
Diet Sierra Mist® (16 fl oz)									
	0	0	0	0	0	0	0	0	50
Diet Sierra Mist® (20 fl oz)									
	0	0	0	0	0	0	0	0	60
Lipton® Brisk® Sweet Iced Tea (16 fl oz)									
	140	0	0	0	40	0	40	0	70
Lipton® Brisk® Sweet Iced Tea (20 fl oz)									
	180	0	0	0	50	0	50	0	90
Lipton® Brisk® Lemon Tea (20 fl oz)									
	180	0	0	0	50	0	50	0	40
Lipton® Brisk® No Calorie Peach Iced Green Tea (16 fl oz)									
	0	0	0	0	0	0	0	0	140
Lipton® Brisk® No Calorie Peach Iced Green Tea (20 fl oz)									
	0	0	0	0	0	0	0	0	175
Lipton® Brisk® Peach Iced Green Tea (16 fl oz)									
	160	0	0	0	42	0	42	0	50

Food Serving size	Cal.	(g) Total Fat	(g) Sat. Fat	(mg) Chol.	(g) Carb.	(g) Fiber	(g) Sug.	(g) Prot.	(mg) Sod.
Lipton® Brisk® Peach Iced Green Tea (20 fl oz)									
	200	0	0	0	53	0	53	0	65
Lipton® Brisk® Raspberry Tea (16 fl oz)									
	160	0	0	0	42	0	42	0	50
Lipton® Brisk® Raspberry Tea (20 fl oz)									
	200	0	0	0	53	0	53	0	65
Mountain Dew® (16 fl oz)									
	220	0	0	0	58	0	58	0	70
Mountain Dew® (20 fl oz)									
	280	0	0	0	73	0	73	0	90
Diet Mountain Dew® (16 fl oz)									
	0	0	0	0	0	0	0	0	80
Diet Mountain Dew® (20 fl oz)									
	0	0	0	0	0	0	0	0	100
Code Red Mountain Dew® (16 fl oz)									
	220	0	0	0	62	0	62	0	70
Code Red Mountain Dew® (20 fl oz)									
	280	0	0	0	78	0	78	0	90
Tropicana® Lemonade (16 fl oz)									
	200	0	0	0	54	0	54	0	210
Tropicana® Lemonade (20 fl oz)									
	250	0	0	0	68	0	68	0	265
Tropicana® Light Lemonade (16 fl oz)									
	10	0	0	0	0	0	0	0	190
Tropicana® Light Lemonade (20 fl oz)									
	10	0	0	0	0	0	0	0	240
Tropicana® Pink Lemonade (16 fl oz)									
	200	0	0	0	54	0	54	0	210
Tropicana® Pink Lemonade (20 fl oz)									
	250	0	0	0	68	0	68	0	265
Tropicana® Fruit Punch (16 fl oz)									
	220	0	0	0	60	0	60	0	50
Tropicana® Fruit Punch (20 fl oz)									
	280	0	0	0	75	0	75	0	65

Food Serving size	Cal.	(g) Total Fat	(g) Sat. Fat	(mg) Chol.	(g) Carb.	(g) Fiber	(g) Sug.	(g) Prot.	(mg) Sod.
Tropicana® Twister® Orange (16 fl oz)									
	220	0	0	0	62	0	62	0	50
Tropicana® Twister® Orange (20 fl oz)									
	280	0	0	0	78	0	78	0	65
Mug Root Beer® (16 fl oz)									
	200	0	0	0	52	0	52	0	30
Mug Root Beer® (20 fl oz)									
	250	0	0	0	65	0	65	0	40
Dr Pepper® (16 fl oz)									
	200	0	0	0	53	0	53	0	80
Dr Pepper® (20 fl oz)									
	250	0	0	0	66	0	64	0	100
Diet Dr Pepper® (16 fl oz)									
	0	0	0	0	0	0	0	0	80
Diet Dr Pepper® (20 fl oz)									
	0	0	0	0	0	0	0	0	100
7UP® (16 fl oz)									
	190	0	0	0	51	0	50	0	55
7UP® (20 fl oz)									
	240	0	0	0	64	0	63	0	70

Long John Silver's

Alaskan Pollock and Seafood

Battered Alaskan Pollock (1 Piece)									
	260	16	4	35	17	0	0	12	790
Battered Shrimp (3 Pieces)									
	130	9	2.5	45	8	0	0	5	480
Breaded Clam Strips (1 Snack Box)									
	320	19	4.5	35	29	2	1	9	1190
Buttered Langostino Lobster Bites (1 Snack Box)									
	230	9	3	60	24	2	0	13	520
Grilled Pacific Salmon (2 Filets)									
	150	5	1	50	2	0	1	24	440

Food Serving size	Cal.	(g) Total Fat	(g) Sat. Fat	(mg) Chol.	(g) Carb.	(g) Fiber	(g) Sug.	(g) Prot.	(mg) Sod.
Grilled Tilapia (1 Filet)									
	110	2.5	1	55	1	0	1	22	250
Langostino Lobster Stuffed Crab Cake (1 Cake)									
	170	9	2	30	16	1	0	6	390
Popcorn Shrimp (1 Snack Box)									
	270	16	4	75	23	1	1	9	570
Shrimp Scampi (8 Pieces)									
	200	13	2.5	135	3	0	1	17	650

Beverages

Food Serving size	Cal.	(g) Total Fat	(g) Sat. Fat	(mg) Chol.	(g) Carb.	(g) Fiber	(g) Sug.	(g) Prot.	(mg) Sod.
Mountain Dew (Small) (20 fl oz)									
	270	0	0	0	72	0	72	0	85
Pepsi (Kids) (12 fl oz)									
	150	0	0	0	42	0	40	0	35
Pepsi (Large) (40 fl oz)									
	500	0	0	0	140	0	135	0	125
Pepsi (Medium) (32 fl oz)									
	400	0	0	0	112	0	108	0	100
Pepsi (Small) (20 fl oz)									
	250	0	0	0	70	0	67	0	60
Sierra Mist (Kids) (12 fl oz)									
	150	0	0	0	40	0	40	0	30
Sierra Mist (Large) (40 fl oz)									
	500	0	0	0	135	0	135	0	100
Sierra Mist (Medium) (32 fl oz)									
	400	0	0	0	108	0	108	0	80
Tropicana Lemonade (Large) (40 fl oz)									
	500	0	0	0	135	0	135	0	525
Wild Cherry Pepsi (Kids) (12 fl oz)									
	150	0	0	0	42	0	42	0	30
Wild Cherry Pepsi (Large) (40 fl oz)									
	500	0	0	0	140	0	140	0	100
Wild Cherry Pepsi (Medium) (32 fl oz)									
	400	0	0	0	112	0	112	0	80

Food Serving size	Cal.	(g) Total Fat	(g) Sat. Fat	(mg) Chol.	(g) Carb.	(g) Fiber	(g) Sug.	(g) Prot.	(mg) Sod.
Wild Cherry Pepsi (Small) (20 fl oz)									
	250	0	0	0	70	0	70	0	50

Chicken Strips

Chicken Strips (1 Piece)									
	140	8	2	20	9	0	0	8	480

Desserts

Chocolate Cream Pie (1 Slice)									
	280	17	10	10	28	1	19	3	230
Pineapple Cream Pie (1 Slice)									
	300	17	11	10	35	0	25	3	250

Iceflow Lemonade

Iceflow Lemonade (16 oz Cup)									
	190	0	0	0	47	0	40	0	15
Iceflow Lemonade (20 oz Cup)									
	240	0	0	0	60	0	50	0	15
Strawberry Iceflow Lemonade (16 oz Cup)									
	240	0	0	0	60	0	48	0	15
Strawberry Iceflow Lemonade (20 oz Cup)									
	310	0	0	0	79	0	62	0	20

Sandwiches and More

Alaskan Pollock Sandwich (1 Sandwich)									
	470	23	5	40	49	3	4	18	1180
Baja Chicken Strip Taco (1 Taco)									
	370	23	5	25	31	3	2	11	890
Baja Fish Taco (1 Taco)									
	360	23	4.5	25	30	3	2	9	810
Chicken Strip Sandwich (1 Sandwich)									
	440	30	6	50	47	4	2	22	1350
Freshside Grille Salmon Entrée (1 Plate)									
	280	7	2	50	27	3	5	27	1010
Freshside Grille Shrimp Scampi (1 Plate)									
	330	15	3.5	135	29	3	5	20	1230

Food Serving size	Cal.	(g) Total Fat	(g) Sat. Fat	(mg) Chol.	(g) Carb.	(g) Fiber	(g) Sug.	(g) Prot.	(mg) Sod.
Freshside Grille Tilapia Entrée (1 Plate)									
	250	4.5	2	60	27	3	4	25	820
Ultimate Alaskan Pollock Sandwich (1 Sandwich)									
	530	27	8	55	50	3	4	21	1500
Zesty Chicken Strip Sandwich (1 Sandwich)									
	380	19	4	25	39	3	2	14	880

Sauces/Condiments

Food Serving size	Cal.	(g) Total Fat	(g) Sat. Fat	(mg) Chol.	(g) Carb.	(g) Fiber	(g) Sug.	(g) Prot.	(mg) Sod.
BBQ (1 Dipping Cup)									
	40	0	0	0	10	0	6	0	230
Cocktail Sauce (1 oz)									
	25	0	0	0	6	0	5	0	250
Honey Mustard (1 Dipping Cup)									
	100	6	1.5	0	12	0	6	0	170
Ketchup (1 Packet)									
	10	0	0	0	2	0	2	0	100
Lemon Juice (1 Packet)									
	0	0	0	0	0	0	0	0	0
Louisiana Hot Sauce (1 Teaspoon)									
	0	0	0	0	0	0	0	0	140
Malt Vinegar (0.5 oz)									
	0	0	0	0	0	0	0	0	35
Marina (1 Dipping Cup)									
	15	0	0	0	4	1	2	1	125
Ranch (1 Dipping Cup)									
	160	17	2.5	15	2	0	1	0	240
Sweet and Sour (1 Dipping Cup)									
	45	0	0	0	12	0	7	0	120
Tartar Sauce (1 oz)									
	100	9	1.5	15	4	0	3	0	250

Sides

Food Serving size	Cal.	(g) Total Fat	(g) Sat. Fat	(mg) Chol.	(g) Carb.	(g) Fiber	(g) Sug.	(g) Prot.	(mg) Sod.
Breaded Mozzarella Sticks (3 Pieces)									
	150	9	3.5	10	13	1	0	5	350
Breadstick (1 Breadstick)									
	170	3.5	1	0	29	1	2	6	290

Food Serving size	Cal.	(g) Total Fat	(g) Sat. Fat	(mg) Chol.	(g) Carb.	(g) Fiber	(g) Sug.	(g) Prot.	(mg) Sod.
Broccoli Cheese Bites (5 Pieces)									
	230	12	4.5	15	25	2	2	5	550
Broccoli Cheese Soup (1 Bowl)									
	220	18	8	30	8	1	2	5	650
Cole Slaw (4 oz)									
	200	15	2.5	20	15	3	10	1	340
Corn Cobbette with Butter Oil (1 Cobbette)									
	150	10	2	0	14	3	6	3	30
Corn Cobbette Without Butter Oil (1 cobbette)									
	90	3	0.5	0	4	3	6	3	0
Crumblies (1 oz)									
	170	12	2.5	0	14	1	0	1	410
Fries - Basket Combo Portion (4 oz)									
	310	14	3.5	0	45	4	0	3	460
Fries - Platter Portion (3 oz)									
	230	10	2.5	0	34	3	0	3	350
Hushpuppy (1 Pup)									
	60	2.5	0.5	0	9	1	1	1	200
Jalapeno Cheddar Bites (5 Pieces)									
	240	14	5	15	23	2	2	6	730
Jalapeno Peppers (1 Whole Pepper)									
	15	0	0	0	2	0	1	1	190
Rice (5 oz)									
	180	1	0.5	0	37	2	1	4	470
Vegetable Medley (4 oz)									
	50	2	0.5	0	8	3	3	1	360

McDonald's

Burgers & Sandwiches

Bacon Clubhouse Burger									
	740	41	16	125	51	4	14	40	1480

Food Serving size	Cal.	(g) Total Fat	(g) Sat. Fat	(mg) Chol.	(g) Carb.	(g) Fiber	(g) Sug.	(g) Prot.	(mg) Sod.
Premium Grilled Chicken Bacon Clubhouse Sandwich									
	610	26	8	125	50	3	14	45	1750
Premium Buttermilk Crispy Chicken Bacon Clubhouse Sandwich									
	790	40	11	110	67	5	15	40	1620
McChicken®									
	370	17	3.5	40	40	2	5	14	650
Buffalo Ranch McChicken									
	370	17	3.5	40	41	2	5	14	850
Bacon Buffalo Ranch McChicken									
	440	21	5	55	41	2	6	20	1120
Bacon Cheddar McChicken									
	490	25	7	70	43	2	6	22	1120
Southern Style Buttermilk Crispy Chicken Sandwich									
	470	21	4.5	65	46	2	5	25	800
Filet-O-Fish									
	390	19	4	40	39	2	5	15	590
McRib®									
	500	26	10	70	44	3	11	22	980
Premium McWrap Chicken & Bacon (Buttermilk Crispy)									
	690	34	10	100	58	4	6	36	1450
Premium McWrap Chicken & Bacon (Grilled)									
	500	19	8	115	41	3	5	41	1570
Premium McWrap Chicken & Ranch (Buttermilk Crispy)									
	660	34	9	85	59	4	6	31	1250
Premium McWrap Chicken & Ranch (Grilled)									
	470	19	7	100	41	3	5	35	1370
Premium McWrap Chicken Sweet Chili (Buttermilk Crispy)									
	590	25	5	65	64	4	12	27	1160
Premium McWrap Chicken Sweet Chili (Grilled)									
	400	10	3	80	46	3	11	31	1250
Big Mac									
	540	28	10	80	47	3	9	25	970
Quarter Pounder® with Cheese									
	540	28	13	100	42	3	10	31	1110

Food Serving size	Cal.	(g) Total Fat	(g) Sat. Fat	(mg) Chol.	(g) Carb.	(g) Fiber	(g) Sug.	(g) Prot.	(mg) Sod.
Double Quarter Pounder with Cheese									
	780	45	21	175	43	3	10	50	1310
Hamburger									
	250	8	3	30	32	1	6	12	490
Cheeseburger									
	300	12	6	40	33	2	7	15	680
BBQ Ranch Burger									
	350	15	6	45	37	3	7	15	670
Grilled Onion Cheddar									
	310	13	6	45	32	2	6	15	640
Double Cheeseburger									
	440	22	11	85	35	2	7	25	1050
McDouble									
	390	18	8	70	34	2	7	22	850
Bacon McDouble									
	460	23	10	85	34	2	7	28	1120
Daily Double									
	440	24	9	75	34	2	7	22	770
Ranch Snack Wrap® (Buttermilk Crispy)									
	380	21	6	45	33	2	2	16	760
Ranch Snack Wrap® (Grilled)									
	290	13	4.5	55	25	1	2	19	820
Mac Snack Wrap									
	330	19	7	45	26	1	3	14	670
Jalapeño Double									
	440	24	9	75	35	2	6	23	990
Premium Crispy Chicken Deluxe Sandwich									
	530	22	4	45	59	3	13	25	1000
Quarter Pounder Deluxe									
	600	33	14	105	44	3	11	31	1200
Artisan Grilled Chicken Sandwich									
	360	6	1.5	75	43	3	10	33	960
Premium Buttermilk Crispy Chicken Deluxe Sandwich									
	580	24	4.5	65	62	4	11	29	900

Food Serving size	Cal.	(g) Total Fat	(g) Sat. Fat	(mg) Chol.	(g) Carb.	(g) Fiber	(g) Sug.	(g) Prot.	(mg) Sod.
## Chicken & Fish									
Premium Grilled Chicken Bacon Clubhouse Sandwich									
	610	26	8	125	50	3	14	45	1750
Premium Buttermilk Crispy Chicken Bacon Clubhouse Sandwich									
	790	40	11	110	67	5	15	40	1620
McChicken®									
	370	17	3.5	40	40	2	5	14	650
Buffalo Ranch McChicken									
	370	17	3.5	40	41	2	5	14	850
Bacon Buffalo Ranch McChicken									
	440	21	5	55	41	2	6	20	1120
Bacon Cheddar McChicken									
	490	25	7	70	43	2	6	22	1120
Southern Style Buttermilk Crispy Chicken Sandwich									
	470	21	4.5	65	46	2	5	25	800
Filet-O-Fish									
	390	19	4	40	39	2	5	15	590
Premium McWrap Chicken & Bacon (Buttermilk Crispy)									
	690	34	10	100	58	4	6	36	1450
Premium McWrap Chicken & Bacon (Grilled)									
	500	19	8	115	41	3	5	41	1570
Premium McWrap Chicken & Ranch (Buttermilk Crispy)									
	660	34	9	85	59	4	6	31	1250
Premium McWrap Chicken & Ranch (Grilled)									
	470	19	7	100	41	3	5	35	1370
Premium McWrap Chicken Sweet Chili (Buttermilk Crispy)									
	590	25	5	65	64	4	12	27	1160
Premium McWrap Chicken Sweet Chili (Grilled)									
	400	10	3	80	46	3	11	31	1250
Chicken McNuggets® (10 piece)									
	470	30	5	65	30	2	0	22	900
Ranch Snack Wrap® (Buttermilk Crispy)									
	380	21	6	45	33	2	2	16	760
Chicken McNuggets® (20 piece)									
	940	59	10	135	59	3	0	44	1800

Food Serving size	Cal.	(g) Total Fat	(g) Sat. Fat	(mg) Chol.	(g) Carb.	(g) Fiber	(g) Sug.	(g) Prot.	(mg) Sod.
Chicken McNuggets® (6 piece)									
	280	18	3	40	18	1	0	13	540
Artisan Grilled Chicken Sandwich									
	360	6	1.5	75	43	3	10	33	960
Premium Buttermilk Crispy Chicken Deluxe Sandwich									
	580	24	4.5	65	62	4	11	29	900
Bacon Clubhouse Crispy Chicken Sandwich									
	750	38	10	90	65	4	16	36	1720
Premium McWrap Chicken & Bacon (Crispy)									
	640	32	9	80	56	4	7	33	1550
Premium McWrap Chicken & Ranch (Crispy)									
	610	31	8	65	56	4	7	27	1350
Premium McWrap Chicken Sweet Chili (Crispy)									
	540	23	4.5	50	61	4	13	24	1260
Ranch Snack Wrap® (Crispy)									
	360	20	5	40	32	1	3	15	810
Premium Bacon Ranch Salad with Crispy Chicken									
	450	26	8	85	23	3	6	30	1100
Premium Southwest Salad with Crispy Chicken									
	470	24	6	60	41	7	11	25	890

Breakfast

Food Serving size	Cal.	(g) Total Fat	(g) Sat. Fat	(mg) Chol.	(g) Carb.	(g) Fiber	(g) Sug.	(g) Prot.	(mg) Sod.
Fruit 'n Yogurt Parfait									
	150	2	1	5	30	1	23	4	80
Steak, Egg & Cheese Bagel †									
	650	33	14	285	56	4	8	32	1460
Steak & Egg Biscuit (Regular Biscuit)									
	530	32	15	260	37	2	3	25	1420
Sausage McMuffin with Egg									
	470	30	12	275	29	1	2	21	830
Hotcakes and Sausage									
	510	25	8	55	55	2	13	15	830
Bacon, Egg & Cheese McGriddles									
	450	21	9	230	48	2	15	19	1240

Food Serving size	Cal.	(g) Total Fat	(g) Sat. Fat	(mg) Chol.	(g) Carb.	(g) Fiber	(g) Sug.	(g) Prot.	(mg) Sod.
Sausage McGriddles®									
	440	25	9	40	44	2	15	11	990
Sausage, Egg & Cheese McGriddles®									
	570	34	13	250	47	2	15	19	1270
Bacon, Egg & Cheese Bagel with Egg Whites									
	520	22	10	65	55	4	8	26	1280
Big Breakfast® (Regular Size Biscuit)									
	740	48	17	445	50	3	2	25	1480
Big Breakfast with Hotcakes (Regular Size Biscuit)									
	1050	56	19	465	105	5	15	33	2010
Cinnamon Melts									
	460	19	9	15	66	3	32	6	370
Hotcakes									
	320	7	1.5	20	54	2	13	8	530
Egg White Delight									
	250	8	4.5	30	29	1	3	17	740
Hash Browns									
	150	9	1.5	0	15	2	0	1	310
Bacon, Egg & Cheese Biscuit (Large Size Biscuit)									
	530	31	15	230	43	3	4	19	1420
Big Breakfast with Hotcakes (Large Size Biscuit)									
	1130	61	21	465	111	7	16	33	2170
Big Breakfast® (Large Size Biscuit)									
	810	54	19	445	57	4	3	25	1640
Sausage Biscuit (Large Size Biscuit)									
	520	35	14	40	40	3	3	11	1160
Sausage Biscuit with Egg (Large Size Biscuit)									
	600	41	16	235	41	3	3	17	1240
Southern Style Chicken Biscuit (Large Size Biscuit)									
	480	25	10	35	46	3	4	17	1300
Bacon, Egg & Cheese Biscuit with Egg Whites (Large Biscuit)									
	480	26	13	40	42	3	4	19	1410
Sausage McMuffin with Egg Whites									
	430	25	10	60	29	1	2	20	830

Food Serving size	Cal.	(g) Total Fat	(g) Sat. Fat	(mg) Chol.	(g) Carb.	(g) Fiber	(g) Sug.	(g) Prot.	(mg) Sod.
Bacon, Egg & Cheese McGriddles with Egg Whites									
	400	16	7	35	47	2	15	19	1240
Bacon, Egg & Cheese Biscuit with Egg Whites (Regular Biscuit)									
	400	20	11	40	35	2	3	19	1250
Big Breakfast with Egg Whites (Large Size Biscuit)									
	730	46	16	50	55	4	4	24	1630
Big Breakfast with Egg Whites (Regular Size Biscuit)									
	650	40	14	50	49	3	3	24	1470
Big Breakfast with Hotcakes and Egg Whites (Large Biscuit)									
	1050	53	18	70	110	7	16	33	2160
Big Breakfast with Hotcakes and Egg Whites (Regular Biscuit)									
	970	47	16	70	103	5	15	33	2000
Fruit & Maple Oatmeal									
	290	4	1.5	5	58	5	32	5	160
Fruit & Maple Oatmeal without Brown Sugar									
	260	4	1.5	5	49	5	18	5	115
Sausage Biscuit with Egg Whites (Large Size Biscuit)									
	550	35	15	45	40	3	3	17	1240
Sausage Biscuit with Egg Whites (Regular Size Biscuit)									
	470	30	13	45	33	1	2	17	1080
Sausage, Egg & Cheese McGriddles with Egg Whites									
	520	29	11	55	47	2	15	20	1260
Bacon, Egg & Cheese Bagel									
	570	27	12	255	55	4	7	26	1290
Steak, Egg & Cheese McMuffin									
	430	23	10	285	30	2	2	26	970
Sausage McMuffin									
	400	25	10	60	28	1	2	14	750

Salads

Side Salad									
	15	0	0	0	3	2	1	1	10
Premium Bacon Ranch Salad (Without Chicken)									
	190	12	6	40	8	3	3	14	530

Food Serving size	Cal.	(g) Total Fat	(g) Sat. Fat	(mg) Chol.	(g) Carb.	(g) Fiber	(g) Sug.	(g) Prot.	(mg) Sod.
Premium Southwest Salad (Without Chicken)									
	160	7	3	15	18	5	4	8	190
Premium Bacon Ranch Salad with Buttermilk Crispy Chicken									
	490	29	8	100	26	4	4	34	1000
Premium Bacon Ranch Salad with Grilled Chicken									
	310	14	6	115	9	3	3	38	1120
Premium Southwest Salad with Buttermilk Crispy Chicken									
	510	26	6	75	43	7	9	28	790
Premium Southwest Salad with Grilled Chicken									
	330	11	4	90	26	6	9	33	920

Snacks & Sides

Food Serving size	Cal.	(g) Total Fat	(g) Sat. Fat	(mg) Chol.	(g) Carb.	(g) Fiber	(g) Sug.	(g) Prot.	(mg) Sod.
Fruit 'n Yogurt Parfait									
	150	2	1	5	30	1	23	4	80
Small French Fries									
	230	11	1.5	0	30	2	0	2	130
Apple Slices									
	15	0	0	0	4	0	3	0	0
Side Salad									
	15	0	0	0	3	2	1	1	10
Large French Fries									
	510	24	3.5	0	67	5	0	6	290
Medium French Fries									
	340	16	2.5	0	44	4	0	4	190
Kids Fries									
	110	5	1	0	15	1	0	1	65
Ranch Snack Wrap® (Buttermilk Crispy)									
	380	21	6	45	33	2	2	16	760
Ranch Snack Wrap® (Grilled)									
	290	13	4.5	55	25	1	2	19	820
Mac Snack Wrap									
	330	19	7	45	26	1	3	14	670
Go-GURT **Strawberry Flavored Low Fat Yogurt Tube**									
	50	0.5	0	5	9	0	6	2	35

Food Serving size	Cal.	(g) Total Fat	(g) Sat. Fat	(mg) Chol.	(g) Carb.	(g) Fiber	(g) Sug.	(g) Prot.	(mg) Sod.
Cuties									
	40	0	0	0	10	1	8	1	0
Mozzarella Sticks (3 Piece)									
	200	10	4	20	18	1	1	9	560

Beverages

Food Serving size	Cal.	(g) Total Fat	(g) Sat. Fat	(mg) Chol.	(g) Carb.	(g) Fiber	(g) Sug.	(g) Prot.	(mg) Sod.
McCafé Mocha (Small)									
	340	11	7	35	49	2	42	10	150
Coffee (Small)									
	0	0	0	0	0	0	0	0	0
Chocolate McCafé Shake (Small)									
	560	16	10	60	91	1	77	12	240
Vanilla McCafé Shake (Small)									
	530	15	10	60	86	0	63	11	160
Strawberry McCafé Shake (Small)									
	550	16	10	60	90	0	79	12	160
Coffee (Large)									
	0	0	0	0	0	0	0	0	0
Premium Roast Iced Coffee (Small)									
	140	4.5	3	15	23	0	22	1	35
McCafé Caramel Mocha (Small)									
	320	11	7	35	45	1	40	10	170
Frappe Mocha (Small)									
	440	18	11	60	64	1	57	7	125
Frappe Caramel (Small)									
	440	18	12	65	63	0	57	7	125
Frappe Chocolate Chip (Small)									
	520	22	14	65	75	1	66	8	130
Blueberry Pomegranate Smoothie (Small)									
	220	0.5	0	5	50	3	44	2	40
Strawberry Banana Smoothie (Small)									
	210	0.5	0	5	47	3	44	3	50
Mango Pineapple Smoothie (Small)									
	210	0.5	0	5	50	1	46	2	40

Food Serving size	Cal.	(g) Total Fat	(g) Sat. Fat	(mg) Chol.	(g) Carb.	(g) Fiber	(g) Sug.	(g) Prot.	(mg) Sod.
McCafé Hot Chocolate (Small)									
	360	13	8	40	50	1	45	11	180
Minute Maid® 100% Apple Juice Box									
	80	0	0	0	21	0	19	0	15
McCafé Latte (Small)									
	170	9	5	25	15	1	12	9	115
Shamrock McCafe® Shake (Small)									
	530	15	10	60	86	0	73	11	160
McCafé Iced Mocha (Small)									
	290	11	6	35	40	1	34	8	125
McCafé Iced Caramel Mocha (Small)									
	270	11	6	35	37	0	32	8	140
McCafé White Chocolate Mocha (Small)									
	320	11	6	35	47	1	43	11	160
Coffee (Medium)									
	0	0	0	0	0	0	0	0	0
Iced Coffee with Sugar Free French Vanilla Syrup (Large)									
	160	9	6	35	18	0	2	2	135
Iced Coffee with Sugar Free French Vanilla Syrup (Medium)									
	120	7	4.5	25	12	0	2	1	90
Iced Coffee with Sugar Free French Vanilla Syrup (Small)									
	80	4.5	3	15	9	0	1	1	65
Iced Coffee—Caramel (Large)									
	260	9	6	35	43	0	42	2	65
Iced Coffee—Caramel (Medium)									
	180	7	4.5	25	29	0	28	1	50
Iced Coffee—Caramel (Small)									
	130	4.5	3	15	22	0	21	1	35
Iced Coffee—French Vanilla (Large)									
	240	9	6	35	41	0	39	2	80
Iced Coffee—French Vanilla (Medium)									
	170	7	4.5	25	27	0	26	1	55
Iced Coffee—French Vanilla (Small)									
	120	4.5	3	15	20	0	19	1	40

Food Serving size	Cal.	(g) Total Fat	(g) Sat. Fat	(mg) Chol.	(g) Carb.	(g) Fiber	(g) Sug.	(g) Prot.	(mg) Sod.
Iced Coffee—Hazelnut (Large)									
	250	9	6	35	43	0	41	2	75
Iced Coffee—Hazelnut (Medium)									
	180	7	4.5	25	29	0	28	1	50
Iced Coffee—Hazelnut (Small)									
	130	4.5	3	15	21	0	20	1	35
Iced Coffee—Regular (Large)									
	270	9	6	35	47	0	45	2	75
Iced Coffee—Regular (Medium)									
	190	7	4.5	25	31	0	30	1	50
Iced Coffee—Regular (Small)									
	140	4.5	3	15	23	0	22	1	35
Premium Roast Iced Coffee (Large)									
	270	9	6	35	47	0	45	2	75
Premium Roast Iced Coffee (Medium)									
	190	7	4.5	25	31	0	30	1	50
Fat Free Chocolate Milk Jug									
	130	0	0	5	23	1	22	9	135
Minute Maid® Orange Juice (Small)									
	150	0	0	0	34	0	30	2	0
Dasani® Water									
	0	0	0	0	0	0	0	0	0
1% Low Fat Milk Jug									
	100	2.5	1.5	10	12	0	12	8	125
Coca-Cola® Classic (Small)									
	140	0	0	0	39	0	39	0	0
Diet Coke® (Small)									
	0	0	0	0	0	0	0	0	10
Dr Pepper® (Small)									
	140	0	0	0	37	0	35	0	45
Sprite® (Small)									
	140	0	0	0	37	0	37	0	30
Hi-C® Orange Lavaburst (Small)									
	160	0	0	0	43	0	42	0	0

Food Serving size	Cal.	(g) Total Fat	(g) Sat. Fat	(mg) Chol.	(g) Carb.	(g) Fiber	(g) Sug.	(g) Prot.	(mg) Sod.
Iced Tea (Small)									
	0	0	0	0	0	0	0	0	10
Sweet Tea (Small)									
	160	0	0	0	40	0	40	0	10
Minute Maid® Orange Juice (Medium)									
	190	0	0	0	44	0	39	3	0
POWERade® Mountain Blast (Small)									
	80	0	0	0	21	0	21	0	75
Sweet Tea (Medium)									
	220	0	0	0	56	0	56	0	15
Coca-Cola® Classic (Extra Small)									
	100	0	0	0	28	0	28	0	0
Coca-Cola® Classic (Medium)									
	200	0	0	0	55	0	55	0	5
Diet Coke® (Extra Small)									
	0	0	0	0	0	0	0	0	15
Diet Coke® (Medium)									
	0	0	0	0	0	0	0	0	20
Diet Dr Pepper® (Extra Small)									
	0	0	0	0	0	0	0	1	50
Diet Dr Pepper® (Medium)									
	0	0	0	0	0	0	0	3	100
Dr Pepper® (Extra Small)									
	100	0	0	0	27	0	26	0	30
Dr Pepper® (Medium)									
	190	0	0	0	53	0	51	0	65
Hi-C® Orange Lavaburst (Extra Small)									
	110	0	0	0	31	0	31	0	0
Hi-C® Orange Lavaburst (Medium)									
	230	0	0	0	61	0	61	0	0
Iced Tea (Extra Small)									
	0	0	0	0	0	0	0	0	5
Iced Tea (Medium)									
	0	0	0	0	0	0	0	0	10

Food Serving size	Cal.	(g) Total Fat	(g) Sat. Fat	(mg) Chol.	(g) Carb.	(g) Fiber	(g) Sug.	(g) Prot.	(mg) Sod.
Minute Maid® Orange Juice (Large)									
	280	0	0	0	65	0	58	4	0
POWERade® Mountain Blast (Extra Small)									
	60	0	0	0	15	0	15	0	55
POWERade® Mountain Blast (Medium)									
	120	0	0	0	30	0	30	0	105
Sprite® (Extra Small)									
	100	0	0	0	27	0	27	0	25
Sprite® (Large)									
	280	0	0	0	74	0	74	0	60
Sprite® (Medium)									
	200	0	0	0	54	0	54	0	45
Sweet Tea (Extra Small)									
	130	0	0	0	32	0	32	0	0
Sweet Tea (Large)									
	280	0	0	0	71	0	71	1	15
McCafé White Hot Chocolate (Small)									
	350	13	8	40	48	0	46	12	180
McCafé White Hot Chocolate (Medium)									
	420	15	9	50	59	0	57	14	230
Red Flash (Extra Small)									
	110	0	0	0	29	0	29	0	0
Red Flash (Small)									
	150	0	0	0	41	0	41	0	0
Red Flash (Medium)									
	220	0	0	0	58	0	58	0	0
Iced Classic Lemonade (Small)									
	100	0	0	0	25	1	21	0	10
Iced Classic Lemonade (Medium)									
	130	0	0	0	32	1	28	0	15
Iced Classic Lemonade (Large)									
	170	0	0	0	43	1	37	1	15
Frozen Classic Lemonade (Small)									
	160	0	0	0	40	0	36	0	10

Food Serving size	Cal.	(g) Total Fat	(g) Sat. Fat	(mg) Chol.	(g) Carb.	(g) Fiber	(g) Sug.	(g) Prot.	(mg) Sod.
Frozen Classic Lemonade (Medium)									
	200	0	0	0	50	0	44	0	15
Frozen Classic Lemonade (Large)									
	250	0	0	0	63	0	56	0	15
Iced Strawberry Lemonade (Small)									
	120	0	0	0	32	1	28	1	10
Iced Strawberry Lemonade (Medium)									
	160	0	0	0	43	1	37	1	15
Southern Style Iced Lemonade (Medium)									
	180	0	0	0	48	0	43	0	135
Oreo Frappe (Small)									
	540	20	12	60	82	1	68	7	170
Oreo Frappe (Medium)									
	650	24	14	75	102	1	84	9	200
Oreo Frappe (Large)									
	810	28	17	90	128	1	106	11	240

McCafé

Food Serving size	Cal.	Total Fat	Sat. Fat	Chol.	Carb.	Fiber	Sug.	Prot.	Sod.
McCafé Mocha (Small)									
	340	11	7	35	49	2	42	10	150
Coffee (Small)									
	0	0	0	0	0	0	0	0	0
Mango Pineapple Smoothie (Small)									
	210	0.5	0	5	50	1	46	2	40
McCafé Hot Chocolate (Small)									
	360	13	8	40	50	1	45	11	180
McCafé Latte (Small)									
	170	9	5	25	15	1	12	9	11
Shamrock McCafe® Shake (Small)									
	530	15	10	60	86	0	73	11	160
McCafé Iced Mocha (Small)									
	290	11	6	35	40	1	34	8	125
McCafé Hot Chocolate (Medium)									
	440	16	9	50	61	1	56	14	220

Food Serving size	Cal.	(g) Total Fat	(g) Sat. Fat	(mg) Chol.	(g) Carb.	(g) Fiber	(g) Sug.	(g) Prot.	(mg) Sod.
McCafé White Chocolate Mocha (Large)									
	480	16	9	50	70	1	65	17	250
McCafé Latte (Medium)									
	210	10	6	30	18	1	15	11	140
McCafé White Chocolate Mocha (Small)									
	320	11	6	35	47	1	43	11	160
Nonfat Latte (Medium)									
	130	0	0	5	19	1	16	12	135
Nonfat Latte with Sugar Free French Vanilla Syrup (Medium)									
	170	0	0	5	30	1	16	12	180
McCafé Caramel Mocha (Medium)									
	390	14	8	40	55	1	50	12	220
Hot Chocolate (Small)									
	360	13	8	40	50	1	45	11	180
Hot Chocolate (Medium)									
	440	16	9	50	61	1	56	14	220
Hot Chocolate (Large)									
	540	20	12	60	73	1	68	17	280
Hot Chocolate with Nonfat Milk (Small)									
	280	3.5	2	15	50	1	46	12	180
Hot Chocolate with Nonfat Milk (Medium)									
	340	3.5	2	15	61	1	57	14	220
Blueberry Pomegranate Smoothie (Medium)									
	260	1	0	5	62	4	54	3	50
Coffee (Medium)									
	0	0	0	0	0	0	0	0	0
Mango Pineapple Smoothie (Medium)									
	260	1	0	5	61	1	56	3	45
Iced Mocha (Medium)									
	340	12	7	40	49	1	43	9	150
Latte (Medium)									
	210	10	6	30	18	1	15	11	140
Caramel Latte (Medium)									
	340	10	6	30	50	1	48	11	140

Food Serving size	Cal.	(g) Total. Fat	(g) Sat. Fat	(mg) Chol.	(g) Carb.	(g) Fiber	(g) Sug.	(g) Prot.	(mg) Sod.
Caramel Latte (Small)									
	270	9	5	·25	40	1	38	9	115
Hazelnut Latte (Small)									
	270	9	5	25	40	1	38	9	115
Nonfat Latte (Small)									
	100	0	0	5	15	1	13	10	110
White Hot Chocolate (Small)									
	350	13	8	40	48	0	46	12	180
White Hot Chocolate (Medium)									
	420	15	9	50	59	0	57	14	230
Nonfat White Hot Chocolate (Small)									
	260	3	2	15	48	0	46	12	180
Nonfat White Hot Chocolate (Medium)									
	320	3	2	20	59	0	58	15	220
Iced Classic Lemonade (Small)									
	100	0	0	0	25	1	21	0	10
Frozen Classic Lemonade (Small)									
	160	0	0	0	40	0	36	0	10
Iced Strawberry Lemonade (Small)									
	120	0	0	0	32	1	28	1	10
Frozen Strawberry Lemonade (Small)									
	180	0	0	0	48	0	43	1	10

Desserts & Shakes

Food	Cal.	Total. Fat	Sat. Fat	Chol.	Carb.	Fiber	Sug.	Prot.	Sod.
Baked Hot Apple Pie									
	230	10	5	0	32	4	13	2	160
Chocolate Chip Cookie									
	160	8	3.5	10	21	1	15	2	90
Oatmeal Raisin Cookie									
	150	6	2.5	10	22	1	13	2	135
Fruit 'n Yogurt Parfait									
	150	2	1	5	30	1	23	4	80
McFlurry® with M&M'S® Chocolate Candies (12 fl oz cup)									
	650	23	14	50	96	1	89	13	180

Food Serving size	Cal.	(g) Total Fat	(g) Sat. Fat	(mg) Chol.	(g) Carb.	(g) Fiber	(g) Sug.	(g) Prot.	(mg) Sod.
McFlurry® with OREO® Cookies (12 fl oz cup)									
	520	17	9	45	80	1	64	12	260
Chocolate McCafé Shake (Small)									
	560	16	10	60	91	1	77	12	240
Vanilla McCafé Shake (Small)									
	530	15	10	60	86	0	63	11	160
Strawberry McCafé Shake (Small)									
	550	16	10	60	90	0	79	12	160
Strawberry Crème Pie									
	310	17	9	10	36	1	15	4	180
Fried Cherry Pie									
	230	10	3.5	0	33	1	15	2	135
Sweet Potato and Creme Pie									
	290	15	9	15	34	2	13	3	170
Pumpkin and Creme Pie									
	270	15	8	10	32	2	12	3	160

Condiments

Food Serving size	Cal.	(g) Total Fat	(g) Sat. Fat	(mg) Chol.	(g) Carb.	(g) Fiber	(g) Sug.	(g) Prot.	(mg) Sod.
Newman's Own® Creamy Southwest Dressing									
	120	8	1.5	20	11	0	3	1	300
Newman's Own® Low Fat Family Recipe Italian Dressing									
	50	1.5	0	0	8	1	2	0	380
Salt Packet									
	0	0	0	0	0	0	0	0	270
Honey									
	50	0	0	0	12	0	11	0	0
Newman's Own® Ranch Dressing									
	200	17	2.5	20	11	1	4	1	530
Sweet 'N Sour Sauce									
	50	0	0	0	12	0	10	0	150
Hotcake Syrup									
	180	0	0	0	44	0	34	0	0
Peanuts (for Sundaes)									
	45	3.5	0.5	0	2	1	0	2	0

Food Serving size	Cal.	(g) Total Fat	(g) Sat. Fat	(mg) Chol.	(g) Carb.	(g) Fiber	(g) Sug.	(g) Prot.	(mg) Sod.
Honey Mustard Sauce									
	60	4	0.5	5	6	1	5	0	115
Tangy Barbeque Sauce									
	50	0	0	0	12	0	10	0	260
Buffalo Ranch McChicken									
	370	17	3.5	40	41	2	5	14	850
Whipped Butter (1 pat)									
	40	4.5	2.5	15	0	0	0	0	35
Tartar Sauce Cup									
	140	15	2.5	10	0	0	0	0	150
Marinara Sauce (Package)									
	15	0	0	0	2	0	2	0	75

All Day Breakfast

Food Serving size	Cal.	(g) Total Fat	(g) Sat. Fat	(mg) Chol.	(g) Carb.	(g) Fiber	(g) Sug.	(g) Prot.	(mg) Sod.
Fruit 'n Yogurt Parfait									
	150	2	1	5	30	1	23	4	80
Sausage McMuffin with Egg									
	470	30	12	275	29	1	2	21	830
Hotcakes and Sausage									
	510	25	8	55	55	2	13	15	830
Egg McMuffin®									
	300	12	6	245	29	1	2	17	730
Fruit & Maple Oatmeal									
	290	4	1.5	5	58	5	32	5	160
Sausage McMuffin									
	400	25	10	60	28	1	2	14	750

Pizza Hut

6" Personal Pan Pizza®

Food Serving size	Cal.	(g) Total Fat	(g) Sat. Fat	(mg) Chol.	(g) Carb.	(g) Fiber	(g) Sug.	(g) Prot.	(mg) Sod.
Pepperoni Lover's®									
	730	37	16	85	69	4	7	31	1980
Sweet Sriracha Dynamite									
	600	21	8	55	77	4	13	28	1690

Food Serving size	Cal.	(g) Total Fat	(g) Sat. Fat	(mg) Chol.	(g) Carb.	(g) Fiber	(g) Sug.	(g) Prot.	(mg) Sod.
Ultimate Cheese Lover's®									
	680	32	14	65	68	3	6	29	1450
Veggie Lover's®									
	550	20	8	35	70	5	8	22	1290

12" Medium Pan Pizza

Food Serving size	Cal.	(g) Total Fat	(g) Sat. Fat	(mg) Chol.	(g) Carb.	(g) Fiber	(g) Sug.	(g) Prot.	(mg) Sod.
7-Alarm Fire™									
	250	11	4	20	29	2	2	9	660
BBQ Bacon Cheeseburger									
	280	13	5	25	32	1	4	11	500
BBQ Lover's™									
	290	13	5	25	31	1	4	11	570
Buffalo State of Mind™									
	250	10	4	20	30	1	1	10	630
Cheese									
	240	10	4.5	20	28	1	1	10	500
Cherry Pepper Bombshell™									
	250	11	4.5	20	29	2	2	10	530
Cock-A-Doodle Bacon™									
	240	9	4	25	27	1	1	12	510
Garden Party™									
	230	9	3.5	15	30	2	3	9	450
Giddy-Up BBQ Chicken™									
	270	11	4	25	31	1	4	11	490
Hot and Twisted™									
	240	10	3.5	15	28	2	2	9	740
Meat Lover's®									
	310	17	6	35	27	1	1	13	750
Old Fashioned Meatbrawl™									
	250	11	4	20	28	2	1	10	500
Pepperoni									
	260	12	4.5	25	27	1	1	10	610
Pepperoni Lover's®									
	310	16	7	35	28	2	1	12	780

Food Serving size	Cal.	(g) Total Fat	(g) Sat. Fat	(mg) Chol.	(g) Carb.	(g) Fiber	(g) Sug.	(g) Prot.	(mg) Sod.
Pretzel Piggy™									
	260	12	4	20	28	1	1	9	590
Supreme									
	270	13	4.5	25	28	2	1	10	570
Sweet Sriracha Dynamite									
	240	9	3	20	32	2	4	10	650
Ultimate Cheese Lover's®									
	270	13	5	25	27	1	1	11	510
Veggie Lover's®									
	220	9	3	15	28	2	1	8	460

12" Medium Hand Tossed Pizza

Food Serving size	Cal.	(g) Total Fat	(g) Sat. Fat	(mg) Chol.	(g) Carb.	(g) Fiber	(g) Sug.	(g) Prot.	(mg) Sod.
7-Alarm Fire™									
	210	8	3.5	20	26	2	2	9	620
BBQ Bacon Cheeseburger									
	250	10	4.5	25	29	1	4	10	460
BBQ Lover's™									
	250	10	4.5	25	28	1	4	11	520
Buffalo State of Mind™									
	210	7	3.5	20	27	1	1	10	590
Meat Lover's®									
	280	15	6	35	25	1	1	12	710
Old Fashioned Meatbrawl™									
	220	9	4	20	26	2	1	9	450
Pepperoni									
	220	9	4	25	25	1	1	9	540
Pepperoni Lover's®									
	270	13	6	35	26	1	1	12	700
Pretzel Piggy™									
	220	9	4	20	25	1	1	9	550
Supreme									
	240	10	4.5	25	26	2	1	10	530
Sweet Sriracha Dynamite									
	210	6	3	20	30	1	4	9	600

Food Serving size	Cal.	(g) Total Fat	(g) Sat. Fat	(mg) Chol.	(g) Carb.	(g) Fiber	(g) Sug.	(g) Prot.	(mg) Sod.
Ultimate Cheese Lover's®	230	10	5	25	25	1	1	10	460
Veggie Lover's®	190	6	3	15	26	2	1	8	430

12" Medium Thin 'N Crispy® Pizza

Food Serving size	Cal.	(g) Total Fat	(g) Sat. Fat	(mg) Chol.	(g) Carb.	(g) Fiber	(g) Sug.	(g) Prot.	(mg) Sod.
7-Alarm Fire™	200	8	3.5	20	23	1	5	8	800
BBQ Bacon Cheeseburger	240	11	5	25	26	1	7	9	580
BBQ Lover's™	240	11	5	30	25	1	7	10	650
Garden Party™	190	7	3	15	24	2	6	8	530
Giddy-Up BBQ Chicken™	220	9	4	25	25	1	7	10	570
Hot and Twisted™	190	8	3.5	15	23	1	5	8	860
Meat Lover's®	270	15	6	35	22	1	4	12	850
Old Fashioned Meatbrawl™	210	9	4	20	23	1	4	8	580
Pepperoni	210	10	4.5	25	21	1	4	9	700
Pepperoni Lover's®	260	14	6	35	22	1	4	11	860
Pretzel Piggy™	220	11	4	20	22	1	4	8	690
Supreme	220	10	4.5	25	23	1	4	9	660
Sweet Sriracha Dynamite	190	6	3	20	26	1	7	9	750
Ultimate Cheese Lover's®	220	11	5	25	21	1	4	10	590

Food Serving size	Cal.	(g) Total Fat	(g) Sat. Fat	(mg) Chol.	(g) Carb.	(g) Fiber	(g) Sug.	(g) Prot.	(mg) Sod.
Veggie Lover's®									
	180	6	3	15	23	2	5	7	570

14" Large Pan Pizza

7-Alarm Fire™									
	360	17	6	25	37	2	3	13	930
BBQ Bacon Cheeseburger									
	410	20	7	35	43	1	7	15	730
BBQ Lover's™									
	410	20	7	40	41	1	6	16	830
Buffalo State of Mind™									
	360	16	6	30	39	1	2	15	940
Cheese									
	350	17	7	30	36	1	1	14	730
Cherry Pepper Bombshell™									
	360	17	6	25	38	2	3	14	750
Cock-A-Doodle Bacon™									
	380	19	7	35	35	1	1	17	730
Garden Party™									
	330	15	5	20	38	2	3	13	630
Giddy-Up BBQ Chicken™									
	380	17	6	35	42	1	6	16	710
Hot and Twisted™									
	350	16	6	25	36	2	2	13	1010
Meat Lover's®									
	460	27	9	50	36	1	1	18	1090
Old Fashioned Meatbrawl™									
	370	18	6	30	37	2	2	14	720
Pepperoni									
	370	19	7	35	35	1	1	14	870
Pepperoni Lover's®									
	440	25	10	50	36	1	1	18	1110
Pretzel Piggy™									
	360	19	6	25	36	1	2	13	810

Food Serving size	Cal.	(g) Total Fat	(g) Sat. Fat	(mg) Chol.	(g) Carb.	(g) Fiber	(g) Sug.	(g) Prot.	(mg) Sod.
Supreme	390	20	7	35	37	2	2	15	840
Sweet Sriracha Dynamite	350	14	5	30	42	1	5	14	920
Ultimate Cheese Lover's®	380	20	8	35	35	1	1	15	720
Veggie Lover's®	320	14	5	20	37	2	2	12	670

14" Large Original Stuffed Crust™ Pizza

Food Serving size	Cal.	(g) Total Fat	(g) Sat. Fat	(mg) Chol.	(g) Carb.	(g) Fiber	(g) Sug.	(g) Prot.	(mg) Sod.
7-Alarm Fire™	320	14	7	40	36	2	3	14	950
BBQ Bacon Cheeseburger	380	17	8	45	42	2	7	15	760
Cherry Pepper Bombshell™	330	14	7	40	37	2	3	15	780
Cock-A-Doodle Bacon™	350	16	7	45	34	2	1	17	750
Garden Party™	300	12	6	30	37	2	4	13	660
Giddy-Up BBQ Chicken™	350	14	7	45	41	2	6	16	740
Hot and Twisted™	310	13	6	35	35	2	2	14	1030
Meat Lover's®	430	24	10	60	35	2	2	19	1120
Old Fashioned Meatbrawl™	340	15	7	40	36	2	2	15	750
Pepperoni	340	16	8	45	34	2	2	14	870
Pepperoni Lover's®	390	21	10	55	35	2	2	17	1070
Pretzel Piggy™	330	15	7	35	35	2	2	14	830

Food Serving size	Cal.	(g) Total Fat	(g) Sat. Fat	(mg) Chol.	(g) Carb.	(g) Fiber	(g) Sug.	(g) Prot.	(mg) Sod.
Supreme									
	360	18	8	45	36	2	2	15	870
Sweet Sriracha Dynamite									
	320	11	6	40	41	2	6	15	940
Ultimate Cheese Lover's®									
	340	16	8	40	34	1	1	15	720
Veggie Lover's®									
	300	12	6	30	36	2	2	13	700

14" Large Hand Tossed Pizza

Food Serving size	Cal.	(g) Total Fat	(g) Sat. Fat	(mg) Chol.	(g) Carb.	(g) Fiber	(g) Sug.	(g) Prot.	(mg) Sod.
7-Alarm Fire™									
	290	11	5	25	35	2	3	12	850
BBQ Bacon Cheeseburger									
	340	14	6	35	40	2	7	14	640
BBQ Lover's™									
	340	15	6	40	39	1	6	15	740
Meat Lover's®									
	390	21	9	50	34	2	1	17	1010
Old Fashioned Meatbrawl™									
	300	12	6	30	35	2	2	13	620
Pepperoni									
	300	13	6	30	33	2	1	13	750
Pepperoni Lover's®									
	370	19	9	50	34	2	1	16	990
Pretzel Piggy™									
	300	13	5	25	34	2	2	12	720
Supreme									
	330	15	6	35	34	2	2	14	750
Sweet Sriracha Dynamite									
	280	8	4	30	40	2	6	13	840
Ultimate Cheese Lover's®									
	310	14	7	35	33	1	1	14	630
Veggie Lover's®									
	260	9	4	20	35	2	2	11	590

Food Serving size	Cal.	(g) Total Fat	(g) Sat. Fat	(mg) Chol.	(g) Carb.	(g) Fiber	(g) Sug.	(g) Prot.	(mg) Sod.
14" Large Thin 'N Crispy® Pizza									
7-Alarm Fire™	270	12	5	25	30	2	7	11	1060
BBQ Bacon Cheeseburger	320	15	7	35	35	1	10	13	800
BBQ Lover's™	330	15	7	40	33	1	9	14	890
Garden Party™	250	9	4	20	31	2	7	10	700
Giddy-Up BBQ Chicken™	300	12	5	35	34	1	10	14	780
Hot and Twisted™	260	11	4.5	25	30	2	6	11	1120
Meat Lover's®	370	22	9	50	28	1	5	16	1180
Old Fashioned Meatbrawl™	280	12	6	30	30	2	6	12	790
Pepperoni	280	14	6	35	28	1	5	12	940
Pepperoni Lover's®	350	19	9	50	29	1	5	15	1180
Pretzel Piggy™	290	14	6	25	28	1	5	11	890
Supreme	300	15	6	35	30	2	6	13	910
Sweet Sriracha Dynamite	260	9	4	30	35	1	10	12	1010
Ultimate Cheese Lover's®	290	15	7	35	28	1	5	13	780
Veggie Lover's®	240	9	4	20	30	2	6	10	760
Skinny Beach™	200	6	3	20	27	2	2	10	440
Skinny Club™	230	9	4	25	25	1	1	12	540

Food Serving size	Cal.	(g) Total Fat	(g) Sat. Fat	(mg) Chol.	(g) Carb.	(g) Fiber	(g) Sug.	(g) Prot.	(mg) Sod.
Skinny Italy									
	220	8	3.5	20	28	2	3	9	460
Skinny Luau™									
	210	6	3	20	27	2	3	11	530
Skinny with a Kick™									
	230	9	4	20	28	2	3	9	680

Rectangular/Dinner Box Pizza

Food	Cal.	Total Fat	Sat. Fat	Chol.	Carb.	Fiber	Sug.	Prot.	Sod.
7-Alarm Fire™									
	250	11	4	20	30	2	2	9	670
Pretzel Piggy™									
	260	12	4	20	29	1	1	9	620
Supreme									
	270	13	5	25	29	2	1	10	600
Sweet Sriracha Dynamite									
	250	9	3.5	20	33	2	4	10	670
Ultimate Cheese Lover's®									
	270	13	5	25	28	1	1	11	540
Veggie Lover's®									
	230	9	3	15	29	2	1	9	490
Creamy Chicken Alfredo									
	510	26	7	40	47	3	3	22	900
Meaty Marinara									
	450	19	8	45	48	3	9	21	1000

Appetizers/Sides

Food	Cal.	Total Fat	Sat. Fat	Chol.	Carb.	Fiber	Sug.	Prot.	Sod.
Baked Hot Wings (2 pieces)									
	100	7	2	55	0	0	0	10	420
Baked Mild Wings (2 pieces)									
	110	7	2	55	1	0	0	10	430
Baked Boneless Wings (2 pieces)									
	100	3	0.5	15	10	0	0	9	450
Breadsticks (each)									
	130	4.5	1	0	19	1	1	4	260
Cheese Sticks (each)									
	160	6	2.5	10	20	1	1	7	370

Food Serving size	Cal.	(g) Total Fat	(g) Sat. Fat	(mg) Chol.	(g) Carb.	(g) Fiber	(g) Sug.	(g) Prot.	(mg) Sod.
Fiery Red Pepper Flavor Sticks (each)									
	140	4.5	1	0	20	1	1	4	220
Honey Sriracha Flavor Sticks (each)									
	120	3	0.5	0	20	1	2	4	240
Hut Favorite Flavor Sticks (each)									
	130	4	1	0	20	1	1	4	230
Toasted Asiago Flavor Sticks (each)									
	140	4.5	1.5	5	19	1	1	5	250
Toasted Cheddar Flavor Sticks (each)									
	140	4	1.5	5	19	1	1	5	220
Toasted Parmesan Flavor Sticks (each)									
	140	4	1	5	19	1	1	5	250
Waffle Fries (side order)									
	660	41	8	10	66	7	0	8	440

Condiments/Dipping Sauces

Ranch Dipping Sauce (1.5 oz)									
	220	23	3.5	10	2	0	1	0	420
Blue Cheese Dipping Sauce (1.5 oz)									
	230	24	4.5	20	2	0	2	1	420
Marinara Dipping Sauce (3 oz)									
	45	0	0	0	9	2	6	1	290
Buffalo Wing Sauce for Baked Boneless Wings (3 oz)									
	20	1	0	0	2	1	0	1	2210
BBQ Wing Sauce for Baked Boneless Wings (3 oz)									
	170	0	0	0	40	1	29	1	870

Desserts

Cinnamon Sticks (2 pieces)									
	160	4.5	0.5	0	26	1	8	4	200
White Icing Dipping Sauce (2 oz)									
	170	0	0	0	44	0	38	0	5
HERSHEY'S® Chocolate Dunkers® (2 pieces)									
	190	8	3	0	26	1	9	5	210
HERSHEY'S® Chocolate Dipping Sauce (1.5 oz)									
	120	2	1	0	25	1	19	1	65

Food Serving size	Cal.	(g) Total Fat	(g) Sat. Fat	(mg) Chol.	(g) Carb.	(g) Fiber	(g) Sug.	(g) Prot.	(mg) Sod.
The Ultimate HERSHEY'S® Chocolate Chip Cookie (1 piece)									
	180	9	4.5	10	24	2	16	2	110

WingStreet® Bone-Out Wings

Food Serving size	Cal.	(g) Total Fat	(g) Sat. Fat	(mg) Chol.	(g) Carb.	(g) Fiber	(g) Sug.	(g) Prot.	(mg) Sod.
Buffalo Burnin' Hot									
	200	9	2	25	18	1	2	10	860
Buffalo Medium									
	200	9	2	25	18	1	2	10	840
Buffalo Mild									
	200	9	2	25	18	1	2	10	870
Garlic Parmesan									
	260	20	3.5	25	11	1	1	10	560
Honey BBQ									
	230	9	1.5	25	27	1	12	10	570
Honey Sriracha									
	190	9	1.5	25	18	1	4	10	620
Naked									
	160	9	1.5	25	11	1	0	10	340
Spicy BBQ									
	210	9	1.5	25	23	1	9	10	640
Sweet Chili									
	220	9	1.5	25	24	1	13	10	540

WingStreet® Breaded Bone-In Wings

Food Serving size	Cal.	(g) Total Fat	(g) Sat. Fat	(mg) Chol.	(g) Carb.	(g) Fiber	(g) Sug.	(g) Prot.	(mg) Sod.
Buffalo Burnin' Hot									
	220	12	2.5	40	19	1	2	9	820
Buffalo Medium									
	220	12	2.5	40	19	1	2	9	800
Buffalo Mild									
	220	12	2.5	40	19	1	2	9	840
Naked									
	180	12	2.5	40	11	1	0	9	300
Spicy BBQ									
	230	12	2.5	40	24	1	9	9	600
Sweet Chili									
	240	12	2.5	40	25	1	13	9	500

Food Serving size	Cal.	(g) Total Fat	(g) Sat. Fat	(mg) Chol.	(g) Carb.	(g) Fiber	(g) Sug.	(g) Prot.	(mg) Sod.
WingStreet® Traditional Wings									
Buffalo Burnin' Hot	130	7	1.5	45	8	0	2	10	770
Buffalo Medium	130	7	1.5	45	8	0	2	10	760
Buffalo Mild	130	7	1.5	45	8	0	2	10	790
Garlic Parmesan	200	17	3.5	45	1	0	0	11	480
Honey BBQ	160	6	1.5	45	16	0	12	11	490
Honey Sriracha	120	6	1.5	45	7	0	4	10	530
Naked	90	6	1.5	45	0	0	0	10	250
Spicy BBQ	140	6	1.5	45	12	0	9	10	550
Sweet Chili	150	6	1.5	45	13	0	13	11	460
Beverages									
Mountain Dew®	110	0	0	0	31	0	31	0	40
Mountain Dew®	290	0	0	0	77	0	77	0	100
Pepsi®	100	0	0	0	28	0	28	0	20
Pepsi®	250	0	0	0	69	0	69	0	55
Diet Pepsi®	0	0	0	0	0	0	0	0	25
Diet Pepsi®	0	0	0	0	0	0	0	0	60
Sierra Mist®	100	0	0	0	27	0	27	0	20

Food Serving size	Cal.	(g) Total Fat	(g) Sat. Fat	(mg) Chol.	(g) Carb.	(g) Fiber	(g) Sug.	(g) Prot.	(mg) Sod.

Subway

Sandwiches

Food Serving size	Cal.	Total Fat	Sat. Fat	Chol.	Carb.	Fiber	Sug.	Prot.	Sod.
6" Black Forest Ham	290	4.5	1	25	46	5	8	18	800
6" Oven Roasted Chicken	320	5	1.5	45	45	5	7	23	610
6" Roast Beef	320	5	1.5	45	45	5	7	24	660
6" Subway Club®	310	4.5	1.5	40	46	5	7	23	840
6" Sweet Onion Chicken Teriyaki	370	4.5	1	50	57	5	16	25	770
6" Turkey Breast	280	3.5	1	20	46	5	7	18	760
6" Turkey Breast & Black Forest Ham	280	4	1	20	46	5	8	18	780
6" Veggie Delite®	230	2.5	0.5	0	44	5	6	8	280
6" Chicken & Bacon Ranch Melt	610	30	10	95	47	5	8	38	1290
6" Cold Cut Combo	360	12	4	45	46	5	7	17	1030
6" Italian B.M.T.®	410	16	6	45	46	5	8	20	1260
6" Meatball Marinara	480	18	7	30	59	8	12	21	920
6" Spicy Italian	480	24	9	50	46	5	8	20	1490
6" Steak & Cheese	380	10	4.5	50	48	5	9	26	1030
6" Tuna	480	25	4.5	40	44	5	7	20	580

Food Serving size	Cal.	(g) Total Fat	(g) Sat. Fat	(mg) Chol.	(g) Carb.	(g) Fiber	(g) Sug.	(g) Prot.	(mg) Sod.
Kids Meal Sandwiches									
Veggie Delite®									
	150	1.5	0	0	29	3	4	6	190
Black Forest Ham									
	180	2.5	0.5	10	30	3	5	10	450
Roast Beef									
	200	3	1	25	30	4	5	14	390
Turkey Breast									
	180	2	0.5	10	30	3	5	10	430
6" Limited Time Offer/Regional Subs									
6" Barbecue Rib Patty									
	430	18	6	50	47	5	8	19	590
6" Big Philly Cheesesteak									
	500	17	9	85	51	6	9	38	1280
6" B.L.T.									
	380	13	5	20	44	5	7	20	1130
6" Buffalo Chicken (with regular Ranch dressing)									
	420	16	3	55	46	6	8	25	1100
6" Chicken Pizziola Melt									
	460	16	6	80	49	6	9	32	1140
6" Pastrami Melt, Big Hot									
	580	28	11	85	47	5	8	29	1470
6" Subway Melt®									
	410	13	5	40	47	5	8	26	1410
6" Subway Seafood Sensation™									
	420	19	3	15	51	5	8	13	780
6" Turkey & Bacon Avocado									
	420	14	3.5	30	50	7	8	24	1190
6" Veggie Patty									
	390	7	1	10	56	8	8	23	800
Salads									
Black Forest Ham									
	110	3	1	25	12	4	6	12	600

Food Serving size	Cal.	(g) Total Fat	(g) Sat. Fat	(mg) Chol.	(g) Carb.	(g) Fiber	(g) Sug.	(g) Prot.	(mg) Sod.
Double Chicken	220	4.5	1.5	100	10	4	4	36	490
Oven Roasted Chicken Breast	130	2.5	0.5	50	10	4	4	19	280
Roast Beef	140	3.5	1	45	11	4	5	19	460
Subway Club®	140	3.5	1	40	12	4	5	18	640
Sweet Onion Chicken Teriyaki (includes sweet onion dressing)	240	3	1	50	34	4	22	20	720
Turkey Breast	110	2	0.5	20	12	4	5	12	560
Turkey Breast & Ham	110	2.5	0.5	20	12	4	5	12	580
Veggie Delite®	50	1	0	0	9	4	4	3	80
Chicken & Bacon Ranch Melt (includes Ranch dressing)	540	40	12	100	14	4	7	32	1290
Cold Cut Combo	180	11	4	45	12	4	5	12	820
Italian B.M.T.®	230	15	6	45	12	4	6	14	1060
Meatball Marinara	310	17	7	30	25	6	10	16	720
Spicy Italian	310	23	9	50	11	4	6	15	1280
Steak & Cheese	210	8	4	50	14	4	6	20	830
Tuna	310	24	4	40	10	4	4	15	370

Salad Dressings (amount mixed into chopped salad)

Food Serving size	Cal.	(g) Total Fat	(g) Sat. Fat	(mg) Chol.	(g) Carb.	(g) Fiber	(g) Sug.	(g) Prot.	(mg) Sod.
Chipotle Southwest	190	20	3.5	15	2	0	1	1	330

Food Serving size	Cal.	(g) Total Fat	(g) Sat. Fat	(mg) Chol.	(g) Carb.	(g) Fiber	(g) Sug.	(g) Prot.	(mg) Sod.
Honey Mustard									
	60	1	0	0	13	0	11	0	240
Oil & Vinegar									
	190	21	1.5	0	0	0	0	0	0
Ranch									
	220	23	3.5	10	2	0	2	0	400
Subway® Vinaigrette									
	110	11	2	0	3	0	2	0	330
Sweet Onion									
	80	0	0	0	18	0	16	0	170

Breakfast

Food Serving size	Cal.	Total Fat	Sat. Fat	Chol.	Carb.	Fiber	Sug.	Prot.	Sod.
6" Egg White & Cheese									
	320	8	3	10	44	4	5	19	910
6" Egg White & Cheese (with Ham)									
	350	9	3.5	25	45	4	6	24	1170
6" Bacon, Egg White & Cheese									
	400	13	5	20	45	4	5	25	1330
6" Mega Melt									
	500	20	7	45	46	4	6	33	1650
6" Sausage, Egg White & Cheese									
	420	15	5	35	45	4	5	27	1220
6" Steak, Egg White & Cheese									
	390	10	4	35	47	4	6	28	1240
6" Turkey, Egg White & Cheese									
	350	8	3	20	45	4	5	24	1150
6" Egg & Cheese									
	360	12	4.5	230	44	5	6	19	860
6" Egg & Cheese (with Ham)									
	390	13	5	240	45	5	7	24	1120
6" Bacon, Egg & Cheese									
	440	17	7	240	45	5	7	25	1280
6" Mega Melt									
	580	28	11	270	46	5	7	35	1800

Food Serving size	Cal.	(g) Total Fat	(g) Sat. Fat	(mg) Chol.	(g) Carb.	(g) Fiber	(g) Sug.	(g) Prot.	(mg) Sod.
6" Sausage, Egg & Cheese									
	500	23	9	265	45	5	7	29	1380
6" Steak, Egg & Cheese									
	430	15	6	255	47	5	7	28	1190
6" Turkey, Egg & Cheese									
	390	13	4.5	240	45	5	6	24	1100

Breakfast Sides

Hash Browns									
	210	10	2.5	0	28	3	0	2	610

Flatizza™

Cheese									
	390	16	8	35	42	2	3	21	810
Pepperoni									
	500	26	12	60	43	2	4	26	1340
Spicy Italian									
	490	25	11	60	43	2	4	25	1290
Veggie									
	410	17	8	35	44	3	4	21	850

8" Pizza

Cheese									
	680	22	9	40	96	4	7	32	1070
Cheese & Veggies									
	740	25	11	50	100	5	9	36	1270
Pepperoni									
	790	32	13	60	96	4	8	38	1350

Breads

6" Italian (White) Bread									
	200	2	0.5	0	38	1	5	7	270
6" 9-Grain Wheat Bread									
	210	2	0.5	0	40	4	5	8	270
6" Parmesan Oregano Bread									
	220	2.5	1	0	40	2	5	8	420

Food Serving size	Cal.	(g) Total Fat	(g) Sat. Fat	(mg) Chol.	(g) Carb.	(g) Fiber	(g) Sug.	(g) Prot.	(mg) Sod.
6" Honey Oat 9-Grain Wheat Bread									
	230	3	0.5	0	43	4	6	8	280
6" Hearty Italian Bread									
	210	2.5	0.5	0	41	2	5	7	270
6" Monterey Cheddar									
	240	6	2.5	10	38	2	5	10	340
6" Italian Herbs & Cheese									
	250	5	2.5	10	40	2	5	9	470
6" Roasted Garlic									
	230	2.5	0.5	0	45	2	7	8	1240
6" Sourdough									
	190	1.5	0	0	36	1	3	9	310
6" Flatbread, Multigrain									
	220	5	1	0	37	6	3	8	280
6" Flatbread, White									
	220	4.5	1	0	38	2	2	7	340
Mini Italian Bread									
	130	1.5	0	0	25	1	3	5	180
Mini Wheat Bread									
	140	1.5	0	0	27	3	3	5	180
Wrap									
	310	8	2.5	0	51	1	0	8	610

Condiments

Food Serving size	Cal.	(g) Total Fat	(g) Sat. Fat	(mg) Chol.	(g) Carb.	(g) Fiber	(g) Sug.	(g) Prot.	(mg) Sod.
Bacon (2 strips)									
	80	5.5	2	10	1	0	1	6	420
Buffalo Sauce									
	5	0	0	0	<1	0	0	0	400
Chipotle Southwest Sauce									
	100	10	1.5	5	1	0	<1	0	160
Guacamole									
	70	6	1	0	3	2	1	1	100
Vinegar (1 tsp.)									
	0	0	0	0	0	0	0	0	0

Food Serving size	Cal.	(g) Total Fat	(g) Sat. Fat	(mg) Chol.	(g) Carb.	(g) Fiber	(g) Sug.	(g) Prot.	(mg) Sod.
Vegetables									
Avocado	60	5	1	0	3	2	0	1	<5
Banana Peppers (3 rings)	<5	0	0	0	0	0	0	0	60
Cucumbers (3 slices)	<5	0	0	0	<1	0	0	0	0
Green Peppers (3 strips)	0	0	0	0	0	0	0	0	0
Jalapeno Peppers (3 rings)	<5	0	0	0	0	0	0	0	70
Lettuce	<5	0	0	0	0	0	0	0	0
Onions	<5	0	0	0	1	0	0	0	0
Pickles (3 chips)	0	0	0	0	0	0	0	0	115
Olives (3 rings)	<5	0	0	0	0	0	0	0	25
Spinach	2	0	0	0	0	0	0	0	15
Tomatoes (3 wheels)	5	0	0	0	2	0	0	0	0
Cheese									
American, Processed	40	3.5	2	10	1	0	0	2	200
Monterey Cheddar, Shredded	50	4.5	3	15	0	0	0	3	90
Mozzarella, Shredded	40	3	2	10	0	0	0	3	100
Natural Cheddar	60	5	3	15	0	0	0	4	100
Pepperjack	50	4	2.5	15	0	0	0	3	140

Food Serving size	Cal.	(g) Total Fat	(g) Sat. Fat	(mg) Chol.	(g) Carb.	(g) Fiber	(g) Sug.	(g) Prot.	(mg) Sod.
Provolone									
	50	4	2	10	0	0	0	4	125
Swiss									
	50	4.5	2.5	15	0	0	0	4	30

Individual Meats

Food Serving size	Cal.	(g) Total Fat	(g) Sat. Fat	(mg) Chol.	(g) Carb.	(g) Fiber	(g) Sug.	(g) Prot.	(mg) Sod.
Chicken Patty, Roasted									
	90	2.5	0.5	45	2	0	1	15	330
Chicken Strips, Plain									
	80	1.5	0.5	50	0	0	0	16	210
Chicken Strips, Buffalo Chicken									
	90	2	0.5	50	1	0	0	16	620
Chicken Strips, Teriyaki Glazed									
	100	2	0.5	50	5	0	2	16	400
Cold Cut Combo Meats									
	130	10	3	45	2	0	1	9	750
Egg Patty (regular)									
	110	7	2	220	3	1	1	9	380
Egg White Patty									
	70	2	0.5	0	3	0	0	9	430
Ham									
	60	2	0.5	25	2	0	2	9	520
Italian B.M.T.® Meats									
	180	14	5	45	2	0	2	11	990
Meatballs									
	260	16	6	30	16	3	6	13	640
Roast Beef									
	90	2.5	1	45	1	0	1	16	390
Sausage, Breakfast									
	140	11	4.5	35	1	0	1	10	520
Subway Seafood Sensation™									
	190	17	2.5	15	8	0	2	4	500
Steak (no cheese)									
	110	4	1.5	40	4	0	2	15	550

Food Serving size	Cal.	(g) Total Fat	(g) Sat. Fat	(mg) Chol.	(g) Carb.	(g) Fiber	(g) Sug.	(g) Prot.	(mg) Sod.
Subway Club® Meats	90	2.5	1	40	2	0	1	15	560
Tuna	250	23	4	40	0	0	0	12	300
Turkey Breast	50	1	0.5	20	2	0	1	9	480
Veggie Patty	160	5	0.5	10	12	3	2	15	520

Cookies & Desserts

Food Serving size	Cal.	(g) Total Fat	(g) Sat. Fat	(mg) Chol.	(g) Carb.	(g) Fiber	(g) Sug.	(g) Prot.	(mg) Sod.
Chocolate Chip	200	10	5	15	30	1	18	2	130
Chocolate Chunk	210	10	5	10	30	<1	17	2	100
Double Chocolate Chip	210	9	5	15	30	1	20	2	130
M&M®	210	10	5	15	30	<1	18	2	100
Oatmeal Raisin	200	8	3.5	15	30	1	16	3	130
Peanut Butter	220	12	5	10	26	1	16	4	130
Raspberry Cheesecake	200	9	4.5	10	29	0	16	2	120
Sugar	230	12	6	15	28	<1	14	2	130
White Chip Macadamia Nut	220	11	5	15	28	<1	17	2	130
Gingerbread	190	7	3	15	31	<1	17	2	110
Apple Pie	250	10	2	0	37	1	25	0	290
Apple Slices - 1 package	35	0	0	0	9	2	7	0	0

Food Serving size	Cal.	(g) Total Fat	(g) Sat. Fat	(mg) Chol.	(g) Carb.	(g) Fiber	(g) Sug.	(g) Prot.	(mg) Sod.
Chips									
Baked Lay's®									
	130	2	0	0	23	2	2	2	200
Baked Lay's® Sour Cream & Onion									
	140	3.5	0.5	0	24	2	3	3	240
Doritos Nacho									
	250	13	2.5	<5	30	2	2	4	310
Lays® Classic									
	230	15	1.5	0	23	2	0	3	270
Sunchips Harvest Cheddar									
	210	9	1.5	0	29	3	3	4	240
Chips, 1 bag									
	130-340	0-22	0-4.5	0-35	13-36	0-3	0-9	0-7	150-940
Beverages									
Bottled Juice/Drink									
	0-300	0	0	0	54-68	0	48-64	0	40-160
Fountain Drink/Sweetened Tea, Regular - 16 oz, no ice									
	120-240	0	0	0	34-66	0	34-66	0	0-110
Fountain Drink, Diet/Unsweetened Tea - 16 oz, no ice									
	0-10	0	0	0	0	0	0	0	0-60
Fountain Drink, Diet/Unsweetened Tea - 21 oz, no ice									
	0-15	0	0	0	0	0	0	0	0-80
Fountain Drink, Diet/Unsweetened Tea - 30 oz, no ice									
	0-25	0	0	0	0	0	0	0	0-60
Coca Cola®, no ice									
	260	0	0	0	71	0	71	0	15
Diet Coke®, no ice									
	0	0	0	0	0	0	0	0	25
Minute Maid® Light Lemonade, no ice									
	15	0	0	0	3	0	3	0	15
Sprite®, no ice									
	260	0	0	0	68	0	68	0	60

Food Serving size	Cal.	(g) Total Fat	(g) Sat. Fat	(mg) Chol.	(g) Carb.	(g) Fiber	(g) Sug.	(g) Prot.	(mg) Sod.
Juice Box									
	100	0	0	0	24	0	21	0	15
Milk, Low Fat									
	100	2.5	1.5	10	12	0	12	8	120
Milk, Chocolate Flavored Reduced Fat									
	200	5	3.5	25	32	<1	29	10	200

Soup (8 oz bowl)

Food Serving size	Cal.	(g) Total Fat	(g) Sat. Fat	(mg) Chol.	(g) Carb.	(g) Fiber	(g) Sug.	(g) Prot.	(mg) Sod.
Black Bean									
	210	1	0	0	39	15	6	12	860
Broccoli & Cheddar									
	170	9	5	25	18	1	4	5	630
Clam Chowder									
	200	11	7	30	20	2	3	5	850
Creamy Chicken & Dumpling									
	150	4.5	2	35	20	3	3	8	740
Creamy Chicken & Wild Rice									
	180	10	4	35	16	2	4	6	820
Homestyle Chicken Noodle									
	110	3	1.5	30	14	1	2	8	720
Loaded Baked Potato									
	210	13	7	35	15	1	4	5	800
Poblano Corn Chowder									
	150	7	4	20	18	2	7	5	560
Thai Coconut									
	210	13	3	25	17	1	7	5	680
Tomato Basil									
	140	7	4	25	15	2	8	5	750
Poblano Corn Chowder									
	150	7	4	20	18	2	7	5	560
Tomato Basil									
	140	7	4	25	15	2	8	5	750

Food Serving size	Cal.	(g) Total Fat	(g) Sat. Fat	(mg) Chol.	(g) Carb.	(g) Fiber	(g) Sug.	(g) Prot.	(mg) Sod.
Taco Bell									
Fresco									
Fresco Crunchy Taco									
	150	8	2.5	20	13	3	1	7	370
Fresco Soft Taco - Beef									
	180	7	3	20	21	3	2	8	650
Fresco BURRITO SUPREME® - Chicken									
	330	8	2.5	25	49	7	5	18	1360
Fresco BURRITO SUPREME® - Steak									
	330	8	3	20	48	7	5	16	1250
Fresco Fiesta Burrito - Chicken									
	330	8	2.5	25	48	3	4	16	1240
Fresco Zesty Chicken BORDER BOWL® without Dressing									
	350	8	1.5	25	51	10	4	19	1600
Fresco Ranchero Chicken Soft Taco									
	170	4	1.5	25	21	3	3	12	730
Fresco Grilled Steak Soft Taco									
	160	4.5	1.5	20	20	2	3	10	550
Fresco Bean Burrito									
	330	7	2.5	0	54	9	4	12	1200
Tacos									
Crunchy Taco									
	170	10	3.5	25	13	3	1	8	350
Crunchy TACO SUPREME®									
	210	13	6	40	15	3	2	9	370
DOUBLE DECKER® TACO SUPREME®									
	370	17	7	40	40	7	4	14	820
Soft Taco - Beef									
	200	9	4	25	21	3	2	10	630
Soft TACO SUPREME® - Beef									
	250	13	6	40	23	3	3	11	650

Food Serving size	Cal.	(g) Total Fat	Sat. Fat	(mg) Chol.	(g) Carb.	(g) Fiber	(g) Sug.	(g) Prot.	(mg) Sod.
Ranchero Chicken Soft Taco									
	270	14	4	35	21	2	3	14	820
Grilled Steak Soft Taco									
	270	16	4.5	35	20	2	3	12	660

Gorditas

Food Serving size	Cal.	(g) Total Fat	Sat. Fat	(mg) Chol.	(g) Carb.	(g) Fiber	(g) Sug.	(g) Prot.	(mg) Sod.
GORDITA SUPREME® - Beef									
	310	16	6	40	29	3	6	14	620
GORDITA SUPREME® - Chicken									
	290	12	5	45	28	2	6	17	650
GORDITA SUPREME® - Steak									
	290	13	5	40	28	2	6	15	530
GORDITA BAJA® - Beef									
	340	19	5	35	29	4	6	13	780
GORDITA BAJA® - Chicken									
	320	16	3.5	40	28	3	6	17	800
GORDITA BAJA® - Steak									
	320	17	4	35	27	3	5	15	690
Gordita Nacho Cheese - Beef									
	300	14	4	25	31	3	6	12	770
Gordita Nacho Cheese - Chicken									
	280	11	2.5	25	29	2	6	16	800
Gordita Nacho Cheese - Steak									
	270	12	3	20	29	2	6	14	680

Chalupas

Food Serving size	Cal.	(g) Total Fat	Sat. Fat	(mg) Chol.	(g) Carb.	(g) Fiber	(g) Sug.	(g) Prot.	(mg) Sod.
Chalupa Supreme - Beef									
	380	23	7	40	30	3	4	14	620
Chalupa Supreme - Chicken									
	360	20	5	45	29	2	4	17	650
Chalupa Supreme - Steak									
	360	21	6	40	28	2	4	15	530
Chalupa Baja - Beef									
	410	27	6	35	30	4	4	13	780
Chalupa Baja - Chicken									
	390	23	4	40	29	3	4	17	800

Food Serving size	Cal.	(g) Total Fat	(g) Sat. Fat	(mg) Chol.	(g) Carb.	(g) Fiber	(g) Sug.	(g) Prot.	(mg) Sod.
Chalupa Baja - Steak									
	390	24	4.5	35	28	3	3	15	690
Chalupa Nacho Cheese - Beef									
	370	22	4.5	20	32	3	4	12	770
Chalupa Nacho Cheese - Chicken									
	350	18	3	25	30	2	4	16	790
Chalupa Nacho Cheese - Steak									
	340	19	3.5	20	30	2	4	14	680

Burritos

Food Serving size	Cal.	(g) Total Fat	(g) Sat. Fat	(mg) Chol.	(g) Carb.	(g) Fiber	(g) Sug.	(g) Prot.	(mg) Sod.
Bean Burrito									
	350	9	3.5	5	54	8	4	13	1190
7-Layer Burrito									
	490	18	7	25	65	9	5	17	1350
BURRITO SUPREME® - Beef									
	420	17	8	40	51	7	5	17	1340
BURRITO SUPREME® - Chicken									
	400	13	6	45	49	6	5	20	1360
BURRITO SUPREME® - Steak									
	390	14	6	40	49	6	5	18	1250
Fiesta Burrito - Beef									
	370	13	5	25	49	4	4	14	1200
Fiesta Burrito - Chicken									
	350	10	3.5	30	47	3	4	18	1220
Fiesta Burrito - Steak									
	340	11	4	25	47	3	3	15	1110
Grilled Stuft Burrito - Beef									
	680	30	10	55	76	9	6	27	2120
Grilled Stuft Burrito - Chicken									
	640	23	7	65	73	7	6	34	2160
Grilled Stuft Burrito - Steak									
	630	25	8	55	72	7	5	30	1930

Food Serving size	Cal.	(g) Total Fat	(g) Sat. Fat	(mg) Chol.	(g) Carb.	(g) Fiber	(g) Sug.	(g) Prot.	(mg) Sod.
Big Bell Value Menu®									
Grande Soft Taco									
	430	20	8	45	43	5	5	19	1440
DOUBLE DECKER® Taco									
	320	13	5	25	38	6	2	14	810
Spicy Chicken Soft Taco									
	170	6	2	25	20	2	2	10	580
Spicy Chicken Burrito									
	400	17	4	30	48	3	4	14	1190
1/2 lb. Beef Combo Burrito									
	440	18	7	45	51	8	4	21	1630
1/2 lb. Beef & Potato Burrito									
	530	23	7	30	66	6	4	15	1720
1/2 lb. Cheesy Bean & Rice Burrito									
	470	20	6	15	58	6	5	13	1400
Cheesy Fiesta Potatoes									
	290	17	4	15	29	2	2	4	830
Caramel Apple Empanada									
	290	14	2.5	5	37	1	13	3	300
Specialties									
CRUNCHWRAP SUPREME®									
	560	24	8	35	68	5	7	17	1430
Spicy Chicken CRUNCHWRAP SUPREME®									
	540	23	7	40	67	4	7	19	1360
Mexican Pizza									
	530	30	8	40	46	6	3	20	1000
ENCHIRITO® - Beef									
	360	17	8	50	34	7	3	18	1420
ENCHIRITO® - Chicken									
	340	13	7	50	33	6	3	22	1450
ENCHIRITO® - Steak									
	330	14	7	45	33	6	3	20	1330
MEXIMELT®									
	280	14	7	40	22	3	2	15	860

Food Serving size	Cal.	(g) Total Fat	(g) Sat. Fat	(mg) Chol.	(g) Carb.	(g) Fiber	(g) Sug.	(g) Prot.	(mg) Sod.
Fiesta Taco Salad Without Shell									
	470	24	10	65	41	13	9	23	1510
Chicken Fiesta Taco Salad									
	790	38	8	75	77	13	10	37	1830
Steak Quesadilla									
	520	28	13	70	39	3	4	26	1300
Zesty Chicken BORDER BOWL®									
	640	35	6	30	60	10	4	22	1800
Zesty Chicken BORDER BOWL® Without Dressing									
	440	15	2.5	30	57	10	3	21	1540
Southwest Steak BORDER BOWL®									
	600	24	6	55	68	9	3	28	2120

Nachos and Sides

Food Serving size	Cal.	(g) Total Fat	(g) Sat. Fat	(mg) Chol.	(g) Carb.	(g) Fiber	(g) Sug.	(g) Prot.	(mg) Sod.
Nachos									
	330	21	3.5	5	32	2	3	4	530
Nachos Supreme									
	440	26	7	35	41	7	3	12	800
Nachos BELLGRANDE®									
	770	44	9	35	77	12	5	19	1280
Pintos 'n Cheese									
	160	6	3	15	19	7	1	9	670
Mexican Rice									
	180	7	3	15	23	1	0	6	790
Cinnamon Twists									
	170	7	0	0	26	1	12	1	200

Regional Menu Items

Food Serving size	Cal.	(g) Total Fat	(g) Sat. Fat	(mg) Chol.	(g) Carb.	(g) Fiber	(g) Sug.	(g) Prot.	(mg) Sod.
Cheese Quesadilla									
	470	26	12	50	39	2	4	19	1100
Chili Cheese Burrito									
	370	16	8	40	40	3	3	16	1060
Tostada									
	240	10	3.5	15	27	7	2	11	730

Food Serving size	Cal.	(g) Total Fat	(g) Sat. Fat	(mg) Chol.	(g) Carb.	(g) Fiber	(g) Sug.	(g) Prot.	(mg) Sod.

Tasti D-Lite

Blended Coffee and Tea

Green Tea (16 fl oz)

	210	1.5	1	5	38	0	34	6	115

Green Tea (24 fl oz)

	310	2	1.5	10	57	0	51	9	170

Java D-Lite, with Whipped Cream and Caramel (16 fl oz)

	330	1.5	1	5	66	0	39	7	230

Java D-Lite, with Whipped Cream and Caramel (24 fl oz)

	460	2	1.5	10	92	0	58	11	320

Java D-Lite, Without Whipped Cream and Caramel (16 fl oz)

	270	1.5	1	5	66	0	39	7	230

Java D-Lite, Without Whipped Cream and Caramel (24 fl oz)

	410	2	1.5	10	92	0	58	11	320

Mocha D-Lite, Without Whipped Cream and Caramel (24 fl oz)

	480	2	1.5	10	109	1	75	11	340

Cakes

Apple Pie, 6" Round Cake (Serving Size, 102g)

	150	4.5	2.5	5	25	1	19	3	65

Apple Pie, 8" Round Cake (Serving Size, 97g)

	140	4	2.5	5	24	1	18	3	60

Cake Batter Up! 6" Round Cake (Serving Size, 103g)

	130	4	3	5	20	0	17	2	65

Cake Batter Up! 8" Round Cake (Serving Size, 100g)

	120	4	3	5	20	0	17	2	65

Caramel Apple Pie, 6" Round Cake (Serving Size, 120g)

	180	4.5	3	5	31	1	22	3	85

Neapolitan, 6" Round Cake (Serving Size, 110g)

	130	3.5	2.5	5	21	1	19	3	70

Neapolitan, 8" Round Cake (Serving Size, 101g)

	120	3.5	2.5	5	20	0	18	2	70

Oreo Cookie, 6" Round Cake (Serving Size, 97g)

	160	6	3	5	25	0	19	3	115

Food Serving size	Cal.	(g) Total Fat	(g) Sat. Fat	(mg) Chol.	(g) Carb.	(g) Fiber	(g) Sug.	(g) Prot.	(mg) Sod.
Oreo Cookie, 8" Round Cake (Serving Size, 94g)									
	160	6	3	5	24	0	19	3	110
Peanut Buddy, 6" Round Cake (Serving Size, 112g)									
	220	10	5	5	27	1	18	5	120
Peanut Buddy, 8" Round Cake (Serving Size, 109g)									
	210	10	5	5	27	1	17	5	115
Pumpkin Cheesecake, 6" Round Cake (Serving Size, 102g)									
	150	4	3	5	25	0	19	3	95
Pumpkin Cheesecake, 8" Round Cake (Serving Size, 98g)									
	140	4.5	3	5	24	0	19	3	90
Pumpkin Pie, 6" Round Cake (Serving Size, 110g)									
	150	4.5	3	5	25	0	20	3	105
Pumpkin Pie, 8" Round Cake (Serving Size, 106g)									
	150	4.5	3	5	24	0	19	3	100
Raspberry Chocolate Truffle Cake (Serving Size, 120g)									
	240	8	5	0	39	2	23	4	75
Triple Berry D-Lite, 6" Round Cake (Serving Size, 127g)									
	150	3.5	2.5	5	26	0	23	2	65
Triple Berry D-Lite, 8" Round Cake (Serving Size, 123g)									
	140	4	2.5	5	25	1	22	2	60
Vanilla Chip, 6" Round Cake (Serving Size, 109g)									
	180	6	4.5	5	28	0	19	3	75
Vanilla Chip, 8" Round Cake (Serving Size, 108g)									
	190	7	4.5	5	29	0	19	3	75

Dry Toppings

Food Serving size	Cal.	Total Fat	Sat. Fat	Chol.	Carb.	Fiber	Sug.	Prot.	Sod.
Butterfinger Crumbles Topping (1 fl oz)									
	100	4	2	0	16	0	10	1	50
Chocolate Cookie Crunch Topping (1 fl oz)									
	50	1	0	NA	10	0	4	1	50
Chocolate Dipping Sauce Topping (0.5 fl oz)									
	110	9	5	0	8	1	7	0	10
Chocolate Sprinkles Topping (1 fl oz)									
	140	6	4	10	20	NA	NA	2	20

Food Serving size	Cal.	(g) Total Fat	(g) Sat. Fat	(mg) Chol.	(g) Carb.	(g) Fiber	(g) Sug.	(g) Prot.	(mg) Sod.
Chopped Peanuts Topping (1 fl oz)									
	100	8	1	0	3	1	1	4	0
Cinnamon Toast Granola Topping (1 fl oz)									
	60	2	0	0	10	2	3	2	5
Graham Cracker Crunch Topping (1 fl oz)									
	70	1.5	0	0	13	1	4	1	110
Heath Bar Chunk Topping (1 fl oz)									
	110	7	3.5	5	13	0	12	1	70
Honey Nut O's Topping (1 fl oz)									
	15	0	0	0	3	0	1	0	30
Mini Chocolate Chips Topping (1 fl oz)									
	160	8	5	0	20	NA	NA	2	0
Mini M&M's Topping (1 fl oz)									
	140	7	4	10	20	0	18	2	20
Oreo Cookie Pieces Topping (1 fl oz)									
	70	3	0	0	10	0	5	0	80
Peanut Butter Chips Topping (1 fl oz)									
	160	8	8	0	14	NA	12	6	70
Rainbow Sprinkles Topping (1 fl oz)									
	20	0	0	0	5	0	5	0	0
Vanilla Cookie Crunch Topping (1 fl oz)									
	60	2	1	NA	9	1	3	1	55

Fruit Toppings (Serving Size, 1 fl oz)

Food	Cal.	Total Fat	Sat. Fat	Chol.	Carb.	Fiber	Sug.	Prot.	Sod.
Banana Fruit Topping									
	15	0	0	0	4	0	2	0	0
Blackberry Fruit Topping									
	10	0	0	0	2	1	1	0	0
Blueberry Fruit Topping									
	10	0	0	0	3	0	2	0	0
Kiwi Fruit Topping									
	15	0	0	0	3	1	2	0	0
Mango Fruit Topping									
	15	0	0	0	4	0	3	0	0

Food Serving size	Cal.	(g) Total Fat	(g) Sat. Fat	(mg) Chol.	(g) Carb.	(g) Fiber	(g) Sug.	(g) Prot.	(mg) Sod.
Pineapple Fruit Topping	15	0	0	0	4	0	3	0	0
Raspberry Fruit Topping	10	0	0	0	2	1	1	0	0
Strawberry Fruit Topping	5	0	0	0	2	0	1	0	0

Parfaits (Serving Size, 140 g)

Food Serving size	Cal.	(g) Total Fat	(g) Sat. Fat	(mg) Chol.	(g) Carb.	(g) Fiber	(g) Sug.	(g) Prot.	(mg) Sod.
Fruit Parfait - Regular	160	3	1.5	5	29	1	21	4	75

Pies

Food Serving size	Cal.	(g) Total Fat	(g) Sat. Fat	(mg) Chol.	(g) Carb.	(g) Fiber	(g) Sug.	(g) Prot.	(mg) Sod.
Apple Pie Square (Serving Size, 93 g)	160	6	4	5	24	0	19	3	60
Caramel Apple Pie (Square) (Serving Size, 114g)	190	6	4	5	32	1	22	3	90
Caramel Toffee Square Pie (Serving Size, 104g)	190	7	5	5	30	0	22	3	105
Oreo Cookie Square Pie (Serving Size, 106g)	170	7	4	5	25	0	19	2	110
Peanut Buddy Square Pie (Serving Size, 118g)	230	7	4	0	38	1	16	5	125
Pumpkin Cheesecake Pie (Square) (Serving Size, 94g)	160	6	4	5	24	0	19	2	85
Pumpkin Pie Square (Serving Size, 98g)	140	5	4	5	22	1	19	2	70
Triple Berry D-Lite Square Pie (Serving Size, 129g)	130	3.5	2.5	5	23	1	20	2	55

Smoothies

Food Serving size	Cal.	(g) Total Fat	(g) Sat. Fat	(mg) Chol.	(g) Carb.	(g) Fiber	(g) Sug.	(g) Prot.	(mg) Sod.
Acai Smoothie (16 fl oz)	270	4.5	2	5	53	4	41	4	70
Acai Smoothie (24 fl oz)	440	7	3	10	91	8	68	7	105
Blueberry Banana Classic Smoothie (16 fl oz)	190	1.5	1	5	43	3	34	3	70

Food Serving size	Cal.	(g) Total Fat	(g) Sat. Fat	(mg) Chol.	(g) Carb.	(g) Fiber	(g) Sug.	(g) Prot.	(mg) Sod.
Blueberry Banana Classic Smoothie (24 fl oz)									
	330	3	1.5	5	73	5	56	5	100
Goji Smoothie (16 fl oz)									
	260	2	1	5	59	3	34	3	65
Goji Smoothie (24 fl oz)									
	420	3	1.5	5	95	5	54	6	95
Mango Classic Smoothie (16 fl oz)									
	220	1.5	1	5	49	2	45	3	95
Mango Classic Smoothie (24 fl oz)									
	330	2	1	5	74	4	68	4	140
Mangosteen Smoothie (16 fl oz)									
	230	2	1	5	53	5	40	4	75
Mangosteen Smoothie (24 fl oz)									
	380	3	1.5	10	86	8	64	6	115
Mixed Berry Classic Smoothie (16 fl oz)									
	170	1.5	1	5	37	2	31	3	100
Mixed Berry Classic Smoothie (24 fl oz)									
	270	2.5	1	5	58	3	49	4	150
Peanut Butter Banana Smoothie (16 fl oz)									
	370	7	3	10	67	2	54	12	230
Peanut Butter Banana Smoothie (24 fl oz)									
	580	11	4.5	20	107	4	85	18	340
Pineapple Mango Classic Smoothie (16 fl oz)									
	260	1.5	1	5	59	3	48	3	115
Pineapple Mango Classic Smoothie (24 fl oz)									
	440	2.5	1.5	5	102	7	82	6	170
Pineapple Strawberry Classic Smoothie (16 fl oz)									
	250	1.5	1	5	56	3	45	3	105
Pineapple Strawberry Classic Smoothie (24 fl oz)									
	420	2.5	1.5	5	95	5	74	5	160
Pomegranate Smoothie (16 fl oz)									
	250	1.5	1	5	56	4	42	3	65
Pomegranate Smoothie (24 fl oz)									
	400	2.5	1.5	5	91	6	66	5	95

Food Serving size	Cal.	(g) Total Fat	(g) Sat. Fat	(mg) Chol.	(g) Carb.	(g) Fiber	(g) Sug.	(g) Prot.	(mg) Sod.
Strawberry Banana Smoothie (16 fl oz)									
	290	1.5	1	5	64	3	51	3	125
Strawberry Banana Smoothie (24 fl oz)									
	470	2.5	1.5	5	107	5	85	5	190

Sundaes

Food Serving size	Cal.	Total Fat	Sat. Fat	Chol.	Carb.	Fiber	Sug.	Prot.	Sod.
Large Caramel Sundae (8 fl oz)									
	170	2	1	5	44	0	20	4	170
Large Hot Fudge Sundae (8 fl oz)									
	200	2	1.5	5	42	1	35	4	90
Large Strawberry Sundae (8 fl oz)									
	200	2	1	5	43	0	37	3	70
Regular Caramel Sundae (6 fl oz)									
	140	1.5	1	5	37	0	15	3	150
Regular Hot Fudge Sundae (6 fl oz)									
	170	1.5	1	5	35	1	29	3	70
Regular Strawberry Sundae (6 fl oz)									
	170	1.5	1	5	36	0	32	2	45

Tasti Rounds and Bars

Food Serving size	Cal.	Total Fat	Sat. Fat	Chol.	Carb.	Fiber	Sug.	Prot.	Sod.
Chocolate Tasti Bar (7 fl oz)									
	320	19	11	0	36	2	33	4	120
Tasti D-Lite Chocolate Round (74g)									
	180	2.5	1.5	0	36	1	17	3	230
Tasti D-Lite Chocolate Round with Rainbow Sprinkles (97g)									
	200	2.5	1.5	0	41	1	22	3	230
Tasti D-Lite Vanilla Round (71g)									
	180	2.5	1.5	0	36	1	16	3	220
Tasti D-Lite Vanilla Round with Rainbow Sprinkles (94g)									
	200	2.5	1.5	0	41	1	21	3	220
Vanilla Tasti Bar (7 fl oz)									
	310	19	11	5	35	1	31	4	85

Food Serving size	Cal.	(g) Total Fat	(g) Sat. Fat	(mg) Chol.	(g) Carb.	(g) Fiber	(g) Sug.	(g) Prot.	(mg) Sod.
Tropical Smoothie Café									
Breakfast									
All American Wrap	614	28	11	372	50	1	3	36	2015
Buffalo Kick Start Sandwich	569	23	9	374	50	2	6	35	1873
Early Bird Wrap	808	48	14	389	52	2	3	38	1466
Junior All American Wrap	372	18	7	187	33	1	1	19	1179
Junior Early Bird Wrap	494	29	10	207	35	1	2	23	938
Junior Salsa Surprise Wrap	407	20	9	200	35	1	2	22	1159
Salsa Sunrise Wrap	654	30	12	384	53	1	5	38	2100
The Classic Sandwich (Bacon)	642	33	15	382	47	2	5	35	1455
The Classic Sandwich (Ham)	607	28	13	387	48	2	6	38	1582
The Classic Sandwich (Sausage)	809	50	21	404	48	2	6	38	1625
Toasted Bagel with Cream Cheese	410	10	6	30	67	2	8	13	740
Cookies									
Chocolate Chunk	320	15	9	40	42	2	27	4	310
Snickerdoodle	290	11	7	55	43	0	22	5	330
Fresh Salads									
Chicken Caesar Salad	497	40	7	129	11	5	3	28	956

Food Serving size	Cal.	(g) Total Fat	(g) Sat. Fat	(mg) Chol.	(g) Carb.	(g) Fiber	(g) Sug.	(g) Prot.	(mg) Sod.
Loaded Spinach Salad	698	46	10	44	73	5	43	12	694
Southwest Chicken Salad	495	29	4	73	31	10	12	27	1607
Thai Chicken Salad	281	8	1	60	40	4	20	26	1123

Get Nutrified Smoothies

Food	Cal.	Total Fat	Sat. Fat	Chol.	Carb.	Fiber	Sug.	Prot.	Sod.
Caribbean C-burst Smoothie	458	0	0	0	110	6	93	4	87
Island Green Smoothie	377	0	0	0	97	4	83	2	31

Indulgent Smoothies

Food	Cal.	Total Fat	Sat. Fat	Chol.	Carb.	Fiber	Sug.	Prot.	Sod.
Bahama Mama Smoothie	475	4	4	1	122	6	101	7	92
Beach Bum Smoothie	520	4	4	1	122	6	101	7	92
Chocolate Chiller Smoothie	570	7	6	2	125	2	117	6	186
Mocha Madness Smoothie	588	5	4	1	126	3	117	4	128
Peanut Butter Cup Smoothie	693	20	7	1	121	7	99	11	232
Tropi-Colada Smoothie	457	2	2	0	109	3	99	1	18

Kids Food Items

Food	Cal.	Total Fat	Sat. Fat	Chol.	Carb.	Fiber	Sug.	Prot.	Sod.
Cheese Pizza	395	14	6	22	50	4	7	19	1021
Cheese Pizza with Chicken	463	15	6	62	51	4	7	32	1242
Cheese Quesadilla	467	26	13	60	34	1	1	26	1043
Cheese Quesadilla with Chicken	535	27	14	100	35	1	1	39	1264

Food Serving size	Cal.	Total Fat (g)	Sat. Fat (g)	Chol. (mg)	Carb. (g)	Fiber (g)	Sug. (g)	Prot. (g)	Sod. (mg)
Ham & American Wrap	310	12	5	43	34	1	2	19	1375
Junior Chicken Caesar Salad	231	19	3	62	5	2	2	13	402
Turkey & American Wrap	310	11	5	48	34	1	2	23	1265

Kids Smoothies (12 oz)

Food Serving size	Cal.	Total Fat (g)	Sat. Fat (g)	Chol. (mg)	Carb. (g)	Fiber (g)	Sug. (g)	Prot. (g)	Sod. (mg)
Awesome Orange Smoothie	263	3	2	1	59	1	55	2	61
Chocolate Chimp Smoothie	247	2	2	0	58	2	48	2	47
Jetty Junior Smoothie	170	0	0	0	43	2	35	1	2
Lil' Lemonberry Smoothie	211	0	0	0	52	1	50	0	5

Low-Fat Smoothies

Food Serving size	Cal.	Total Fat (g)	Sat. Fat (g)	Chol. (mg)	Carb. (g)	Fiber (g)	Sug. (g)	Prot. (g)	Sod. (mg)
Blimey Limey Smoothie	386	0	0	0	99	1	97	1	15
Blue Lagoon Smoothie	311	1	0	0	78	4	67	1	3
Hawaiian Breeze Smoothie	337	0	0	0	87	1	85	2	40
Jetty Punch Smoothie	341	0	0	0	86	4	70	2	3
Kiwi Quencher Smoothie	430	0	0	0	103	1	100	2	38
Mango Magic Smoothie	368	0	0	0	94	2	88	2	38
Paradise Point Smoothie	401	0	0	0	105	5	88	2	0
Peaches 'N Silk Smoothie	314	0	0	0	79	2	68	1	8

Food Serving size	Cal.	(g) Total Fat	(g) Sat. Fat	(mg) Chol.	(g) Carb.	(g) Fiber	(g) Sug.	(g) Prot.	(mg) Sod.
Pineapple Delight Smoothie	347	0	0	0	0	91	3	83	1
Rockin' Raspberry Smoothie	402	0	0	0	100	6	88	1	3
Strawberry Beach Smoothie	417	0	0	0	103	2	98	3	38
Strawberry Lemonade Smoothie	373	0	0	0	91	1	87	1	9
Sunny Day Smoothie	436	0	0	0	108	4	92	2	5
Sunrise Sunset Smoothie	320	0	0	0	81	2	76	1	5

Supercharged Smoothies

Food Serving size	Cal.	(g) Total Fat	(g) Sat. Fat	(mg) Chol.	(g) Carb.	(g) Fiber	(g) Sug.	(g) Prot.	(mg) Sod.
Acai Berry Boost Smoothie	433	3	1	0	101	3	87	2	10
Get Up and Goji Smoothie	425	0	0	0	104	3	90	2	34
Health Nut with Soy Smoothie	496	5	0	0	88	5	71	31	245
Health Nut with Whey Smoothie	476	5	0	40	88	5	71	25	35
Lean Machine Smoothie	442	0	0	0	112	4	96	2	3
Muscle Blaster with Soy Smoothie	461	2	0	0	88	4	70	30	243
Muscle Blaster with Whey Smoothie	441	2	0	40	88	4	70	24	33
Peanut Paradise with Soy Smoothie	695	18	3	0	101	5	81	38	418
Peanut Paradise with Whey Smoothie	675	18	3	40	101	5	81	32	208
Pomegranate Plunge Smoothie	450	0	0	0	110	3	97	1	16

Food Serving size	Cal.	(g) Total Fat	(g) Sat. Fat	(mg) Chol.	(g) Carb.	(g) Fiber	(g) Sug.	(g) Prot.	(mg) Sod.
Triple Berry Oat+ Smoothie									
	541	3	0	20	116	7	89	16	29

Supplements

Energizer Supplement									
	0	0	0	0	0	0	0	0	0
Fat Burner Supplement									
	0	0	0	0	0	0	0	0	0
Ground Flax Seed Supplement									
	19	1	0	0	1	1	0	1	0
Multi-Vitamin Supplement									
	15	0	0	0	4	0	0	0	3
Pea Protein Supplement									
	148	2	0	0	4	0	0	28	532
Probiotic Supplement									
	29	0	0	0	6	0	0	0	0
Soy Protein Supplement									
	120	2	0	0	2	0	0	28	240
Vitamin B12 Supplement									
	24	0	0	0	6	0	0	0	0
Vitamin-C Immune Complex Supplement									
	20	0	0	0	5	0	5	0	60
Whey Protein Supplement									
	100	2	0	40	2	0	0	22	30
Whole Grain Oats Supplement									
	70	1	0	0	15	3	0	3	0

Toasted Flatbreads

Baja Chicken Toasted Flatbread									
	468	18	6	63	47	2	3	31	1151
Caribbean Luau Toasted Flatbread									
	456	13	5	60	57	3	13	31	1115
Chicken Pesto Toasted Flatbread									
	463	18	6	64	44	2	2	32	1089

Food Serving size	Cal.	(g) Total Fat	(g) Sat. Fat	(mg) Chol.	(g) Carb.	(g) Fiber	(g) Sug.	(g) Prot.	(mg) Sod.
Chipotle Chicken Club Flatbread									
	541	28	8	81	44	2	2	28	1137
Honey Ham and Swiss Toasted Flatbread									
	422	12	5	50	54	2	14	23	1212

Toasted Sandwiches

Food Serving size	Cal.	Total Fat	Sat. Fat	Chol.	Carb.	Fiber	Sug.	Prot.	Sod.
Cranberry Walnut Chicken Salad Toasted Sandwich									
	645	35	5	51	61	5	13	20	673
Turkey Bacon Ranch Toasted Sandwich									
	576	20	7	109	53	2	8	46	1940
Ultimate Club Toasted Sandwich									
	645	28	8	108	52	2	8	44	1994
Turkey Guacamole Toasted Sandwich									
	497	9	1	70	66	7	16	38	1626
Wasabi Caesar Roast Beef Toasted Sandwich									
	482	14	5	91	49	3	5	37	1546

Toasted Wraps

Food Serving size	Cal.	Total Fat	Sat. Fat	Chol.	Carb.	Fiber	Sug.	Prot.	Sod.
Buffalo Chicken Toasted Wrap									
	646	28	10	87	58	4	5	40	2485
Hummus Veggie Toasted Wrap									
	590	23	7	25	78	7	9	22	1526
Jamaican Jerk Chicken Toasted Wrap									
	617	19	8	79	71	2	9	41	1748
King Caesar Toasted Wrap									
	626	31	8	99	53	3	5	35	1555
Southwest Chicken Toasted Wrap									
	607	22	5	66	70	5	8	31	1757
Thai Chicken Toasted Wrap									
	497	14	4	60	66	3	13	32	1613
Totally Turkey Toasted Wrap									
	615	26	8	97	54	3	8	45	2032

Food Serving size	Cal.	(g) Total Fat	(g) Sat. Fat	(mg) Chol.	(g) Carb.	(g) Fiber	(g) Sug.	(g) Prot.	(mg) Sod.

Wendy's

Additional Salad Dressings

Classic Ranch									
	100	10	1.5	10	2	0	1	1	150
Fat-free French									
	40	0	0	0	9	0	8	0	95
Italian Vinaigrette									
	70	6	1	0	4	0	3	0	180
Light Classic Ranch									
	50	4.5	1	10	2	0	1	1	150
Thousand Island									
	160	15	2.5	15	5	0	4	0	290

Beverages

Barq's Root Beer (Small Cup)									
	180	0	0	0	50	0	50	0	40
Coca-Cola (Small Cup)									
	160	0	0	0	44	0	44	0	0
Coke Zero (Small Cup)									
	0	0	0	0	0	0	0	0	5
Diet Coke (Small Cup)									
	0	0	0	0	0	0	0	0	15
Dr Pepper (Small Cup)									
	160	0	0	0	43	0	43	0	40
Fanta Orange (Small Cup)									
	180	0	0	0	49	0	49	0	25
Hi-C Flashin' Fruit Punch (Small Cup)									
	170	0	0	0	46	0	46	0	15
Juicy Juice Apple Juice									
	90	0	0	0	22	0	20	0	5
Minute Maid Light Lemonade (Small Cup)									
	5	0	0	0	1	0	0	0	5
Nestea Sweetened Iced Tea									
	100	0	0	0	28	0	27	0	10

Food Serving size	Cal.	(g) Total Fat	Sat. Fat	(mg) Chol.	(g) Carb.	(g) Fiber	(g) Sug.	(g) Prot.	(mg) Sod.
Nestea Unsweetened Iced Tea	0	0	0	0	0	0	0	0	10
Nestle Pure Life Bottled Water	0	0	0	0	0	0	0	0	0
Pibb Xtra (Small Cup)	160	0	0	0	43	0	43	0	25
Sprite (Small Cup)	160	0	0	0	43	0	43	0	35
TruMoo Low-fat Chocolate Milk	140	2.5	1.5	10	22	0	20	7	170
TruMoo Low-fat White Milk	100	2.5	1.5	10	12	0	11	8	125

Crispy Chicken Nuggets

Food Serving size	Cal.	(g) Total Fat	Sat. Fat	(mg) Chol.	(g) Carb.	(g) Fiber	(g) Sug.	(g) Prot.	(mg) Sod.
10 Piece Chicken Nuggets	450	29	6	65	26	2	1	21	930
4 Piece Kids' Meal Chicken Nuggets	180	11	2.5	25	11	1	1	8	370
5 Piece Chicken Nuggets	220	14	3	35	13	1	1	10	460
Babecue Nugget Sauce	45	0	0	0	11	0	4	0	120
Heartland Ranch Dipping Sauce	120	12	1.5	10	3	0	2	0	240
Honey Mustard Nugget Sauce	80	6	1	10	7	0	3	0	220
Sweet and Sour Nugget Sauce	50	0	0	0	12	0	11	0	120

Frosty Treats

Food Serving size	Cal.	(g) Total Fat	Sat. Fat	(mg) Chol.	(g) Carb.	(g) Fiber	(g) Sug.	(g) Prot.	(mg) Sod.
Caramel Apple Parfait	400	9	5	30	71	1	57	8	180
Caramel Frosty Shake (Small)	680	15	9	50	126	0	102	11	330

Food Serving size	Cal.	(g) Total Fat	(g) Sat. Fat	(mg) Chol.	(g) Carb.	(g) Fiber	(g) Sug.	(g) Prot.	(mg) Sod.
Chocolate Frosty (Small)									
	250	6	4	25	41	0	35	6	115
Chocolate Frosty Shake (Large)									
	890	18	11	55	168	4	151	16	380
Chocolate Frosty Shake (Small)									
	610	14	9	45	109	2	98	12	260
Oreo Frosty Parfait									
	400	10	6	30	68	1	56	8	220
Strawberry Frosty Shake (Large)									
	820	16	10	55	156	1	142	13	240
Strawberry Frosty Shake (Small)									
	580	14	8	45	104	1	94	10	190
Vanilla Bean Frosty Shake (Small)									
	620	14	8	45	115	0	83	10	450
Vanilla Frosty (Small)									
	260	7	4.5	25	43	0	37	7	125
Vanilla Frosty Float with Coca-Cola									
	380	7	4.5	30	75	0	69	7	135
Wild Berry Frosty Shake (Large)									
	750	16	10	55	137	2	120	13	250
Wild Berry Frosty Shake (Small)									
	550	14	8	45	96	1	84	11	190

Garden Sensations Salads

Food Serving size	Cal.	(g) Total Fat	(g) Sat. Fat	(mg) Chol.	(g) Carb.	(g) Fiber	(g) Sug.	(g) Prot.	(mg) Sod.
Apple Pecan Chicken Salad									
	340	11	7	105	28	5	20	35	1150
Apple Pecan Chicken Salad (Half-size)									
	170	6	3.5	50	15	3	11	18	580
Avocado Ranch Dressing									
	100	10	2	10	2	0	1	1	210
Baja Salad									
	550	33	14	90	34	12	12	32	1650
Baja Salad (Half-size)									
	280	17	7	45	18	6	6	16	840

Food Serving size	Cal.	(g) Total Fat	(g) Sat. Fat	(mg) Chol.	(g) Carb.	(g) Fiber	(g) Sug.	(g) Prot.	(mg) Sod.
BLT Cobb Salad	450	25	11	275	9	3	5	46	1610
BLT Cobb Salad (Half-size)	230	13	6	140	5	1	3	23	810
Creamy Red Jalapeno Dressing	100	10	2	10	2	0	1	1	270
Gourmet Croutons	80	3	0	0	12	0	0	2	220
Lemon Garlic Caesar Dressing	110	11	2	10	2	0	1	2	180
Pomegranate Vinaigrette Dressing	60	3	0	0	8	0	7	0	160
Roasted Pecans	110	9	1	0	5	1	4	1	60
Seasoned Tortilla Strips	80	4.5	1.5	0	11	1	0	1	105
Spicy Chicken Caesar Salad	460	25	12	85	27	6	3	33	1410
Spicy Chicken Caesar Salad (Half-size)	240	13	6	40	15	4	3	17	710

Sandwich Components

Food Serving size	Cal.	(g) Total Fat	(g) Sat. Fat	(mg) Chol.	(g) Carb.	(g) Fiber	(g) Sug.	(g) Prot.	(mg) Sod.
1/4 lb. Hamburger Patty	220	15	7	70	0	0	0	19	170
American Cheese	40	3.5	2	10	0	0	0	2	200
Applewood Smoked Bacon - 1 Strip	30	2.5	1	5	0	0	0	2	100
Crispy Chicken Patty	200	12	2.5	30	13	1	0	11	460
Dill Pickles - 4 Each	0	0	0	0	0	0	0	0	150
Homestyle Chicken Fillet	240	11	2	50	16	1	0	19	770

Food Serving size	Cal.	(g) Total Fat	(g) Sat. Fat	(mg) Chol.	(g) Carb.	(g) Fiber	(g) Sug.	(g) Prot.	(mg) Sod.
Honey Mustard Sauce									
	40	3.5	0	5	3	0	2	0	75
Iceberg Lettuce Leaf									
	0	0	0	0	0	0	0	0	0
Junior Hamburger Patty									
	90	7	3	30	0	0	0	8	70
Ketchup									
	10	0	0	0	2	0	2	0	80
Mayonnaise									
	40	3.5	0.5	5	1	0	0	0	55
Mustard									
	5	0	0	0	0	0	0	0	50
Natural Asiago Cheese									
	50	4	2.5	15	1	0	0	3	100
Premium Bun									
	190	2	0	0	36	1	6	6	360
Ranch Sauce									
	40	4	0.5	5	1	0	0	0	55
Red Onion - 2 Rings									
	0	0	0	0	0	0	0	0	0
Sandwich Bun									
	120	1	0	0	24	1	4	4	240
Spicy Chicken Fillet									
	250	11	2.5	50	17	1	0	19	950
Tomato - 1 Slice									
	5	0	0	0	1	0	1	0	0
Tortilla									
	130	3.5	1	0	21	0	0	3	280
Ultimate Chicken Grill Fillet									
	120	1.5	0	80	1	0	0	26	670

Sandwiches

1/2 lb Double									
	770	43	19	160	43	2	10	50	1430

Food Serving size	Cal.	(g) Total Fat	(g) Sat. Fat	(mg) Chol.	(g) Carb.	(g) Fiber	(g) Sug.	(g) Prot.	(mg) Sod.
1/4 lb Single									
	550	28	12	95	43	2	10	30	1270
Asiago Ranch Club with Homestyle Chicken									
	660	33	9	90	56	3	8	34	1650
Asiago Ranch Club with Spicy Chicken									
	670	34	10	90	57	3	8	35	1830
Asiago Ranch Club with Ultimate Chicken Grill									
	540	24	8	120	41	2	8	41	1550
Bacon Deluxe Double									
	850	51	22	180	43	2	11	54	1690
Bacon Deluxe Single									
	640	36	15	110	43	2	11	35	1520
Baconator Double									
	930	58	25	195	41	1	10	59	1840
Baconator Single									
	630	36	15	110	41	1	9	35	1370
Cheeseburger, Kids' Meal									
	260	11	5	40	26	1	6	14	570
Crispy Chicken Caesar Wrap									
	430	25	7	45	35	2	1	17	950
Crispy Chicken Sandwich									
	350	15	3.5	35	38	2	4	15	740
Crispy Chicken Sandwich, Kids' Meal									
	330	13	3	30	36	2	4	15	700
Double Junior Bacon Cheeseburger									
	440	25	11	85	26	1	5	26	820
Double Stack									
	360	18	8	70	27	1	6	23	740
Grilled Chicken Go Wrap									
	260	10	3.5	50	25	1	3	19	730
Hamburger, Kids' Meal									
	220	8	3	30	26	1	5	12	370
Homestyle Chicken Fillet Sandwich									
	470	16	3	55	55	3	7	26	1190

Food Serving size	Cal.	(g) Total Fat	(g) Sat. Fat	(mg) Chol.	(g) Carb.	(g) Fiber	(g) Sug.	(g) Prot.	(mg) Sod.
Homestyle Chicken Go Wrap									
	320	16	4.5	35	30	1	1	15	770
Junior Bacon Cheeseburger									
	350	19	8	55	26	1	5	18	750
Junior Cheeseburger									
	270	11	5	40	27	1	6	15	670
Junior Cheeseburger Deluxe									
	300	14	6	45	29	2	7	15	710
Junior Hamburger									
	230	8	3	30	26	1	6	12	470
Spicy Chicken Fillet Sandwich									
	480	17	3.5	55	56	3	7	26	1370
Spicy Chicken Go Wrap									
	330	16	4.5	40	31	1	1	16	860
Ultimate Chicken Grill Sandwich									
	360	7	1.5	80	42	2	9	33	1110

Side Selections

Food Serving size	Cal.	(g) Total Fat	(g) Sat. Fat	(mg) Chol.	(g) Carb.	(g) Fiber	(g) Sug.	(g) Prot.	(mg) Sod.
Buttery Best Spread									
	50	5	1	0	0	0	0	0	95
Caesar Side Salad									
	60	3.5	2.5	10	5	2	2	4	115
Cheddar Cheese, Shredded									
	70	6	3.5	15	1	0	0	4	110
Garden Side Salad									
	25	0	0	0	5	2	3	1	30
Gourmet Croutons									
	80	3	0	0	12	0	0	2	220
Gourmet Croutons									
	80	3	0	0	12	0	0	2	220
Small Chili									
	210	6	2.5	40	21	6	6	17	880
Small Natural-cut Fries									
	320	16	3	0	42	4	0	4	350

Food Serving size	Cal.	(g) Total Fat	(g) Sat. Fat	(mg) Chol.	(g) Carb.	(g) Fiber	(g) Sug.	(g) Prot.	(mg) Sod.
Sour Cream and Chives Baked Potato									
	320	3.5	2	10	63	7	4	8	50
Value Natural-cut Fries									
	230	11	2.5	0	30	3	0	3	250

White Castle

Breakfast Sliders on a Bun

Food Serving size	Cal.	(g) Total Fat	(g) Sat. Fat	(mg) Chol.	(g) Carb.	(g) Fiber	(g) Sug.	(g) Prot.	(mg) Sod.
Bacon									
	130	6	2	10	12	1	1	5	330
Bacon, Cheese									
	150	9	3.5	15	12	1	2	7	460
Bacon, Egg									
	200	11	3.5	220	12	1	2	12	400
Bacon, Egg, Cheese									
	190	11	4	225	13	1	2	12	430
Bologna, Cheese - Louisville and Nashville Regions									
	240	15	6	35	14	1	3	10	760
Bologna, Egg - Louisville and Nashville Regions									
	290	18	6	240	14	1	3	15	690
Bologna, Egg, Cheese - Louisville and Nashville Regions									
	310	20	7	250	15	1	3	16	830
Egg									
	140	6	2	210	12	1	2	9	190
Egg, Cheese									
	160	8	3	220	13	1	2	10	330
Hamburger, Egg									
	200	11	4	220	12	1	2	13	210
Hamburger, Egg, Cheese									
	230	14	6	225	13	1	2	14	350
Huevos Rancheros with Bacon Slider (Cincinnati Region)									
	190	11	4.5	225	14	1	2	12	500
Huevos Rancheros with Sausage Slider (Cincinnati Region)									
	310	23	9	245	14	1	2	15	710

Food Serving size	Cal.	(g) Total Fat	(g) Sat. Fat	(mg) Chol.	(g) Carb.	(g) Fiber	(g) Sug.	(g) Prot.	(mg) Sod.
Sausage									
	220	15	6	25	12	1	1	8	430
Sausage, Cheese									
	250	17	7	30	13	1	2	9	570
Sausage, Egg									
	290	20	7	240	13	1	2	14	500
Sausage, Egg, Cheese									
	320	22	9	245	13	1	2	15	640

Buffalo Chicken Rings

6 Rings									
	540	48	8	105	14	1	1	18	870
9 Rings									
	810	71	12	160	22	1	1	26	1390

Buffalo Chicken Rings - New Jersey Region

6 Rings									
	540	48	9	110	14	1	1	18	870
9 Rings									
	810	71	14	160	22	1	1	26	1390

Cheese Fries

Cheese Fries (Medium)									
	410	28	4.5	0	35	3	2	4	350
Cheese Fries (New Jersey Region) (Medium)									
	410	28	5	0	35	3	2	4	350
Loaded Fries (Cheddar, Bacon, Ranch) - New Jersey Region (Medium)									
	460	38	8	20	20	2	3	4	900
Loaded Fries (Cheddar, Bacon, Ranch) (Medium)									
	470	38	6	20	21	2	3	4	990
6 Rings									
	530	47	10	105	12	0	0	18	610
9 Rings									
	790	71	12	160	18	1	0	26	910

Food Serving size	Cal.	(g) Total Fat	(g) Sat. Fat	(mg) Chol.	(g) Carb.	(g) Fiber	(g) Sug.	(g) Prot.	(mg) Sod.
Chicken Rings - New Jersey Region									
6 Rings	530	47	9	105	12	0	0	18	610
Clam Strips									
Regular	210	17	2	15	5	0	1	8	620
Sack	410	34	4	35	9	0	2	16	1250
Clam Strips - New Jersey Region									
Medium	210	17	2.5	15	5	0	1	8	620
Sack	410	34	5.5	35	9	0	2	16	1250
Coffee									
Large	5	0	0	0	0	0	0	1	10
Medium	5	0	0	0	0	0	0	1	10
Small	5	0	0	0	0	0	0	0	5
Coffee (Decaffeinated)									
Large	0	0	0	0	0	0	0	1	10
Medium	0	0	0	0	0	0	0	0	10
Small	0	0	0	0	0	0	0	0	5
Condiments									
BBQ Sauce - 1 Packet	10	0	0	0	3	0	2	0	130

Food Serving size	Cal.	(g) Total Fat	(g) Sat. Fat	(mg) Chol.	(g) Carb.	(g) Fiber	(g) Sug.	(g) Prot.	(mg) Sod.
Fat-free Honey Mustard Sauce - 1 Packet									
	20	0	0	0	5	0	3	0	50
Hot Sauce - 1 Packet									
	5	0	0	0	1	1	0	0	170
Ketchup - 1 Packet									
	10	0	0	0	2	0	2	0	100
Lemon Juice - 1 Packet									
	5	0	0	0	1	0	0	0	0
Mayonnaise - 1 Packet									
	60	7	1	5	0	0	0	0	55
Mustard - Columbus, Detroit, Minneapolis, Nashville, NE Ohio, New Jersey and New York Regions - 1 Packet									
	5	0	0	0	<1	0	0	0	85
Mustard - Dusseldorf - Chicago, Cincinnati, Louisville and Nashville Regions - 1 Packet									
	5	0	0	0	0	0	0	0	65
Mustard - Horseradish - Indianapolis and St. Louis Regions - 1 Packet									
	5	0	0	0	0	0	0	0	65
Tartar Sauce - 1 Packet									
	25	1.5	0	0	1	0	1	0	85

Condiments Delivered on Sliders

Food	Cal.	Total Fat	Sat. Fat	Chol.	Carb.	Fiber	Sug.	Prot.	Sod.
Golden BBQ Sauce									
	15	0	0	0	3	0	3	0	80
Hamburger Sauce (1 1/2 tsp) Detroit Region									
	0	0	0	0	0	0	0	0	75
Ketchup - Chicago, Cincinnati, Columbus, Detroit, Louisville, Minneapolis, Nashville, New York, New Jersey and NE Ohio Regions (1 tbsp)									
	5	0	0	0	1	0	1	0	50
Marinara Sauce									
	5	0	0	0	2	0	1	0	105
Mustard (1 tsp) - Indianapolis Region									
	0	0	0	0	0	0	0	0	85
Mustard (1 tsp) - Minneapolis, Columbus, Detroit & NE Ohio Regions									
	0	0	0	0	0	0	0	0	60

Food Serving size	Cal.	(g) Total Fat	(g) Sat. Fat	(mg) Chol.	(g) Carb.	(g) Fiber	(g) Sug.	(g) Prot.	(mg) Sod.
Ranch Dressing									
	90	9	1.5	0	1	0	1	0	140
Spicy Hamburger Sauce (1 1/2 tsp) - Chicago Region									
	0	0	0	0	1	- 0	0	0	45

Crave Coolers

Food Serving size	Cal.	(g) Total Fat	(g) Sat. Fat	(mg) Chol.	(g) Carb.	(g) Fiber	(g) Sug.	(g) Prot.	(mg) Sod.
Crave Cooler Coke - Kids									
	40	0	0	0	12	0	12	0	0
Crave Cooler Coke - Large									
	200	0	0	0	56	0	56	0	20
Crave Cooler Coke - Medium									
	140	0	0	0	39	0	39	0	15
Crave Cooler Coke - Saver									
	90	0	0	0	24	0	24	0	10
Crave Cooler Coke - Small									
	110	0	0	0	29	0	29	0	10
Crave Cooler Fanta Wild Cherry - Kids									
	40	0	0	0	12	0	12	0	0
Crave Cooler Fanta Wild Cherry - Large									
	210	0	0	0	56	0	56	0	15
Crave Cooler Fanta Wild Cherry - Medium									
	140	0	0	0	39	0	39	0	10
Crave Cooler Fanta Wild Cherry - Saver									
	90	0	0	0	24	0	24	0	5
Crave Cooler Fanta Wild Cherry - Small									
	110	0	0	0	29	0	29	0	10

Desserts

Food Serving size	Cal.	(g) Total Fat	(g) Sat. Fat	(mg) Chol.	(g) Carb.	(g) Fiber	(g) Sug.	(g) Prot.	(mg) Sod.
Chocolate Chunk Cookie (Select Regions)									
	170	8	4	10	23	1	13	2	130
Oatmeal Raisin Cookie (Select Regions)									
	160	6	2.5	10	23	1	12	2	115
White Chocolate Macadamia Cookie (Select Regions)									
	180	9	4	10	22	1	14	2	125

Food Serving size	Cal.	(g) Total Fat	(g) Sat. Fat	(mg) Chol.	(g) Carb.	(g) Fiber	(g) Sug.	(g) Prot.	(mg) Sod.
Doubles									
Bacon Cheddar	370	23	10	50	21	1	2	17	1240
Bacon Cheeseburger	350	22	10	40	21	1	2	18	1050
Cheeseburger	300	17	8	30	20	1	3	15	940
Fish Slider with Cheese	610	48	9	45	25	23	2	19	700
Fish Slider Without Cheese	550	43	6	30	24	23	1	17	420
Jalapeno Cheeseburger	280	17	8	30	21	1	2	15	860
Original Slider	240	12	5	20	21	1	2	12	660
Smokey Bacon Ranch	420	29	8	40	22	1	4	13	1100
French Fries									
Medium	370	25	4	0	33	3	2	3	50
Saver	350	24	4	0	32	3	2	3	50
French Fries (New Jersey Region)									
Medium	360	22	5	0	36	3	2	5	40
Sack	810	49	11	0	81	8	4	12	95
Saver	350	21	5	0	34	3	1	5	40
Home-style Onion Rings - Chicago, Louisville and St. Louis Regions									
Medium	480	33	4.5	0	40	2	7	6	580

Food Serving size	Cal.	(g) Total Fat	(g) Sat. Fat	(mg) Chol.	(g) Carb.	(g) Fiber	(g) Sug.	(g) Prot.	(mg) Sod.
Saver	290	19	2.5	0	25	1	5	4	360

Onion Rings - New Jersey Region

Medium	340	22	4	0	33	3	5	2	310
Sack	640	41	7	0	62	6	9	4	580
Saver	220	14	2.5	0	21	2	3	1	190

Ranch Chicken Rings

6 Rings	540	48	8	107	14	1	1	18	820
9 Rings	810	71	12	160	21	1	1	27	1300

Ranch Chicken Rings - New Jersey Region

6 Rings	540	48	.9	110	14	1	1	18	820

Shakes

Chocolate Shake - Chicago Region - Kids	260	4.5	2.5	15	51	1	43	6	160
Chocolate Shake - Chicago Region - Saver	420	8	4	25	81	2	69	9	250
Chocolate Shake - Chicago Region - Small	550	10	5.5	35	106	2	90	12	330
Chocolate Shake - Cincinnati Region - Kids	310	8	5	15	53	0	42	7	170
Chocolate Shake - Cincinnati Region - Saver	490	13	8	25	85	0	67	11	270
Chocolate Shake - Cincinnati Region - Small	650	17	11	35	111	0	88	14	350
Chocolate Shake - Columbus Region - Kids	240	6	3.5	20	42	0	39	6	220

Food Serving size	Cal.	(g) Total Fat	(g) Sat. Fat	(mg) Chol.	(g) Carb.	(g) Fiber	(g) Sug.	(g) Prot.	(mg) Sod.
Chocolate Shake - Columbus Region - Medium									
	710	18	11	65	126	0	117	19	670
Chocolate Shake - Columbus Region - Saver									
	380	9	6	35	67	0	62	10	360
Chocolate Shake - Columbus Region - Small									
	500	12	8	45	88	0	82	13	470
Chocolate Shake - Detroit Region - Kids									
	210	6	3	20	32	0	32	6	190
Chocolate Shake - Detroit Region - Medium									
	620	17	9	55	96	0	96	17	570
Chocolate Shake - Detroit Region - Saver									
	330	9	4.5	30	52	0	52	9	300
Chocolate Shake - Detroit Region - Small									
	440	12	6	40	68	0	68	12	400
Chocolate Shake - Indianapolis Region - Kids									
	230	7	4.5	35	42	1	32	6	170
Chocolate Shake - Indianapolis Region - Saver									
	370	12	7	60	67	2	51	9	270
Chocolate Shake - Indianapolis Region - Small									
	490	15	9	75	88	3	67	12	350
Chocolate Shake - Louisville Region - Kids									
	230	7	4.5	35	42	1	32	6	170
Chocolate Shake - Louisville Region - Saver									
	370	12	7	60	67	2	51	9	270
Chocolate Shake - Louisville Region - Small									
	490	15	9	75	88	3	67	12	350
Chocolate Shake - Minneapolis Region - Kids									
	200	4	2	20	37	0	30	4	200
Chocolate Shake - Minneapolis Region - Medium									
	590	13	7	65	111	0	91	13	590
Chocolate Shake - Minneapolis Region - Saver									
	310	7	3.5	35	59	0	49	7	310
Chocolate Shake - St. Louis Region - Saver									
	370	9	6	30	66	3	49	9	120

Food Serving size	Cal.	(g) Total Fat	Sat. Fat	(mg) Chol.	(g) Carb.	(g) Fiber	(g) Sug.	(g) Prot.	(mg) Sod.
Strawberry Shake - Cincinnati Region - Saver									
	480	12	8	25	83	0	67	11	270
Strawberry Shake - Cincinnati Region - Small									
	630	16	11	35	109	0	88	14	350
Strawberry Shake - Columbus Region - Kids									
	230	5	3.5	20	41	0	39	6	220
Strawberry Shake - Columbus Region - Medium									
	690	16	11	65	122	0	117	19	670
Strawberry Shake - Columbus Region - Saver									
	370	9	6	35	65	0	62	10	360
Strawberry Shake - Columbus Region - Small									
	480	11	8	45	85	0	81	13	470
Vanilla Shake - Chicago Region - Kids									
	220	4	2.5	15	41	1	34	6	170
Vanilla Shake - Chicago Region - Saver									
	360	6.5	4	25	65	2	55	9	270
Vanilla Shake - New Jersey Region - Kids									
	210	6	4	25	31	0	26	8	220
Vanilla Shake - New Jersey Region - Saver									
	330	9	6	40	50	0	42	12	350
Vanilla Shake - New Jersey Region - Small									
	440	12	8	55	65	0	54	16	460

Side Sauces

Food Serving size	Cal.	Total Fat	Sat. Fat	Chol.	Carb.	Fiber	Sug.	Prot.	Sod.
Apple Sauce (Select Regions) - 1 Container									
	100	0	0	0	24	2	19	0	10
BBQ Sauce - 1 Container									
	35	0.5	0	0	8	0	8	0	390
Cheese Sauce - Nashville and Louisville Regions									
	130	10	3.5	10	6	0	3	3	560
Cheese Sauce (Nacho) - Cincinnati, Chicago, Indianapolis, Minneapolis, New Jersey and St. Louis Regions									
	50	4	1	0	3	0	0	0	400
Cinnamon Sauce - 1 Container									
	110	4	0.5	0	20	0	17	0	85

Food Serving size	Cal.	(g) Total Fat	(g) Sat. Fat	(mg) Chol.	(g) Carb.	(g) Fiber	(g) Sug.	(g) Prot.	(mg) Sod.
Fat-free Honey Mustard Sauce - 1 Container									
	50	0	0	0	13	0	7	0	70
Marinara Sauce - 1 Container									
	15	0	0	0	4	0	2	0	80
Ranch Dressing - 1 Container									
	150	17	2.5	10	1	0	1	0	210
Seafood Sauce - 1 Container									
	30	0	0	0	7	0	3	0	340
Tartar Sauce - Chicago, Minneapolis and New Jersey Regions - 1 Conta									
	90	8	1	10	4	0	2	0	220
White Castle Zesty Zing Sauce - 1 Container									
	120	11	1.5	15	4	0	3		190

Slider Alterations

American Cheese Slice									
	30	2	2	5	0	0	0		140
Bacon									
	30	3	1	4	0	0	0		105
Bacon Topping									
	40	2.5	1	10	0	0			180
Cheddar Cheese Slice									
	30	2.5	1.5	10	0	0			160
Jalapeno Cheese Slice									
	20	3	2	5	1	0	1		140
Traditional Bun									
	70	1	0	0	12		2		120

Sliders

Bacon Cheddar									
	200	12	5	25	13		9		650
Bacon Cheeseburger									
	190	11	5	20	13		9		550
Bacon Jalapeno Cheeseburger									
	190	12	5	20			9	5	
Bacon Ranch									
	260	18	5	20		7			

Food Serving size	Cal.	(g) Total Fat	(g) Sat. Fat	(mg) Chol.	(g) Carb.	(g) Fiber	(g) Sug.	(g) Prot.	(mg) Sod.
Cleese Supreme Slider - Detroit and Cincinnati Regions									
	420	31	6	30	20	1	2	14	750
Geeseburger									
	170	9	4	15	15	1	3	8	550
Cken Breast Slider									
	360	26	3.5	20	20	1	1	11	510
Clen Breast Slider with Cheese									
	390	28	5	25	20	1	2	13	650
Chn Ring Slider									
	350	28	4.5	35	16	1	1	8	320
Chi Ring Slider with Cheese									
	380	30	6	40	16	1	2	10	460
Fish									
	310	22	3	15	18	12	1	9	270
Fish with Cheese									
	340	24	4.5	20	18	12	2	11	410
Jalap eseburger									
	160	9	4	15	14	1	2	8	460
Mush ddar (Select Regions)									
	170	9	4.5	20	14	1	1	8	600
Origin									
	140	6	2.5	10	13	1	1	7	360
Pulled Slider									
	0	4.5	1	25	25	1	12	9	460
Surf an									
		33	8	35	26	13	2	19	720
rf an heese									
		38	11	45	27	13	2	22	990
heese									
			1.5	5	12	1	2	4	260
ted)									
	640		0	0	29	0	29	0	20

Food Serving size	Cal.	(g) Total Fat	(g) Sat. Fat	(mg) Chol.	(g) Carb.	(g) Fiber	(g) Sug.	(g) Prot.	(mg) Sod.
Barq's Red Cream Soda - Large									
	480	0	0	0	130	0	130	0	80
Barq's Red Cream Soda - Medium									
	320	0	0	0	87	0	87	0	50
Barq's Red Cream Soda - Saver									
	170	0	0	0	47	0	47	0	30
Coca-Cola Classic - Small									
	210	0	0	0	57	0	57	0	15
Coke Zero - Kids									
	0	0	0	0	0	0	0	0	25
Coke Zero - Large									
	5	0	0	0	0	0	0	0	115
Coke Zero - Medium									
	0	0	0	0	0	0	0	0	80
Coke Zero - Saver									
	0	0	0	0	0	0	0	0	40
Coke Zero - Small									
	0	0	0	0	0	0	0	0	60
Diet Coke - Kids									
	0	0	0	0	0	0	0	0	10
Diet Coke - Large									
	0	0	0	0	0	0	0	0	40
Diet Coke - Medium									
	0	0	0	0	0	0	0	0	25
Diet Coke - Saver									
	0	0	0	0	0	0	0	0	15
Diet Coke - Small									
	0	0	0	0	0	0	0	0	20
Diet Coke, Caffeine Free - Kids									
	0	0	0	0	0	0	0	0	10
Diet Coke, Caffeine Free - Large									
	0	0	0	0	0	0	0	0	40
Diet Coke, Caffeine Free - Medium									
	0	0	0	0	0	0	0	0	30

Food Serving size	Cal.	(g) Total Fat	(g) Sat. Fat	(mg) Chol.	(g) Carb.	(g) Fiber	(g) Sug.	(g) Prot.	(mg) Sod.
Diet Coke, Caffeine Free - Saver									
	0	0	0	0	0	0	0	0	15
Diet Coke, Caffeine Free - Small									
	0	0	0	0	0	0	0	0	20
Fanta Grape Soda - Kids									
	110	0	0	0	31	0	31	0	30
Fanta Grape Soda - Large									
	510	0	0	0	138	0	138	0	125
Fanta Grape Soda - Medium									
	340	0	0	0	93	0	93	0	85
Fanta Orange Soda - Medium									
	310	0	0	0	99	0	99	0	100
Fanta Orange Soda - Saver									
	170	0	0	0	53	0	53	0	55
Fanta Orange Soda - Small									
	240	0	0	0	74	0	74	0	75
Fanta Strawberry Soda - Kids									
	110	0	0	0	31	0	31	0	30
Fanta Strawberry Soda - Large									
	500	0	0	0	138	0	138	0	125
Fanta Strawberry Soda - Medium									
	340	0	0	0	93	0	93	0	85
Fanta Strawberry Soda - Saver									
	180	0	0	0	50	0	50	0	45
Fanta Strawberry Soda - Small									
	260	0	0	0	70	0	70	0	65
Sprite - Kids									
	90	0	0	0	24	0	24	0	20
Sprite - Large									
	410	0	0	0	109	0	109	0	90
Sprite - Medium									
	270	0	0	0	73	0	73	0	60
Sprite - Saver									
	150	0	0	0	39	0	39	0	30

Food Serving size	Cal.	(g) Total Fat	(g) Sat. Fat	(mg) Chol.	(g) Carb.	(g) Fiber	(g) Sug.	(g) Prot.	(mg) Sod.
Sprite - Small									
	210	0	0	0	55	0	55	0	45
Vault - Kids									
	100	0	0	0	26	0	26	0	10
Vault - Large									
	450	0	0	0	117	0	117	0	40
Vault - Medium									
	300	0	0	0	79	0	79	0	25
Vault - Saver									
	160	0	0	0	42	0	42	0	15
Vault - Small									
	230	0	0	0	60	0	60	0	20

Soft Drinks (Noncarbonated)

Food Serving size	Cal.	(g) Total Fat	(g) Sat. Fat	(mg) Chol.	(g) Carb.	(g) Fiber	(g) Sug.	(g) Prot.	(mg) Sod.
Hi-C Flashing Fruit Punch - Kids									
	100	0	0	0	26	0	26	0	10
Hi-C Flashing Fruit Punch - Large									
	440	0	0	0	117	0	117	0	40
Hi-C Flashing Fruit Punch - Medium									
	290	0	0	0	79	0	79	0	25
Hi-C Flashing Fruit Punch - Saver									
	160	0	0	0	42	0	42	0	15
Hi-C Flashing Fruit Punch - Small									
	220	0	0	0	60	0	60	0	20
Hi-C Orange Lavaburst - Kids									
	100	0	0	0	28	0	28	0	0
Hi-C Orange Lavaburst - Large									
	470	0	0	0	126	0	126	0	0
Hi-C Orange Lavaburst - Medium									
	310	0	0	0	85	0	85	0	0
Hi-C Orange Lavaburst - Saver									
	170	0	0	0	45	0	45	0	0
Hi-C Orange Lavaburst - Small									
	240	0	0	0	64	0	64	0	0

Food Serving size	Cal.	(g) Total Fat	(g) Sat. Fat	(mg) Chol.	(g) Carb.	(g) Fiber	(g) Sug.	(g) Prot.	(mg) Sod.
Hi-C Poppin' Pink Lemonade Pink - Kids									
	90	0	0	0	23	0	23	0	38
Hi-C Poppin' Pink Lemonade Pink - Large									
	400	0	0	0	101	0	101	0	170
Hi-C Poppin' Pink Lemonade Pink - Medium									
	270	0	0	0	68	0	68	0	115
Hi-C Poppin' Pink Lemonade Pink - Saver									
	140	0	0	0	36	0	36	0	60
Hi-C Poppin' Pink Lemonade Pink - Small									
	200	0	0	0	51	0	51	0	85

Sweet Potato Fries

Medium									
	480	30	3	0	47	6	13	4	380
Saver									
	420	26	3	0	41	5	12	3	330

Sweet Potato Fries (New Jersey Region)

Medium									
	480	30	4	0	47	6	13	4	380
Sack									
	900	56	7	0	89	11	25	7	710
Saver									
	420	26	3	0	41	5	12	3	330